Nutrition in Clinical Practice

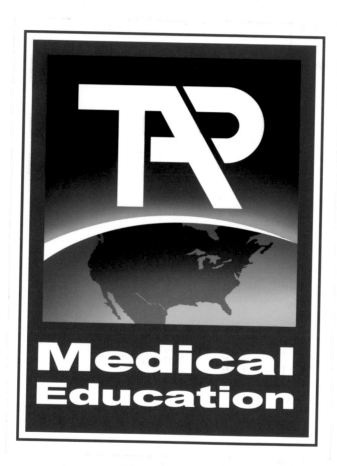

Nutrition in Clinical Practice

A Comprehensive, Evidence-Based Manual
for the Practitioner

David L. Katz, M.D., M.P.H.
Associate Clinical Professor of Public Health and Medicine
Director of Medical Studies in Public Health
Yale University School of Medicine
New Haven, Connecticut

Director, Preventive Medicine Residency Program and
Department of Preventive Medicine
Yale-Griffin Prevention Research Center
Griffin Hospital
Derby, Connecticut

LIPPINCOTT WILLIAMS & WILKINS
A **Wolters Kluwer** Company
Philadelphia • Baltimore • New York • London
Buenos Aires • Hong Kong • Sydney • Tokyo

Acquisitions Editor: Timothy Y. Hiscock
Developmental Editor: Sarah Fitz-Hugh
Supervising Editor: Mary Ann McLaughlin
Manufacturing Manager: Tim Reynolds
Production Service: Colophon
Cover Designer: Mark Lerner
Cover Illustration: Nancy Howell
Compositor: The PRD Group, Inc.
Printer: Edwards Brothers

© 2001 by Lippincott Williams & Wilkins
530 Walnut Street
Philadelphia, PA 19106
LWW.com

Printed in the USA

Library of Congress Cataloging-in-Publication Data

Katz, David L.
    Nutrition in clinical practice / David L. Katz.
       p. ; cm.
    Includes bibliographical references and index.
    ISBN 0-683-30638-3
    1. Diet therapy. 2. Diet in disease. 3. Nutrition. I. Title.
    [DNLM: 1. Nutrition. 2. Evidence-Based Medicine. QU 145 K193n 2000]
  RM216.K37 2000
  615.5′8—dc21
                                                                00-55875

Care has been taken to confirm the accuracy of the information presented and to describe generally accepted practices. However, the authors, editors, and publisher are not responsible for errors or omissions or for any consequences from application of the information in this book and make no warranty, expressed or implied, with respect to the currency, completeness, or accuracy of the contents of the publication. Application of this information in a particular situation remains the professional responsibility of the practitioner.

The authors, editors, and publisher have exerted every effort to ensure that drug selection and dosage set forth in this text are in accordance with current recommendations and practice at the time of publication. However, in view of ongoing research, changes in government regulations, and the constant flow of information relating to drug therapy and drug reactions, the reader is urged to check the package insert for each drug for any change in indications and dosage and for added warnings and precautions. This is particularly important when the recommended agent is a new or infrequently employed drug.

Some drugs and medical devices presented in this publication have Food and Drug Administration (FDA) clearance for limited use in restricted research settings. It is the responsibility of health care providers to ascertain the FDA status of each drug or device planned for use in their clinical practice.

10 9 8 7 6 5 4 3 2 1

With pride and more love than sons tend to talk about, I dedicate this book to my parents, Dr. Donald I. Katz and Susan A. Katz.

My father—a man of admirable principle, compelling intellect, and great ability, whose accomplishments have always and only been limited by the bounds of his will, and the high wall of his unshakable humility. My mother—a woman with boundless creativity, insight, love, and the capacity to dream.

Dad, you have always shown me the way. Mom, you have enabled me to believe I could follow it.

Contents

Foreword

Rare is the day that the newspaper does not report some new finding or claim about a diet, nutrient, or supplement that is purported to improve health, prevent disease, or help people lose weight. No other area of health has so much written about it in the scientific literature as nutrition has; yet, in this same area where so much is known with reasonable surety much is also touted as truth without a firm scientific base.

The net effects on the public are widespread appreciation of the importance of nutrition for health, confusion about how it all fits together, and expectation of breakthroughs they can easily take advantage of. Often individuals look to their health care providers for advice on what to do or, failing that, muddle through on their own.

This high public visibility, coupled with voluminous claims and counterclaims, sense, nonsense, and speculation, falls on a clinical community that often is badly undertrained in nutrition and its underlying science. It is high time for a book like *Nutrition in Clinical Practice.*

In this text, Dr. David Katz has undertaken separating the dross from the gold by succinctly summarizing the quality of the evidence as it applies specifically to human health. Therein lies the book's uniqueness. It is summative, not encyclopedic, and more practical than theoretical. It offers the unifying perspective of the sole author rather than the unconnected views of many. Its perspective is clearly and tightly tied to the science. As medicine moves into the twenty-first century, the volume of data and information is overwhelming. Increasingly, the practitioner will require credible sources to help synthesize and summarize nutrition information, so that conclusions and actions are easily discernible.

Most people and their clinicians cannot readily separate the proven and the possible from the preposterous. In this useful book, the prose is lean, easily digestible, portion-controlled with few empty phrases, and loaded with nutritional knowledge. It is not light—but, read carefully—it is satisfying and sticks with you. This is a tremendous effort in a much-needed area beneficial to all who are struggling to systematically add a sturdy, but easily borne, layer of nutritional science and advice to their life's armor against illness. The nation's health will be better if clinicians consistently apply the lessons in this text.

James S. Marks, M.D., M.P.H.
Assistant Surgeon General
Director, National Center for Chronic
Disease Prevention and Health
Promotion
Centers for Disease Control and Prevention
Atlanta, Georgia

About the Author

David L. Katz, M.D., M.P.H., is Associate Clinical Professor of Epidemiology and Public Health & Medicine, and Director of Medical Studies in Public Health at the Yale University School of Medicine. He is board certified in Internal Medicine and Preventive Medicine/Public Health. He earned his B.A. from Dartmouth College, his M.D. from the Albert Einstein College of Medicine, and an M.P.H. from the Yale University School of Medicine. He directs courses in public health, epidemiology, preventive medicine, biostatistics, health policy, and nutrition at the Yale School of Medicine. He is director of the Preventive Medicine Residency Program and co-director of the Integrated Training Program in Internal and Preventive Medicine at Griffin Hospital, a Yale affiliate in Derby, Connecticut. He also is director of the CDC-funded Yale-Griffin Prevention Research Center and of the Integrative Medicine Center at Griffin Hospital. Dr. Katz has authored scientific articles and books covering topics in epidemiology and public health, chronic disease prevention, clinical epidemiology, cardiovascular disease, and nutrition.

Preface

While compiling this text, I have been as committed to what it excludes as to what it includes. Excellent, comprehensive textbooks, even encyclopedias, of nutrition have been written. I have made use of a good many of them in this effort. But as it may, in fact, be considered true that we "are" what we eat, such books cover a vast array of topics in agonizing detail. Agonizing, that is, for the clinician seeking the answers to clinical questions, but quite appropriate for the nutritional biochemist.

First among the principles to which this text is devoted is *clinical relevance*. If material seemed likely to be of use to the clinician interacting with a patient, even occasionally, it was included. If such an application seemed far-fetched, or if the material did not support an understanding that would enhance such an exchange, it was left out. The range of nutrition topics germane to clinical care is quite expansive. Thus, a fairly selective inclusion process resulted in leaving quite a lot still to be said.

The second principle governing the compilation of this text is *consistency of application*. Only in books do states of health and disease, and the underlying factors that promote them, stay neatly in their own columns and rows. In reality, these states coexist in single patients, often in complex abundance. Therefore, mutually exclusive, disease-specific nutrition recommendations are apt to be of limited clinical utility. Conversely, if dietary recommendations never change in accommodation to varying states of health and clinical objectives, a book of many chapters seems an excessive effort to portray this set of uniform guidelines. I have sought the middle ground between the subtle applications of nutritional management that pertain to the occasional disease or risk factor, and the unifying features of diet that may be universally applied to promote health.

The third principle governing this effort is that to be of use, material intended for clinical application must be described in terms of the extent, consistency, and quality, of *the underlying evidence*. This may be considered a text of evidence-based medicine, with the literature reviewed for each chapter considered to represent preliminary, suggestive, or definitive evidence of any association described.

I strove to be consistent in the application of such terms, but found myself sometimes using, for example, "conclusive" rather than "definitive." Despite such variation, the character of the evidence base should generally be clear. Associations supported by animal or *in vitro* or observational evidence only were considered *preliminary*; associations supported by a combination of basic science studies as well as observational studies in humans, or by limited interventional studies in humans, were considered *suggestive*; and associations subtended by the results of either large-scale human intervention trials (particularly randomized, controlled trials), or the aggregation of consistent results from numerous less rigorous studies were considered *definitive*.

The fourth principle, related to the third, is that for a subject of scrutiny to be well understood, it must be *viewed in its entirety* (or some approximation thereof). There is a risk (although certainly, too, a benefit) when each of many experts elaborates one particular aspect of nutrition as it pertains to health. That risk was perhaps never better expressed than in the allegorical poem, *The Blind Men and the Elephant,* by John Godfrey Saxe. I in no way wish to suggest that the expert authors of detailed chapters in the standard nutrition texts suffer any semblance of blindness, but rather that something of the overall character of nutrition and health is missed when only a small part is examined in great detail. I have become convinced, for example, that nominal n-3 fatty acid deficiency is likely widespread in the United States and contributing to adverse health outcomes. This conclusion is reached less on the basis of definitive evidence in any one area and more on the basis of remarkably consistent and voluminous evidence in the aggregate, across the expanse of many subjects. Only one author, struggling through each of many chapters in turn, may infuse the characterization of each topic with understanding derived from the others. As I cannot dispute the potential disadvantages of solo authorship, I have sought instead to capitalize fully on any potential advantages. I have therefore freely shared what insights I have gained in the sequential review of so many topics, endeavoring at all times to be clear about the sources of my opinion and the nature of the evidence.

The final principle to which this text is devoted is the notion that there should be a *theoretical model* in which the complex interplay of human behavior, food, and health outcomes is decipherable. In much the same way that unifying threads of evidence have led me to specific recommendations for nutrition management, I have come through this labor convinced of the utility of the *evolutionary biology model* of human dietary behavior. This argument is elaborated in Chapter 39. The behavior and physiology of all animals are largely governed by the environments to which they adapted; there is both reason and evidence to suggest that, with regard to nutrition, the same is true of us.

While there is some interpretation offered in this text, it is only that which a devotee and teacher of evidence-based principles of medicine could abide and not avoid. In the inescapable need to convey to you my interpretations, I have endeavored to cleave as close and consistently to fact as possible. In the time-honored medical tradition of blending the best of available science with just the requisite art, I submit this work to you as a platform for the clinical practice of nutrition.

Following the introduction, a concise but comprehensive overview of dietary influences on the organ system or pathology under discussion is provided. The overview is generally divided into the influence of the overall dietary pattern (*Diet*) and the influence of specific nutrient (*Nutrients/Nutriceuticals*). As indicated, other topics are included in the overview, such as pathophysiology, epidemiology, and other issues of clinical relevance and/or general interest. The overview section uses the scheme above to rate the available evidence for each practice. Unpublished and non-peer-reviewed literature has been accessed as required to facilitate preparation of this text, but the assessment of evidence is based only on the peer-reviewed literature; references are to be found at the end of each chapter. Following the overview, other *Topics of Interest* not related directly to dietary management are provided as indicated (e.g., surgical management of severe obesity). Chapters conclude with *Clinical Highlights*, a summary of those nutritional interventions of greatest clinical utility and for which the evidence is decisive, convincing, or suggestive. Each chapter is cross-referenced with other chapters and with pertinent *Nutrient/Nutriceutical Reference Tables* and other *Nutrition Resource Materials* in Section III.

Claims, Disclaimers, and Acknowledgments

Solo authorship of a text on nutrition may seem an act of either brash imprudence or unpardonable hubris. At times, poring over references and painstakingly compiling chapters, I have been tempted to think it both. But, please accept my assurances that it is neither. There is very definitely method in the potential madness of this project.

I am a clinician with an active practice in primary care internal medicine. Every day in the office I am confronted by the abiding interest of my patients in their own nutritional practices and by the innumerable attendant questions. And to be of use to my patients, to offer guidance when guidance is needed, I must have the answers at hand. I can certainly refer to a dietitian for counseling in support of clinical goals, but hardly as a means of answering each question that comes along.

So the clinician in practice, encountering what I in my practice encounter every day, must be able to answer a range of questions about nutrition and health, nutrition and disease. If unable to do so, the clinician misses a crucial opportunity to influence favorably the role of dietary behavior in the mitigation of chronic disease. On the list of the leading causes of death in the United States, dietary practices rank number 2, just behind smoking.

My nutrition expertise, cultivated by training, research, and teaching over the past fifteen years, is appropriate for this project. But I certainly cannot claim to have the consummate knowledge in each of the diverse content areas of this text that is owned by that field's luminaries. To those experts, far too numerous to mention here, I owe a monumental debt. I have endeavored to make their work accessible to an audience of clinicians, but, in doing so, I have traveled the many trails they so painstakingly blazed.

My legitimacy, or perhaps my excuse, then, is not so much my claim to expertise in everything from lipid metabolism to ergogenic aids, but rather my dual devotion to nutrition and to clinical practice. The experts to whom I am indebted have made their contributions to the literature, yet the accessibility of that literature to the busy practitioner is suspect. This text is as much translation as original work, the translation of current nutrition knowledge into a form useful to the clinician. This text of nutrition is both by, and for, the practicing clinician. If any one practitioner is to access all of this information and apply it to clinical practice, it is only reasonable that one clinician has been able to write it.

And so that is why I have written this text and justified the interminable hours of effort to myself. To those whose work has guided me, I offer thanks. For any omissions, or worse still, misrepresentations, I accept full responsibility (who else could I blame?). Yet even this solo effort has depended, and greatly benefited, from the direct and indirect contributions of many individuals. I owe debts of gratitude I have little hope to repay to those who made this book possible.

D.L.K.

Acknowledgments

I am grateful to Professor Linda Bartoshuk of the Yale School of Medicine. I suspect Dr. Bartoshuk will be surprised to find her name here, because her capacity to motivate and inspire is so much a part of who she is that she may overlook it. I have not, and am grateful for the exposures, far too limited, that have left an indelible impression.

For similar reasons, I am grateful to Professor Kelly Brownell of Yale University. Dr. Brownell's thoughtful, meticulous intelligence, profound knowledge, and refined teaching ability have benefited me, as they have countless others privileged to call themselves his students.

I am grateful to Professor James Jekel of the Yale School of Public Health who helped set me on the academic path.

I am deeply indebted to Joan Tichy, Anastasia Timpko, and the staff of the Griffin Hospital Resource Center. I cannot imagine many authors demanding more of a library resource, nor of receiving a more gracious, accommodating, and tireless response. I am not sure whether I, or staff at the Resource Center, put more hours into this book. I am sure that I could not have done my part without their assistance.

In all that I do, and particularly whatever I manage to do well, I am indebted to Jennifer Ballard, administrator of the Yale-Griffin Prevention Research Center. Despite what should by all rights be an unmanageable schedule, Jen assists me with every endeavor, this one included. Her hours of typing, filing, and generally keeping me on track, are deeply appreciated.

I am indebted to the editorial staff at Lippincott Williams & Wilkins who converted my initial passion and subsequent effort into a book. In particular, I would like to acknowledge the acquisitions editor, Tim Hiscock, and the developmental editor Sarah Fitz-Hugh.

I am truly awed by the depth and breadth of nutrition literature. To the countless contributors to so vast a sea of knowledge and insight, I am thankful for the vistas and the challenge of the crossing.

Finally, and most of all, I am grateful to my family. To my wife, Catherine, I am thankful for her capacity to keep the faith when I lost mine, and to help me keep going when the finish line seemed impossibly far away. Without her constancy and love, I would not have completed this project, nor would doing so mean as much to me. To my children, Rebecca, Corinda, Valerie, Natalia, and Gabriel, I owe thanks that they have kept me in their hearts while I, for several years, have found so little time for them in my schedule. That has been the highest price of all, and one for which I eagerly look forward to making amends.

To my fellow clinicians, I offer the sincere hope that this effort is ultimately validated as a meaningful contribution to our efforts at optimizing the health of our patients.

David L. Katz

Sources for All Chapters

Bendich A, Deckelbaum RJ, eds. *Preventive nutrition. The comprehensive guide for health professionals.* Totowa, NJ: Humana Press, 1997.

Committee on Diet and Health, Food and Nutrition Board, Commission on Life Science, National Research Council. *Diet and health. Implications for reducing chronic disease risk.* Washington, DC: National Academy Press, 1989.

Craig SY, Haigh J, Harrar S, eds. *The complete book of alternative nutrition.* Emmaus, PA: Rodale Press, 1997.

Eaton SB, Eaton SB III, Konner MJ. Paleolithic nutrition revisited: a twelve-year retrospective on its nature and implications. *Eur J Clin Nutr* 1997;51:207–216.

Ensminger AH, Ensminger ME, Konlande JE, Robson, JRK. *The concise encyclopedia of foods and nutrition.* Boca Raton, FL: CRC Press, Inc., 1995.

Haas EM. *Staying healthy with nutrition.* Berkeley, CA: Celestial Arts, 1992.

Institute of Medicine. *Improving America's diet and health: from recommendations to action.* Washington, DC: National Academy Press, 1991.

Lutz CA, Przytulski KR. *Nutrition and diet therapy,* 2nd ed. Philadelphia: FA Davis Co., 1997.

Margen S, ed., and the editors of the University of California at Berkeley Wellness Letter. *The wellness encyclopedia of food and nutrition.* New York: Rebus, 1992.

Margen S. *The wellness nutrition counter.* New York: Health Letter Associates, 1997.

Morgan SL, Weinsier RL. *Fundamentals of clinical nutrition.* St. Louis, MO: Mosby-Year Book, 1998.

Murray MT. *Encyclopedia of nutritional supplements.* Rocklin, CA: Prima Publishing, 1996.

National Research Council. *Recommended dietary allowances,* 10th ed. Washington, DC: National Academy Press, 1989.

Price WWA. *Nutrition and physical degeneration. 50th anniversary edition.* New Canaan, CT: Keats Publishing, 1989.

Rinzler CA. *The new complete book of food. A nutritional, medical, and culinary guide.* New York: Facts on File, 1999.

Sardesai VM. *Introduction to clinical nutrition.* New York: Marcel Dekker, 1998.

Shils ME, Olson JA, Shike M, eds. *Modern nutrition in health and disease,* 8th ed. Philadelphia: Lea & Febiger, 1994.

Tannahill R. *Food in history.* New York: Three Rivers Press, 1988.

Temple NJ, Burkitt DP, eds. *Western diseases. Their dietary prevention and reversibility.* Totowa, NJ: Humana Press, 1994.

Thomas B. *Nutrition in primary care. A handbook for health professionals.* Oxford, England: Blackwell Science, 1996.

United States Department of Agriculture. *USDA Nutrient Database for Standard Reference,* Release 12, 1998.

Von Hippel A. *Human evolutionary biology.* Anchorage, AK: Stone Age Press, 1994.

Werbach MR. *Nutritional influences on illness. A sourcebook of clinical research.* New Canaan, CT: Keats Publishing, 1990.

Ziegler EE, Filer LJ Jr., eds. *Present knowledge in nutrition,* 7th ed. Washington, DC: ILSI Press, 1996.

SECTION I

Clinical Nutrition

PART A

Clinically Relevant Nutrient Metabolism

1

Clinically Relevant Carbohydrate Metabolism

Carbohydrate represents the principal source of dietary energy for humans in virtually every culture, largely because carbohydrate constitutes the bulk of all living matter. Generally between 50% and 70% of calories are derived from carbohydrate. Maintaining relatively stable levels of glucose in plasma to meet energy needs is the primary goal of the various components of carbohydrate metabolism. The principal metabolic function of dietary carbohydrate is to provide energy. From a dietary standpoint, carbohydrate functions primarily to sweeten food.

Carbohydrates are so named because their chemical structure consists of carbon and water molecules in a 1:1 ratio. Digestible carbohydrates include polysaccharides and the sugars of the disaccharide and monosaccharide classes. Polysaccharides include cellulose and starches, of which only starch is digestible. Starches are glucose polymers. Starch is relatively resistant to digestion unless cooked, as heat and moisture rupture the plant cell wall, rendering the carbohydrate accessible to enzymatic degradation.

Disaccharides include sucrose, a molecule each of glucose and fructose; lactose, a molecule each of glucose and galactose; and maltose, two molecules of glucose. Monosaccharides of dietary importance include glucose, which is derived principally from the hydrolysis of dietary starch, fructose, and galactose. The five-carbon monosaccharides, ribose and deoxyribose, are synthesized endogenously for the production of nucleic acids. Sorbitol is the alcohol of glucose. The alcohol of xylose, xylitol, also is used as a sweetener.

Carbohydrate is absorbed only in the form of monosaccharides. Therefore, all more complex carbohydrates must undergo hydrolysis in the gut. This process begins in the mouth with the release of salivary amylase. Amylose is a glucose polymer occurring in straight chains, as opposed to amylopectin, the other primary constituent of plant starch, which is branched. Amylase disrupts the α-1,4-glucosidic bonds of amylose, breaking it down to maltose and oligosaccharides. The α-1,6-glucosidic bonds of amylopectin are resistant to amylase and are broken by isomaltase in the intestinal brush border.

The glucose linkages in cellulose are derived from a β-1,4 bond for which no enzyme is available, which accounts for the indigestibility of cellulose. The products of the action of salivary and pancreatic amylase are maltose and maltotriose from amylose, and maltose, maltotriose, limit dextrin (a composite of 1,4-α and 1,6-α glucose molecules), and some glucose from amylopectin. Serum glucose levels rise more rapidly after the ingestion of amylopectin than of amylose.

Anaerobic glucose metabolism in muscle leads to the production of pyruvate, which can be metabolized further to CO_2 in muscle or transported to the liver. During vigorous physical activity, there is insufficient oxygen in muscle to permit the metabolism of pyruvate to CO_2. The conversion of pyruvate to lactate ensues, which is necessary to reoxidize NADH formed during glycolysis. The accumulation of lactate during vigorous activity is responsible for the muscle pain that develops.

The rate of glycolysis can be altered by as much as 90-fold in response to the metabolic needs of working muscle and the availability of substrate to muscle and liver. Abundant carbohydrate intake induces glycolysis and inhibits gluconeogenesis, whereas fasting does the opposite. Energy stores within the cell act as signals to influence metabolism. When ATP levels are high, the tricarboxylic acid cycle is slowed and glycolysis is inhibited. High levels of ADP and AMP induce glycolysis and the regeneration of ATP.

When carbohydrate intake is very high, the glucose load can be handled in one of two ways. Either excess glucose can be permitted to enter the circulation, creating a situation analogous to diabetes mellitus any time a large carbohydrate load is ingested, or the carbohydrate can be disposed so as to avoid hyperglycemia. The latter occurs in nondiabetic individuals. Glucose is transported to liver and muscle to fully replenish glycogen stores.

As glucose continues to enter the circulation, glycolysis is induced, resulting in energy release and oxidative phosphorylation, with the generation of ATP. High levels of ATP tend to inhibit glycolysis by inhibiting the enzyme phosphofructokinase. An intermediate product of glycolysis, fructose-6-phosphate, then accumulates. The accumulation of fructose-6-phosphate activates an enzyme that converts it to fructose-2,6-biphosphate, which reactivates phosphofructokinase.

The marked rises in ATP and citrate that result in turn lead to increases in oxaloacetic acid and acetyl CoA. These increases, in turn, stimulate fatty acid synthesis. Consequently, the metabolism of a high carbohydrate load results in body fat deposition as a means of preventing the excess glucose from circulating and storing it for future use. Insulin release stimulates glycogen formation, whereas glucagon and epinephrine stimulate glycogenolysis in liver. Epinephrine also stimulates glycogenolysis in skeletal muscle, whereas glucagon does not.

Carbohydrate in cytosol glycosylates proteins in a specific manner under enzymatic control. When blood glucose levels are abnormally high, however, abnormal glycosylation, or glycation, can occur. Proteins exposed to the circulating glucose include those in the glomerular basement membrane, those in the vascular endothelium, and those in the lens of the eye, which appear to be particularly vulnerable. Glucose and galactose are metabolized in the lens of the eye, and elevated serum levels of either are associated with cataract formation. Thus, both diabetes mellitus and galactosemia are risk factors for cataract formation.

A sugar called D-tagatose glycates proteins much less than does glucose, and it is being studied as a possible replacement sweetener with health benefits. Fructose glycates nearly ten times as efficiently as glucose. Even at high intake, fructose levels in blood are only about 10% that of glucose. Thus, fructose may contribute as much to glycation as glucose when intake is high. Glycation is one of the cumulative injuries to cells associated with aging, linking high consumption of sugar to premature or accelerated aging of cells.

Starch degradation continues in the intestine with exposure to pancreatic amylase and intestinal brush border enzymes in the upper and middle portions of the jejunum. Brush border enzymes include isomaltase, sucrase, and lactase. An excess of enzyme is available for oligosaccharide digestion, with the exception of lactose. Lactase availability limits the rate at which glucose and galactose are cleaved from lactose. Brush border enzymes are inhibited as levels of monosaccharides rise in the intestinal lumen, preventing an accumulation of monosaccharides that could cause osmotic diarrhea. Dietary sucrose induces the enzymes sucrase and maltase. Lactase levels, however, are not influenced by the quantity of dietary lactose.

The starches resistant to enzymatic digestion are fermented by bacteria in the large bowel, providing 50% to 80% of the available energy in the form of fatty acids, and resulting in the formation of carbon dioxide and methane. The fatty acids produced in the large bowel include butyric, isobutyric, propionic, and acetic acids. Cells of the large bowel apparently derive energy from butyric acid and isobutyric acid in particular, and a role for these molecules in lowering the bowel's susceptibility to carcinogens has been described.

Monosaccharides are absorbed by simple diffusion, facilitated diffusion, and active transport. The monosaccharides absorbed exclusively via passive diffusion include the sugar alcohols and the L-isomers of glucose and galactose. Ingestion at one time of more than approximately 50 g of any of these sugars will exceed the rate of diffusion and generally produce gastrointestinal discomfort. Passive diffusion is slowed by the movement of water into the gut lumen as a result of the osmotic effect of ingested sugars. Proteins participate in the transport of carbohydrate molecules across lipophilic cell membranes. Active absorption of the D-stereoisomers of glucose and galactose permits more rapid uptake into the blood than passive diffusion could support. Fructose, a monosaccharide derived from sucrose, is absorbed via facilitated diffusion. Osmotic diarrhea is induced by the acute ingestion of approximately 100 g of fructose; more sugar is tolerated if ingested as sucrose, with the digestion of the disaccharide slowing the rate of absorption.

Lactase deficiency, the most common enzyme deficiency that has an impact on carbohydrate metabolism, affects approximately half of all adults worldwide. Variation by ethnic background appears to correlate with the practice of dairying over centuries or millennia, although a causal association in either direction has not been elucidated. Lactose-intolerant adults generally can tolerate approximately 5 g of lactose at a time without symptoms (see Chapter 17). This amount is found in approximately 100 mL of milk. Lactose tolerance can be assessed by administering 50 g of lactose and measuring the serum glucose. If glucose rises more than 1.4 mmol/L, the lactose has been hydrolyzed.

Glucose is the principal source of nutrient energy. It is metabolized to carbon dioxide and water via the tricarboxylic acid cycle. Alternative uses of glucose include formation of glycogen and conversion to fatty acids for deposition in adipose tissue. Approximately 5% of the available energy from oxidation is lost when glucose is converted to glycogen, and more than 25% is lost when glucose is stored as fat. Glycogen stores in muscle and liver account for approximately 300 g, or 1,200 kcal, which is enough to meet the energy needs of a fasting adult on a 2,000-kcal diet for approximately 14 hours. Nearly 100 times as much energy, or 120,000 kcal, is stored in the adipose tissue of a lean adult. However, only a small portion of this energy is readily expendable, generally enough to support energy needs for up to 10 days. Once glycogen stores are full, excess dietary carbohydrate is converted to fatty acids and stored in adipose tissue. The efficiency with which various sugars are converted to fat may be variable.

After carbohydrate ingestion, most of the glucose in the circulation escapes first-pass removal by the liver, whereas fructose is largely cleared by the liver. Fructose in the liver is used to produce glucose, lipid, or lactate. Fructose ingestion may raise serum levels of both lactic acid and uric acid. Galactose is metabolized principally in liver; the administration of galactose and measurement of the serum levels have been used as an assay of liver function. Galactose rises in serum in proportion to the dose ingested, although serum levels of galactose are blunted by concomitant administration of glucose, either orally or intravenously.

Most tissues can use glucose or other nutrients for fuel, but the brain and red blood cells utilize glucose exclusively, with the capacity to convert to ketone body metabolism during a protracted fast. Congenital deficiency of the enzyme glucose-6-phosphate dehydrogenase principally affects the red blood cell, occurring in populations with historical exposure to malaria. The inability to maintain reduced glutathione in the presence of various drugs, such as sulfonamides, renders such individuals susceptible to hemolysis.

The brain of an adult requires approximately 140 g of glucose per day, accounting for 560 kcal. Glucose needs increase during pregnancy and lactation, where it is used in the production of lactose. Both amino acids and triglycerides can be used to manufacture glucose. Gluconeogenesis can produce approximately 130 g of glucose per day in the absence of carbohydrate ingestion if other nutrients are abundant. Although the glucose deficit can be made up by ketone-body metabolism, fat oxidation also requires glucose. Once glycogen stores are depleted, therefore, a minimal intake of 50 g of glucose in any form appears to be desirable. Because glucose can be produced endogenously, it is not considered an essential nutrient, and no recommended daily allowance has been established.

A diet rich in fructose tends to raise serum triglycerides, although levels tend to normalize over a period of weeks unless the association is compounded by obesity. High-carbohydrate diets lower levels of high-density lipoproteins, and this effect too seems to be particularly strong for fructose. Consequently, a diet high in sucrose has deleterious effects on the lipid profile, whereas these effects are to some degree mitigated if complex carbohydrates predominate. Polyunsaturated fat in the diet also blunts the fasting triglyceride rise induced by sucrose. Individuals with hypertriglyceridemia tend to have a particularly brisk rise in triglycerides in response to high carbohydrate intake.

BIBLIOGRAPHY

See "Sources for All Chapters."

2

Clinically Relevant Fat Metabolism

INTRODUCTION

Lipids are categorized broadly as compounds that are soluble in organic solvents, but not water. They include both plant and animal products. Cholesterol, a nutritionally important lipid compound, is found exclusively in animal tissues.

Most of the fat energy in the diet is derived from triglycerides, molecules formed by linkage via ester bonds of three fatty acid molecules to a molecule of glycerol. Fat serves as an energy source and as a source of precursors in prostaglandin metabolism, and it contributes essential structural components of cells. Polyunsaturated fatty acids (PUFAs) are precursors of eicosanoids, including prostaglandins, thromboxanes, and leukotrienes.

Cholesterol and phospholipids are constituents of all cell membranes and of myelin. Cholesterol is utilized in the production of adrenal and gonadal steroid hormones and of bile acids. Among the three principal classes of macronutrients (carbohydrate, protein, and fat), lipids provide the greatest energy density—approximately 9 kcal/g. In addition to providing concentrated energy, dietary lipids enhance the palatability and absorption of fat-soluble micronutrients, such as vitamins A, D, E, and K (see Chapter 4).

ABSORPTION AND TRANSPORT

Lipases produced by the tongue and stomach act on triglycerides in the upper gastrointestinal tract; both require an acid environment. For the most part, lipases are active at the 1- and 3-ester bonds in a triglyceride molecule, but not at the no. 2 linkage. The transport of hydrophobic lipids in an aqueous medium is accomplished through emulsification, the dispersal of fat into tiny droplets. Bile salts contribute to the stabilization of lipid micelles, preventing them from reaggregating. In addition to fatty acids, micelles are rich in 2-monoglycerides, owing to the resistance of the fatty acid at the 2 position on glycerol to lipolysis.

Emulsification and chemical digestion of fat are accelerated in the duodenum; mechanical digestion in the stomach serves to decrease droplet size and increase exposed surface area. The presence of fatty acids and amino acids and release of hydrochloric acid in the stomach trigger release of cholecystokinin-pancreozymin as well as secretin. The acidity of the gastric chyme is reversed by the buffering effects of the duodenal mucosa, the secretin-induced release of bicarbonate from the pancreas, and the release of alkaline bile from the gall bladder induced by cholecystokinin.

Emulsified fat droplets are acted on by pancreatic lipase in the upper small bowel. Pancreatic lipase is activated only in an alkaline environment. Lipase is held to the droplets by colipase, which is secreted concurrently from the pancreas. Pancreatic lipase also cleaves fatty acids from the 1 and 3 positions of a triglyceride, producing two molecules of free fatty acid and one of monoglyceride (a fatty acid bound to glycerol in the 2 carbon position). Fat absorption then occurs predominantly in the proximal portion of the small bowel.

Free fatty acids and monoglycerides as well are readily absorbed in the upper small intestine. Short-chain fatty acids are absorbed into portal blood, bound to albumin, and transported to the liver. Longer-chain fatty acids are reesterified to triglyceride, as is cholesterol. They are packaged into chylomicrons that are transported via lymph.

Bile salts separate from the lipid droplets at the mucosa and ultimately are reabsorbed in the lower small bowel as part of the enterohepatic circulation. Bile acid sequestrants lower cholesterol by interrupting this circulation, causing bile acids to be lost in stool and depleted; their reconstitution requires consumption of cholesterol.

Absorption of ingested triglyceride is facilitated by phospholipid, which is present in the diet in much smaller quantities. Phospholipids serve to emulsify triglyceride in the stomach. They are structurally important in separating hydrophobic lipids from water in the cell membrane.

Fatty acids and monoglycerides are absorbed almost completely, whereas cholesterol absorption ranges from 30% to 70%. Fatty acids can be used as an energy source by most cells, with erythrocytes and cells of the central nervous system being notable exceptions. The brain uses glucose for fuel exclusively unless the supply is depleted, at which time ketone bodies produced from the catabolism of fatty acids are substituted. The mitochondrial transport of long-chain fatty acids requires a carrier, carnitine transferase. The fixed metabolic needs for fat can be met with an intake level of as little as 20 to 25 g per day.

Energy consumed in excess of needs is stored principally as triglycerides in adipose tissue, predominantly as palmitic (saturated) and oleic (monounsaturated) acids. The energy reserves in body fat even in lean individuals are generally 100-fold greater than glycogen stores, providing a depot of approximately 120,000 kcal.

The longer the chain length of fatty acids, the less readily they are absorbed. There are virtually no short-chain fatty acids (two to four carbons) of nutritional significance. Medium-chain triglycerides, which have six to 12 carbons, are absorbed more readily than longer-chain triglycerides because of more efficient emulsification and greater water solubility. They also tend to be absorbed, bound to albumin, without reesterification by enterocytes, directly into the portal circulation, whereas the micelles are absorbed via lymphatics.

Portal flow is considerably faster than lymphatic flow. Thus, medium-chain triglycerides are relatively unaffected by deficiencies of bile salts, require minimal pancreatic lipase activity, are relatively unaffected by impaired enterocyte function, and are absorbed far faster than long-chain trigylcerides (see Chapters 22 and 24). Long-chain triglycerides of the n-3 variety from marine sources are more readily absorbed than saturated or monounsaturated fatty acids of comparable length.

Cholesterol in the bowel, whether of endogenous or exogenous origin, is incompletely absorbed. There is debate regarding the upper limit of cholesterol absorption in adults. Although some authorities believe it to be maximal at approximately 500 mg per day, others believe 40% of up to 2 g of intestinal cholesterol will be absorbed daily. Ingested cholesterol affects serum cholesterol, but to a limited extent because of limited absorption. A high cholesterol intake may raise serum cholesterol by as much as 15%. The bacterial degradation of unabsorbed cholesterol in the large bowel may contribute to the increased risk of colon cancer associated with diets high in animal fat.

Average stool fat in adults is in the range from 4 to 6 g per day. With very high fat intake, fat absorption continues more distally in the small bowel. Of note, human infants have a similar capacity to absorb fat when fed human milk, because of the presence of lipase in breast milk. Lipase is absent from bovine milk, and bottle-fed infants are subject to some degree of fat malabsorption.

Adults have a reserve capacity to absorb even twice the amount of fat typically present in even high-fat diets. Although neonates have low levels of bile salts and thus are poor at forming micelles, the lipase present in human milk can cleave even the fatty acid at the 2 position on glycerol, producing free fatty acids that are relatively readily absorbed, independent of micelle formation. Capacity for fat absorption tends to decline with age in older adults. Vitamin D deficiency appears to be one consequence of clinical importance.

Partial gastric resections tend to produce some degree of fat malabsorption, with fecal fat increasing from 4 to 6 g up to 15 g per day. Exocrine pancreatic insufficiency results in fat malabsorption. Disease or resection of the ileum may result in bile acid deficiency, which leads to fat malabsorption.

LIPOPROTEIN METABOLISM

Triglycerides are the principal source of fuel from fat and the principal source of energy stored in adipose tissue. Cholesterol and phospholipid act primarily as membrane constituents. In the fasting state, fatty acids for energy production are derived from adipose tissue stores. In the fed state, fatty acids are available from chylomicrons and very-low-density lipoprotein (VLDL); the extraction of triglyceride from these particles is mediated by the enzyme lipoprotein lipase. Most fat is transported via triglycerides resynthesized in enterocytes.

Fatty acids with chain lengths shorter than 14 carbons are bound to albumin and transported directly to the liver via the portal vein. Endothelial cells can take up lipoprotein particles, as well as free fatty acid bound to albumin; triglyceride from lipoprotein particles is the predominant source.

Several enzymatic pathways are involved. The triglycerides are packaged in chylomicrons, which contain unesterified cholesterol in the outer layer and esterified cholesterol in the core. There is some evidence that the ingestion of fat of any type stimulates endogenous production of primarily saturated fatty acids, which are released into the circulation along with the fat from exogenous sources.

Enterocytes package ingested fat into chylomicrons and VLDL, both of which contain apoprotein B-48. High-density lipoprotein (HDL), manufactured in the liver and rich in apoproteins C (apo C) and E (apo E), interacts with the lipoproteins of intestinal origin. HDL transfers apo C and apo E to chylomicrons. Apo C serves as a cofactor that activates lipoprotein lipase, whereas apo E in the chylomicron remnant core facilitates the particle's uptake by hepatocytes.

The activity of lipoprotein lipase is stimulated by heparin and insulin. The hypertriglyceridemia seen in poorly controlled diabetes mellitus is associated with reduced insulin action leading to reduced lipoprotein lipase activity (see Chapter 10). Niacin activates lipoprotein lipase, which explains its utility in treating hypertriglyceridemia. Lipoprotein lipase is inhibited by glucagon, thyroid-stimulating hormone, catecholamines, and adrenocorticotrophic hormone; these hormones generally also stimulate the release of free fatty acids from adipose tissue reserves.

Free fatty acids are used to produce ATP in muscle and adipose tissue; if not used immediately for energy generation, they are reesterified to triglyceride. This process requires the enzyme glycerol-3-phosphate, which requires both glucose and insulin for synthesis. Therefore, carbohydrate feeding has the tendency to drop the concentration of free fatty acids in circulation by augmenting the availability of glucose and the levels of insulin. Insulin action promotes reesterification of free fatty acid into triglyceride and opposes lipolysis. Free fatty acid taken up from plasma by the liver is predominantly incorporated into VLDL. High levels of VLDL production in the liver lead to hypertriglyceridemia.

Fatty acids from chylomicrons and VLDL are used for fuel by the heart, smooth muscle, red muscle fibers, kidneys, and platelets in particular. In addition, they serve as substrate for the formation and function of biomembranes. The fatty acid composition of lipid particles formed by enterocytes influences cellular and subcellular membrane integrity and function, as well as the synthesis of prostaglandins and leukotrienes (see Chapters 15 and 18). Extracted fatty acids from lipoprotein particles of intestinal origin contribute to the energy stored in adipose tissue. The fatty acid composition of VLDL synthesized by the liver is influenced by dietary fat composition, which influences the composition of adipose tissue. Both VLDL and the LDL produced when VLDL is acted on by lipoprotein lipase, are atherogenic, and are taken up by macrophages and subendothelial smooth muscle cells.

Uptake of HDL by the liver is influenced by the interaction of apo E and its receptor. There are several isoforms of apo E, encoded by various mutations in the apo E allele. Apo E-II is associated with the accumulation of chylomicrons and VLDL in blood due to impaired hepatic uptake. Although the concentration of HDL in plasma is lower than that of LDL, HDL particles are present in larger numbers. HDL particles transfer apoproteins and surface lipids with chylomicrons and VLDL. Cholesterol acquired by HDL is esterified by the enzyme lecithin cholesterol acyltransferase (LCAT). The esterified cholesterol moves to the core of the HDL particle, facilitating additional uptake of cholesterol from other lipoprotein particles. HDL is largely taken up by the liver, but also by the adrenals, and in women by the ovaries; all are tissues with a high cholesterol requirement.

Cholesterol can by synthesized by virtually all human tissues from acetate. The rate-limiting step in cholesterol biosynthesis involves the enzyme beta-hydroxy-beta-methylglutaryl coenzyme A (HMG-CoA) reductase. HMG-CoA reductase is stimulated by insulin and inhibited by glucagon. High cholesterol feeding can inhibit endogenous cholesterol synthesis, whereas gastrointestinal loss of cholesterol, such as induced by bile acid sequestrant drugs, can actually stimulate endogenous production.

When LDL receptors are deficient, as in familial hyperlipidemia type IIA, rising levels of LDL do not inhibit cholesterol biosynthesis, as they do normally. Under conditions of homeostasis, an adult in a westernized country may consume a daily average of 335 mg of cholesterol. An additional 800 mg per day is synthesized endogenously.

Approximately 400 mg is lost daily in bile acids, another 600 mg in biliary cholesterol, 50 mg in the production of steroid hormones, and 85 mg is excreted as sterols from skin. Thus, 1,135 mg of cholesterol is exchanged daily. Most cholesterol in circulation is in the esterified form, produced through the action of LCAT, which is produced by the liver. Esterification of cholesterol is also mediated by acyl-CoA cholesterol acyltransferase (ACAT), particularly in liver. The esterifying enzymes have different preferences for fatty acid substrate.

FATTY ACIDS

Fatty acids, carbon chains with the basic formula $CH_3(CH_2)_nCOOH-$, are short, medium, or long chain, and saturated, monounsaturated, or polyunsaturated. Short-chain fatty acids have less than six carbons; medium-chain fatty acids have six to ten; and long-chain fatty acids have 12 or more carbons. Saturated fatty acids contain no carbon-to-carbon double bonds, whereas monounsaturates contain one and polyunsaturates contain more than one. PUFAs are further divided into those with the initial double-bond 3 carbons from the methyl terminus of the molecule (n-3 or ω-3 fatty acids) and those with the initial double-bond 6 carbons from the methyl terminus (n-6 or ω-6 fatty acids). The synthesis of cholesterol, saturated fatty acids, and unsaturated fatty acids from acetyl coenzyme A occurs endogenously; thus, none of these nutrients is essential in the diet. Certain PUFAs cannot be synthesized endogenously and therefore are considered essential. Naturally occurring fatty acids tend to have even numbers of carbons, to be unbranched, and to be in the cis configuration relative to double bonds.

Naturally occurring monounsaturates are predominantly of the cis configuration relative to the single double bond. The partial hydrogenation of polyunsaturated fat produces a preponderance of trans monounsaturates. The trans configuration allows for tighter packing of the molecules, with resultant heat resistance. The melting point of a triglyceride is the product of carbon chain length of its constituent fatty acids, the configuration of the fatty acids (cis or trans), and the position of the fatty acid with regard to the glycerol. Saturation of fatty acids raises the melting point and decreases water solubility. While providing the favorable properties to industry of longer shelf life and higher melting point, the physiologic effects of trans fat are more comparable to those of saturated fats than to those of monounsaturates in the cis configuration (see Chapter 6).

ESSENTIAL FATTY ACIDS

Most fatty acids can be synthesized endogenously from excess energy of any source or from other fatty acids; those that are required for metabolic functions and cannot be synthesized endogenously are essential nutrients. Fatty acids of the n-3 and n-6 polyunsaturated classes are referred to as essential fatty acids (EFAs). Fatty acid synthesis occurs primarily in the liver. Enzymes involved in fatty acid synthesis have a high affinity for fatty acid of the n-3 PUFA class, with successively lesser affinity for fatty acids of the n-6 PUFA, n 9, and n-7 classes. Affinity in general is greater the less saturated the fatty acid. The composition of fatty acids in cell membranes can provide evidence of EFA deficiency, as the end products of fatty acid metabolism vary with the substrate. EFAs of the n-3 and n-6 classes are substrate for the lipoxygenase and cyclooxygenase enzymes. The products of EFA metabolism are referred to collectively as eicosanoids.

The eicosanoid products of EFA metabolism clearly vary with the distribution of n-3 and n-6 fatty acids in the diet, with implications for immune function, hemostasis, and metabolism discussed in more detail elsewhere (see Chapters 8, 15, and 18). Deficiency of EFAs is associated with impaired growth, abnormal skin, and infertility. EFAs of the n-3 class are preferentially incorporated into the brain and the retina. The requirement for n-3 fatty acid is not reliably known, but various lines of evidence support greater proportional intake of n-3 fatty acids than the Western diet generally provides (see Chapters 6, 15, 27, and 39). High intake of saturated or trans fat increases requirements for EFAs.

Animals and humans are deficient in an enzyme needed to convert oleic acid to linoleic acid and therefore require linoleic acid, an ω-6 fatty acid, in the diet. Linoleic acid can be converted to the 20-carbon arachidonic acid, also ω-6. Therefore, arachidonic acid is essential in the diet only when linoleic acid intake is inadequate. Thus, one n-6 fatty acid is truly essential, whereas a second is conditionally essential. The third polyunsaturate considered essential is α-linolenic acid, an 18-carbon ω-3. The importance of ω-3 fatty acids to homeostasis and a variety of physiologic states is discussed throughout the text (see especially Chapters 6, 8, 15, and 18). Linolenic acid can be metabolized to docosahexaenoic acid (22 carbons, n-3) or eicosapentaenoic acid (20 carbons, n-3), both of which are important constituents of cell membranes and are particularly abundant in the retina and brain. The longer-chain n-3 fatty acids may be obtained directly from consumption of fish and seafood.

PUFAs of the n-6 class are particularly important in cell and subcellular membranes throughout the body; both linoleic and arachidonic acid are abundant in structural phospholipids. Additionally, as noted, polyunsaturates of both n-6 and n-3 classes are important eicosanoid precursors. As discussed elsewhere (see Chapters 8, 15, and 18), the relative abundance of each class of EFA in the diet influences the distribution of prostaglandins and leukotrienes, with important implications for platelet function and inflammatory reactions. In general, the n-6 fatty acids promote both platelet aggregation and inflammatory activity, whereas the n-3 fatty acids are inhibitory. At present, intake of linoleic acid not less than 1% to 2% of total daily calories (3 to 6 g per day for an adult) is recommended, as is intake of α-linolenic acid (or other n-3 fatty acids) at not less than 10% to 25% the level of n-6 fatty acids. As of 1989, when the last formal edition of the recommended dietary allowance (RDAs) was published (1), no RDA had been established for either n-6 or n-3 fatty acids.

CURRENT INTAKE PATTERNS AND RECOMMENDATIONS

Dietary fat constitutes as little as 10% of total ingested energy in some Asian countries, as much as 45% in some European countries, and between 30% and 40% in the United States. The National Health and Nutrition Examination Surveys suggest that fat ingestion as a proportion of total calories is declining in the United States, from more than 40% to a current level of approximately 34% (2,3). However, total fat intake has remained relatively constant, owing to an increase in total energy consumption (4). Principal sources of fat in the US diet include red meat, other meats, and dairy products. The proportion of fat contributed by vegetable oils has increased over recent years, because of consumption of fast foods cooked with such oils, as well as dressings, spreads, condiments, and processed foods incorporating vegetable fat.

The health effects of dietary fat in the United States are predominantly those of excess rather than deficiency, although the contributions of n-3 fatty acid deficiency to chronic disease may be considerable. Saturated fat in the diet is the principal exogenous determinant of serum cholesterol levels, which in turn influence risk of cardiovascular events (see Chapter 6). Dietary cholesterol contributes as well to serum cholesterol, but it is consumed in milligram rather than gram amounts and therefore contributes relatively less (see Chapter 6, and Hegsted and Keys equations, Section IIIA).

Conventional recommendations regarding dietary fat are that the total not exceed 30% of calories; saturated fat intake not exceed 10% of calories; and cholesterol intake not exceed 300 mg per day. There is on-going debate, however, about both optimal quantity and distribution of dietary fat (5,6). On the basis of confluent lines of evidence, recommendations may be made for approximately 25% of total calories from fat; less than 5% of total calories derived from the combination of saturated and trans fat; approximately 10% to 15% of calories from polyunsaturated fat, divided between n-6 and n-3 fatty acids in a ratio of between 4:1 and 1:1; and the remaining 10% to 15% of calories from monounsaturated fat (see Chapters 6 and 40). Of note, the requirement for vitamin E and other antioxidants rises with consumption of polyunsaturated fat, as fatty acids with double bonds are particularly subject to oxidation and rancidification.

Saturated fats derived from both animal and plant sources constitute approximately 12% of calories in the prevailing US diet. Most naturally occurring oils and fats contain a variety of fatty acids. Butter fat, beef fat, and coconut oil are all highly saturated, although the distribution of saturated fatty acids is considerably variable (see Section IIIF). The average intake of trans fatty acid in the United States, from processed and snack foods, spreads, and dressings, is approximately 5% to 8% of calories and has been increasing. A potential hazard of efforts to reduce fat intake is that visible fat in oils may be eliminated, resulting in the fat hidden in processed foods accounting for a higher percentage of total fat intake. Oils (and some spreads) are apt to be the main sources of EFAs, whereas the fat added during food processing is predominantly either saturated or trans hydrogenated.

Triglycerides, the principal dietary fat, are composed of three fatty acid molecules esterified with one glycerol molecule. The diverse combinations of fatty acids with glycerol result in a great variety of dietary fat. Fatty acids in the saturated class include stearic (18 carbons), palmitic (16 carbons), myristic (14 carbons), lauric (12 carbons), and medium-chain fatty acids (8 to 10 carbons). The principal dietary monounsaturate derived from nature is oleic acid (18 carbons, cis configuration), whereas the trans stereoisomer, elaidic acid, is derived primarily from industrial hydrogenation of fat. PUFAs include the n-6 linoleic acid (18 carbons), and the n-3 fatty acids linolenic (18 carbons), eicosapentaenoic (20 carbons), and docosahexaenoic (22 carbons). In the US diet, the major saturated fatty acids are palmitic and stearic acids. The predominant monounsaturated fatty acid is oleic. The principal sources of polyunsaturates in the diet are plants, which provide predominantly linoleic acid (18-carbon n-6 fatty acid) and linolenic acid (18-carbon n-3), and seafoods, which are rich in eicosapentaenoic acid and docosahexaenoic acid.

Linoleic acid is found in a variety of commonly used vegetable oils, including corn, sunflower, and safflower. Evening primrose oil provides γ-linoleic acid, a form that bypasses an intermediate metabolic step. Plant sources particularly rich in linolenic acid (n-3) include flaxseed, soy, rapeseed (canola), and walnuts. Long-chain n-3 fatty acids are abundant in salmon, mackerel, sardines, and scallops. Farm-raised fish may provide less n-3 fatty acid than wild fish, as the source of n-3 PUFAs in fish is the vegetation and plankton on which they feed. Similarly, the flesh of wild ungulates contains n-3 PUFAs in appreciable amounts, whereas the flesh of domesticated feed animals does not.

EFAs are derived from either vegetable sources or the flesh of herbivorous animals consuming plant matter that contains these nutrients. EFAs modified during processing, with resultant formation of trans isomers or movement of double bonds, may act as metabolic competitors of the EFAs in their native state. During processing of vegetables for the production of vegetable oils, much of the sterols and phospholipids are removed. Sterols interfere with cholesterol absorption; for this reason, cholesterol absorption may increase as a result of processed vegetable oil in the diet. The plant sterol, β-sitosterol, has been used to lower serum cholesterol modestly by interfering with cholesterol absorption. Phosphatidylcholine, a phospholipid, also interferes with cholesterol absorption.

REFERENCES

1. National Research Council. *Recommended dietary allowances,* 10th ed. Washington, DC: National Academy Press, 1989.
2. MMWR. Daily dietary fat and total food-energy intakes—Third National Health and Nutrition Examination Survey, Phase I, 1988–1991. *MMWR* 1994; 43:116.
3. Katz DL, Brunner RL, St. Jeor ST, et al. Dietary fat consumption in a cohort of American adults, 1985–1991: covariates, secular trends, and compliance with guidelines. *Am J Health Promot* 1998;12:382.
4. Kennedy ET, Bowman SA, Powell R. Dietary-fat intake in the US population. *J Am Coll Nutr* 1999; 18:207.
5. Connor WE, Connor SL. Should a low-fat, high-carbohydrate diet be recommended for everyone? The case for a low-fat, high-carbohydrate diet. *N Engl J Med* 1997;337:562.
6. Katan MB, Grundy SM, Willett WC. Should a low-fat, high-carbohydrate diet be recommended for everyone? Beyond low-fat diets. *N Engl J Med* 1997; 337:563.

BIBLIOGRAPHY

See "Sources for All Chapters."

3

Clinically Relevant Protein Metabolism

OVERVIEW

Protein represents one of three principal classes of macronutrients; the other classes are carbohydrate and fat. Dietary protein is required as a source of amino acids, both essential and nonessential, and for use in the synthesis of structural and functional body proteins. The need for amino acids is driven by the constant turnover of body tissues. In its function as a source of fuel, protein is the least energy-dense of the macronutrient classes, providing between 3 and 4 kcal/g.

Ingested proteins are broken down by pepsin in the stomach and further by pancreatic enzymes activated on release into the duodenum. Pancreatic enzyme release is stimulated by the presence of protein in the stomach and inhibited when the level of trypsin exceeds the available protein to which it can bind. Unbound trypsin inhibits the release of trypsinogen. The pancreatic proteases are specific to peptide bonds adjacent to particular amino acids or amino acid classes. Amino acids and dipeptides are absorbed through the mucosa of the small bowel. The amount of protein absorbed daily is derived from that ingested, as well as the protein from gastrointestinal secretions and the sloughing of gastrointestinal cells into the bowel lumen.

Once absorbed, amino acids are transported to the liver via the portal vein. The liver is the principal site of catabolism for all of the essential amino acids, except those with branched chains. The branched-chain amino acids are catabolized principally in muscle and kidney, which provides a ratio-

nale for their use in selected cases of advanced liver disease (see Chapter 21).

The liver responds to varying levels of intake of the essential amino acids by inducing or inhibiting specific enzymatic pathways. Metabolism of essential amino acids consumed in excess of need is accelerated to eliminate the excess. The degree of regulation is less strict for nonessential amino acids, the metabolism of which is simply proportional to the amount ingested. The synthetic functions of the liver relying on metabolized protein as substrate vary daily according to the availability of amino acids from the circulation.

Plasma levels of amino acids are influenced by dietary intake to varying degrees. The liver controls the release of specific amino acids into the peripheral circulation, but the levels of some amino acids rise as intake exceeds metabolic demand. Conversely, levels in plasma fall as intake falls, but only as low as the level needed to satisfy the demand of body tissues. At that level, called the point of inflection, plasma levels are maintained as intake falls, barring frank deficiency. This level has been used to determine the dietary requirements for certain amino acids, although it is not a reliable index for all of them.

Carbohydrate ingestion stimulates insulin release, and insulin facilitates the entry of amino acids into muscle. The levels of branched-chain amino acids in particular fall after a carbohydrate meal. Branched-chain amino acids (leucine, isoleucine, and valine) compete with tryptophan for uptake by brain cells. Following insulin release, the levels of circulating branched-chain amino acids fall, resulting in preferential uptake of tryptophan by the brain. Tryptophan is used in the production of serotonin, which is thought to induce sleepiness. Tryptophan is rate limiting in the synthesis of serotonin, and thus serotonin levels depend largely on hepatic regulation of protein degradation and the release of tryptophan.

During a fast, the prototypical 70-kg man loses approximately 50 g of protein per day from skeletal muscle, the largest depot in the body. The principal amino acids released from muscle are alanine and glutamine, which are the main carriers of nitrogen from muscle to liver. Alanine is transported directly to the liver, whereas glutamine is transported to the intestine and transaminated to alanine before reaching the liver through the portal circulation.

In the liver, the carbon chain of alanine is used in gluconeogenesis, whereas the amino group is metabolized to urea or recycled to other amino acids. Under carefully controlled conditions, 3-methylhistidine, a product of protein catabolism in muscle, can be measured in urine to assess the extent of amino acid release from muscle to liver.

The most readily accessible, and therefore measurable, pool of proteins is that circulating in plasma. Plasma proteins are predominantly glycoproteins and albumin. The levels of plasma proteins fall and rise with nutritional status. Albumin levels decline with significant malnutrition, but they are relatively insensitive to minor or short-term aberrations in dietary intake. Prealbumin and retinol-binding protein are better indicators of short-term deficits of dietary protein or energy (see Chapter 24).

For a 70-kg man, daily dietary protein intake in the United States is approximately 100 g, augmented by approximately 70 g secreted or sloughed into the bowel. Roughly 160 of these 170 g is absorbed as amino acids or dipeptides, whereas 10 g is lost in stool. Approximately 300 g of protein is synthesized each day, utilizing nearly 200 g of recycled protein in addition to the 100 g ingested.

Recycled proteins are derived from intestinal secretions and cells, plasma proteins, muscle, and senescent blood cells. A 100-g pool of free amino acids, predominantly nonessential, is maintained as well. A total of 400 g of amino acids is exchanged daily. Protein intake is 100 g, and 300 g of protein is derived daily from body-tissue turnover. Of this pool, 300 g is used for protein synthesis, and 100 g is consumed in catabolism.

Dietary protein provides amino acids for the synthesis of cells in all body tissues. Amino acids are essential if they cannot be synthesized endogenously. There are nine essential amino acids in humans: histidine, isoleucine, leucine, lysine, methionine, phenylalanine, threonine, tryptophan, and valine. Two other amino acids, cysteine and tyrosine, become essential if intake of their precursors, methionine and phenylalanine, respectively, is limited. The nonessential amino acids include arginine, alanine, aspartic acid, asparagine, glutamic acid, glutamine, glycine, proline, and serine. Other amino acids are derived from these 20.

Ingested amino acids serve one of four purposes. They are used in the synthesis of tissue proteins, catabolized to meet energy needs, incorporated into energy stores as glycogen or adipose tissue, or used to synthesize other nitrogen containing moieties, such as other amino acids, catecholamines, or purine bases. Amino acid degradation in the liver results in the formation of urea, most of which is secreted into urine. In the gut, about 20% of urea is converted to ammonia, which in turn is cleared by the liver via the enterohepatic circulation.

Amino acids are used in the synthesis of the purine bases, adenine and guanine, and the pyrimidine bases, uracil and cytosine. These ribonucleotides serve as precursors for DNA synthesis. Glutamine is important in the biosynthesis of purines. The initial step in pyrimidine biosynthesis involves carbamoyl phosphate, which also serves as a substrate for urea synthesis. When arginine intake is deficient, or in individuals with deficiency of ornithine-carbamoyl transferase, excessive carbamoyl phosphate is diverted to the pyrimidine synthesis pathway. The result is the spillage of orotic acid in the urine, which is therefore a marker of arginine deficiency.

Arginine and glycine are metabolized in the kidney and liver to produce creatine. Creatine is transported to muscle, where it is stored as creatine and creatine phosphate. A dehydration reaction in muscle converts creatine and creatine phosphate to creatinine, which is released from muscle into the pool of total body water. Slightly less than 2% of creatine in the body is converted to creatinine each day. Urinary creatinine is a product of muscle mass, the concentration of creatine in muscle, and dietary intake of creatine in meat.

Ammonia is formed in the kidney as an end product of glutamine metabolism. The glutamine ultimately is metabolized to α-ketoglutarate, which is used in gluconeogenesis during a protracted fast. Acidosis and starvation accelerate ammonia production.

Protein metabolism is linked to carbohydrate and fat metabolism. In the fasted state, insulin levels are low, and glucagon levels are elevated. Lipases in adipose tissue release fatty acids and glycerol. Glycogen stores in the liver are consumed to meet energy needs for the first 12 to 18 hours of fasting. With more protracted fasting, energy needs are met by the release of protein from muscle and intestine serving as a substrate for gluconeogenesis in the liver. Free fatty acids are used in the liver to produce ketone bodies. Muscle uses free fatty acids, and subsequently ketone bodies, as an alternative fuel to glucose. With feeding, insulin levels rise and glucagon levels subside. Glucose is carried into liver and muscle, both to reconstitute glycogen and to be used as fuel. Insulin suppresses the action of lipases in adipose tissue and inhibits the release of fatty acids.

NITROGEN BALANCE

Nitrogenous wastes are removed from the body in urine as urea, ammonia, uric acid, and creatinine, and in stool as unabsorbed proteins. Minor losses occur through skin and in the form of shed integument and the secretions of mucous membranes. Ordinarily, urea accounts for approximately 80% of the nitrogenous waste in urine. During a protracted fast, the proportion of urine nitrogen lost in the form of ammonia rises, particularly in response to acidosis.

Proteins typically contain approximately 16% nitrogen, therefore, 1 g of nitrogen corresponds to 6.25 g of total protein. Nitrogen balance (B) is measured as the difference between intake (I) and all losses, including urine (U), feces (F), skin (S), and miscellaneous minor losses (M):

$$B = I - (U + F + S + M).$$

B may be positive, negative, or zero. (For additional pertinent formulas, see Section IIIA.)

Nitrogen balance is affected by total energy intake. When ingested calories exceed need, protein needs fall, and nitrogen balance remains positive. When energy intake falls to near or below requirements, protein needs rise, and nitrogen balance tends to become negative unless protein intake increases substantially. Amino acid requirements in men have been estimated to range from 0.5 g/kg/day when energy intake is high (57 kcal/kg/day), to over 1 g/kg/day when energy intake is low (40 kcal/kg/day). Even with high intake of energy, however, essential amino acid consumption below required levels will result in negative nitrogen balance. In a state of normal health and dietary adequacy in an adult, nitrogen balance is maintained, with intake matching losses.

DIETARY PROTEIN REQUIREMENTS

Protein requirements have been estimated on the basis of replacing obligate nitrogen losses (i.e., those losses that persist on a protein-free diet) and on the basis of maintaining healthy adults in nitrogen balance. For children, estimates have been based on the maintenance of optimal growth.

Requirements during pregnancy and lactation have been estimated on the basis of optimal fetal and neonatal growth.

Obligate nitrogen losses on a protein-free diet have been estimated at approximately 54 g/kg. To replace this amount of nitrogen, 340 g of protein is required (nitrogen is multiplied by 6.25 to give an average relative protein mass). Therefore, 0.34 g/kg/day of protein is required to replenish obligate losses of sedentary adults. The World Health Organization increases that value to 0.45 g/kg/day to account for individual variation. Replacement studies have further demonstrated that as protein is replenished, the efficiency of its utilization declines as intake approaches requirements. This inefficiency adds 30% to required intake, increasing the estimate for adults to 0.57 g/kg/day. In situations where energy intake is not clearly in excess of need, this estimate is further raised to 0.8 g/kg/day.

In the United States, the average daily requirement for total protein has been estimated at 0.6 g/kg/day, given the availability of both abundant nutrient energy for most of the population and of protein of high biologic quality. This figure was increased by two standard deviations to 0.75 g/kg/day, then rounded up to 0.8 g/kg/day to establish the recommended dietary allowance (RDA) for adult men and women in the United States. Pregnancy adds approximately 10 g to daily protein needs, and lactation adds nearly 15 g for the first 6 months, then in the range of 12 g thereafter. Rapid growth in early childhood results in substantially higher needs for protein. The RDA for infants up to 6 months of age is 2.2 g/kg/day; between 6 months and 1 year, it is 1.6 g/kg/day; and by the age of 7, it declines to approximately 1.0 g/kg/day. The adult RDA of 0.8 g/kg/day pertains beginning at age 15 in females and 19 in males. Higher intake levels may be indicated with vigorous physical activity (see Chapter 30).

Estimates are available of the required daily intake of each of the essential amino acids for both children and adults (see Section III). The proportion of daily protein intake that must be made up of essential amino acids declines from over 40% in infancy, to approximately 35% in children, and further to 20% in adults. When protein losses attributable to acute illness or injury are being made up during the convalescent period, protein with 35% to 40% essential amino acids generally is favored. Protein restriction is required during acutely decompensated hepatic insufficiency (see Chapter 21) and uremia (see Chapter 11).

For protein synthesis to occur, all essential amino acids must be available simultaneously in the serum. If there is a deficit in any of the essential amino acids, its generation to permit protein synthesis will require catabolism. Thus, the ingestion of balanced protein is necessary to prevent negative nitrogen balance. Protein synthesis occurs within the first several postprandial hours; therefore, the distribution of incomplete but complementary protein meals over a day is of less utility in the maintenance of nitrogen balance than the ingestion of balanced protein during a single meal.

High doses of single amino acids may be toxic; this is particularly true for methionine and tyrosine. Antagonism also may occur, in which high doses of an amino acid interfere with the metabolism of another; this is true for the branched-chain amino acids. An imbalance in amino acids refers to situations where tissue growth is impaired on account of limiting amounts of one or more amino acids, despite adequate total protein intake.

PROTEIN QUALITY/ BIOLOGIC VALUE

The quality of dietary protein refers to the array of amino acids provided. The more completely food protein provides essential amino acids, the greater its biologic quality. A variety of methods have been used to gauge the biologic value of protein, the favored of which is to determine the proportion of a protein used in metabolism without raising nitrogen losses. A formula used to indicate the degree to which ingested nitrogen is retained is a common measure of protein quality, or biologic value:

Biologic value =
$$[food\ N - (fecal\ N + urinary\ N)]/\\(food\ N - fecal\ N).$$

The value for egg albumin, which represents a complete source of amino acids, is 100; other proteins are compared with this reference standard. Alternative measures of protein quality also are in use; the biologic value of protein may be expressed as the ratio of the limiting amino acid per gram of a particular food to its quantity per gram of egg. Lysine, sulfur-containing amino acids, or tryptophan tend to be limiting.

Proteins used more completely in metabolism are considered to be of higher biologic value. In general, meat and eggs provide protein of high biologic value, whereas protein of plant origin tends to be of lower quality. However, certain beans and legumes provide very high biologic quality protein (see Section IIIF). The higher the biologic quality of ingested protein, the less required to meet metabolic needs, and vice versa.

Plants contain a wide variety of amino acids not used in protein synthesis in humans, some of which are actually toxic. The biologic value of plant protein may be modified further by other constituents interfering with digestion. The soybean, for example, contains an inhibitor of trypsin, although it is inactivated by cooking. Whereas egg, dairy products, and meats provide protein of high biologic value when consumed alone, other foods do so in combinations. Vegetables combined with legumes or beans, and cereal grains combined with nuts, seeds, or legumes, comprise complete protein sources. Good examples are rice and beans, or peanut butter on bread. Generally, a well-balanced diet in the United States provides ample protein of high biologic value. Strict vegetarians (vegans) need to be particularly attentive to food combinations to be assured of optimal protein intake (see Chapter 37).

PROTEIN DEFICIENCY

Malnutrition develops when protein needs are not met. In the developing world, this typically occurs when children are weaned from breast milk, resulting in a condition known as kwashiorkor. Infants and children with this condition are bloated and edematous, but are severely malnourished. A condition of wasting and emaciation due to a deficit of total dietary energy is known as marasmus.

In the United States during the 1970s, the use of very-low-calorie liquid diets that did not provide adequate protein was associated with sudden cardiac death due to the leaching of amino acids from viscera, including the heart. Susceptibility to this effect may be greater during such diets than during complete starvation, because of other metabolic effects of total starvation (see Chapter 24). During starvation, approximately 25% of structural proteins can be turned over before life is threatened, often enough to sustain a fast for as long as 30 to 50 days. Very-low-calorie liquid diets now provide complete protein, to allow for a so-called protein-sparing modified fast (see Chapter 5), considerably mitigating the risks involved.

FOOD PROCESSING

Heating food can reduce the availability of lysine in particular. If exposed to high heat, proteins become less readily digestible. Oxidation may deplete methionine.

BIBLIOGRAPHY

See "Sources for All Chapters."

4

Overview of Clinically Relevant Micronutrient Metabolism

Needs for nutrient energy are met by the macronutrient classes discussed in Chapters 1 through 3. Macronutrients—protein, carbohydrate, and fat—are consumed in quantities measured in grams and are plainly visible to the naked eye. In contrast, specific metabolic needs are met by various classes of micronutrients that typically are consumed in milligram or microgram amounts invisible to the naked eye.

Micronutrients include vitamins and vitamin-like substances, minerals, and specific subclasses of macronutrients essential for survival. This chapter provides an overview of clinically relevant micronutrients and micronutrient classes. More detailed information for specific nutrients of interest can be found in the nutrient reference tables in Section IIIE.

VITAMINS

By definition, vitamins are organic compounds the body requires in small amounts for metabolic processes but cannot produce endogenously. In some instances, some endogenous production occurs but either is inadequate for metabolic demand or requires ingestion of a precursor. Vitamins are divided into water-soluble and fat-soluble groups. In addition, there are vitamin-like compounds, nutrients that meet some but not all of the defining criteria for vitamins. Some of these compounds are subject to re-

classification if and when an essential role in metabolism is established.

The letter designations of vitamins are something of an anachronism, reflecting the sequence in which essential dietary "factors" were discovered in the early part of the twentieth century. The essential functions of vitamin B, for example, came over time to be attributed to a variety of nutrients that then took on numerical designations as well. In some instances, the numerical designations came into wide use (e.g., vitamins B_6 and B_{12}), whereas in other instances the chemical name supplanted the alphanumeric. Further subdivisions have been identified over time, so that certain vitamins (e.g., vitamins A, D, and B_6) actually each comprise a group of related compounds. Therefore, although the chemical name is preferred in most instances, the alphanumeric designation retains value in reference to a group of compounds with a shared biologic function.

WATER-SOLUBLE VITAMINS

Water-soluble vitamins are generally readily available in the food supply, are well absorbed, and are stored to a very limited extent in the body. The water-soluble vitamins include the B complex—thiamine (B_1), riboflavin (B_2), niacin (B_3), pantothenic acid (B_5), pyridoxine (B_6), folate, biotin, cyanocobalamin (B_{12})—and ascorbic acid, or vitamin C. Vitamins included in the B complex are not chemically related to one another, but rather represent discrete nutrients initially (1910–1920) thought to be a single water-soluble vitamin.

Thiamine (B₁)

Thiamine functions as a cofactor in the decarboxylation of keto acids and plays a role in the pentose phosphate pathway, essentially serving to generate accessible energy. Because thiamine releases energy from ingested macronutrients, requirements vary with total energy intake.

Overt deficiency manifests as beriberi and occurs at an intake below 0.12 mg per 1,000 kcal in adults. Deficiency of thiamine often occurs in alcoholism and manifests as the Wernicke-Korsakoff syndrome. The administration of dextrose to thiamine-deficient patients can further deplete thiamine and induce an acute encephalopathic state; therefore, alcoholics seen for acute care should receive thiamine before dextrose.

A recommended dietary allowance (RDA) of 0.5 mg per 1,000 kcal, or at least 1 mg per day, has been established for adults. Thiamine is innocuous in high doses. Paleolithic intake is estimated to have been nearly 4 mg per day in adults. Thiamine is widely found in foods but is abundant in relatively few, including grains and seeds with intact bran, and pork.

Riboflavin (B₂)

Riboflavin catalyzes oxidation–reduction reactions in intermediate metabolism as a component of flavin mononucleotide and flavin adenine dinucleotide. The metabolic functions of vitamin B₆ and niacin require adequate riboflavin. Riboflavin deficiency manifests as pathology of the skin and mucous membranes, particularly glossitis and stomatitis. The RDA for riboflavin is 0.6 mg per 1,000 kcal, or at least 1.2 mg per day. Higher intake is not associated with known toxicity. Paleolithic intake is estimated to have been upwards of 6 mg per day. Riboflavin is natu-

rally abundant in meat and dairy products, and in grain products in the United States as a result of fortification.

Niacin (B₃)

Niacin refers to both nicotinic acid and nicotinamide. The vitamin functions in glycolysis, cellular respiration, and fatty acid metabolism as a component of nicotinamide adenine dinucleotide and nicotinamide adenine dinucleotide phosphate. Niacin can be synthesized from the amino acid tryptophan; therefore, niacin ingestion is not essential when tryptophan is available in sufficient amount. The efficiency with which tryptophan is converted to niacin is enhanced by the action of estrogens. In general, approximately 60 mg of tryptophan can be used to produce 1 mg of niacin; therefore, either is considered one niacin equivalent (NE).

Overt deficiency of niacin manifests as pellagra, a syndrome comprising dermatitis, diarrhea, and, when advanced, dementia. The RDA for niacin is 6.6 NE per 1,000 kcal, or a minimum of 13 NE for adults. High-dose niacin is used pharmacologically to treat hyperlipidemia and is associated with vasodilation and flushing. A paleolithic intake estimate is not available. Niacin is widely distributed in nature and is especially abundant in meat, dairy products, eggs, as well as fortified grain products.

Pantothenic Acid (B₅)

Pantothenic acid is a component of coenzyme A and the acyl carrier protein of fatty acid synthetase. As such, the vitamin is vital to the metabolism of, and energy release from, carbohydrate, protein, and fat. It plays a role in the synthesis of acetylcholine, functions in cholesterol and steroid hormone biosynthesis, and is required for protoporphyrin production.

Deficiency induced under experimental conditions induces a wide range of manifestations, but a naturally occurring deficiency syndrome is not known to exist.

Malnourished prisoners of war have been known to develop paresthesias of the feet (burning foot syndrome) relieved by administration of pantothenic acid. An intake of between 4 and 7 mg per day is thought to be adequate for adults, but the RDA has not been established. An estimate of paleolithic intake is not available. High doses of pantothenic acid are apparently safe, but can cause diarrhea. Pantothenic acid is found in fish and poultry, organ meats, legumes, and whole grains.

Pyridoxine (B$_6$)

Vitamin B$_6$ refers to pyridoxine, pyridoxal, and pyridoxamine, which function in transamination reactions. Vitamin B$_6$ is therefore of fundamental importance to amino acid metabolism, and B$_6$ requirements rise as protein intake rises. Overt deficiency manifests as dermatitis, anemia, and seizures. The RDA for vitamin B$_6$ is 0.016 mg per gram of protein, resulting in a recommendation of between 1.5 and 2.0 mg per day for most adult women and men, respectively. An estimate of paleolithic intake is not available. High doses well above the RDA, generally used for treating neuropathies, are relatively safe, but may induce a transient dependency on higher intake and may be neurotoxic. Fish, poultry and other meats are good sources of B$_6$.

Folic Acid

Folate is converted to the biologically active tetrahydrofolic acid, which functions as a coenzyme in the transfer of one-carbon units. Folate is essential in the metabolism of many amino acids and in the biosynthesis of nucleic acids. All rapidly dividing tissues are dependent on folate for viability.

Deficiency, which may be more common in developed countries than previously believed and is known to be common in developing countries, manifests as macrocytic anemia, gastrointestinal disturbances, and glossitis. Folate deficiency has been identified as the most common nutrient deficiency in the United States.

The RDA for folate has been set at 200 μg per day for men and 180 μg per day for women. The RDA in pregnancy is 400 μg per day; however, the recognition that intake at this level at the time of conception greatly reduces the risk of neural tube defects has resulted in fortification of grain products. The approximation of this higher intake by the estimated paleolithic intake of 360 μg per day is noteworthy. The principal risk of high-dose intake of folate is the masking of B$_{12}$ deficiency. Folate is abundant in fruits and vegetables, particularly green leafy vegetables, and in fortified grains.

Biotin

Biotin functions as a component of several enzymes involved in the transfer of carboxyl units. These enzymes participate in fatty acid synthesis, gluconeogenesis, and the citric acid cycle. Biotin deficiency is unusual but can be induced by the ingestion of sufficient raw egg albumin, which contains avidin, a biotin antagonist. Deficiency is characterized by nausea and vomiting, dermatitis, depression, alopecia, and glossitis.

The RDA is not established, but the National Research Council has recommended intake in the range from 30 to 100 μg per day in adults. Paleolithic intake has not been estimated. High doses are not associated with any known toxicity. Good sources of biotin include yeast, soybeans, eggs (yolk), peanut butter, and mushrooms.

Vitamin B$_{12}$

Vitamin B$_{12}$ refers to a group of cobalamin-containing compounds; the commercially available form is cyanocobalamin. Vitamin B$_{12}$ is required to produce the active form of folate and participates in most aspects of folate metabolism. Vitamin B$_{12}$ is required to convert methylmalonyl CoA to succinyl CoA. Methylmalonyl CoA accumulates when B_{12} is deficient; this deficiency impairs myelin formation and results in neuropathy.

Unlike other water-soluble vitamins, which are replenished frequently from diverse dietary sources, B_{12} is stored in the liver in reserves that can last up to 30 years. Therefore, deficiency results when either dietary intake is deficient for protracted periods or absorption is impaired. The former situation occurs rarely due to strict vegetarianism, the latter usually because of gastric atrophy and lack of intrinsic factor, a protein required for B_{12} absorption.

Deficiency of B_{12} due to lack of intrinsic factor is pernicious anemia. The deficiency syndrome consists of macrocytic anemia and neuropathy, which consists of paresthesias and/or deficits of memory and cognition. Sufficient folate intake can overcome the effects of B_{12} deficiency on the bone marrow, but not the nervous system. The RDA for adults is 2 μg per day. Paleolithic intake of B_{12} has not been estimated. There is no known toxicity associated with high doses. Vitamin B_{12} is found in meats, dairy products, shellfish, and eggs; it is absent in all plant foods.

Vitamin C (Ascorbic Acid)

Vitamin C is a cofactor in hydroxylation reactions that are particularly important in the production of collagen. Diverse roles of the nutrient suggest that it is of importance in immune function and wound healing, and possibly allergic reactions. Vitamin C functions as a potent antioxidant, generating interest in its potential to combat disease and retard the aging process. The serum level of vitamin C peaks at an intake in the range of 150 mg per day.

The RDA, previously set at 60 mg per day for adults, is being revised upward to 200 mg per day by the National Research Council as the importance of antioxidants to health becomes increasingly clear. High doses of vitamin C are relatively innocuous, but toxic effects, particularly gastrointestinal discomfort, at doses in excess of 500 mg per day have

been reported. Overt deficiency manifests as scurvy and occurs at an intake level of approximately 10 mg per day in adults. Paleolithic intake of vitamin C is estimated to have been slightly above 600 mg per day. Ascorbate is abundant in fruits, especially citrus fruits, and a variety of vegetables.

FAT-SOLUBLE VITAMINS

In general, fat-soluble vitamins are stored in the body in sufficient reserves so that daily intake is not required. The fat-soluble vitamins include A, D, E, and K.

Vitamin A

Vitamin A refers to a group of compounds known as retinoids with varying degrees of vitamin A activity; the predominant compound is retinol. Active vitamin A can be synthesized endogenously from carotenoid precursors. More than 500 carotenoids are known, but only approximately 10% of them have provitamin A activity. Among that 10% are β-carotene, α-carotene, and cryptoxanthin.

Vitamin A is incorporated into the rod and cone cells of the retina; in the rods, it is a structural constituent of rhodopsin and functions in night vision. Vitamin A also functions in the generation of epithelial cells, in the growth of bones and teeth, in reproduction (by several mechanisms), and in immune function.

Deficiency of vitamin A, due to malnutrition or fat malabsorption, results in night blindness and, in more extreme cases, more severe eye injury and visual impairment resulting from drying of the eye, or xerophthalmia. Deficiency also is associated with increased susceptibility to infectious disease. The RDA for vitamin A is measured in retinol equivalents (RE), so called because of the various nutrients that can be used to produce active vitamin A. One RE is equal to 1 μg of all-trans retinol. An intake of 1,000 RE is recommended daily for adult men and 800 RE for adult women.

Paleolithic intake is estimated to have been three to four times the RDA and approximately twice the current intake among adults in the United States. Symptoms of vitamin A toxicity include headache, vomiting, visual disturbances, desquamation, liver damage, and birth defects. Symptoms may result from single doses greater than 100,000 RE in adults or 60,000 RE in children. Sustained supplementation with more than 4,000 RE daily in children or 10,000 daily in adults may be toxic. Toxicity does not result from the ingestion of provitamin A carotenoids. Preformed vitamin A is found in organ meats, especially liver, and in fish, egg yolks, and fortified milk. Carotenoids are abundant in brightly colored fruits and vegetables.

Vitamin D

Vitamin D refers to calciferol and related chemical compounds. Unique among vitamins, vitamin D is essential in the diet only when the skin is not exposed to sufficient ultraviolet light, which acts to produce vitamin D from a precursor stored in skin. Melanin in skin impedes vitamin D synthesis, so that dark-skinned people in temperate climates are particularly subject to deficiency without adequate dietary intake. After synthesis or ingestion, vitamin D undergoes two hydroxylation reactions, one each in the liver and the kidney, to the metabolically active 1,25-dihydroxycholecalciferol, or calcitriol. Calcitriol functions as a hormone regulating the metabolism of calcium and phosphorus. Fundamentally, vitamin D promotes the intestinal absorption of calcium.

Deficiency occurs with inadequate dietary intake and inadequate sun exposure and manifests as rickets in children and osteomalacia in adults. When sun exposure is abundant, there is no requirement for dietary vitamin D; therefore, the RDA is predicated on the inconsistency of population exposure to sunlight. The RDA for vitamin D is 10 μg daily during childhood and adolescence and 5 μg daily in adulthood. An estimate of paleolithic intake is unavailable. Sun exposure cannot result in vitamin D toxicity, but high-dose supplements can. Intake five times greater than the RDA is associated with soft tissue calcification and hypercalcemia. Vitamin D is found in fatty fish, but the principal source in the United States is milk, which generally is fortified with 5 μg (100 IU) per cup.

Vitamin E

Vitamin E refers to a group of compounds collectively known as tocopherols and tocotrienols. The most abundant and biologically active is α-tocopherol. Vitamin E functions as a lipid antioxidant, protecting and preserving the integrity of cellular and subcellular membranes. Overt deficiency is rare because of the distribution of vitamin E in the food supply. Deficiency is thought to manifest as muscle weakness, hemolysis, ataxia, and impaired vision.

The RDA is expressed in α-tocopherol equivalents (TE) and is 10 mg per day for men and 8 mg per day for women. Higher intakes are required when the diet is rich in polyunsaturated fatty acids (PUFAs) that are subject to rancidification. Vitamin E is found in vegetable oils, so intake tends to rise with intake of PUFAs.

A variety of health benefits have been claimed for doses between 200 and 800 IU daily, representing between 10 and 50 times the RDA (see table, Section IIIE). High doses are thought to be safe, but vitamin E interferes somewhat with vitamin K metabolism and therefore can prolong the prothrombin time at high doses. High-dose supplementation in patients on anticoagulants or platelet-inhibiting drugs is apt to be particularly hazardous. Paleolithic intake is estimated to have been approximately 33 mg per day, or between three and four times the RDA. Vitamin E is found in vegetable oils and seeds. Owing to its distribution in fat, high dietary intake is unusual and not recommended. For the putative benefits offered by high doses, supplementation is required.

Vitamin K

Vitamin K refers to a group of compounds derived from naphthoquinone that are essential in the production of prothrombin, clotting factors VII, IX, and X, and proteins C and S. Vitamin K appears to have other functions as well, particularly related to bone and kidney metabolism. Limited amounts of vitamin K are stored in the body. Needs are met partly but not completely by synthesis of the vitamin by intestinal bacteria.

Deficiency of vitamin K results in coagulopathy. Newborns, who are particularly susceptible to deficiency owing to a lack of intestinal flora, receive a prophylactic parenteral dose soon after birth. The RDA for an adult man is 80 μg per day and for an adult woman is 65 μg per day. An estimate of paleolithic intake is not available. There is no particular toxicity associated with high-dose vitamin K. The vitamin is abundant in leafy green and cruciferous vegetables.

VITAMIN-LIKE SUBSTANCES

Certain organic nutrients for which a true requirement remains uncertain have vitamin-like properties. The nutrients listed here, and others, could come to be considered vitamins if and when an essential biologic function is identified along with a need for dietary intake.

Choline

Choline is a water-soluble compound known to be essential for several mammalian species, but not humans. It is a constituent of phosphatidylcholine (lecithin), sphingomyelin, and acetylcholine. Choline is a component of molecules that are vital to the structural integrity of biologic membranes and lipoprotein particles. Humans can synthesize choline when both serine and methionine are available in adequate supply along with vitamin B_{12} and folate. A deficiency syndrome in humans has not been identified. Choline is widely distributed in the food supply.

Taurine

Taurine, an amino acid, functions in a variety of metabolic activities, including neuromodulation, the stabilization of cell membranes, and osmotic regulation. It is required for the production of certain bile salts. Taurine is not considered an essential nutrient because it can be synthesized from cysteine or methionine. Dietary taurine may be essential in formula-fed infants, but this need has not been reliably established. There is no clear evidence of a deficiency syndrome or evidence of toxicity associated with high doses. Taurine is relatively abundant in meat and seafood.

Carnitine

Carnitine is a nitrogenous compound synthesized from lysine and methionine in the liver and kidney. It functions in transesterification reactions and in the transport of long-chain fatty acids into mitochondria. Synthesis is adequate in the adult, but may not be in newborns. Whereas human milk delivers adequate carnitine, the same may not be true of formula.

Deficiency in humans has been established, generally resulting from inborn errors of metabolism. Deficiency is predominantly manifest as muscle weakness, cardiomyopathy, and hypoglycemia. Supplementation is inconsistently beneficial in deficiency syndromes. Carnitine is abundant in meats and dairy products.

Myo-inositol

Myo-inositol is an alcohol, structurally similar to glucose. It functions as a constituent of phospholipids in biologic membranes and has been found to be essential for the replication of many human cell lines. To date, human deficiency has not been established.

Myo-inositol is found in cereal grains and can be synthesized from glucose.

Bioflavonoids

Bioflavonoids are water-soluble, brightly colored phenolic compounds found in plants. They are believed to influence capillary permeability and fragility. Bioflavonoids are found in wine, beer, and tea, and particularly in citrus fruits. A deficiency has not been defined in humans.

Lipoic Acid

Lipoic acid is fat soluble and related to B vitamins. It functions as a coenzyme, transferring acyl groups. A deficiency state is not known to exist in humans.

Coenzyme Q (Ubiquinone)

Coenzyme Q refers to a group of lipid-like compounds, structurally related to vitamin E. Members of the group all contain an isoprenoid side chain off a quinone ring; the number of units in the side chain varies from six to ten. Coenzyme Q_{10}, the group member of greatest interest to date, is the variety native to human mitochondria.

Coenzyme Q functions in mitochondrial electron transport. Coenzyme Q is widely distributed in the food supply, and a true deficiency state has not been established. Interest in the potential benefits of higher doses than are generally provided by diet is considerable (see Section III, nutrient reference tables).

MINERALS AND TRACE ELEMENTS

Although the term "mineral" often is applied to essential dietary inorganic elements, some of this group are not minerals, and "elements" is the proper designation. Nonetheless, those elements found most abundantly in human tissue are minerals and, given their abundance, are referred to as dietary macrominerals. They include calcium, phosphorus, magnesium, potassium, sodium, chloride, and sulfur. These substances are present in the body in amounts upward of 100 mg, up to as much as hundreds of grams. In contrast, trace elements are present in the body in milligram or even microgram quantities. Trace elements essential to human health include iron, copper, zinc, cobalt, molybdenum, selenium, manganese, iodine, chromium, fluoride, silicon, nickel, boron, arsenic, tin, and vanadium.

MACROMINERALS

Calcium

Healthy adults store more than 1 kg of calcium in the body, predominantly in bones and teeth. Calcium, a vital structural component of the skeleton, is essential for muscular contraction and participates in a variety of other biologic processes including coagulation. Calcium deficiency results in osteopenia, with the skeletal depot serving to maintain serum levels under most circumstances. The RDA for calcium varies throughout the lifecycle; 1,200 mg per day is recommended for most adults. Paleolithic intake is estimated to have been nearly 2 g per day, more than twice the typical intake in the United States. Excessive intake accompanied by vitamin D supplementation may lead to soft tissue calcification and hypercalcemia, although these outcomes are not associated with high intake from whole-food sources. Dairy products are the best dietary source of readily bioavailable calcium.

Phosphorus

Phosphorus is primarily incorporated along with calcium into the hydroxyapatite of bones and teeth. Phosphorus also functions in the synthesis of nucleic acids and phospholipids and in the formation of high-energy phosphate bonds in ATP. Phosphorus intake should approximate calcium intake, and the RDA for the two nutrients is matched. Phosphorus deficiency is not known to occur in humans. Paleolithic intake has not been estimated but likely corresponds with the higher calcium intake. Excess dietary phosphorus, exceeding the calcium intake by more than two-fold, can lead to hypocalcemia and possibly secondary hyperparathyroidism. Foods rich in protein are generally rich in phosphorus as well; thus, meat and dairy products are good sources.

Magnesium

The 20 to 30 g of magnesium stored in an adult body are principally in bone and muscle. Magnesium is vital to the integrity of the mitochondrial membrane and functions as a cofactor in diverse metabolic pathways involving more than 300 enzymes. Deficiency, generally the result of malabsorption or alcoholism, is manifest as anorexia, irritability, psychosis, and seizures. The RDA is 350 mg per day for adult men and 280 mg per day for adult women. Paleolithic intake has not been estimated. Excess intake of magnesium appears dangerous only in individuals with impaired renal function; toxicity is manifest as nausea, vomiting, and hypotension. Severe hypermagnesemia is life threatening. Dietary sources of magnesium include green vegetables, grains, beans, and seafood.

Potassium

Potassium is the principal cation of the intracellular space. It functions in osmotic regulation, acid–base balance, and muscle cell depolarization. The cardiac muscle is particularly sensitive to potassium concentrations. Dietary deficiency of potassium is uncommon, but conditions producing fluid shifts, such as surgery, or metabolic imbalances, such as diabetic ketoacidosis, can produce life-threatening derangements of the serum potassium. High dietary potassium intake is not associated with toxicity when renal function is normal. There is no RDA for potas-

sium, but a daily intake by adults of at least 3 g per day is advised. Paleolithic intake is estimated to have been more than 10 g per day, exceeding current intake levels by a factor of four. Potassium is abundant in grains, legumes, vegetables, and fruits. Citrus fruits, raisins, and bananas are particularly good sources.

Sodium

Sodium is the major extracellular cation. The body of an adult stores approximately 100 g of sodium; more than half is in the extracellular space and much of the remainder is in bone. Sodium functions to regulate the distribution of water in the body, regulate acid–base balance, and maintain transmembrane potential. Sodium deficiency, resulting in hyponatremia, causes weakness, fatigue, anorexia, and confusion; if severe, hyponatremia can cause seizures and be life threatening.

There is no RDA for sodium, but a daily intake of at least 115 mg is thought to be essential, and an intake of at least 500 mg is advised. Excess intake may play a role in hypertension and osteoporosis. Intake should be limited to not more than 2,400 mg per day; typical daily intake in the United States is nearly 4,000 mg. Paleolithic intake of sodium is estimated to have been less than 1,000 mg per day. Of note, potassium intake exceeded sodium intake by a factor of more than ten in the prehistoric diet of humans, whereas in the modern diet of developed countries sodium intake exceeds that of potassium by a factor of two. Sodium is abundant in foods of animal origin, but it is present in the food supply principally as seasoning or preservatives added to processed foods.

Chloride

Chloride is distributed with sodium in the extracellular fluid where it functions to maintain fluid and acid–base balance. Chloride functions in digestion as a constituent of hydrochloric acid in the stomach. Chloride deficiency does not generally occur under normal circumstances, but it can accompany sodium deficiency in the context of volume depletion or result from metabolic derangements. Chloride deficiency results in alkalosis and impaired cognition. The RDA for chloride has not been established; dietary deficiency is not considered a health threat. Chloride toxicity has not been reported. Paleolithic intake has not been estimated to date, but likely corresponds to the lower sodium intake. Dietary chloride is derived largely from salt, with the sources those of sodium.

Sulfur

Sulfur is present in all cells, principally as a component of the amino acids cystine, cysteine, methionine, and taurine. Sulfur functions in collagen synthesis and in energy transfer. A deficiency syndrome has not been described. Sulfur is derived in the diet from the amino acids in which it is incorporated; therefore, intake corresponds with the quality and quantity of protein intake.

TRACE ELEMENTS

Iron

Approximately 4 g of iron is stored in the body of a typical adult male and slightly less than 3 g in the body of a typical adult female. The primary function of iron is to transport oxygen as a component of hemoglobin, and the bulk of stored iron is in red blood cells. Iron also is incorporated in myoglobin, mitochondrial cytochromes, and several enzyme systems such as peroxidase and catalase. Iron-containing enzyme systems generally function in oxidation reactions.

Iron deficiency manifests in sequence as depleted ferritin, impaired erythropoiesis, and then anemia, and develops over time because of blood losses or inadequate intake. Iron deficiency is associated with impaired immunity and impaired cognition in children. The RDA for iron is 10 mg per day for men and 15 mg per day for women, with variations over the lifecycle. Paleolithic intake is estimated to have been nearly 90 mg per day, which is six- to nine-fold higher than the RDA.

Toxicity from dietary iron in healthy individuals is virtually unknown, although a role in oxidative injury to cells has been proposed. Ferrous sulfate can be lethal at a dose of 3,000 mg in children and 200 to 250 mg/kg in adults. Iron is accumulated, producing multiorgan system failure in individuals with hemochromatosis, a genetic disease resulting in enhanced iron absorption.

Iron is absorbed in the upper small intestine. Absorption is enhanced by ascorbic acid and impaired by fiber, phytates, and oxalates in plant foods. Heme iron in meat is more readily absorbed than nonheme iron in plants. Good sources of iron include beef, lamb, and liver, and the dark meat of poultry. Beans, peas, nuts and seeds, and green leafy vegetables are good sources of nonheme iron.

Copper

The store of copper—approximately 80 mg—in an adult body functions in at least 15 enzyme systems, largely involved in oxidation and energy production. Copper participates in enzymes influencing immune cell function, collagen and elastin synthesis, and neurotransmitter generation. Dietary intake of copper generally readily exceeds requirements, and deficiency is rare. Deficiency manifestations documented in malnourished children include anemia, neutropenia, and bone demineralization.

Excess zinc intake can chelate ingested copper and prevent its absorption. The RDA for copper has not been established, but an intake range from 1.5 to 3 mg per day for adults is considered appropriate. An estimate of paleolithic intake is not available.

Copper toxicity from whole-food ingestion is unknown. Copper toxicity can occur with supplement ingestion in the range from 10 to 30 mg. Severe neurocognitive effects of copper toxicity are seen in Wilson's disease, a recessive genetic defect in copper metabolism. Copper is found in shellfish, legumes, nuts, seeds, and liver.

Zinc

The amount of zinc stored in the adult human body, approximately 2 to 2.5 g, resides primarily in bone, but it is distributed to all body tissues. Zinc functions in nearly 100 enzyme systems and plays prominent roles in CO_2 transport and digestion. Zinc also influences DNA and RNA synthesis, immune function, collagen synthesis, olfaction, and taste. Zinc deficiency manifests as anorexia, impaired growth, impaired immune function, impaired wound healing, and impaired taste sensation.

Although overt deficiency is rare in the absence of malnutrition, mild deficiency may be prevalent in the United States, particularly among the elderly. The RDA for zinc is 15 mg per day for adult men and 12 mg per day for adult women. Paleolithic intake is estimated to have been three to four times the RDA. High-dose zinc supplementation can result in vomiting; over time, zinc supplementation can interfere with copper metabolism. Supplementation in excess of 15 mg per day is controversial. Zinc is found in meat, shellfish (especially oysters), legumes, nuts, and, to a lesser extent, grains.

Cobalt

Cobalt is an integral component of vitamin B_{12}, and a normal adult body contains approximately 1 mg of the element. Toxicity, manifesting as cardiomyopathy, has been observed in heavy drinkers of beer to which cobalt was added to improve foaming. There is no RDA for cobalt. Seafood represents the best dietary source.

Molybdenum

Molybdenum is a component of several enzyme systems that function in uric acid formation and in fluoride, iron, copper, and sulfur metabolism. Deficiency under natural conditions is unknown, but it has been observed in individuals with inborn errors of metabolism and following long-term total parenteral nutrition lacking the element. Manifestations of deficiency are principally neurocognitive, including irritability and eventually coma. The recommended intake range for adults is 75 to 250 μg per day. An estimate of paleolithic intake is not available. Toxicity occurs at intakes in the range from 10 to 15 mg per day and manifests as diarrhea, anemia, and gout. High intake of molybdenum interferes with copper metabolism. Molybdenum is found in dairy products, cereal grain, and legumes; concentration in food varies with concentration in soil.

Selenium

Selenium is a constituent of glutathione peroxidase, an important antioxidant, and enzyme systems involved in the synthesis of thyroid hormones. Selenium deficiency is associated with two diseases endemic to areas of China with low soil selenium content: Keshan disease is a cardiomyopathy, and Kashin-Beck syndrome is an inflammatory arthritis. Overt selenium deficiency in the United States is unknown. Low selenium intake, however, is suspected to increase the risk of atherosclerotic heart disease and several cancers. The RDA is 70 μg per day for adult men and 55 μg per day for adult women. Estimates of paleolithic intake of selenium have not been reported.

Toxicity can occur with intake above 200 μg per day and manifests as nausea, diarrhea, fatigue, neuropathy, and potentially cirrhosis. Selenium is widely distributed in the food supply, with concentrations varying with soil content. Brazil nuts are the most concentrated source.

Manganese

Approximately 12 to 20 mg of manganese is stored in the body of an adult, with most found in bone, liver, and the pituitary gland. Manganese is concentrated in mitochondria. It functions as a component of numerous enzyme systems involved in connective tissue formation, urea synthesis, and energy release. Manganese deficiency has not been observed in humans under natural conditions. The RDA has not been established, but an intake of 2 to 5 mg per day is recommended for adults. Estimates of paleolithic intake have not been reported. Toxicity due to ingestion is rare; dementia and psychosis have been seen in manganese miners with heavy inhalation exposure. Dietary sources of manganese include nuts, grains, shellfish, coffee, and tea.

Iodine

The adult body contains approximately 20 to 50 mg of iodine, virtually all of which is incorporated into thyroid hormones (thyroxine and triiodothyronine). Iodine deficiency, common in regions with low soil iodine and lack of food supply fortification, results in endemic goiter. Maternal iodine deficiency during pregnancy and deficiency in infancy are associated with the syndrome of cretinism. Iodine metabolism is impeded by goitrogens contained in cabbage, cassava, and peanuts. Dietary pattern can influence susceptibility to goiter.

The RDA for adults is 150 μg per day. In the United States, this level is met through fortification of salt. Paleolithic intake of iodine has not been reported. Dietary iodine intake in excess of the RDA is rarely toxic. Supplementation in excess of 50 mg per day can interfere with thyroid function and lead to an acne-like skin condition termed iododerma. Fish and shellfish are good sources of iodine, although fortified salt is the most reliable dietary source.

Chromium

The adult body contains 6 to 10 mg of chromium that is widely distributed throughout the body. The principal function of chro-

mium is as a component of glucose tolerance factor, a complex that apparently facilitates binding of insulin to its receptors. Chromium also functions in macronutrient oxidation and lipoprotein metabolism. Deficiency is associated with glucose intolerance, peripheral neuropathy, and, if severe, encephalopathy. The RDA for chromium has not been established, but the Food and Nutrition Board has advised an intake between 50 and 200 μg per day for adults. Estimates of paleolithic intake of chromium have not been reported. Toxicity from dietary sources is unknown. Sources include yeast, grains, nuts, prunes, potatoes, and seafood.

Fluoride

An adult body contains less than 1 g of fluoride, virtually all of which is in the bones and teeth. Definitive evidence that fluoride is an essential nutrient is lacking, but a role for fluoride in preventing dental caries and strengthening bone is well established. Fluoride deficiency is associated with increased susceptibility to dental caries and osteoporosis. The RDA has not been established, but an intake range from 1.5 to 4.0 mg per day for adults is recommended by the Food and Nutrition Board. Estimates of paleolithic intake have not been reported.

Fluoride intake in the range from 2 to 8 mg/kg/day in childhood can produce mottling of the teeth known as fluorosis. Intake of 20 to 80 mg per day in adults can adversely affect bone, muscle, kidney, and nerve tissue. Fluoride is ubiquitous in the food supply, but in very small amounts, varying with the concentration in soil and ground water. The principal source in the Unites States is supplemented water supplies.

Silicon

Silicon is present in all tissues in trace amounts, functioning in calcification, cell growth, and mucopolysaccharide formation. Deficiency in humans has not been established. There is no RDA, and optimal intake is unknown. Good dietary sources include barley and oats.

Nickel

Approximately 10 mg of nickel is widely distributed in the adult body. Nickel appears to play a role in nucleic acid metabolism. A deficiency state in humans has not been elucidated, although deficiency is well established in animal models. Intake of approximately 30 μg per day for adults is thought to be appropriate. A toxicity state is unknown. Cereal grains and most vegetables contain nickel.

Boron

Boron is thought to influence calcium and estrogen metabolism, and consequently to play a role in bone mineralization. Boron also may function in cell membrane formation. An overt deficiency state has not been defined, but low levels are associated with osteoporosis in particular. The RDA has not been established, but expert opinion supports an intake of approximately 1 mg per day for adults. Toxicity due to supplementation apparently occurs at levels above 50 mg per day and manifests as nausea, vomiting, diarrhea, dermatitis, and cognitive impairment. Boron is found in beans, nuts, vegetables, beer, and wine.

Arsenic

The adult body is thought to contain approximately 20 mg of arsenic, widely distributed in all tissues and concentrated in skin, hair, and nails. The physiologic role of arsenic remains uncertain, although it can influence the function of many enzyme systems. Deficiency in humans has not been established. No RDA exists, but an intake of 12 to 15 μg per day is thought to be appropriate for adults. Toxicity from food sources is unknown; arsenic toxicity results from ingestion of concentrated arsenic or industrial exposure. Manifestations of toxicity include a burning sensation in the mouth, abdominal pain, nausea, vomiting, and diarrhea. Seafood is the richest source of dietary arsenic.

Tin

Approximately 14 mg of tin is widely distributed in the tissues of adult humans, although none is found in brain tissue. Tin is thought to function in oxidation–reduction reactions, but its exact role is unknown. Tin deficiency in humans has not been elucidated. The RDA has not been established, and the range of optimal intake is unknown. Tin is thought to be minimally toxic, as it is poorly absorbed. Tin is widely distributed in the food supply, but in very small amounts. Dietary intake rises as much as 30-fold when food stored in tin cans is eaten frequently.

Vanadium

Approximately 25 mg of vanadium is widely distributed in the tissues of adult humans. The element is concentrated in serum, bones, teeth, and adipose tissue. Vanadium appears to influence several important enzyme systems, including that of ATPase. Vanadium may inhibit cholesterol biosynthesis. Deficiency in humans has not been established. There is no RDA, and optimal intake levels are unknown. Toxicity is low owing to poor absorption. Shellfish, mushrooms, and several spices including pepper and dill are relatively rich sources of vanadium.

Other

Restrictions of dietary cadmium, lead, and lithium have produced abnormalities in laboratory animals, but there is as yet no evidence of human requirements.

ESSENTIAL AMINO ACIDS

Dietary proteins are composed predominantly of a group of 20 amino acids. Of these, humans can readily synthesize eleven. The remaining nine—histidine, isoleucine,

leucine, lysine, methionine, phenylalanine, threonine, tryptophan, and valine—must be ingested to meet metabolic demand and therefore are referred to as essential. An absolute dependence on dietary histidine in adults is uncertain. Infants also may require dietary arginine. Cystine and tyrosine are synthesized endogenously from methionine and phenylalanine, respectively, and therefore are semiessential. The need for dietary intake varies inversely with the ingestion of their precursors.

The RDA for protein in adults has been established at or near 0.8 g/kg/day. Paleolithic intake is thought to have been much higher, in the range from 2.5 to 3.5 g/kg/day. Essential amino acid needs are met when protein of high biologic value is consumed. The four least abundant essential amino acids—lysine, methionine/cystine, threonine, and tryptophan—are used to gauge the quality of dietary protein. Sources of high-quality protein include egg white, milk, meat, soybeans, beans, and lentils.

ESSENTIAL FATTY ACIDS

The PUFAs required for normal metabolism that cannot be synthesized endogenously are essential dietary nutrients. Two such fatty acids, linoleic acid (C18, ω-6) and α-linolenic acid (C18, ω-3), are unconditionally essential, whereas arachidonic acid (C20, ω-6), which can be synthesized from linoleic acid, is essential when supplies of its precursor are deficient. Essential fatty acids participate in a wide variety of metabolic functions, including eicosanoid synthesis and biomembrane development.

Overt deficiency of essential fatty acids has not been observed in free-living adults, but its manifestations, including hair loss, desquamative dermatitis, and impaired wound healing, are known from cases of deficient parenteral nutrition. The RDA has not been established for essential fatty acids, but an intake of linoleic acid at 1% to 2% of total calories is advised. Of note, the ω-6:ω-3 ratio in the typical US diet is more than 10:1, whereas the ratio estimated for the paleolithic diet is between 4:1 and 1:1.

Dietary sources of linoleic acid include most vegetable oils; evening primrose oil is a particularly rich source. Sources of α-linolenic acid include linseeds and flaxseeds and their oils, and marine foods, especially salmon, mackerel, sardines, scallops, and oysters. The ω-3 content of fish is derived from phytoplankton and algae, so that farmed fish generally are lower in ω-3 than their free-living counterparts.

BIBLIOGRAPHY

See "Sources for All Chapters."
Standing Committee on the Scientific Evaluation of Dietary Reference Intakes, Food and Nutrition Board, Institute of Medicine. *Dietary reference intakes for calcium, phosphorus, magnesium, vitamin D, and fluoride.* Washington, DC: National Academy Press, 1997.

Dietary Management in Clinical Practice: Diet and Disease

5

Diet, Obesity, and Weight Regulation

INTRODUCTION

Obesity and overweight, affecting more than 50% of the adult population in the United States and increasing proportions of the adolescent and pediatric populations, may be the most common conditions seen in primary care. Evidence, long convincing, continues to accrue that obesity contributes to a range of morbidities and increases the risk of premature mortality. The link between dietary pattern and weight regulation is more than decisive; it is self-evident. However, the myriad factors governing the complex relationship among caloric intake, energy expenditure, energy metabolism, and energy storage as body fat remain considerably unresolved. Although it is clear that a balance between energy ingestion and energy consumption is the principal determinant of weight maintenance in an individual, the factors responsible for the wide variations in the setpoint for that equilibrium are uncertain. Genetic factors apparently play both a direct (i.e., by influencing levels of leptin) and indirect (i.e., by influencing levels of thyroid hormone, the degree of postprandial thermogenesis, the mass of brown fat) role in establishing the propensity for weight gain or loss in an individual. Environmental influences, such as the prevailing food supply and accessibility of opportunities for physical activity, are comparably important. The rising prevalence of obesity throughout the industrialized world makes clear that far from being a problem of impaired self-restraint in an individual, obesity may be seen as a public health threat mediated by a "toxic" nutritional environ-

ment. An appreciation for the public health importance of obesity, its complex pathogenesis, and principles of management are supportive of optimal interventions by clinicians.

OVERVIEW

Overweight and Obesity: Definitions

The definitions of obesity and overweight remain subject to some controversy. This is partly due to the fact that weight is used as a surrogate measure of fatness, or adiposity, which is more difficult and costlier to measure. An individual heavy on the basis of a well-developed musculature naturally is not subject to the same health outcomes as an individual with excess body fat. As the prevalence of excess adiposity is far greater than the prevalence of heaviness on the basis of muscular development, measures of weight function well as surrogates of adiposity on a population basis. The other controversial issue has been the need for a clinically valid referent. To define overweight relative to an ideal requires validation of the ideal, preferably on the basis of morbidity and mortality risk. This has largely been achieved.

On the basis of advances in research clarifying the relationship between weight and health outcomes, the National Institutes of Health has adopted a body mass index (BMI; weight in kilograms divided by height in meters squared; see Section IIIA) of 25 as the threshold for defining overweight (1). A BMI greater than 30 and less than 35 is defined as stage I obesity; a BMI greater than or equal to 35 and less than 40 is defined as stage II obesity; and a BMI of 40 or greater is defined as stage III obesity (2). The risks of complications of excess adiposity may, in general, be considered low, moderate, and high as BMI rises through overweight to stage III obesity, but the actual risk in an individual will vary with comorbidity (3).

Alternatives to the BMI for classifying obesity vary in complexity and suitability for the clinical setting. Of most potential value is the waist-to-hip ratio (WHR). This measure requires looping a tape measure about the waist at the narrowest point and the hips at the widest point. The WHR is an index of body fat distribution of established importance and potential clinical utility (4). A WHR greater than 0.9 in men or 0.85 in women is consistent with central or abdominal obesity, also known as android obesity, and descriptively as the "apple" pattern of obesity. An elevated BMI with a normal WHR is consistent with peripheral obesity, also referred to as gynoid or the "pear" pattern. Although in general men are more subject to abdominal obesity and women to peripheral obesity, the patterns are not gender specific. Following menopause in particular, women are increasingly subject to abdominal obesity (5).

Abdominal obesity is distinct from peripheral obesity with regard to physiology and complications. Central obesity correlates with the accumulation of visceral adipose tissue. This body habitus is linked to the insulin resistance syndrome (see Chapter 10). As a result, there is a strong association between central obesity and cardiovascular disease risk (see Chapters 6 and 10); this association is much less apparent for peripheral obesity. One mediating mechanism of cardiovascular risk in central obesity appears to be an association with high sympathetic tone (6–8). This, in turn, may be related to the density of adrenergic receptors in centrally distributed and visceral adipose tissue. Although associated with metabolic complications of obesity, central fat tissue tends to be more readily lost than peripheral fat, in part because adrenergic receptors facilitate fat oxidation during catabolism. Thus, the frequently reported complaint of women that men lose weight more readily often is valid.

Other anthropometric measures, such as skin-fold thickness, are unlikely to be of use in the clinical practice setting. Body density can be measured by the administration of "heavy" (tritiated) water, with evaluation of adiposity based on the volume of distribution (9). Underwater weighing permits assessment of body density as well (10). Bioelectrical impedance also is used to calculate fat mass. Dual-energy X-ray absorptiometry or dual-photon absorptiometry may be the best available method for measuring total body fat (10). Computed tomography and magnetic resonance imaging may be used to quantify body fat, with particular utility for visualizing visceral fat (10). Although such sophisticated techniques offer advantages in research settings, there is satisfactory evidence that even simple observation is a fairly reliable gauge of excess body fat in the clinical setting.

Epidemiology

As obesity is well established in the US population and has been at high levels for decades, it may be considered endemic. However, as prevalence continues to rise beyond historical precedent, it may be considered epidemic as well (11). In 1994, Kuczmarski and colleagues (12) published a widely cited report on the prevalence of obesity in the United States. Based on nationally representative data gathered by the *National Health and Nutrition Examination Surveys* (NHANES), the authors reported a prevalence of overweight of over 33% among adults in the United States as of 1991. This figure represented an 8% increase in the prevalence of overweight between the second *National Health and Nutrition Examination Survey* (NHANES II; 1976–1980) and the third (NHANES III; 1988–1994) (see Section IIIC) (12).

The definition of overweight applied by Kuczmarski and colleagues (12), then in common use, was a BMI of 27.3 or greater for women, and 27.8 or greater for men. As noted, this measure has since been revised downward to 25 kg/m² for both men and women. Simply by applying a new definition, the prevalence of overweight in the United States has been increased by some 29 million (13). Applying current criteria to the most recently analyzed NHANES data reveals a prevalence of overweight among US adults of more than 50% (14). That the prevalence of obesity is rising independent of the definition applied has been confirmed as well; approximately 18% of the adult population has a BMI ≥30 (15). Although the figures are lower, available data indicate a steady rise in the prevalence of childhood and adolescent obesity as well (16).

Obesity in children has been linked to higher risk of developing hypertension (17,18), hypercholesterolemia (19), hyperinsulinemia (19), insulin resistance (20), hyperandrogenemia (20), gallstones (21,22), hepatitis (23–25), sleep apnea (26–28), orthopedic abnormalities (e.g., slipped capital epiphyses) (29–32), and increased intracranial hypertension (33–36). Obese children suffer from poor self-esteem (37) and are subjected to teasing, discrimination, and victimization (38). Obesity during adolescence increases rates of cardiovascular disease (39–43) and diabetes (40) in adulthood, in both men and women. In women, adolescent obesity is associated with completion of fewer years of education, higher rates of poverty, and lower rates of marriage and household income (40). In men, obesity in adolescence is associated with increased all-cause mortality and mortality from cardiovascular disease and colon cancer (40,44). Adults who were obese as children have increased mortality and morbidity independent of adult weight (38,40,45).

The prevalence of obesity is rising worldwide, especially as countries are westernized (46). The spread of obesity is sufficiently uncontrolled to constitute a global epidemic (47). Universal dietary preferences evidently predominate over cultural patterns as nutri-

ent-dilute, energy-dense foods become available (48,49).

Obesity is associated with increased risk of cardiovascular disease, diabetes, cancer, arthritis, and a wide range of other morbidities (50). A recent 1999 report, based on computer modeling, highlights the health and economic consequences of obesity, suggesting that greater efforts at prevention and treatment would likely be both beneficial and cost effective (51). In a related study, the authors again used computer modeling to estimate the health and economic benefits of sustained, modest (10%) weight loss in subjects with varying degrees of obesity. The results are consistent with meaningful improvements in health, along with health care cost reductions ranging from $2,200 to $5,300 per patient (52).

In 1993, McGinnis and Foege (53) identified the combination of dietary pattern and sedentary lifestyle as the second leading cause of preventable, premature death in the United States, accounting for some 300,000 deaths per year. Obesity contributes to the majority of these deaths and now is considered to be directly or indirectly responsible for approximately 300,000 annual deaths (54). Calle and colleagues (55) reported a linear relationship between BMI and mortality risk based on an observational cohort of more than one million subjects followed for 14 years. In this cohort, high BMI was less predictive of mortality risk in blacks than in whites. Manson et al. (56) found a linear relationship between BMI and mortality risk in women from the Nurses' Health Study; the lowest risk of all-cause mortality occurred in women with a BMI 15% below average with stable weight over time. Including women with a smoking history in the analysis yielded a J-shaped mortality curve, with a higher mortality rate among the leanest women. In a study of Seventh Day Adventists, Singh and colleagues (57) found a linear relationship between BMI and all-cause mortality in all groups except postmenopausal women not taking hormone replacement therapy (HRT). In this group, the relationship was

J-shaped, with higher mortality associated with a BMI below 20.7. The authors suggest that mortality risk might rise in estrogen-deficient women.

Data supporting the relationship between obesity and mortality risk come from a variety of sources and generally are consistent (58,59). There is evidence that obesity in adolescence, at least in males, is predictive of increased all-cause mortality (44). Data from the Iowa Women's Health Study suggest that the WHR may be a superior predictor of mortality risk than the BMI in women. Whereas BMI produced a J-shaped curve, WHR and mortality were linearly related (60). Although earlier studies consistently demonstrated a J-shaped relationship between BMI and mortality, correction for several biases has resulted in increasing consensus that the relationship is linear (61).

Finally, reports that weight cycling may be independently associated with morbidity or mortality are of uncertain significance (62,63). There is some evidence that when other risk factors are adequately controlled in the analysis, weight cycling does not predict mortality independently of obesity (64). There is also evidence that cardiovascular risk factors are dependent on the degree of obesity, rather than weight regain following loss (65). The benefits of weight loss are thought to override any potential hazards of weight regain (66); therefore, efforts at weight loss generally should be encouraged even in obese individuals with a prior history of weight cycling (67). However, repeated cycles of weight loss and regain may render subsequent weight loss more difficult by affecting metabolic rate. For this reason, as well as others, weight loss efforts should be predicated on sustainable adjustments to diet and lifestyle whenever possible, rather than extreme modifications over the short term.

Often overlooked, but of clear relevance to office-based dietary counseling, is the relationship between obesity and mental health. Body image, adversely affected and even distorted by obesity, is important to self-esteem (68). Thus, poor self-esteem is a common consequence of obesity (the converse often also being true, with poor self-esteem adversely affecting diet; see Chapter 32). This has important implications for dietary modification efforts (see Chapter 41). Repeated cycles of weight loss and regain may have particularly adverse effects on psychological well-being, although research in this area is limited (63). Evidence is consistent and clear that obesity engenders antipathy, resulting in stigma, social bias, and discrimination (68,69).

The metabolic effects, psychosocial sequelae, management, and, to some extent, etiology of obesity vary with its severity (70). Although more than 50% of adults in the United States are overweight, far fewer have severe degrees of obesity. Approximately 4% of adults have a BMI greater than 35, considered severe obesity. A BMI $\geq$40 is considered very severe, or "morbid" obesity, and accounts for approximately 3% of the population (71).

Pathogenesis

The complexity of the pathogenesis of obesity is increasingly appreciated, with a wide range of genetic, physiologic, psychologic, and sociologic factors implicated. Although the process may be complex, the ultimate determinant of obesity in an individual is, in fact, simple: greater energy consumed than expended. Efforts to control weight, prevent gain, or facilitate loss must address this imbalance to be successful. Control of body weight relies on achieving a balance between energy input and energy consumption at a desired level of energy storage.

Working against this goal is the natural tendency to accumulate body fat. The storage of energy in the form of adipose tissue is adaptive in all species with variable and unpredictable access to food. In humans, only 1,200 kcal of energy is stored as glycogen in the prototypical 70-kg man, enough to last 12 to 18 hours at most. Our ability to survive a more protracted fast depends on energy reserves in body fat, which average 120,000 kcal in the same, lean prototype. The natural tendency to store available energy as body fat persists, although the constant availability of nutrient energy has rendered this tendency maladaptive.

The development of obesity appears to be related to an increase in both the size and number of adipocytes. Excess energy intake in childhood leads more readily to increases in fat cell number. In adults, excess energy consumption leads initially to increases in adipocyte size and only with more extreme imbalance to increased number. Childhood obesity does not lead invariably to adult obesity, as the total number of adipocytes in a lean adult generally exceeds the number in an obese child. Thus, correction for early energy imbalance can restore the number of adipocytes to the normal range. In general, lesser degrees of obesity are more likely to be due to increased fat cell size, whereas more severe obesity often suggests increased fat cell number as well. Obesity due exclusively to increased adipocyte size is hypertrophic, whereas that due to increased fat cell number is hyperplastic. Weight loss apparently is more difficult to maintain in hyperplastic as compared to hypertrophic obesity, because it requires reducing an abnormally high number of total adipocytes down to an abnormally low size. By some as yet uncertain signaling mechanism, adipocytes may regulate their size so that it is maintained within the normal range. Such signaling may pertain to various chemical messengers released from adipose tissue, including angiotensinogen, tissue necrosis factor, and/or leptin. Adipocytes also produce lipoprotein lipase, which acts on circulating lipoprotein particles, especially very-low-density lipoprotein, to extract free fatty acids, which then are stored in the adipocyte as triglyceride. The effects on metabolism or weight over time of surgical resection of subcutaneous fat in hyperplastic obesity (i.e., liposuction) have not been reported to date, although adverse effects are possible (72).

The imbalance between energy consumption and expenditure that leads to excess weight gain can be mediated by either and generally is mediated by both in the United States. Relative inactivity and abundantly available calories both contribute. Energy expenditure is comprised of basal, or resting, metabolic rate (BMR), the thermic effect of food, and physical activity (Table 5.1). BMR accounts for approximately 70% of total energy expenditure, thermogenesis approximately 15%, and physical activity approximately 15% on average. The contribution of physical activity to energy expenditure is, of course, quite variable. Resting energy expenditure can be measured by various methods, with the doubly labeled water method representing the prevailing standard in research settings (73). In clinical settings, basal energy requirements for weight maintenance can be estimated by use of the Harris-Benedict equation (see Section IIIA). A rough estimate of calories needed to maintain weight at an average level of activity is derived by multiplying the ideal weight of a woman (in pounds) by 12 to 14, and that of a man by 14 to 16.

BMR is lower in women than in men when matched for height and weight due to the higher body fat content in women. A strong genetic component to the BMR results in familial clustering, as well as clustering within ethnic groups predisposed to obesity (74,75). BMR is largely explained by lean body mass, but among subjects matched for lean body mass, age, and sex, a variation of as much as 30% may be seen. This explains, at least in part, why comparable energy intake will produce obesity in some individuals but not others. Total body weight correlates positively with BMR, so that weight loss reduces BMR (76). BMR may fall by as much as 30% with dieting, although sustained reductions tend to be smaller, which explains why the maintenance of weight loss becomes increasingly difficult over time after initial success. This may contribute as well to increasing difficulty in losing weight after successive attempts (77). As muscle is more metabolically active than fat, the conversion of body fat to muscle at a stable weight will increase BMR. Energy expenditure per unit

TABLE 1. *Energy expenditure of some representative physical activities[a]*

Activity	METs[b] (multiples of RMR)	kcal/min
Resting (sitting or lying down)	1.0	1.2–1.7
Sweeping	1.5	1.8–2.6
Driving (car)	2.0	2.4–3.4
Walking slowly (2 mph)	2.0–3.5	2.8–4
Bicycling slowly (6 mph)	2.0–3.5	2.8–4
Horseback riding (walk)	2.5	3–4.2
Volleyball	3.0	3.5
Mopping	3.5	4.2–6.0
Golf	4.0–5.0	4.2–5.8
Swimming slowly	4.0–5.0	4.2–5.8
Walking moderately fast (3 mph)	4.0–5.0	4.2–5.8
Baseball	4.5	5.4–7.6
Bicycling moderately fast (12 mph)	4.5–9.0	6–8.3
Dancing	4.5–9.0	6–8.3
Skiing	4.5–9.0	6–8.3
Skating	4.5–9.0	6–8.3
Walking fast (4.5 mph)	4.5–9.0	6–8.3
Swimming moderately fast	4.5–9.0	6–8.3
Tennis (singles)	6.0	7.7
Chopping wood	6.5	7.8–11
Shoveling	7.0	8.4–12
Digging	7.5	9–12.8
Cross-country skiing	7.5–12	8.5–12.5
Jogging	7.5–12	8.5–12.5
Football	9.0	9.1
Basketball	9.0	9.8
Running	15	12.7–16.7
Running, 4-minute mile pace	30	36–51
Swimming (crawl) fast	30	36–51

[a] All values are estimates and based on a prototypical 70-kg male; energy expenditure is generally lower in women and higher in larger individuals. MET and kcal values derived from different sources may not correspond exactly.

[b] A MET is the rate of energy expenditure at rest, attributable to the resting (or basal) metabolic rate (RMR). Although resting energy expenditure varies with body size and habitus, a MET is generally accepted to equal approximately 3.5 mL/kg/min of oxygen consumption. The energy expenditure at one MET generally varies over the range from 1.2 to 1.7 kcal/min. The intensity of exercise can be measured relative to the RMR in METs.

Derived from: Ensminger AH, et al. The concise encyclopedia of foods and nutrition. In: Wilmore JH, Costill DL, eds. *Physiology of sport and exercise. Human kinetics.* Champaign, IL: 1994; American College of Sports Medicine. *Resource manual for guidelines for exercise testing and prescription,* 2nd ed. Philadelphia: Williams & Wilkins, 1993; Burke L, Deakin V, eds. *Clinical sports nutrition.* Sydney, Australia: McGraw-Hill Book Company, 1994; McArdle WD, Katch FI, Katch VL. *Sports exercise nutrition.* Baltimore: Lippincott Williams & Wilkins, 1999.

body mass peaks in early childhood due to the metabolic demands of growth. Total energy expenditure generally peaks in the second decade as, often, does energy intake. Thereafter, energy requirements decline with age, as does energy consumption. Energy expenditure tends to decline more than energy intake, so that weight gain, and increasing adiposity, often are characteristic of aging (see Chapter 29).

Thermogenesis

Food ingestion increases sympathetic tone, raising levels of catecholamines as well as insulin. Brown fat (brown adipose tissue;

BAT), concentrated in the abdomen and present in varying amounts, functions principally in the regulation of energy storage and wastage by inducing heat generation, in response to stimulation by catecholamines, insulin, and thyroid hormone. The increase in sympathetic tone postprandially results in thermogenesis (heat generation), which may consume up to 15% of ingested calories. A reduced thermic effect of food may contribute to the development of obesity, although this is controversial (78). Approximately 7% to 8% of total energy expenditure is accounted for by obligatory thermogenesis, but up to an additional 7% to 8% is facultative and may vary between the lean and obese. Insulin resistance may be associated with reduced postprandial thermogenesis. However, obesity apparently precedes reduced thermogenesis, suggesting that impaired thermogenesis is unlikely as an explanation for susceptibility to obesity. Thermogenesis is related to the action of β_3-adrenergic receptors, the density of which varies substantially. Reduced thermogenesis may contribute to weight gain with aging, as thermogenesis apparently declines with age, at least in men (79).

Physical Activity

Energy consumption generally has risen in industrialized countries over recent decades as both the energy density of the diet and portion sizes have increased. During the same period, energy expenditure generally has fallen, largely due to changes in the environment and the patterns of work and leisure activity. A majority of Americans are sedentary (80) as a result both of reduced work-related activity and limited leisure-time activity (81). A reduction in exercise-related energy expenditure contributes to energy imbalance and weight gain. The attribution of weight gain to physical inactivity is compounded by the associations between activity and dietary patterns. For example, data from the *Behavioral Risk Factor Surveillance System* indicate that relative inactivity correlates with a high dietary fat intake (82). Although there is consensus that physical activity is essential to long-term weight maintenance, the mechanisms of benefit remain controversial. Evidence that physical activity reduces food intake or results in extended periods of increased oxygen consumption is lacking, and there is evidence to the contrary. Exercise has the potential to increase the BMR by increasing muscle mass. Energy consumption during exercise can help maintain energy balance. For example, a pound of weight loss per week requires a daily deficit of approximately 500 kcal; at a constant level of dietary intake, such a deficit could be achieved by 45 minutes of jogging or 75 minutes of brisk walking per day. The efficiency for linking energy consumption to physical work of contracting muscle is approximately 30%; 70% of the available energy is wasted as heat. There is little evidence that the efficiency of work-related energy metabolism differs between the lean and obese.

A strong national emphasis on the health benefits of physical activity, as evidenced by release of the Surgeon General's Report in 1996, has produced some clear benefits, such as increased availability of worksite exercise facilities (83). Overall, however, little progress has been made toward *Healthy People 2000/2010* objectives in this category. Although the utility of physical activity per se in promoting weight loss is uncertain, lifetime physical activity apparently mitigates age-related weight gain and clearly is associated with important health benefits (84). The contribution of physical activity to weight maintenance may vary among individuals on the basis of genetic factors that are as yet poorly understood (85). There is recent (1999) encouraging evidence that lifestyle activity, as opposed to structured aerobic exercise, may be helpful in both achieving and maintaining weight loss (86). Such unobtrusive physical activity may be more readily accepted by exercise-averse patients. Physical activity is among the best predictors of long-term weight maintenance (87–90). It has been estimated that the expenditure of approximately 12 kcal per kilogram body weight per day in physical activity is the minimum protective against increasing body fat over time (90) (see Table 5.1 for the energy expenditure associated with representative physical activities).

Genetics of Human Obesity

The physiologic determinants of obesity are increasingly associated with candidate genes. Not fewer than 20 genes have been implicated as candidates for explaining, at least partly, susceptibility to obesity in different individuals; gene–gene interactions are highly probable in most cases (91,92). As many as 200 genes are under investigation (93). Among the potential genetic factors mediating susceptibility to obesity, the Ob gene and its product leptin have received particular attention (94). Leptin, produced in adipose tissue, binds to receptors in the hypothalamus, apparently providing information about the state of energy storage and affecting satiety (95). Binding of leptin inhibits secretion of neuropeptide Y, which is a potent stimulator of appetite.

The Ob gene originally was identified in mice, and Ob/Ob mice are deficient in leptin and obese (96). The administration of leptin to Ob/Ob mice results in weight loss. In humans, obesity is associated with elevated leptin levels (97). Nonetheless, the administration of leptin to obese humans has been associated with modest weight loss (98), suggesting that leptin resistance rather than deficiency may be an etiologic factor in human obesity (99). The relative contribution of leptin to human obesity remains uncertain.

Macronutrient Metabolism

There is some degree of metabolic control over the consumption and distribution of macronutrients. Cortisone, galanin, and endogenous opioid peptides stimulate the medial hypothalamus to promote fat intake. Dopamine has antagonistic effects, suppressing desire for fat intake. Amphetamines act as do-pamine precursors and thereby tend to reduce fat intake. Drugs such as neuroleptics (e.g., phenothiazines) that antagonize dopamine often are associated with excess fat intake and weight gain. Endogenous opioid peptides and growth hormone releasing factor may play a role in the regulation of protein intake. Carbohydrate intake and craving is mediated by effects of γ-aminobutyric acid, norepinephrine, neuropeptide Y, and cortisol on the paraventricular nucleus of the medial hypothalamus. Activity of this system tends to be high when serum glucose and/or glycogen stores are low. Suppression of carbohydrate craving apparently is mediated by serotonin (see Chapter 32) and cholecystokinin. Insulin resistance may be associated with carbohydrate craving due to elevations of norepinephrine, cortisone, and neuropeptide Y.

Sociocultural Factors

The imbalance between energy intake and energy expenditure fundamental to obesity is largely the product of an interaction between physiologic traits and sociocultural factors. Human metabolism is the product of nearly 4 million years of natural selection, the overwhelming majority of which occurred in an environment demanding vigorous physical activity and providing access to a largely nutrient-dense but energy-dilute diet (100). In such an environment characterized by cyclical feast and famine, metabolic efficiency would be favored, as would a capacity to store nutrient energy in the body against the advent of famine. Such an environment likely would shape behavioral responses as well. The tendency to binge eat, characteristic of modern-day hunter gatherers and many animal species, is adaptive when food is occasionally abundant but often deficient; therefore, such a tendency may be nearly universal in humans (100). With food abundantly and constantly available, this tendency is conducive to excess energy consumption.

An innate preference for sweet foods has been well documented in humans and other animals (101). Such a preference would likely be adaptive in a primitive environment, as naturally sweet foods (e.g., fruit, honey) provide readily metabolizable energy and rarely are toxic. There is evidence of a strong pleasure response to dietary fat, mediated in part by opioid receptors (102). A strong affinity for dietary fat would have been adaptive in an environment where dietary fat was scarce, yet represented a source of concentrated energy and essential nutrients. Similarly, the need for a range of micronutrients and the potential difficulty in consistently finding a variety of foods would likely have cultivated a strong preference for dietary variety. This trait, sensory-specific satiety, becomes maladaptive in an environment providing food in constant variety as well as abundance, favoring excessive intake (103). The imbalance between energy intake and expenditure is compounded by modern conveniences that have led to a decline in physical activity associated with daily activities (104). The global spread of modern technology is associated with the emergence of obesity as a global public health problem (46). Prevailing patterns of behavior, including use of convenience devices that minimize physical activity (e.g., elevators, remote control devices) and consumption of an energy-dense diet, generally are reinforced at the societal level, often taking on culturally normative implications (105). Sociocultural influences are powerful determinants of dietary patterns (106,107) and, in the modern context, of obesity.

Both obese and lean individuals generally underreport calorie intake, but the degree of underreporting is greater in the obese. Generally, calorie consumption is higher in obese than in lean individuals (108,109). Endocrinopathy, such as Cushing's syndrome or hypothyroidism, is a rare cause of obesity. Relatively few obese patients have hypothyroidism, and most previously lean patients with hypothyroidism do not become obese as a result of the thyroid disease.

Diet

Energy intake varies with the macronutrient composition of the diet. Each gram of dietary carbohydrate releases 4 kcal of energy when metabolized; each gram of protein releases slightly less then 4 kcal; and each gram of fat releases approximately 9 kcal.

Despite significant variability in basal metabolism, it is possible to estimate energy requirements. Several formulas are available to approximate energy needs based on age, body mass, and state of health. The most widely cited of these is the Harris-Benedict Equation and simplifications of it (see Section IIIA). Such formulas typically are used to determine the caloric requirements of inpatients receiving total parenteral nutrition, but they are equally applicable to the ambulatory setting. Although it is relatively straightforward to estimate caloric needs, the utility of doing so in the outpatient setting is debatable. Unless a patient is willing to carefully count calories, there is likely to be a substantial discrepancy between a formulaic recommendation and actual practice. The availability of software for tracking calorie intake may render determination of energy needs more useful.

Because approximately 70% of calories are spent on basal metabolism, even vigorous physical activity may be insufficient to control weight when caloric intake substantially exceeds the needs of resting metabolism. Although the number of calories required to maintain weight varies substantially among individuals, the degree of caloric restriction, relative to habitual intake, required to produce weight loss is more predictable. Each pound of body fat represents a repository of approximately 4,000 kcal (454 g multiplied by 9 kcal/g). To lose a pound of fat requires that energy expenditure be increased by 4,000 kcal, or that intake be restricted by a comparable amount. To reduce caloric intake by 4,000 kcal over a week requires a daily restriction of between 500 and 600 kcal. In a 2,000 kcal diet, this represents a 25% reduction in total calorie intake. Therefore, whatever the baseline calorie intake required to maintain weight, a reduction of 500–600 kcal per day will generally result in approximately 1 pound of weight loss per week initially. As basal metabolism declines, further reductions may be required to sustain the weight loss.

Achieving the requisite restriction in calorie intake to promote weight loss is exceedingly difficult for most patients. While an imbalance between energy intake and expenditure is inevitably the cause of excess body weight, the marked variation in basal metabolism causes some patients to gain weight at a level of calorie intake that would result in weight loss in other, comparably active or inactive individuals. In addition to the vagaries of resting metabolism, individuals differ with regard to facultative and postprandial thermogenesis. Finally, all patients must contend with powerful physiologic, sociologic, and anthropologic forces that protect us all against energy deficiency, but render us susceptible, and undefended against, energy excess (see Chapters 39 and 41).

Macronutrient Classes

Dietary Fat

There is an intuitive rationale for restricting dietary fat in efforts to control weight: it is the most calorically dense macronutrient. Per gram, fat contains at least twice as much energy as protein or carbohydrate. Consequently, every gram of fat removed from the diet would need to be replaced with twice the mass of these other macronutrients to replace the lost calories. In addition, because carbohydrate sources in particular are apt to contain at least some fiber that is noncaloric, the volume differential between fat and carbohydrate to achieve the same calorie load is even greater than the mass difference. At a certain point, volume becomes limiting in calorie intake.

However, there is evidence that fat restriction has important limitations in achieving weight control. Although NHANES III data suggest that the proportion of total calories consumed as fat has declined, total fat intake has been stable due to increases in the intake of calories from other macronutrient sources, particularly carbohydrate (110). There is evidence that, in general, portion sizes have been increasing in the United States for several decades at least, leading to an increase in total calories consumed regardless of the source. The booming low-fat and nonfat food industry has capitalized on the expectation of the public that fat restriction will facilitate weight control and promote health. For many, the result is excessive intake of nutrient-poor foods that are high in simple sugars and low in fiber. Although these foods are less calorically dense than their higher-fat predecessors, they often are consumed in excess due to the ostensible "guiltlessness" of the consumer and possibly to lesser effects on satiety.

Restrictions of dietary fat, and alterations in the type of fat consumed in the United States, are strongly supported by an extensive literature (111). An association between dietary fat intake and obesity is similarly supported by an extensive literature, including observational and interventional studies (111,112). In a study of nearly 80 adults who volunteered for dietary analysis, Miller and colleagues (113) found dietary fat intake to correlate with obesity. High levels of added sugar and low dietary fiber were associated with high intake of dietary fat. King and Blundell (114) showed that *ad libitum* consumption of high-fat food following vigorous exercise exceeds the energy expended, whereas low-fat food preserves an energy deficit. Alfieri and colleagues (115) surveyed 150 subjects evenly divided into lean, moderately obese, or severely obese groups. They found total fat intake to be significantly higher in the obese groups and the degree of obesity to correlate with fat intake. Degree of obesity was negatively correlated with the carbohydrate intake and the carbohydrate-to-fat ratio of the diet (115). There is evidence from blinded experiments that the energy density of food is an important determinant of energy intake, indicating that abundant dietary fat is likely to play a role in positive energy balance (116). Dietary fat tends to be less satiating than carbohydrate (117). Although there is general agreement that restricting fat intake in isolation is insufficient to control or prevent obesity, fat restriction is considered by most experts to be an essential aspect of the dietary management of obesity (118).

The emphasis on fat restriction in weight control efforts has resulted in recommendations to increase carbohydrate intake as a proportion of total calories. This paradigm has been challenged recently in two ways. First, concern has been expressed that, in insulin-resistant individuals, dietary carbohydrate may lead to the development of obesity by driving up insulin levels; this theory was disseminated on the front page of the *New York Times*. The second challenge to the low-fat, high-carbohydrate model was raised by those advocating a higher protein intake. In particular, the popularity of *The Zone* (119) has generated interest in high-protein intake as a means to control weight.

Overall, the evidence is consistent that dietary fat correlates with body fat, and that the reduction of dietary fat is associated with weight loss (120). Studies suggest that although carbohydrate ingestion induces carbohydrate oxidation, fat consumption does not induce its own oxidation (121). Decreased or constant fat oxidation with increasing fat consumption would favor positive energy balance with increasing intake of fat as a proportion of total calories. Uncertain at present is the optimal distribution of protein and carbohydrate, and the potential role of fat substitutes, in facilitating and maintaining weight loss (120). The mainstream literature examining the role of carbohydrate versus protein in weight loss is focusing on a range of protein fairly close to that espoused in the prevailing dietary guidelines. Evidence available to date suggests that restriction of dietary fat to 30% of calories is safe in well-nourished infants as young as 7 months (122), although guidelines in the US call for no restriction of dietary fat prior to age 2 (see Chapter 27).

Dietary Protein

Despite the proliferation of highly successful diet books advocating low-carbohydrate, high-protein diets for weight loss (119,123–125), the evidence in support of this view in the peer-reviewed medical literature is virtually nonexistent. In a recent (1999) pertinent study, Baba and colleagues (126) divided 13 obese, insulin-resistant male subjects into two groups that received hypoenergetic diets either high in protein or high in carbohydrate. Subjects in both groups lost weight. Subjects in the high-protein group lost more total weight (an average difference of approximately 1.5 kg) over 4 weeks, but also lost significantly more body water, accounting for much of the weight difference. Resting energy expenditure declined more on the high-carbohydrate than high-protein diet. Serum lipids fell in both groups, but only the high-protein diet induced a significant fall in high-density lipoprotein. Fasting insulin levels fell significantly in both groups. Although the authors conclude that their findings suggest that a hypoenergetic, high-protein diet could be the preferred method of producing weight loss in obese, hyperinsulinemic patients, the evidence is far from compelling. Skov and colleagues (127) studied the effects of high-protein (25% of energy) and low-protein (12% of energy) diets on renal function over a 6-month period in 65 overweight adults. The authors concluded that the high-protein diet had no adverse effects on renal function because neither group developed albuminuria. However, the high-protein diet was associated with increased glomerular filtration rate and kidney volume, consistent with hyperfiltration.

In one of the more rigorous studies reported to date, Skov and colleagues (128) randomly assigned 65 overweight and obese adults to fat-restricted diets with either 12% or 25% of energy from protein, or control condition, and followed them for 6 months. Subjects on the higher-protein diet lost significantly more weight (3.7 kg on average) than subjects in the lower-protein group, and both of these groups did significantly better than controls. Noteworthy is that subjects were free to choose the foods providing the protein or carbohydrate and thus were not preferentially steered toward complex carbohydrates. Also important was the range of protein studied; the low-protein diet provided slightly less protein than stipulated by conventional dietary guidelines (15% to 20% of calories), whereas the high-protein diet provided only slightly more protein than called for by the same guidelines. Nonetheless, the study suggests a possible benefit of slightly more protein than is customarily recommended in a freely chosen, fat-restricted diet used for weight loss (128).

Although not specifically germane to the issue of weight control, it is worth noting that the claimed ergogenic effects of the Zone diet have been challenged in the peer-reviewed literature (129).

Dietary Carbohydrate

A diet with approximately 60% of calories from carbohydrate is the standard recommendation for purposes of health promotion (see Chapter 40) and is consistent with most recommendations for weight control. However, the uncertain causal relationship between obesity and insulin resistance has raised concerns that carbohydrate might contribute to weight gain in susceptible individuals. The weight of evidence suggests that obesity exacerbates insulin resistance in susceptible individuals and no clear evidence that insulin resistance is a precursor of obesity. Nonetheless, genetic and physiologic factors contributing to insulin resistance might readily contribute to obesity, and vice versa.

The plausibility of a link between obesity and insulin resistance, as well as evidence linking weight gain to the development of diabetes (Chapter 10) has raised concerns that carbohydrate might facilitate weight gain in susceptible individuals. The putative mechanism is a brisk rise in postprandial insulin levels resulting from foods with a relatively high glycemic index. However, there is increasing appreciation for the limited clinical relevance of the glycemic index, given that foods generally are consumed in combinations (see Chapter 10); the concept of the "glycemic load" imposed by the diet is currently evoking interest

(129a). Further, the total daily insulin production rises over time in response to weight gain, an effect of greater magnitude than that attributable to the glycemic index of individual foods. Although further work in this area is required, to date there is no evidence to support the contention that carbohydrate should be avoided to facilitate weight control, even in patients with the cardinal features of the insulin resistance syndrome. Counseling to promote intake of complex rather than simple carbohydrates, and thereby to increase consumption of fiber, is warranted generally for health promotion and specifically for weight control.

In a review of the literature, Bolton-Smith (130) found no evidence to suggest that dietary carbohydrate, including simple sugar intake, is positively associated with obesity. In general, diets high in carbohydrate but not high in fat content are based largely on grains, vegetables, and fruits and are naturally energy dilute and high in fiber. High-carbohydrate diets based on processed foods tend to be relatively high in fat content as well.

Golay and colleagues (131) reported that energy restriction produces comparable degrees of weight loss over a wide range of carbohydrate intake. In a randomized study of 68 obese adults assigned to hypocaloric diets with low or moderate carbohydrate content, Golay et al. reported no differences in most outcome measures, including weight and fat loss; the low-carbohydrate group had slightly lower fasting insulin levels at the end of the 12-week intervention (132). Both diets, however, reduced fasting insulin and improved the glucose-to-insulin ratio comparably. Reaven (133) has argued that high dietary carbohydrate intake exacerbates the metabolic complications of the insulin-resistance syndrome (see Chapter 10). However, there is evidence that energy restriction leads to comparable weight loss in insulin-resistant and noninsulin-resistant obese subjects (134). A potential advantage of energy-restricted diets relatively high in protein is that they may tend to preserve energy expenditure due to resting metabolism during and following weight loss (135). To date, the duration of such an effect and its impact on long-term weight maintenance are unreported and unknown. Literature on the potential for relatively high-protein diets to spare lean body mass during weight loss is inconsistent and therefore inconclusive.

Nutrients and Nutriceuticals

There are, in general, no substantiated claims for micronutrients that can be consumed in conventional or megadoses to facilitate weight loss. There is evidence that fat-reduced diets recommended to promote weight loss do not compromise the micronutrient profile of the diet and may result in some improvements (136).

Chromium

Chromium is a cofactor in insulin metabolism, and its supplementation may lower insulin levels in insulin-resistant individuals (see Chapter 10). There is no convincing evidence of a role for chromium in weight management per se, but an argument for supplementation in the insulin-resistant obese patient could be made on theoretical grounds and often is by alternative practitioners.

Alcohol

Ethanol provides 7 kcal/g; therefore it is more energy dense than either carbohydrate or protein and only slightly less so than fat. As a result of this energy density, ethanol consumption may contribute to obesity. There is some evidence that ethanol may increase resting energy expenditure while reducing fat oxidation (137). These effects may contribute preferentially to lipid storage.

Olestra

Olestra, or sucrose polyester, is used as a fat substitute in commercially available snack foods; it is discussed in detail in Chapter 38. To date there is no convincing evidence that olestra in the food supply leads to sustainable weight loss or prevents weight gain. However, the evidence that high intake of dietary fat is linked to obesity is convincing in the aggregate, and the use of olestra is one potential means of reducing fat intake. Its use for purposes of weight control can neither be encouraged nor discouraged with great enthusiasm on the basis of the available evidence (see Chapter 38).

RELATED TOPICS OF INTEREST

Surgery

Surgery generally is indicated only for the management of severe obesity, and then only if other therapies have been tried and have proved ineffective (138). A BMI greater than 40, previously referred to as "morbid" obesity and preferably referred to as stage III obesity or "severe" obesity, should raise the consideration of surgical management. Patients with lesser degrees of obesity may be candidates for surgery if refractory to other interventions and experiencing loss of quality of life due to the obesity (138). Vertical gastroplasty is the prevailing method, but laparoscopic gastric banding is now increasingly common (139); the Roux-en-Y gastric bypass is less commonly used than previously (138). The banding procedure is less invasive, less dangerous, and reversible. Surgery reduces the gastric chamber size, thereby diminishing capacity at any given meal. Surgery is of limited benefit if not reinforced by behavioral interventions, but as part of a multidisciplinary approach to severe obesity can produce very substantial weight loss. Weight loss of up to 33% has been maintained after gastric bypass surgery for up to 10 years, an outcome superior to nonsurgical approaches (140). Surgical mortality in skilled hands generally is less than 1% (140). Lipectomy, and even liposuction, may be appropriate interventions for some patients, although the metabolic effects of these approaches are not fully known and are potentially adverse.

Candidates for bariatric surgery require thorough preparation for the effects of such surgery on lifestyle and dietary pattern. The benefits of surgery are generally only well maintained in those patients receiving supportive behavioral counseling. Because of the considerable impact of severe obesity on morbidity and mortality, surgery should be given consideration in all patients with a BMI maintained above 40, or those with a BMI above 35 with metabolic and or functional complications (140). Although the advent of less invasive surgical techniques is promising, advances in the nonsurgical management of obesity are widely acknowledged as preferable. The cost effectiveness of obesity surgery apparently has not been adequately evaluated to date (141), but is considered appropriate for carefully selected patients. For more detailed information on surgical alternatives, readers are referred to the excellent review by Greenway (140).

Pharmacotherapy

Amphetamines, noradrenergic agents, and serotinergic agents have received Food and Drug Administration (FDA) approval for weight loss, principally by means of suppressing appetite (142,143). Selective serotonin reuptake inhibitors, such as fluoxetine, as well as compounds such as caffeine and ephedrine, are not FDA approved for weight loss but are used for that purpose.

Fenfluoramine stimulates the release and inhibits the reuptake of serotonin, whereas phentermine stimulates the release of norepinephrine (142). Although both drugs were FDA approved for the treatment of obesity, the combination, "Fen-Phen," was never approved per se but was widely used until 1997, when an association with valvular heart disease was reported (144). The use of fenfluoramine, or dex-fenfluoramine, is more convincingly associated with a risk of pulmonary hypertension when therapy continues beyond 3 months, although the occurrence is rare (142). The drugs have been withdrawn from the market, although controversy persists as to whether a causal link to valvular heart disease truly exists, and, if so, what is the magnitude of associated risk. The use, apparent toxicity, and withdrawal of Fen-Phen focused attention on the inappropriate use of pharmacotherapy to achieve cosmetic outcomes in mild obesity; under such circumstances, the potential toxicity of even fairly safe medication may well outweigh the benefits (145).

Since the withdrawal of fenfluoramine, sibutramine, a reuptake inhibitor of both serotonin and norepinephrine, has been FDA approved for the treatment of obesity. The limiting side effect associated with use of sibutramine is hypertension, mediated by the effects on norepinephrine levels. In randomized trials, sibutramine is clearly effective in facilitating modest weight loss up to 12 months, but weight is regained if the drug is discontinued, and data on long-term use are not available (146). Sibutramine facilitates weight loss by suppressing appetite (inducing satiety) and increasing energy expenditure by augmenting thermogenesis, and it appears to induce a preferential loss of visceral fat (147).

Orlistat is a drug recently approved by the FDA for obesity treatment that works by inhibiting lipases in the gastrointestinal tract (148). In clinical trials, orlistat has been shown to induce clinically significant weight loss (149). The drug must be taken in advance of meals containing fat and is limited by gastrointestinal side effects related to fat malabsorption.

Advances in the understanding of the pathophysiology of obesity offer the promise of new pharmacologic approaches to its control. Growth hormone secretion is abnormally low in obesity, possibly due to leptin resistance (150). The administration of growth hormone improves body composition in obese subjects during energy restriction and weight loss; therefore, there is interest in the potential therapeutic use of either growth hormone or growth hormone releasing peptides in the treatment of obesity (150). Agents under current investigation include

β_3-adrenergic receptor agonists, corticotropin-releasing factor-binding protein ligand inhibitor, leptin. and neuropeptide Y receptor antagonists (151,152).

Pharmacotherapy is increasingly viewed as a potentially important adjunct to lifestyle interventions in the control of obesity (143,153). As weight generally is regained when pharmacologic agents are discontinued, the need for agents that are safe in the long term and/or robust behavioral interventions that can sustain the weight loss achieved with short-term medication use is clear. Clinicians should be prepared to consider long-term use of pharmacologic agents, as is commonly done with other conditions somewhat responsive to diet, such as hypertension and hyperlipidemia. Weight loss during pharmacotherapy should perhaps not be considered an indication for cessation of treatment, any more than the treatment of diabetes, hypertension, or hyperlipidemia to goal levels of glucose, blood pressure, or low-density lipoprotein result in discontinuation of therapy. However, to apply the same standard in obesity treatment, the long-term safety of pharmacologic agents will need to be assessed. In the mean time, pharmacotherapy generally should be reserved for more severe obesity or obesity associated with metabolic, psychological, or functional complications, so that pharmacotherapy is likely to be associated with greater net benefit than risk. The use of prescription pharmacotherapy for purely cosmetic weight control is, on the basis of currently available evidence, generally ill advised.

Low- and Very-low-energy Diets

Low-calorie diets typically restrict energy intake to between 1,000 and 1,200 kcal/day. Such diets can be constructed to provide balanced nutrition or to be unbalanced in favor of a particular macronutrient class. Evidence of a benefit of unbalanced low-energy diets is, for the most part, lacking, and differences in weight loss are largely attributable to differences in diuresis (154). Evidence for emphasizing a particular macronutrient class is discussed elsewhere in this chapter. Generally, low-calorie diets pose a threat of micronutrient deficiency, and a multivitamin/mineral supplement is appropriate. As a balanced, energy-restricted diet is compatible with both weight control and health promotion goals, such an approach to obesity is widely applicable.

Very-low-energy diets used in the 1970s provided inadequate protein and resulted in visceral protein losses. Cardiac protein mobilization was associated with dysrhythmia and sudden death (154). With attention to the quantity and quality of protein provided, very-low-energy diets can be administered safely; such diets typically are referred to as "protein-sparing modified fasts" and provide approximately 600 kcal/day (154). Very-low-calorie diets (VLCDs) can be based on a narrow range of proteinaceous solid foods (i.e., lean meat, fish, poultry) or a commercial liquid formula. These diets are indicated only in the management of severe obesity and may be a final noninvasive effort prior to bariatric surgery. There is limited evidence of the feasibility of managing VLCDs in primary care practice (155) and some evidence of their utility in reducing weight preoperatively in severely obese patients considered at high risk for elective surgery because of their obesity (156). Kansanen and colleagues (157) reported the effectiveness of VLCD in treating the sleep apnea syndrome in a small group of obese adults followed for 3 months. Micronutrient supplementation and extensive behavioral support are required; therefore, such diets should be undertaken only when the requisite supervision and multidisciplinary support are established. Although very-low-energy diets induce substantial weight loss (e.g., 20 kg in 12 weeks), they generally are ineffective at maintaining such losses over the long term (154). Ryttig and colleagues (158) compared two 24-month weight loss programs in obese university students, one commencing with a very-low-calorie induction diet and the other relying on a balanced, energy-restricted diet throughout.

Although the initial weight loss was substantially greater in the VLCD group, weight loss at 2-year follow-up did not differ.

Commercial Weight Loss Programs

Overall, there is limited evidence that any commercial weight loss programs produce sustainable weight loss. In a study of nearly 200 participants in a Sandoz weight loss program, few had maintained initial weight loss at 3 years (159). Regular physical activity was the best predictor of sustained weight loss. Concerns have been expressed about the costs of commercial programs relative to the sustainable weight loss achieved (160).

Due in part to congressional investigation of the commercial weight loss industry in the early 1990s, credible programs now generally provide information to prospective clients about results achieved. The industry is evolving as the understanding of obesity advances, and results from older programs may or may not pertain to newer ones. Wadden and Frey (161) reported promising results of a proprietary weight loss program beginning with a VLCD at 5-year follow-up. A recent (1999) short-term study of a Weight Watchers program also produced favorable results, but with follow-up limited to 4 weeks (162). A study sponsored by Jenny Craig, Inc., suggests that the high relapse rate of commercial weight loss programs may be an artifact of premature cessation of treatment (163).

Overall, the literature on outcomes in commercial weight loss programs is suspiciously sparse. A multibillion dollar industry would doubtless be supporting the generation of publications were there good news to report. However, as programs adopt new methods, they may be contributory to efforts to achieve lasting changes in lifestyle that help control weight. Thus, at present the clinician is well advised to consider such programs with an open-minded skepticism. Assessment should be based in part on whether the program provides knowledge or skills that will support lifelong efforts to control weight, rather than the short-term management of the patient's diet.

Complementary and Alternative Medicine

Roles for nutriceutical agents, hypnotherapy, and acupuncture in the management of obesity have been claimed, but interpretable evidence of benefit is lacking to date (164).

Dieting Practices

Worth noting in societies such as the United States, which has both highly prevalent obesity and preoccupation with slimness, is a tendency for even normal weight individuals to "diet." In addition, such injudicious practices as smoking may be used as a means to maintain body weight (165). The clinician should be equally prepared to discourage ill-advised weight control practices as to encourage salutary ones.

Physician Counseling

There is suggestive evidence that physician counseling of overweight patients is supportive of weight loss and of the use of appropriate methods to achieve such weight loss (166). Overall, evidence in support of counseling is limited, largely because such counseling is limited. The topic of dietary counseling is addressed extensively in Chapter 41. Of note, the US Preventive Services Task Force recommends routine dietary counseling by physicians, both to prevent and manage obesity, as well as other diet-related health outcomes (167).

Breast-feeding

Obesity is increasingly common in children, and childhood obesity anticipates the development of obesity and its complications in adulthood. There is preliminary evidence that protracted breast-feeding may provide some protection against the later development of obesity (168). The importance of establishing judicious dietary patterns early in life is discussed in Chapters 36 and 41.

Pregnancy

Women with normal weight generally should gain between 11.5 and 13.5 kg during pregnancy (169). Normal weight is defined as a BMI between 90% and 120% of the 1959 Metropolitan Life Insurance Standards, or an absolute BMI between 19.8 and 26.0. The basis of a minimum weight gain recommendation in pregnancy is to reduce the risk of low birth weight in the neonate (169). There is agreement that, in overweight women, weight gain during pregnancy should be of a lesser magnitude. Authorities differ on the absolute amount of recommended weight change during pregnancy in the overweight woman, but most recommend a gain between 7 and 11 kg in women with a BMI greater than 26.1 (170–173). It has been suggested that in women with a prepregnancy BMI greater than 29 or weight more than 135% of ideal, no minimum weight gain is necessary (174). In the United States, each pregnancy is associated with the retention of as much as 5.5 lb; therefore, pregnancies contribute to the development of lifelong obesity in women (175). The prevention of excessive pregnancy-related weight gain and its retention in the postpartum period are important to efforts at controlling the rising prevalence of overweight/obesity in women (176).

Pregnant women who are obese have a higher incidence of gestational diabetes (173,177,178), preeclampsia (173,177–181), fetal macrosomia (172,182–186), induction of labor (173,187), primary cesarean (180, 188–190), postpartum infection (189,191, 192), and neural tube defects in offspring (193–195). Obesity in pregnancy may increase the risk of preeclampsia and pregnancy-induced hypertension (196,197). Little is known about the health care costs related to obesity during pregnancy (198). In a small study comparing 89 overweight women with 54 normal weight women, the cost at care during pregnancy was 3.2 times higher for the severely obese women (177). Hood and Dewan (199) found that hospital stay was longer for obese compared with nonobese women at delivery. Based on data from the 1988 *National Maternal and Infant Health Survey,* Cogswell et al. (182) reported the incidence of obesity in pregnancy as 17%; slightly lower estimates have been reported by others.

Obesity Management in Children

Most weight loss programs available for children are similar to adult treatment programs (45). Long-term weight losses are achieved more successfully in children than in adults (45,200,201). Evidence supports the inclusion of dietary change, behavior modification, parental involvement, and follow-up in a pediatric obesity program (202,203). Programs have emphasized both reduction in sedentary behaviors (204) and dietary modification (45). Childhood food preferences are greatly influenced by parents' food choices and eating habits (see Chapter 36); therefore, family-based approaches are encouraged (38). A recent randomized controlled trial designed to reduce television, video tape, and video game use among third and fourth grade children showed statistically significant decreases in BMI in the intervention group as compared with controls after the 6-month intervention (205). Experience with pharmacotherapy for obesity in children is limited (45).

Summary of Recommended Management Strategies

The concept of the "ideal" body weight and efforts to reach it may be both unrealistic and harmful for most overweight patients. The benefits of moderate weight loss are sufficiently clear to justify efforts to induce a loss of 5% to 10% of total weight, which is apt to be much more readily achievable. Perhaps better still is an emphasis on the means of achieving weight loss, namely changes in diet and activity pattern, rather than weight per se, as the patient has control over the former but can only indirectly influence the latter. Most adult patients concerned about weight regulation will have made multiple attempts at weight control, with at best transient success. Above all, clinicians must not submit to "blame the victim" temptations in this setting.

Temporary weight loss is no more a definitive resolution of the metabolic factors that promote obesity than transient euglycemia is a resolution of diabetes. Therefore, diets designed for short-term weight loss offer no convincing benefit either in terms of sustained weight loss or health outcomes. Because dietary and lifestyle management of weight must be permanent, it is essential that the dietary patterns applied be compatible with recommendations for health promotion in general. Fad diets promoted for purposes of rapid weight loss are unsubstantiated in the peer-reviewed literature. Even if conducive to weight management over time, such diets would be ill advised unless shown to promote health and prevent disease. There is overwhelming consensus that a diet rich in complex carbohydrates, particularly whole grains, fruits, and vegetables, is conducive to optimal health outcomes (see Chapter 40). So that patients are not offered a choice between health promotion and weight control, a health-promoting diet should be recommended for purposes of weight control. Such a diet is nutrient dense, fiber dense, and energy dilute, all properties supportive of weight loss and maintenance.

Several general modifications of the overall dietary pattern are likely to facilitate weight control. Some benefit may derive from frequent, small meals or snacks rather than the conventional three meals a day. Physiologically, there is some evidence that distributing the same number of calories in small snacks ("nibbling") rather than larger meals ("gorging") may reduce 24-hour insulin production, at least in insulin-resistant individuals (206) (see Chapter 10). Speechly and colleagues (207) recently reported evidence that snacking attenuates appetite relative to larger meals spaced farther apart. A

group of seven obese men was provided an *ad libitum* lunch following a morning "preload" provided as a single meal or multiple snacks with the same total nutrient and energy composition. Subjects ate significantly (27%) less following multiple small meals than after a single larger one. Insulin peaked at higher levels following the single meal, but was sustained above baseline for longer with the multiple small meals. Total area under the insulin curves was similar in both groups (207).

Evidence in support of "snacking" as a means of controlling weight or improving insulin metabolism is preliminary and not undisputed (208,209). However, there is generally a profound psychological component to disturbances of weight regulation, and the distribution of meals and calories may be germane. Most patients trying to control their weight are both tempted by, and afraid of, preferred foods. Consequently, many such patients resist eating for protracted periods during the day, only to overindulge in a late-day or evening binge. This pattern perpetuates a dysfunctional and tense relationship between the patient and his or her diet.

Patients caught up in this pattern should be advised to bring healthful and calorically dilute foods with them every day (see Chapter 41) and systematically to resist foods made available by others. Patients should be encouraged to eat whenever they want, but only those foods chosen in advance. By having free access to low-calorie foods (e.g., fresh fruits, fresh vegetables, nonfat dairy, dried fruit, whole grain breads or cereals), patients may overcome their fear of needing to "go hungry" for extended periods each day. In addition, frequent snacking during the day obviates the need and desire for a compulsive and binge-like meal at the end of the day. Finally, for many patients the ideal time for exercise is after work. Overweight patients who have avoided food much of the day may simply be too hungry after work to exercise. A meal at such a time often is prepared impulsively and eaten to satisfy not only energy needs but also to assuage the pent-up frustrations of the day. On questioning, many overweight patients acknowledge that they often eat, and overeat, for reasons having nothing to do with hunger.

There are multiple benefits to physical activity after work and/or prior to the evening meal. Exercise is an effective means of moderating psychological stress (210) and may attenuate the need to resolve such stress with food. Additionally, exercise may temporarily suppress appetite and generally enhances self-esteem, both of which are conducive to more thoughtful choices as the evening meal is prepared. Finally, and most evident, is the additional caloric expenditure resulting from the added activity. A meta-analysis of weight loss studies published in 1997 reveals important limitations in the field of obesity management, but suggests that best results to date have been achieved by combining energy-restricted diets with aerobic exercise (211).

In conjunction with redistribution of calories, several other specific recommendations may be made in the context of primary care encounters that may facilitate weight loss. Dietary fat restriction generally should be recommended, with sufficient detail provided to facilitate food choices (see Chapter 41). Although evidence for weight loss and/or maintenance with fat restriction is only suggestive, there are other, compelling reasons to advise fat restriction to no more than 30% of total calories. The best available evidence indicates that mean intake in the United States is currently 34% of calories (NHANES III). All other evidence aside, the caloric density of fat, and the obvious link between calorie intake and weight control, justifies efforts to moderate dietary fat intake in all efforts at weight loss or maintenance.

Along with fat restriction, patients should be advised to liberalize or increase their intake of fruits and vegetables and whole grain products. In addition to being calorically dilute, these foods tend to be rich in fiber, which is noncaloric yet satiating, at least in the short term (see Chapter 1). Foods such as dried fruits, which are relatively dense in calories, are nonetheless useful in weight loss efforts due to the high fiber content and their capacity to induce satiety with limited intake.

FDA approval of olestra (marketed as *Olean* by Procter and Gamble) has spurred particular interest in the potential utility of fat substitutes in the management of obesity. There is suggestive evidence that noncaloric fat substitutes reduce calorie intake. However, there is some evidence that compensation for lost calories occurs, particularly in the overweight. Thus, the role of fat substitutes in weight regulation is uncertain (see Chapter 38).

Among the more successful strategies for changing the overall dietary pattern is the substitution of ingredients in otherwise familiar dishes. Familiarity is among the principal factors governing dietary preference, and resistance to changing the diet can be formidable. Attempts at reducing dietary fat intake in the Women's Health Trial were most successfully sustained when they relied on substituting lower fat ingredients in recipes that preserved the appearance and taste of familiar foods (212). Although this advice can be offered in the primary care setting, patients will need detailed information on ingredient substitutions to implement such recommendations successfully. Referral to a dietitian, and referral to appropriate literature, are often both necessary (see Section III).

Difficulty in treating obesity has led to increased emphasis on the importance of prevention. However, effective and practical methods of prevention have yet to be demonstrated.

CLINICAL HIGHLIGHTS

The majority of patients with a weight control problem seen in primary care either will be overweight or have nonsevere obesity (BMI between 25 and 35). Evidence is lacking that pharmacotherapy is beneficial in this group. Clinicians should be prepared to consider long-term use of pharmacologic agents, as is commonly done with other diet-sensitive conditions such as hypertension and hyperlipidemia, as an adjunct to lifestyle in the management of obesity. Such decisions should be reached in consideration of the degree and duration of obesity, its refractoriness to lifestyle interventions, its physical and or psychological sequelae, and the risk-to-benefit ratio of pharmacotherapy to the extent it can be determined. The use of pharmacotherapy for minimal overweight without sequelae is generally not indicated.

There is no evidence that commercial weight loss programs are successful in the long term, but such programs are modifying their methods over time and may yet prove to be of value. Although the results of dietary counseling often are disappointing, there is suggestive evidence that physician counseling can be an important factor both in achieving weight loss and in encouraging patients to apply safe and appropriate methods. It is noteworthy that obesity may be the single most common condition encountered in primary care, yet it is often not addressed by primary care providers. There is convincing evidence that severe obesity can be managed effectively in the short term with low- and very-low-calorie liquid diets; evidence is little more than suggestive that such benefits can be sustained. Evidence is decisive that surgery is beneficial in carefully selected patients with severe obesity, but intensive behavioral intervention is required to sustain the weight loss achieved. Such patients make up less than 2–3% of the total population of overweight individuals.

The weight of evidence favoring fat as well as total energy restriction to achieve and maintain weight loss is convincing, if not definitive. There is limited evidence that, within the context of a fat- and energy-restricted diet, relatively more protein and relatively less carbohydrate may result in lower fasting insulin levels. However, weight loss consistently lowers insulin as well. Further, studies have generally varied carbohydrate and protein content within close proximity to the recommended levels of intake. Thus, there is no meaningful evidence that extreme alterations of the basic health-promoting diet (see Chapter 40) are indicated to achieve or maintain weight loss. On the contrary, weight loss is promoted by a diet consistent with recommendations for health promotion. Such recommendations include portion control to restrict energy intake; restriction of fat intake to reduce the energy density of the diet; abundant intake of vegetables, fruits, and whole grains; and consistent physical activity (see Chapter 40). The advisable dietary pattern is rich in complex carbohydrates, but liberal intake of protein is reasonable and may be advantageous provided the protein is from sources (e.g., beans, legumes, fish, poultry, egg white) low in fat. The application of such a diet permits weight loss and the promotion of health to be addressed conjointly; alternative weight loss diets, whether or not they facilitate short-term weight loss, are not consistent with the long-term dietary pattern advised for health maintenance and the prevention of disease. Physical activity is among the best predictors of long-term weight maintenance. Given the many impediments to long-term compliance with such guidelines (see Chapters 36, 39, and 41), the ultimate control of epidemic obesity in developed countries almost certainly will require environmental changes that facilitate consistent physical activity and consumption of a nutrient-dense but relatively energy-dilute diet.

REFERENCES

1. Ikeda J, Hayes D, Satter E, et al. A commentary on the new obesity guidelines from NIH. *J Am Diet Assoc* 1999;99:918–919.
2. Weinsier R. Clinical assessment of obese patients. In: Brownell KD, Fairburn CF, eds. *Eating disorders and obesity. A comprehensive handbook.* New York: Guilford Press, 1995:463–468.
3. Franz M. Managing obesity in patients with comorbidities. *J Am Diet Assoc* 1998;98:s39–s43.
4. Bjorntorp P. The importance of body fat distribution. In: Brownell KD, Fairburn CF, eds. *Eating disorders and obesity. A comprehensive handbook.* New York: Guilford Press, 1995:445–449.
5. Astrup A. Physical activity and weight gain and

fat distribution changes with menopause: current evidence and research issues. *Med Sci Sports Exerc* 1999;31:s564–s567.

6. Reaven G, Lithell H, Landsberg L. Hypertension and associated metabolic abnormalities—the role of insulin resistance and the sympathoadrenal system. *N Engl J Med* 1996;334:374–381.

7. Lamarche B. Abdominal obesity and its metabolic complications: implications for the risk of ischemic heart disease. *Coron Art Dis* 1998;9:473–481.

8. Egan B. Neurohumoral, hemodynamic and microvascular changes as mechanisms of insulin resistance in hypertension: a provocative but partial picture. *Int J Obes* 1991;15:133–139.

9. Pi-Sunyer F. Obesity. In: Shils M, Olson J, Shike M, eds. *Modern nutrition in health and disease*, 8th ed. Philadelphia: Lea & Febiger, 1994.

10. Bray G. Obesity. In: Ziegler EE, Filer LJ, Jr., ed. *Present knowledge in nutrition*, 7th ed. Washington, DC: ILSI Press, 1996.

11. Jekel J, Elmore J, Katz D. *Epidemiology, biostatistics, and preventive medicine*. Philadelphia: WB Saunders, 1996.

12. Kuczmarski RJ, Flegel KM, Campbell SM, Johnson CL. Increasing prevalence of overweight among US adults. The National Health and Nutrition Examination Surveys, 1960 to 1991. *JAMA* 1994;272:205–211.

13. Schwartz L, Woloshin S. Changing disease definitions: implications for disease prevalence. Analysis of the Third National Health and Nutrition Examination Survey, 1988–1994. *Effect Clin Pract* 1999; 2:76–85.

14. Must A, Spadano J, Coakley EH, et al. The disease burden associated with overweight and obesity. *JAMA* 1999;282:1523–1529.

15. Mokdad AH, Serdula MK, Dietz WH, et al. The spread of the obesity epidemic in the United States, 1991–1998. *JAMA* 1999;282:1519–1522.

16. Flegal KM. The obesity epidemic in children and adults: current evidence and research issues. *Med Sci Sports Exerc* 1999;31 (11 suppl):s509–s514.

17. Rames LK, Clarke WR, Connor WE, et al. Normal blood pressure and the evaluation of sustained blood pressure elevation in childhood: the Muscatine study. *Pediatrics* 1978;61:245–251.

18. Figueroa-Colon R, Franklin FA, Lee JY, et al. Prevalence of obesity with increased blood pressure in elementary school-aged children. *South Med J* 1997;90:806–813.

19. Falkner B, Michel S. Obesity and other risk factors in children. *Ethn Dis* 1999;9:284–289.

20. Richards GE, Cavallo A, Meyer WJd, et al. Obesity, acanthosis nigricans, insulin resistance, and hyperandrogenemia: pediatric perspective and natural history. *J Pediatr* 1985;107:893–897.

21. Friesen CA, Roberts CC. Cholelithiasis. Clinical characteristics in children. Case analysis and literature review. *Clin Pediatr (Phila)* 1989;28:294–298.

22. Holcomb GW Jr., O'Neill JA Jr., Holcomb GWD. Cholecystitis, cholelithiasis and common duct stenosis in children and adolescents. *Ann Surg* 1980; 191:626–635.

23. Kinugasa A, Tsunamoto K, Furukawa N, et al. Fatty liver and its fibrous changes found in simple obesity of children. *J Pediatr Gastroenterol Nutr* 1984;3:408–414.

24. Tominaga K, Kurata JH, Chen YK, et al. Prevalence of fatty liver in Japanese children and relationship to obesity. An epidemiological ultrasonographic survey. *Dig Dis Sci* 1995;40:2002–2009.

25. Tazawa Y, Noguchi H, Nishinomiya F, et al. Serum alanine aminotransferase activity in obese children. *Acta Paediatr* 1997;86:238–241.

26. Silvestri JM, Weese-Mayer DE, Bass MT, et al. Polysomnography in obese children with a history of sleep-associated breathing disorders. *Pediatr Pulmonol* 1993;16:124–129.

27. Marcus CL, Curtis S, Koerner CB, et al. Evaluation of pulmonary function and polysomnography in obese children and adolescents. *Pediatr Pulmonol* 1996;21:176–183.

28. Mallory GB Jr., Fiser DH, Jackson R. Sleep-associated breathing disorders in morbidly obese children and adolescents. *J Pediatr* 1989;115:892–897.

29. Kelsey JL. The incidence and distribution of slipped capital femoral epiphysis in Connecticut. *J Chronic Dis* 1971;23:567–578.

30. Kelsey JL, Acheson RM, Keggi KJ. The body build of patients with slipped capital femoral epiphysis. *Am J Dis Child* 1972;124:276–281.

31. Loder RT, Aronson DD, Greenfield ML. The epidemiology of bilateral slipped capital femoral epiphysis. A study of children in Michigan. *J Bone Joint Surg Am* 1993;75:1141–1147.

32. Wilcox PG, Weiner DS, Leighley B. Maturation factors in slipped capital femoral epiphysis. *J Pediatr Orthop* 1988;8:196–200.

33. Scott IU, Siatkowski RM, Eneyni M, et al. Idiopathic intracranial hypertension in children and adolescents. *Am J Ophthalmol* 1997;124:253–255.

34. Durcan FJ, Corbett JJ, Wall M. The incidence of pseudotumor cerebri. Population studies in Iowa and Louisiana. *Arch Neurol* 1988;45:875–877.

35. Corbett JJ, Savino PJ, Thompson HS, et al. Visual loss in pseudotumor cerebri. Follow-up of 57 patients from five to 41 years and a profile of 14 patients with permanent severe visual loss. *Arch Neurol* 1982;39:461–474.

36. Sugerman HJ, DeMaria EJ, Felton WL 3rd, et al. Increased intra-abdominal pressure and cardiac filling pressures in obesity-associated pseudotumor cerebri. *Neurology* 1997;49:507–511.

37. Hill AJ, Draper E, Stack J. A weight on children's minds: body shape dissatisfactions at 9-years old. *Int J Obes Relat Metab Disord* 1994;18:383–389.

38. Strauss R. Childhood obesity. *Curr Probl Pediatr* 1999;29:1–29.

39. Willett WC, Manson JE, Stampfer MJ, et al. Weight, weight change, and coronary heart disease in women. Risk within the "normal" weight range [see comments]. *JAMA* 1995;273:461–465.

40. Dietz WH. Childhood weight affects adult morbidity and mortality. *J Nutr* 1998;128:411S–414S.

41. Srinivasan SR, Bao W, Wattigney WA, et al. Adolescent overweight is associated with adult overweight and related multiple cardiovascular risk factors: the Bogalusa Heart Study. *Metabolism* 1996; 45:235–240.

42. Lauer RM, Clarke WR. Childhood risk factors for

high adult blood pressure: the Muscatine Study. *Pediatrics* 1989;84:633–641.

43. Mossberg HO. Forty-year follow-up of overweight children. *Lancet* 1989;2:491–493.

44. Must A, Jacques P, Dallal G, et al. Long-term morbidity and mortality of overweight adolescents. *N Engl J Med* 1992;327:1350–1355.

45. Schonfeld-Warden N, Warden CH. Pediatric obesity. An overview of etiology and treatment. *Pediatr Clin North Am* 1997;44:339–361.

46. James W, Ralph A. New understanding in obesity research. *Proc Nutr Soc* 1999;58:385–393.

47. Khan L, Bowman B. Obesity: a major global public health problem. *Annu Rev Nutr* 1999;19:xiii–xvii.

48. Lands W, Hamazaki T, Yamazaki K, et al. Changing dietary patterns. *Am J Clin Nutr* 1990;51:991–993.

49. Drewnowski A, Popkin B. The nutrition transition: new trends in the global diet. *Nutr Rev* 1997;55:31–43.

50. Pi-Sunyer F. Comorbidities of overweight and obesity: current evidence and research issues. *Med Sci Sports Exerc* 1999;31:s602–s608.

51. Thompson D, Edelsberg J, Colditz G, et al. Lifetime health and economic consequences of obesity. *Arch Intern Med* 1999;159:2177–2183.

52. Oster G, Thompson D, Edelsberg J, et al. Lifetime health and economic benefits of weight loss among obese persons. *Am J Public Health* 1999;89:1536–1542.

53. McGinnis J, Foege W. Actual causes of death in the United States. *JAMA* 1993;270:2207–2212.

54. Allison DB, Fontaine KR, Manson JE, et al. Annual deaths attributable to obesity in the United States. *JAMA* 1999;282:1530–1538.

55. Calle E, Thun M, Petrelli J, et al. Body weight and mortality. A 27-year follow-up of middle-aged men. *JAMA* 1993;270:2823–2828.

56. Manson J, Willett W, Stampfer M, et al. Body weight and mortality among women. *N Engl J Med* 1995;333:677–685.

57. Singh P, Lindsted K, Fraser G. Body weight and mortality among adults who never smoked. *Am J Epidemiol* 1999;150:1152–1164.

58. Lee I, Manson J, Hennekens C, et al. Body weight and mortality: a 27 year follow up of middle aged men. *JAMA* 1993;270:2823–2828.

59. Garrison R, Castelli W. Weight and thirty-year mortality of men in the Framingham study. *Ann Intern Med* 1985;103:1006–1009.

60. Folsom A, Kaye S, Sellers T, et al. Body fat distribution and 5-year risk of death in older women. *JAMA* 1993;269:483–487.

61. Manson J, Stampfer M, Hennekens C, et al. Body weight and longevity. A reassessment. *JAMA* 1987;257:353–358.

62. Lissner L, Odell P, D'Agostino R, et al. Variability of body weight and health outcomes in the Framingham population. *N Engl J Med* 1991;324:1839–1844.

63. Brownell K. Effects of weight cycling on metabolism, health, and psychological factors. In: Brownell KD, Fairburn CF, eds. *Eating disorders and obesity. A comprehensive handbook.* New York: Guilford Press, 1995:56–60.

64. Iribarren C, Sharp D, Burchfiel C, et al. Association of weight loss and weight fluctuation with mortality among Japanese American men. *N Engl J Med* 1995;333:686–692.

65. Wing R, Jeffery R, Hellerstedt W. A prospective study of effects of weight cycling on cardiovascular risk factors. *Arch Intern Med* 1995;155:1416–1422.

66. National task force on the prevention and treatment of obesity. Weight cycling. *JAMA* 1994;272:1196–1202.

67. Jeffery RW. Does weight cycling present a health risk? *Am J Clin Nutr* 1996;63:452S–455S.

68. Stunkard A, Sobal J. Psychosocial consequences of obesity. In: Brownell KD, Fairburn CF, eds. *Eating disorders and obesity. A comprehensive handbook.* New York: Guilford Press, 1995:417–421.

69. Gortmaker S, Must A, Perrin J, et al. Social and economic consequences of overweight in adolescence and young adulthood. *N Engl J Med* 1993;329:1008–1012.

70. Maddi S, Khoshaba D, Persico M, et al. Psychosocial correlates of psychopathology in a national sample of the morbidly obese. *Obes Surg* 1997;7:397–404.

71. VanItallie T. Prevalence of obesity. *Endocrinol Metab Clin North Am* 1996;25:887–905.

72. Matarasso A, Kim R, Kral J. The impact of liposuction on body fat. *Plast Reconstr Surg* 1998;102:1686–1689.

73. Schoeller D. Recent advances from application of doubly labeled water to measurement of human energy expenditure. *J Nutr* 1999;129:1765–1768.

74. Rush E, Plank L, Robinson S. Resting metabolic rate in young Polynesian and Caucasian women. *Int J Obes Relat Metab Disord* 1997;21:1071–1075.

75. Ravussin E, Gautier J. Metabolic predictors of weight gain. *Int J Obes Relat Metab Disord* 1999;23:37–41.

76. Leibel R, Rosenbaum M, Hirsch J. Changes in energy expenditure resulting from altered body weight. *N Engl J Med* 1995;332:621–628.

77. Astrup A, Gotzsche P, Werken Kd, et al. Meta-analysis of resting metabolic rate in formerly obese subjects. *Am J Clin Nutr* 1999;69:1117–1122.

78. Stock M. Gluttony and thermogenesis revisited. *Int J Obes Relat Metab Disord* 1999;23:1105–1117.

79. Kerckhoffs D, Blaak E, Baak MV, et al. Effect of aging on beta-adrenergically mediated thermogenesis in men. *Am J Physiol* 1998;274:E1075–E1079.

80. US Department of Heath and Human Services. *Physical activity and health. A report of the Surgeon General.* Washington, DC: US Government Printing Office, 1996.

81. Crespo C, Keteyian S, Heath G, et al. Leisure-time physical activity among US adults. *Arch Intern Med* 1996;156:93–98.

82. Simoes E, Byers T, Coates R, et al. The association between leisure-time physical activity and dietary fat in American adults. *Am J Public Health* 1995;85:240–244.

83. Francis K. Status of the year 2000 health goals for physical activity and fitness. *Phys Ther* 1999;79:405–414.

84. Dipietro L. Physical activity in the prevention of

obesity: current evidence and research issues. *Med Sci Sports Exerc* 1999;31:s542–s546.

85. Heitmann B, Kaprio J, Harris J, et al. Are genetic determinants of weight gain modified by leisure-time physical activity? A prospective study of Finnish twins. *Am J Clin Nutr* 1997;66:672–678.

86. Andersen R, Wadden T, Bartlett S, et al. Effects of lifestyle activity vs structured aerobic exercise in obese women: a randomized trial. *JAMA* 1999; 281:335–340.

87. Zachwieja J. Exercise as a treatment for obesity. *Endocrinol Metab Clin North Am* 1996;25:965–988.

88. Doucet E, Imbeault P, Almeras N, et al. Physical activity and low-fat diet: is it enough to maintain weight stability in the reduced-obese individual following weight loss by drug therapy and energy restriction? *Obes Res* 1999;7:323–333.

89. Rippe J, Hess S. The role of physical activity in the prevention and management of obesity. *J Am Diet Assoc* 1998;Oct:s31–s38.

90. Saris W. Exercise with or without dietary restriction and obesity treatment. *Int J Obes Relat Metab Disord* 1995;Oct:s113–s116.

91. Echwald S. Genetics of human obesity: lessons from mouse models and candidate genes. *J Intern Med* 1999;245:653–666.

92. Perusse L, Bouchard C. Genotype-environment interaction in human obesity. *Nutr Rev* 1999;57: s31–s37.

93. Perusse L, Chagnon Y, Weisnagel J, et al. The human obesity gene map: the 1998 update. *Obes Res* 1999;7:111–129.

94. Clement K. Leptin and the genetics of obesity. *Acta Paediatr Suppl* 1999;88:51–57.

95. Marti A, Berraondo B, Martinez J. Leptin: physiological actions. *J Physiol Biochem* 1999;55:43–49.

96. Lonnquist F, Nordfors L, Schalling M. Leptin and its potential role in human obesity. *J Intern Med* 1999;245:643–652.

97. Ronnemaa T, Karonen S-L, Rissanen A, et al. Relation between plasma leptin levels and measures of body fat in identical twins discordant for obesity. *Ann Intern Med* 1997;126:26–31.

98. Heymsfield S, Greenberg A, Fujioka K, et al. Recombinant leptin for weight loss in obese and lean adults: a randomized, controlled, dose-escalation trial. *JAMA* 1999;282:1568–1575.

99. Hamann A, Matthaei S. Regulation of energy balance by leptin. *Exp Clin Endocrinol Diabetes* 1996; 104:293–300.

100. Eaton S, Konner M. Paleolithic nutrition revisited: a twelve-year retrospective on its nature and implications. *Eur J Clin Nutr* 1997;51:207–216.

101. Mennella J, Beauchamp G. Early flavor experiences: research update. *Nutr Rev* 1998;56:205–211.

102. Drewnowski A. Why do we like fat? *J Am Diet Assoc* 1997;97[Suppl]:s58–s62.

103. Rolls B. Sensory-specific satiety. *Nutr Rev* 1986; 44:93–101.

104. Hill J, Melanson E. Overview of the determinants of overweight and obesity: current evidence and research issues. *Med Sci Sports Exerc* 1999;31[11 Suppl]::s515–s521.

105. Nestle M, Wing R, Birch L, et al. Behavioral and social influences on food choice. *Nutr Rev* 1998; 56:s50–s74.

106. Glanz K, Basil M, Maibach E, et al. Why Americans eat what they do: taste, nutrition, cost, convenience, and weight control concerns as influences on food consumption. *J Am Diet Assoc* 1998; 98:1118–1126.

107. Axelson M. The impact of culture on food-related behavior. *Ann Rev Nutr* 1986:6345–6363.

108. Lichtman S, Pisarska K, Berman E, et al. Discrepancy between self-reported and actual caloric intake and exercise in obese subjects. *N Engl J Med* 1992;327:1893–1898.

109. Braam L, Ocke M, Bueno-de-Mesquita H, et al. Determinants of obesity-related underreporting of energy intake. *Am J Epidemiol* 1998;147:1081–1086.

110. Astrup A. The American paradox: the role of energy-dense fat-reduced food in the increasing prevalence of obesity. *Curr Opin Clin Nutr Metab Care* 1998;1:573–577.

111. Lichtenstein AH, Kennedy E, Barrier P, et al. Dietary fat consumption and health. *Nutr Rev* 1998; 56:s3–s28.

112. Lissner L, Heitman B. Dietary fat and obesity: evidence from epidemiology. *Eur J Clin Nutr* 1995;49:79–90.

113. Miller W, Niederpruem M, Wallace J, et al. Dietary fat, sugar, and fiber predict body fat content. *J Am Diet Assoc* 1994;94:612–615.

114. King N, Blundell J. High-fat foods overcome the energy expenditure induced by high-intensity cycling or running. *Eur J Clin Nutr* 1995;49:114–123.

115. Alfieri M, Pomerleau J, Grace D. A comparison of fat intake of normal weight, moderately obese and severely obese subjects. *Obes Surg* 1997;7: 9–15.

116. Rolls B, Bell E. Intake of fat and carbohydrate: role of energy density. *Eur J Clin Nutr* 1999;53: s166–s173.

117. Blundell J, Stubbs R. High and low carbohydrate and fat intakes: limits imposed by appetite and palatability and their implications for energy balance. *Eur J Clin Nutr* 1999;53:s148–s165.

118. Bray G, Popkin B. Dietary fat intake does affect obesity! *Am J Clin Nutr* 1998;68:1157–1173.

119. Sears B, Lawren B. *Enter the zone.* New York: Regan Books, 1995.

120. Astrup A, Toubro S, Raben A, et al. The role of low-fat diets and fat substitutes in body weight management: what have we learned from clinical studies? *J Am Diet Assoc* 1997;97:s82–s87.

121. Larson D, Tataranni P, RT, et al. Ad libitum food intake on a "cafeteria diet" in Native American women: relations with body composition and 24-h energy expenditure. *Am J Clin Nutr* 1995; 62:911–917.

122. Koletzko B. Response to and range of acceptable fat intakes in infants and children. *Eur J Clin Nutr* 1999;53:s78–s83.

123. Atkins DR. *Atkins' new diet revolution.* New York: M. Evans & Company, Inc., 1999.

124. Heller R, Heller R. *The carbohydrate addict's lifespan program.* New York: Plume, 1998.

125. Steward H, Bethea M, Andrews S, et al. *Sugar*

busters! Cut sugar to trim fat. New York: Ballantine Books, 1998.

126. Baba N, Sawaya S, Torbay, et al. High protein vs. high carbohydrate hypoenergetic diet for the treatment of obese hyperinsulinemic subjects. *Int J Obes Relat Metab Disord* 1999;23:1202–1206.

127. Skov A, Toubro S, Bulow J, et al. Changes in renal function during weight loss induced by high vs. low-protein low-fat diets in overweight subjects. *Int J Obes Relat Metab Disord* 1999;23:1170–1177.

128. Skov A, Toubro S, Ronn B, et al. Randomized trial on protein vs. carbohydrate in ad libitum fat reduced diet for the treatment of obesity. *Int J Obes Relat Metab Disord* 1999;23:528–536.

129. Cheuvront S. The zone diet and athletic performance. *Sports Med* 1999;27:213–228.

129a. Liu S, Willett WC, Stampfer MJ, Hu FB, Sampson L, Hennekens CH, Manson JE. A prospective study of dietary glycemic load, carbohydrate intake, and risk of coronary heart disease in US women. *Am J Clin Nutr* 2000;71:1455–1461.

130. Bolton-Smith C. Intake of sugars in relation to fatness and micronutrient adequacy. *Int J Obes Relat Metab Disord* 1996;20:s31–s33.

131. Golay A, Allaz A, Morel Y, et al. Similar weight loss with low- and high-carbohydrate diets. *Am J Clin Nutr* 1996;63:174–178.

132. Golay A, Eigenheer C, Morel Y, et al. Weight-loss with low or high carbohydrate diet? *Int J Obes Relat Metab Disord* 1996;20:1067–1072.

133. Reaven G. Do high carbohydrate diets prevent the development or attenuate the manifestations (or both) of syndrome X? A viewpoint strongly against. *Curr Opin Lipidol* 1997;8:23–27.

134. McLaughlin T, Abbasi F, Carantoni M, et al. Differences in insulin resistance do not predict weight loss in response to hypocaloric diets in healthy obese women. *J Clin Endocrinol Metab* 1999;84:578–581.

135. Whitehead J, McNeill G, Smith J. The effect of protein intake on 24-h energy expenditure during energy restriction. *Int J Obes Relat Metab Disord* 1996;20:727–732.

136. Swinburn B, Woollard G, Chang EC, et al. Effects of reduced-fat diets consumed ad libitum on intake of nutrients, particularly antioxidant vitamins. *J Am Diet Assoc* 1999;99:1400–1405.

137. Suter P, Schutz Y, Jequier E. The effect of ethanol on fat storage in healthy subjects. *N Engl J Med* 1992;326:983–987.

138. Consensus development conference panel. Gastrointestinal surgery for severe obesity. *Ann Intern Med* 1991;115:956–961.

139. Oria H. Gastric banding for morbid obesity. *Eur J Gastroenterol Hepatol* 1999;11:105–114.

140. Greenway F. Surgery for obesity. *Endocrinol Metab Clin North Am* 1996;25:1005–1027.

141. Hauri P, Horber F, Sendi P. Is bariatric surgery worth its costs? *Obes Surg* 1999;9:480–483.

142. Ryan D. Medicating the obese patient. *Endocrinol Metab Clin North Am* 1996;25:989–1004.

143. Aronne L. Modern medical management of obesity: the role of pharmacological intervention. *J Am Diet Assoc* 1998;98:s23–s26.

144. Connolly HM, Crary JL, McGoon MD, et al. Valvular heart disease associated with fenfluramine-

phentermine [see comments] [published erratum appears in *N Engl J Med* 1997;337:1783]. *N Engl J Med* 1997;337:581–588.

145. Curfman G. Diet pills redux. *N Engl J Med* 1997; 337:629–630.

146. McNeely W, Goa KL. Sibutramine. A review of its contribution to the management of obesity. *Drugs* 1998;56:1093–1124.

147. Gaal LV, Wauters M, Leeuw ID. Anti-obesity drugs: what does sibutramine offer? An analysis of its potential contribution to obesity treatment. *Exp Clin Endocrinol Diabetes* 1998;106:35–40.

148. Hvizdos K, Markham A. Orlistat: a review of its use in the management of obesity. *Drugs* 1999; 58:743–760.

149. Sjostrom L, Rissanen A, Andersen T, et al. Randomized placebo-controlled trial of orlistat for weight loss and prevention of weight regain in obese patients. *Lancet* 1998;352:167–173.

150. Scacchi M, Pincelli A, Cavagnini F. Growth hormone in obesity. *Int J Obes Relat Metab Disord* 1999;23:260–271.

151. Leonhardt M HB, Langhans W. New approaches in the pharmacological treatment of obesity. *Eur J Nutr* 1999;38:1–13.

152. Carek P, Dickerson L. Current concepts in the pharmacological management of obesity. *Drugs* 1999;57:883–904.

153. Astrup A, Lundsgaard C. What do pharmacological approaches to obesity management offer? Linking pharmacological mechanisms of obesity management agents to clinical practice. *Exp Clin Endocrinol Diabetes* 1998;106:29–34.

154. Council on scientific affairs. Treatment of obesity in adults. *JAMA* 1988;260:2547–2551.

155. Molokhia M. Obesity wars: a pilot study of very low calorie diets in obese patients in general practice. *Br J Gen Pract* 1998;48:1251–1252.

156. Pekkarinen T, Mustajoki P. Use of very low-calorie diet in preoperative weight loss: efficacy and safety. *Obes Res* 1997;5:595–602.

157. Kansanen M, Vanninen E, Tuunainen A, et al. The effect of a very low-calorie diet-induced weight loss on the severity of obstructive sleep apnoea and autonomic nervous function in obese patients with obstructive sleep apnoea syndrome. *Clin Physiol* 1998;18:377–385.

158. Ryttig K, Flaten H, Rossner S. Long-term effects of a very low calorie diet (Nutrilett) in obesity treatment. A prospective, randomized, comparison between VLCD and a hypocaloric diet + behavior modification and their combination. *Int J Obes Relat Metab Disord* 1997;21:574–579.

159. Grodstein F, Levine R, Troy L, et al. Three year followup of participants in a commercial weight loss program. *Arch Intern Med* 1996;156:1302–1306.

160. Spielman A, Kanders B, Kienholz M, et al. The cost of losing: an analysis of commercial weight-loss programs in a metropolitan area. *J Am Coll Nutr* 1992;11:36–41.

161. Wadden T, Frey D. A multicenter evaluation of a proprietary weight loss program for the treatment of marked obesity: a five-year follow-up. *Int J Eat Disord* 1997;22:203–212.

162. Lowe M, Miller-Kovach K, Frye N, et al. An initial

evaluation of a commercial weight loss program: short-term effects on weight, eating behavior, and mood. *Obes Res* 1999;7:51–59.

163. Wolfe B. Long-term maintenance following attainment of goal weight: a preliminary investigation. *Addict Behav* 1992;17:469–477.

164. Mulhisen L, Rogers J. Complementary and alternative modes of therapy for the treatment of the obese patient. *J Am Osteopath Assoc* 1999;99: s8–s12.

165. Biener L, Heaton A. Women dieters of normal weight: their motives, goals, and risks. *Am J Public Health* 1995;85:714–717.

166. Nawaz H, Adams M, Katz DL. Weight loss counseling by health care providers. *Am J Public Health* 1999;89:764–767.

167. US Preventive Services Task Force. *Guide to clinical preventive services,* 2nd ed. Baltimore: Williams & Wilkins, 1996.

168. von Kries R, Koletzko B, Sauerwald T, et al. Breast feeding and obesity: cross sectional study. *BMJ* 1999;319:147–150.

169. Institute of Medicine. *Nutrition during pregnancy.* National Academy of Sciences. Washington, DC: National Academy Press, 1990.

170. Butman M. *Prenatal nutrition: a clinical manual. WIC program, Massachusetts.* Boston, Department of Public Health, 1982.

171. Dimperio D. *Prenatal nutrition. Clinical guidelines for nurses.* White Plains, NY: March of Dimes Birth Defects Foundation, 1988.

172. Bracero L, Byrne D. Optimal weight gain during singleton pregnancy. *Gynecol Obstet Invest* 1998; 46:9–16.

173. Edwards LE, Hellerstedt WL, Alton IR, et al. Pregnancy complications and birth outcomes in obese and normal-weight women: effects of gestational weight change. *Obstet Gynecol* 1996;87: 389–394.

174. Abrams B, Laros R. Prepregnancy weight, weight gain, and birth weight. *Am J Obstet Gynecol* 1986; 155:918.

175. Lovelady C, Garner K, et al. The effect of weight loss in overweight, lactating women on the growth of their infants. *N Engl J Med* 2000;342:449–453.

176. Butte N. Dieting and exercise in overweight, lactating women. *N Engl J Med* 2000;342:502–503.

177. Galtier-Dereure F, Montpeyroux F, Boulot P, et al. Weight excess before pregnancy: complications and cost. *Int J Obes Relat Metab Disord* 1995;19: 443–448.

178. Ratner RE, Hamner LHd, Isada NB. Effects of gestational weight gain in morbidly obese women: I. Maternal morbidity. *Am J Perinatol* 1991;8: 21–24.

179. Tomoda S, Tamura T, Sudo Y, et al. Effects of obesity on pregnant women: maternal hemodynamic change. *Am J Perinatol* 1996;13:73–78.

180. Parker JD, Abrams B. Prenatal weight gain advice: an examination of the recent prenatal weight gain recommendations of the Institute of Medicine. *Obstet Gynecol* 1992;79:664–669.

181. Morin KH. Obese and nonobese postpartum women: complications, body image, and perceptions of the intrapartal experience. *Appl Nurs Res* 1995;8:81–87.

182. Cogswell ME, Serdula MK, Hungerford DW, et al. Gestational weight gain among average-weight and overweight women—what is excessive? *Am J Obstet Gynecol* 1995;172:705–712.

183. Edwards LE, Dickes WF, Alton IR, et al. Pregnancy in the massively obese: course, outcome, and obesity prognosis of the infant. *Am J Obstet Gynecol* 1978;131:479–483.

184. Garbaciak J, Richter M, Miller S, et al. Maternal weight and pregnancy complications. *Am J Obstet Gynecol* 1985;152:238–245.

185. Kliegman R, Gross T, Morton S, et al. Intrauterine growth and postnatal fasting metabolism in infants of obese mothers. *J Pediatr* 1984;104:601–607.

186. Kliegman R, Gross T. Perinatal problems of the obese mother and her infant. *Obstet Gynecol* 1985;66:299–306.

187. Ekblad U, Grenman S. Maternal weight, weight gain during pregnancy and pregnancy outcome. *Int J Gynaecol Obstet* 1992;39:277–283.

188. Crane SS, Wojtowycz MA, Dye TD, et al. Association between pre-pregnancy obesity and the risk of cesarean delivery. *Obstet Gynecol* 1997;89: 213–216.

189. Isaacs JD, Magann EF, Martin RW, et al. Obstetric challenges of massive obesity complicating pregnancy. *J Perinatol* 1994;14:10–14.

190. Perlow JH, Morgan MA, Montgomery D, et al. Perinatal outcome in pregnancy complicated by massive obesity. *Am J Obstet Gynecol* 1992;167: 958–962.

191. Calandra C, Abell DA, Beischer NA. Maternal obesity in pregnancy. *Obstet Gynecol* 1981;57:8–12.

192. Martens MG, Kolrud BL, Faro S, et al. Development of wound infection or separation after cesarean delivery. Prospective evaluation of 2,431 cases. *J Reprod Med* 1995;40:171–175.

193. Werler MM, Louik C, Shapiro S, et al. Prepregnant weight in relation to risk of neural tube defects [see comments]. *JAMA* 1996;275:1089–1092.

194. Shaw GM, Velie EM, Schaffer D. Risk of neural tube defect-affected pregnancies among obese women [see comments]. *JAMA* 1996;275:1093–1096.

195. Prentice A, Goldberg G. Maternal obesity increases congenital malformations. *Nutr Rev* 1996; 54:146–150.

196. Carter JP, Furman T, Hutcheson HR. Preeclampsia and reproductive performance in a community of vegans. *South Med J* 1987;80:692–697.

197. Baker PN. Possible dietary measures in the prevention of pre-eclampsia and eclampsia. *Baillieres Clin Obstet Gynaecol* 1995;9:497–507.

198. Morin KH. Perinatal outcomes of obese women: a review of the literature. *J Obstet Gynecol Neonatal Nurs* 1998;27:431–440.

199. Hood DD, Dewan DM. Anesthetic and obstetric outcome in morbidly obese parturients. *Anesthesiology* 1993;79:1210–1218.

200. Epstein LH, Valoski A, McCurley J. Effect of weight loss by obese children on long-term growth. *Am J Dis Child* 1993;147:1076–1080.

201. Epstein LH, Valoski AM, Kalarchian MA, et al. Do children lose and maintain weight easier than adults: a comparison of child and parent weight

changes from six months to ten years. *Obes Res* 1995;3:411–417.
202. Dietz WH. Therapeutic strategies in childhood obesity. *Horm Res* 1993;39:86–90.
203. Williams CL, Bollella M, Carter BJ. Treatment of childhood obesity in pediatric practice. *Ann NY Acad Sci* 1993;699:207–219.
204. Glenny AM, O'Meara S, Melville A, et al. The treatment and prevention of obesity: a systematic review of the literature. *Int J Obes Relat Metab Disord* 1997;21:715–737.
205. Robinson TN. Reducing children's television viewing to prevent obesity: a randomized controlled trial. *JAMA* 1999;282:1561–1567.
206. Jenkins D, Wolever T, Vuksan V, et al. Nibbling versus gorging: metabolic advantages of increased meal frequency. *N Engl J Med* 1989;321:929–934.
207. Speechly D, Rogers G, Buffenstein R. Acute appetite reduction associated with an increased frequency of eating in obese males. *Int J Obes Relat Metab Disord* 1999;23:1151–1159.
208. Bellisle F, McDevitt R, Prentice A. Meal frequency and energy balance. *Br J Nutr* 1997;77:s57–s70.
209. Drummond S, Crombie N, Kirk T. A critique of the effects of snacking on body weight status. *Eur J Clin Nutr* 1996;50:779–783.
210. Fox K. The influence of physical activity on mental well-being. *Public Health Nutr* 1999;2:411–418.
211. Miller W, Koceja D, Hamilton E. A meta-analysis of the past 25 years of weight loss research using diet, exercise or diet plus exercise intervention. *Int J Obes Relat Metab Disord* 1997;21:941–947.
212. Kristal A, White E, Shattuck A, et al. Long-term maintenance of a low-fat diet: durability of fat-related dietary habits in the Women's Health Trial. *J Am Diet Assoc* 1992;92:553–559.

BIBLIOGRAPHY

See "Sources for All Chapters."
Arner P. The β-3 adrenergic receptor-a cause and cure of obesity? *N Engl J Med* 1995;333:382–383.
Blundell JE, Stubbs RJ. High and low carbohydrate and fat intakes: limits imposed by appetite and palatability and their implications for energy balance. *Eur J Clin Nutr* 1999;53(1 suppl):s148–s165.
Bray GA. Health hazards of obesity. *Endocrin Metab Clinics North Am* 1996;25:907–919.
Brolin RE. Gastrointestinal surgery for severe obesity. *Nutrition* 1996;12:403–404.
Brownell KD, Fairburn CG (eds.). *Eating disorders and obesity. A comprehensive handbook.* New York: The Guilford Press, 1995.
Drewnowski A. Intense sweeteners and energy density of foods: implications for weight control. *Eur J Clin Nutr* 1999;53:757–763.
Executive summary of the clinical guidelines on the identification, evaluation, and treatment of overweight and obesity in adults. *Arch Intern Med* 1998; 158:1855–1867.
Flegal KM, Carroll MD, Kuczmarski RJ, Johnson CL. Overweight and obesity in the United States: prevalence and trends, 1960–1994. *Int J Obes Relat Metab Disord* 1998;22:39–47.
Gibney MJ. Optimal macronutrient balance. *Proc Nutr Soc* 1999;58:421–425.
Grundy SM. Multifactorial causation of obesity: implications for prevention. *Am J Clin Nutr* 1998;67 (3 suppl):s563–s572.
Grundy SM. The optimal ratio of fat-to-carbohydrate in the diet. *Annu Rev Nutr* 1999;19:325–341.
Institute of Medicine. *Improving America's diet and health. From recommendations to action.* Washington, DC: National Academy Press, 1991.
Jebb SA, Moore MS. Contribution of a sedentary lifestyle and inactivity to the etiology of overweight and obesity: current evidence and research issues. *Med Sci Sports Exerc* 1999;31(11 suppl):s534–s541.
Jequier E, Tappy L. Regulation of body weight in humans. *Physiol Rev* 1999;79:451–480.
Kirk SF. Treatment of obesity: theory into practice. *Proc Nutr Soc* 1999;58:53–58.
Lonnquist F, Nordors L, Schalling M. Leptin and its potential role in human obesity. *J Int Med* 1999; 245:643–652.
Mantzoros CS. The role of leptin in human obesity: a review of current evidence. *Ann Intern Med* 1999; 130:671–680.
Marti A, Berraondo B, Martinez JA. Leptin: physiological actions. *J Physiol Biochem* 1999;55:43–49.
Meisler JG, St. Jeor S. Summary and recommendations from the American Health Foundation's Expert Panel on Healthy Weight. *Am J Clin Nutr* 1996;63(suppl): s474–s477.
Pasman WJ, Saris WH, Westerterp-Plantenga MS. Predictors of weight maintenance. *Obes Res* 1999;7: 43–50.
Pellett PL. Food energy requirements in humans. *Am J Clin Nutr* 1990;51:711–722.
Perusse L, Bouchard C. Genotype-environment interaction in human obesity. *Nutr Rev* 1999;57(5 pt 2): s31–s37.
Popkin BM. The nutrition transition and its health implications in lower-income countries. *Public Health Nutr* 1998;1:5–21.
Poston WS II, Foreyt JP. Obesity is an environmental issue. *Atherosclerosis* 1999;146:201–209.
Robinson TN. Behavioral treatment of childhood and adolescent obesity. *Int J Obes Relat Metab Disord* 1999;(23 suppl)2:s52–s57.
Rogers PJ. Eating habits and appetite control: a psychobiological perspective. *Proc Nutr Soc* 1999;58:59–67.
Rolls BJ, Bell EA. Intake of fat and carbohydrate: role of energy density. *Eur J Clin Nutr* 1999;53 suppl 1:s166–s173.
Wadden TA, Van Itallie TB, Blackburn GL. Responsible and irresponsible use of very-low-calorie diets in the treatment of obesity. *JAMA* 1990;263:83–85.
Weinsier RL, Hunter GR, Heini AF, Goran MI, Sell SM. The etiology of obesity: relative contribution of metabolic factors, diet, and physical activity. *Am J Med* 1998;105:145–150.
Wing RR. Physical activity in the treatment of adulthood overweight and obesity: current evidence and research issues. *Med Sci Sports Exerc* 1999;31(11 suppl): s547–s552.

6

Diet, Atherosclerosis, and Ischemic Heart Disease

INTRODUCTION

The evidence for associations between both macronutrients and micronutrients and the pathogenesis of coronary artery disease is decisive, deriving from multiple, large observational studies, randomized trials, and *in vitro* studies. Total dietary fat intake has been linked to hyperlipidemia and coronary disease for at least 40 years. Recently, evidence has been mounting that although intake of saturated and trans fat should be restricted, intake of monounsaturated fat, and particularly n-3 polyunsaturated fat (see Chapter 2), should be liberalized. There is decisive evidence of an inverse association between dietary fiber and serum lipid levels, and of associations between specific micronutrients and both atherogenesis and endothelial function. Evidence for the role of nutrition in primary, secondary, and tertiary prevention of acute coronary events is definitive as well. Dietary counseling is an essential component in the primary prevention of heart disease and in the clinical management of all patients with established coronary disease, as well as those with risk factors.

OVERVIEW

Diet

Cardiovascular disease remains the leading cause of death in the United States, although cancer deaths are expected to exceed heart disease deaths by approximately the year 2020 if present trends continue. Diet influences the pathogenesis of coronary artery disease in a variety of ways. The initial development of fatty streaks in coronary arteries is mediated by serum lipid levels, as well as free-radical oxidation, both of which are modified by nutrients. Progression of coronary lesions is affected by serum lipids, hypertension (see Chapter 7), hyperinsulinemia (see Chapter 10), possibly obesity (see Chapter 5), and oxidation, all of which are mediated by both macronutrient and micronutrient intake. Once coronary artery atherosclerosis is established, diet plays a role in determining both progression of plaque deposition and the reactivity of the endothelium, both of which may be predictive of cardiac events. Dietary manipulations have been shown to modify all of the known, modifiable coronary risk factors (1) and, when extreme, to induce regression of established lesions (2,3). The role of diet in the management of coronary disease and risk factors is determined by the efficacy of dietary interventions and their complementarity with pharmacologic interventions of proven benefit.

The link between diet and heart disease has been apparent since at least the 1930s, when food shortages in the United States due to the Great Depression were observed to reduce the incidence of cardiovascular events. Similar observations were made in western Europe during World War II. These "natural experiments" were found to be consistent with global patterns of dietary fat intake and served to establish a link between dietary fat and heart disease risk. Original evidence of the strong association between diet and coronary artery disease derived from transcultural studies and natural experiments.

Since the 1950s, an ever-expanding pool of data derived from a wide variety of study types has overwhelmingly linked dietary pattern to atherosclerotic disease of the coronary arteries and the risk of cardiovascular morbidity and mortality. The seminal work of Ancel Keys in the 1960s revealed a linear relationship between the total mean per capita fat intake of a country and the incidence of cardiovascular events (4). Keys' work has since been criticized for not including all of the countries originally surveyed and for retaining only those that most supported the proposed association. However, numerous other studies subsequently corroborated the association between total fat intake and atherogenesis, both within and among different populations. Although total dietary fat intake remains an important predictor of cardiac risk, work over recent years has been focused increasingly on the contribution of specific dietary fats to the atherogenic process. The relative cardiovascular benefits of total fat restriction versus modifying diet to promote monounsaturated fat intake relative to saturated and polyunsaturated fat intake is an area of particular interest at present (5,6).

The role of total caloric intake in cardiovascular disease is somewhat less clear than is the role of dietary fat. When caloric expenditure is high, caloric intake is not thought to represent a cardiac risk factor. Caloric intake in excess of caloric expenditure results in weight gain, and obesity is associated with heart disease risk (see Chapters 5 and 10). A calorie-restricted diet has been consistently associated with longevity in laboratory animals, including primates. The benefits of calorie restriction, if relevant to humans, apply to a wide variety of diseases, as well as aging, rather than to cardiovascular risk in particular.

Intake of fruits, vegetables, and cereal grains is inversely correlated with cardiovascular risk, as is total fiber intake (7). The intake of soluble fiber in particular appears to have cardiovascular benefits attributable to a hypolipidemic effect (8). On a population basis, separating the effects of soluble and insoluble fiber, fruit, vegetable, cereal, and fat intake is complicated by the tendency of dietary behaviors to cluster (9,10). Diets low in fat tend to be relatively high in fiber of both types, and vice versa. Nonetheless, convincing epidemiologic associations exist between both low-fat, predominantly vegetarian diets and the monounsaturated fatty acid (MUFA)-rich Mediterranean diet and a low incidence of cardiovascular events.

Dietary prevention and management of hypertension can contribute to the prevention of cardiovascular disease; this topic is discussed in Chapter 7. Diet and hemostasis is covered in Chapter 8. The effects of diet on peripheral vascular disease and cerebrovascular disease are discussed in Chapter 9. Other topics pertinent to the link between nutrition and cardiovascular disease risk include obesity (see Chapter 5) and diabetes (see Chapter 10).

Dietary Fat

Total Fat

Principal among the dietary factors influencing coronary atherogenesis is total dietary fat intake. Excess dietary fat produces predictable elevations in serum cholesterol and lipoproteins (Hegsted and Keys equations; see Section IIIA), which translate into predictable increases in the risk of events (11). Dietary guidelines in the United States (12) have been based, in large measure, on secure evidence linking diet to heart disease. The current guideline for total fat intake is 30% of total calories, and excess fat intake is defined relative to this reference. The contribution of excess fat and calorie intake to heart disease was emphasized in the 1988 Surgeon General's report (13).

Dietary fat contributes to atherogenesis primarily by inducing a rise in serum lipid levels. The principal mechanism by which fat and cholesterol ingestion translate into increased cardiovascular risk is the induced elevation of serum lipoproteins, especially low-density lipoprotein (LDL). Elevations of LDL result in saturation of the receptor-mediated uptake by hepatocytes (14,15) and the consequent uptake of LDL by tissue-fixed macrophages. This process of so-called "foam cell" formation is accelerated by the oxidation of LDL. The ingestion of polyunsaturated fat, although not associated with elevations of serum lipids, has been increasingly implicated in the promotion of lipoprotein oxidation. The deposition of foam cells in the coronary intima and media induces smooth muscle cell hyperplasia and the growth of obstructing lesions (16,17).

In addition to the chronic effects of fat intake on atherogenesis, there is recent evidence that the acute ingestion of a high-fat meal may represent a cardiac stressor (18). An interest in postprandial atherogenesis dates back to at least the 1970s (19). Although the postprandial rise in triglycerides may contribute to the progression of coronary atherosclerosis, the magnitude of lipid changes seems insufficient to explain the observed increase in events; there are a variety of concomitant metabolic responses (20). The acute ingestion of particularly, and perhaps exclusively, saturated or trans fat may destabilize coronary plaque and impair endothelial function (18,21). Evidence is rapidly increasing that endothelial function is a fundamental index of cardiac risk, and that it is modified in response to a variety of nutritional influences.

Saturated Fat

Saturated fatty acids, those with no carbon-carbon double bonds, in particular raise total cholesterol and LDL. Foods rich in saturated fatty acids include the flesh of most domestic mammals raised for human consumption, dairy products, and several vegetable oils, notably coconut, palm, and palm kernel. The evidence that excessive intake of saturated

fat, specifically C14 myristic and C16 palmitic acids, raises serum lipids and promotes atherogenesis is decisive (see Chapter 2). Evidence linking diets high in saturated fats to cardiovascular events is convincing, but is limited by difficulties in conducting long-term studies requiring assignment of subjects to dietary interventions. Current recommendations call for reducing the intake of saturated fat to 10% or less of calories (National Cholesterol Education Program [NCEP]) and ideally to less than 7% to 8%. Average US adult intake of these fats is approximately 13% to 14%. Prehistoric adaptations may be informative; paleolithic intake of saturated fat was approximately 5% of calories (22).

Apparently unique among the highly saturated fatty acids, stearic acid, C18, is neutral with regard to serum lipids. This fat is found abundantly in beef and in chocolate. (It should be noted that although stearic acid is the predominant fat in dark or bittersweet chocolate, milk chocolate also contains milk fat, rich in palmitic acid, and therefore is likely to be contributory to elevated serum lipid levels). For further discussion of dietary fats, see Chapter 2.

In counseling patients to modify intake of saturated fat, a consideration of all sources of such fat in the diet is essential. The prevailing notion that dietary fat, and saturated fat in particular, derives predominantly from red meat is only partly true. The primary source of dietary fat and saturated fat in the diets of American men is red meat; in the diets of American children it is milk; and in the diets of American women, it is a combination of dairy products, including cheese, and processed foods (23,24). Studies demonstrate that even subjects educated to be fat averse, in attempting to reduce dietary fat intake in general, and saturated fat intake in particular, tend to substitute fat from one source (e.g., meat) with comparable fat from another source (e.g., dairy) (24). When counseling subjects in an effort to reduce total and saturated fat intake, a reasonably detailed dietary history is essential. The contribution to total fat intake of often overlooked and unreported constituents of diet, such as sauces, dressings, and spreads, can be substantial (24). Assertions by patients that they are eating a low-fat diet because they have reduced or eliminated red meat are unreliable.

Cholesterol

The relative contribution of dietary cholesterol to serum lipids is confounded to some extent by the highly correlated distribution of saturated fat and cholesterol in the diet. The meat of domestic mammals, dairy products, and organ meats are rich in both nutrients and are associated with elevated serum lipids. The contribution of cholesterol from eggs to the risk of heart disease is somewhat uncertain, as high-cholesterol diets often are high in total fat, and there is some evidence that egg consumption is unrelated to cardiovascular risk (25). Shellfish, while relatively high in cholesterol content, is low in total and saturated fat, are not convincingly linked to an increase in cardiovascular risk. Conversely, coconut, palm, and palm kernel oils are highly saturated, but are derived from vegetable sources free of cholesterol. Of note, cholesterol is a constituent of cell membranes and is found only in animal products; the common "cholesterol free" on the label of processed foods not of animal origin is therefore a given and often presented to distract from the product's fat content.

The Keys and Hegsted equations (see Section IIIA), indicate that cholesterol contributes relatively less to serum lipids than does saturated fat intake, in part because while fat intake is measured in grams, cholesterol intake is measured in milligrams. The recommended intake of cholesterol is up to 300 mg per day, with restrictions below 200 mg encouraged in patients with hyperlipidemia or established coronary disease. To comply with this recommendation, patients must eliminate or minimize their intake of egg yolks and restrict their intake of red meat, deli meats, cheese, and whole milk and its products.

Trans Fatty Acids

Modern food preparation techniques have greatly increased human exposure to trans fatty acids, which occur naturally in small quantities in milk. Trans fats are produced commercially by bombarding partially unsaturated fatty acids (i.e., fatty acids with some preserved carbon-carbon double bonds; see Chapter 2). The hydrogenation process saturates most of the double bonds in polyunsaturated fats. The trans isomeric configuration about the remaining double bond results in molecules that pack tightly together, limiting the fluidity of the fat and producing a higher melting point. The stability of these fats at room temperature results in products that retain shape (e.g., margarine in stick form as opposed to liquid vegetable oil) and increases product shelf life. Although they are advantageous to the food industry, trans fats influence serum lipids similarly to saturated fats (26). Many processed foods contain trans fats; they can be detected on labels by looking for "partially hydrogenated" before an oil is listed. Commonly hydrogenated oils are soy, cottonseed, and corn. The federal policy that resulted in more informative food labels does not require that trans fats be listed, and therefore they are readily overlooked by even health-conscious patients. (This policy, however, is potentially subject to revision as this text goes to press.) In addition to scanning food labels for "partially hydrogenated," patients should be advised to avoid fatty spreads, sauces, dressings, and creamers that appear solid at room temperature. As an example, tub margarine is generally lower in trans fat than margarine in stick form.

Polyunsaturated Fat

The two essential fatty acids in the human diet, linoleic (18:2n-6) and 2-linolenic (18:3n-3) (see Chapter 2) are both polyunsaturated. Humans, along with other mammals, share the capacity to synthesize saturated fatty acids, as well as unsaturated fatty acids of the n-9 and n-7 series, but lack the requisite enzymes to manufacture n-6 and n-3 polyunsaturates. The metabolism of these fats is discussed in greater detail in Chapter 2. Linoleic acid serves as precursor to arachidonic acid, whereas α-linolenic acid serves as a precursor for eicosapentaenoic acid (20:6n-3) and docosahexaenoic acid (22:5n-3). Collectively, the products of essential fatty acid metabolism are known as eicosanoids, and include prostaglandins, thromboxanes, and leukotrienes. A topic generating considerable interest at present is the optimal intake of n-3 fatty acids. These are polyunsaturated fats with the first double bond after the third carbon molecule (see Chapter 2). Of particular importance to human health appears to be the ratio of n-6 to n-3 fatty acids. An extensive literature has developed linking high intakes of n-3 polyunsaturates, particularly from marine sources, to low rates of heart disease (27–30). Evidence to date is suggestive that increased consumption of n-3 fatty acids may lower cardiovascular risk. Whereas n-6 polyunsaturates are readily available in commonly consumed vegetable oils, including soybean, safflower, sunflower, and corn, n-3 fatty acids are less widely distributed. Oils rich in n-3 fatty acids include flaxseed, linseed, marine oils, and, to a lesser degree, canola oil (29). Fat-restricted diets may result in relative, if not overt, deficiency of n-3 intake, as well as less than optimal intake of monounsaturated fat (31–34). A diet rich in n-3 fatty acids has been linked to reduced levels of serum triglycerides, reduced platelet aggregation, and lower blood pressure; the evidence to date for a protective role of n-3 fatty acids against heart disease is suggestive. The recently reported (1999) GISSI-Prevenzione Trial lends strong support to the practice of n-3 fatty acid supplementation. In a factorial design trial of over 11,000 patients status post myocardial infarction (MI), nearly 3,000 patients received fish oil capsules containing approximately 850 mg eicosapentaenoic acid and approximately twice the dose of docosahexaenoic acid, and another nearly 3,000 patients received matching placebo. At 42-month follow-up, n-3 polyunsaturated fatty acid (PUFA) supplementation had significantly reduced the cardiovascular event and mortality rates and all-cause mortality (35).

Some discord over the optimal level of fat intake has recently arisen as a result of insight into the benefits of n-3 polyunsaturates and monounsaturates. This controversy was conveyed in a recent "clinical debate" in the *New England Journal of Medicine* (31,36). The beneficial effects of monounsaturated fats, and certain polyunsaturates, especially n-3 fatty acids, on cardiovascular health may be sufficiently strong that an intake of total fat in excess of 30% of calories is desirable, provided the fat is predominantly of these types (6). Of note to primary care providers is that either the recommended reduction in total fat intake or the consumption of predominantly monounsaturated fat and n-3 polyunsaturated fat both represent significant dietary changes for most patients seen in the United States (37,38).

In a recent review of the diets of preagricultural humans, Eaton et al. (22) suggested that the diet to which humans adapted during millions of years of evolution be used as an arbiter until or unless disputes about optimal intake can be resolved in prospective intervention trials (see Chapter 39). Paleolithic humans (N.B.: The Stone Age is divided into Paleolithic, Mesolithic, and Neolithic periods; the *Paleolithic* began approximately 2.5 million years ago when our ancestors first started to use rough stone implements, and lasted until approximately 8000 B.C., thereby constituting the major portion of human evolution; the use of more refined stone implements ushered in the Mesolithic period; the use of finely polished stone implements ushered in the Neolithic period) apparently consumed approximately 20% to 25% of total calories from fat, well below average intake in the United States and intermediate between the recommendations of low-fat and Mediterranean diet advocates. The flesh of wild animals, although containing markedly less total fat than the flesh of domestic cattle, is notably richer in n-3 fatty acids, suggesting that our ancestors consumed this class of nutrient in relative abundance (22).

Monounsaturated Fat

Studies in the 1960s suggested that monounsaturates were neutral with regard to serum lipids, resulting in greater interest in the potential health benefits of polyunsaturates. The cardioprotective effects of MUFAs have come to light largely through cross-cultural epidemiologic studies. Rates of heart disease are low in populations with high consumption of monounsaturated fat, even when total fat intake is consequently high, leading to interest in the so-called "Mediterranean diet" (39). There is some evidence suggesting that monounsaturates' apparent neutral effects on serum cholesterol are due to reductions in LDL and concomitant elevations of HDL, both of which reduce cardiovascular risk (40–42). A meta-analysis in 1995, however, reported that monounsaturates lower HDL (from Ziegler and Filer; Gardner and Kraemer 1995). Perhaps of greater importance is the apparent link between monounsaturated fat intake and inhibition of LDL oxidation (43).

Monounsaturates are abundant in traditional diets of the countries bordering the Mediterranean Sea. The so-called "Mediterranean diet," consisting of abundant fresh fruit and vegetables, olives, olive oil, wine, fish, and grains, particularly wheat in the form of pasta, has received increasing attention as a means of lowering cardiovascular risk. Various aspects of this diet may contribute to its cardioprotective properties. As discussed earlier, n-3 polyunsaturated fat in fish may favorably affect serum lipids and inhibit platelet aggregation. Alcohol, discussed later, favorably influences serum lipids and raises endogenous tissue plasminogen activator (44). Fruit and vegetable consumption, discussed later, is likely to be cardioprotective by a variety of mechanisms, as is consumption of grains, seeds, and certain nuts (45). Therefore, transcultural studies are inadequate to provide decisive evidence of the benefits of monounsaturates.

Further evidence supporting a role for monounsaturates in modifying cardiovascular risk derives from recent intervention studies. Garg and colleagues (46,47) showed that the Mediterranean diet results in greater improvements in glycemic control than does a diet rich in carbohydrate. The area under 24-hour insulin curves is known to correlate with cardiac risk. Decreased levels of insulin in patients with manifestations of the insulin resistance syndrome (truncal obesity, hypertension, hypertriglyceridemia) may result in reduced cardiovascular risk by several mechanisms, including modification of the lipid profile and declines in norepinephrine levels (48,49). The Lyon Diet Heart Study, a controlled trial in patients following a first MI, showed convincing evidence of event reduction with a Mediterranean diet (50–52).

A variety of nuts and seeds are rich in monounsaturates, including walnuts, almonds, peanuts, and sesame seeds. Olives and avocados, both fruits, are excellent sources.

Dietary Fat Conclusions

The optimal level of dietary fat intake for primary prevention of heart disease, or for the management of established heart disease, is somewhat controversial. Opinion is divided between total fat restriction and more liberal intake of n-3 PUFAs and MUFAs (53). The weight of evidence appears to be accumulating in support of the latter (54). The prehistoric human diet apparently provided approximately 20% to 25% of calories from fat, with about 5% from saturated and naturally occurring trans fat and the remainder a combination of MUFA and PUFA. The ratio of n-6 to n-3 PUFA, which is approximately 11:1 in the United States and western European diets, was between 4:1 and 1:1 for our ancestors (22). Until intervention studies further elucidate the optimally cardioprotective diet, recommendations consistent with both current evidence and evolutionary theory are appropriate. Saturated and trans fat should be restricted to below 7% of total calories in all cardiac patients and is appropriate primary prevention in willing patients. Intake of fish, nuts, soy, olives, avocados, seeds, olive oil, canola oil, and linseed oil should be encouraged to raise n-3 PUFA and MUFA intake. However, these items should substitute in the diet for other sources of fat to avoid raising total fat and/or calorie intake. The best available evidence indicates that average fat intake in the United States is now 34% of total calories (National Health and Nutrition Examination Survey III); therefore, a reduction in total fat intake appears indicated for virtually all patients. A reduced-fat diet will reduce serum lipid levels by up to 16% in half of hyperlipidemic patients; about 40% show a less than 10% decline in response to diet; and about 10% are unresponsive to diet. Dietary fat and cholesterol reduction is best achieved by restricting intake of red meats; deli meats; whole fat dairy products, especially cheese; cheese- and cream-based sauces and dressings; fatty spreads; and processed foods with more than trivial amounts of partially hydrogenated oils. Particular attention to detail is necessary to prevent substituting of lipid-raising fats from one source for fats from other sources.

Optimal management of dietary fat intake appears capable of lowering LDL by as much as 20% and total cholesterol by as much as 30%, although lesser reductions usually are seen. Although dietary manipulation produces benefits other than lipid lowering, more aggressive lipid lowering is indicated for virtually all hyperlipidemic patients with coronary disease. Statin drugs can lower LDL by up to 60%; the effects of these agents are enhanced by dietary therapy.

Fruit and Vegetable Intake

Whereas the nutrients responsible for the health-promoting properties of fruits and vegetables are a source of ongoing investigation and controversy, the cardioprotective influence of fruit and vegetable intake is decisive. Population-based studies consistently demonstrate health benefits of high fruit and vegetable intake (55). This dietary pattern is strongly associated with a reduced cancer risk as well (see Chapter 12). The constituents of produce contributing to a cardioprotective effect may include a variety of antioxidant micronutrients, essential micronutrients such as vitamins and minerals, and fiber, both soluble and insoluble. Cereal grains have been associated with a reduced risk of both cancer and cardiovascular disease (7,56–58). Establishing a causal relationship between specific food types and cardiovascular risk is confounded by the foods that are replaced; diets high in fruits, vegetables, and cereal products tend to be low in fat, and some of the apparent benefits may derive from fat restriction (59). The evidence for specific nutrient effects is less convincing than is evidence for the effect of a produce-rich dietary pattern.

The extreme expression of fruit and vegetable intake is a strict vegetarian diet. Although some vegetarians exclude meat, (lacto-ovo-vegetarians), vegans exclude all animal products, including dairy and eggs. The latter group may be at risk for certain micronutrient deficiencies, especially fat-soluble vitamins of the B group. The association between vitamin B deficiency and elevated levels of homocysteine raises concern that this dietary pattern might be associated with increased cardiovascular risk. To date, however, population-based studies suggest that vegetarianism is associated with less than average cardiovascular risk in developed countries. Strict vegetarians, for a variety of reasons, should become knowledgeable about dietary sources of both macronutrients and micronutrients of importance to ensure proper balance. A daily multivitamin is a prudent practice in this group.

Nutrients and Nutriceuticals

Antioxidants (Vitamins E and C, Carotenoids, and Flavonoids)

Evidence linking antioxidation to a reduced risk of cardiovascular disease is convincing; evidence in support of specific nutrients is generally not better than suggestive. This may be because antioxidants are most effective in as yet unidentified combinations, or because other nutrient-mediated reactions are equally important. The principal mechanism by which antioxidants confer cardiovascular benefit is thought to be inhibition of LDL oxidation (60,60a). A diet rich in fruits and vegetables typically provides abundant antioxidants, including carotenoids, tocopherols, flavonoids, and ascorbate, and has been decisively linked to reduced cardiac risk.

A variety of antioxidants have been studied for cardioprotective effects (61). The overall weight of evidence does not support a protective role for β-carotene, although observational studies suggest that foods rich in β-carotene are almost certainly protective (62,63). The literature to date is supportive of protective effects of bioflavonoids, found particularly in tea, red wine, and grape juice, as well as the skins of many fruits and vegetables (64–66). There currently is no convincing evidence of a cardioprotective effect of vitamin C, although diets naturally high in ascorbate appear to be protective (67,68). One potential explanation for the inability to elucidate an independent benefit of vitamin C is that its mechanism of action may require interaction with fat-soluble antioxidants (69). Timimi and colleagues (70) reported a beneficial effect of acute vitamin C infusion on endothelial function in diabetic subjects. Plotnick and colleagues (18) reported prevention of dietary fat-induced endothelial dysfunction with concomitant vitamin C and E supplementation in healthy subjects. Such findings tend to perpetuate interest in the potential cardioprotective role of vitamin C despite the paucity of clear evidence to date.

In the aggregate, evidence is strongest for a cardioprotective effect of vitamin E (71–76), although it is not definitive, and there is some contradictory evidence as well (77). Data from the Cambridge Heart Antioxidant Study suggest a benefit of supplemental vitamin E in the prevention of second MI, although evidence of a mortality benefit was not found (78). Beneficial effects of acute vitamin E supplementation on endothelial function have been reported (18).

However, in the GISSI-Prevenzione trial, patients with recent MI (n = 11,324) randomly assigned to vitamin E supplementation (300 mg) did no better than those assigned to placebo with regard to MI or death (35). Similarly, the HOPE trial demonstrated a significant benefit of angiotensin-converting enzyme inhibition with regard to both MI and death in high-risk coronary patients, whereas vitamin E (400 IU) failed to reveal such benefit (79,80). Thus, the most definitive trial to date fails to support a cardioprotective role of supplemental vitamin E, at least as an isolated intervention.

B Vitamins

Accumulating evidence points to the importance of elevations of serum homocysteine in up to one third of all patients with coronary artery disease (81). Hyperhomocysteinemia is particularly likely to occur in patients with coronary disease and normal serum lipids (82). Vitamins B_6 and B_{12}, and folate participate in the metabolism of methionine. Specific metabolic steps beyond the production of homocysteine are dependent on several B complex vitamins. Folate levels apparently are most likely to contribute to elevated homocysteine (83). There is some evidence that intake of B vitamins above levels currently recommended may offer protection against cardiovascular disease (84). Because B complex supplementation is unlikely to be harmful and the preliminary evidence of cardiovascular benefit is provocative, recommendations for multivitamin supplementation (or at least B complex supplementation) to all patients attempting to reduce their risk of heart disease are reasonable (85).

Coenzyme Q_{10}

Coenzyme Q_{10} is a benzoquinone, also known as ubiquinone because of its remarkably widespread distribution in nature. Minute quantities are found in virtually all plant-based foods. Coenzyme Q_{10} functions within the mitochondrion, where it facilitates electron transport and oxidative phosphorylation (86–88). Given the fundamental role of this coenzyme in energy metabolism, it is perhaps not surprising that its putative health effects are protean. An overview of the role of coenzyme Q_{10} is provided in Section IIIE.

With regard to cardiovascular disease, evidence is strongest for a beneficial role of coenzyme Q_{10} in heart failure and cardiomyopathy, where supplementation has been associated with improvement in left ventricular function, quality of life, and functional status (88,89). There is evidence of reduced complications post MI (90); improved hemodynamics post bypass grafting (91); and improved functional status and symptom relief in patients with angina (92). Coenzyme Q_{10} has been shown to have antihypertensive effects as well (93–95). Antioxidant effects of coenzyme Q_{10} apparently preserve levels of both ascorbate and α-tocopherol, enhancing both extracellular and intracellular antioxidant function (96,97). Finally, supplementation with coenzyme Q_{10} appears to reduce levels of lipoprotein (a) (98) and preserve serum levels depleted by statin therapy (99).

In the aggregate, evidence supporting a role for coenzyme Q_{10} in the amelioration of cardiovascular disease and the modification of risk factors is convincing. Large-scale trials are absent from the literature, but this may be due to the nonproprietary nature of the compound and the inability of an industry sponsor of such trials to generate correspondingly large profits as a result. More widespread use of coenzyme Q_{10} in cardiology and primary care practice appears to warrant serious consideration. The usual doses in trials range from 100 to 300 mg per day, dosed b.i.d. Such doses appear safe, with virtually no reports of significant toxicity.

Alcohol

Epidemiologic evidence, both among and within populations, links moderate alcohol consumption to a reduced risk of cardiovas-

cular disease (100,101). Observational data in the United States suggest a reduction in relative risk for angina or MI of as much as 30% in those consuming one drink per day compared to those who abstain (102). Results of a recently (1999) reported observational cohort study in France suggest that moderate alcohol consumption reduces all-cause mortality (103); evidence of benefit was stronger and more consistent for wine than beer. Although there is general consensus that ethanol is partly responsible for the cardioprotective effects of alcoholic beverages, red wine may confer additional benefit due to the polyphenolic compounds in the skin of the grape. A recent (2000) small study demonstrated enhanced endothelial function following consumption of dealcoholized red wine, with no improvement following consumption of an equivalent amount of red wine with alcohol (104). Mechanisms by which alcohol may attenuate cardiovascular risk include elevation of high-density lipoprotein, elevation of tissue plasminogen activator, and inhibition of platelet aggregation. At doses above 30 to 45 g per day, alcohol raises blood pressure and is associated with increased cardiac risk, as well as increased risk of other morbidity and mortality. Consumption of one to at most two drinks per day, preferably red wine, is reasonable with regard to cardiovascular risk reduction. Whether or not the practice should be advocated to a particular patient is dependent on other considerations. Despite the generally consistent evidence of cardiovascular benefit with moderate alcohol consumption, concern regarding the adverse effects of heavier drinking generally mitigates enthusiasm for recommending alcohol consumption for health promotion (105,106).

Iron

Iron may act as a prooxidant, generating speculation that it might contribute to the risk of cardiac disease in men, and that its depletion in menstruating women might contribute to risk reduction. Epidemiologic evidence supports a potential role for high iron levels in cardiovascular disease risk, but the evidence to date is inconclusive (107).

Magnesium

Serum magnesium concentrations have been found to be inversely associated with cardiovascular disease risk (108). However, serum levels may merely be a measure of overall dietary pattern, including intake of fruits and vegetables. Magnesium is known to have antiarrhythmic properties and has corresponding therapeutic applications beyond the scope of this discussion. Any beneficial effects of magnesium on cardiovascular disease risk may be mediated by its association with reduced blood pressure (see Chapter 7). Magnesium is discussed further in Section IIIE.

Calcium and Potassium

Cardiovascular benefit of calcium and potassium is associated with blood pressure-lowering effects, discussed in Chapter 7 (see also Chapter 4 and Section IIIE).

Other

Interest is intense in the development of nutriceutical agents with cardioprotective effect. Among compounds of current interest is Chinese red yeast, which has lipid-lowering effects (109), the antioxidant pycnogenol (110), and the herb hawthorne, also thought to have antioxidant properties. Many other compounds and nutrients have received attention in the lay media. Evidence is insufficient to recommend clinical applications of most such compounds at present. Resources for remaining abreast of evolving options in the nutriceutical management of cardiac risk factors are discussed in Section III.

The pace of developments in this area is so rapid that no print text can be fully current.

CLINICAL HIGHLIGHTS

Data and opinions pertaining to the nutritional mitigation of cardiovascular risk are scattered throughout a staggeringly vast literature. Within this body of work is room for diverging opinions, both on the basis of data and the current absence thereof. Nonetheless, diverse lines of research and observation are converging on a discrete set of dietary recommendations.

The typical American diet suffers from both excesses and deficiencies relative to the ideal diet for cardiovascular health. Although total fat intake is often excessive, maldistribution of fat calories may be at least as important. A total fat intake below 30% of calories is appropriate. The combination of saturated and trans fat should be restricted to below 10% of calories at least and to below 5% for purposes of secondary and tertiary prevention. The absence of data regarding trans fat on nutrition labels requires diligent patient education. The remaining 20% to 25% of calories derived from fat should be more or less equally divided between polyunsaturated and monounsaturated fat. Polyunsaturated fat should be divided between n-6 and n-3 fatty acids in a ratio between 4:1 and 1:1 rather than the prevailing ratio of 11:1 (n-6:n-3). In patients consuming relatively little fish, consistent use of flaxseed oil may be recommended to supplement n-3 fat (α-linolenic acid). Some controversy persists as to the relative health benefits of short-chain versus long-chain n-3 fatty acid consumption (see Chapters 2 and 4 and Section IIIE). The importance of supplementing n-3 fatty acids may be even greater in patients with established coronary disease.

Benefits of dietary fiber are well established, and prevailing intake is deficient. A daily intake of at least 30 g of fiber is appropriate and is readily achievable if whole grains, vegetables, and fruits are the principal sources of food energy. This dietary pattern will similarly serve to raise intake of diverse micronutrients, including antioxidants. The benefits of specific micronutrients are suggested, while the health advantages, and specific cardiovascular benefits, of generous intake of plant foods are conclusively established. Incipient micronutrient deficiencies are readily prevented by daily supplementation with a multivitamin/mineral tablet, a practice that may be generally recommended provided it is recognized as complementary rather than alternative to a balanced diet. Supplementation with vitamin C (up to 500 mg per day) and vitamin E (up to 800 IU per day) is consistent with available evidence and appears likely to be both safe and potentially beneficial, but is not supported by definitive evidence. Data are least available to support this practice in primary prevention. The most recent, and most definitive, trial data argue against a benefit of vitamin E supplementation, but these data fail to address the potential importance of combining lipid- and water-soluble antioxidants. Arguments for a variety of other micronutrients and nutriceuticals can be made with available evidence; many of these are discussed elsewhere in the text (see, in particular, the Nutrient Reference Tables in Section IIIE).

Barring alcohol-related health problems or contraindications such as liver disease, moderate alcohol consumption (30 to 45 g per day) appears to confer cardiovascular benefit the lower end of this range is more appropriate for women. Restriction of cholesterol to less than 300 mg per day appears justified, although its importance when fat intake is optimized is uncertain. Restriction of dietary sodium to 3 g per day is of variable importance, but appropriate. Maintenance of near-optimal weight by moderating total energy intake is of clear cardiovascular benefit.

In general, most dietary recommendations for the primary prevention of cardiovascular disease in adults appear to be safe and appropriate for children over the age of 2 years (111,112) (see Chapter 27). Application of a heart-healthy dietary pattern is appropriate for primary, secondary, and tertiary prevention of heart disease. This pattern is consistent with prevailing and emerging recommendations for health promotion in general (see Chapter 40) and can be expected to confer noncardiovascular health benefits as well. Of note, the American Medical Association has estimated that a diet low in total and saturated fat costs on average $230 *less* per year than the typical American diet.

REFERENCES

1. McCarron D, Oparil S, Chait A, et al. Nutritional Management of cardiovascular risk factors. *Arch Intern Med* 1997;157:169–177.
2. Ornish D, Brown S, Scherwitz L. Can lifestyle changes reverse coronary heart disease? The lifestyle heart trial. *Lancet* 1990;336:129–133.
3. Temple N. Dietary fats and coronary heart disease. *Biomed Pharmacother* 1996;50:261–268.
4. Keys A, Aravanis C, Blackburn H, et al. Epidemiological studies related to coronary heart disease: characteristics of men aged 40–59 in seven countries. *Acta Med Scand Suppl* 1966:460:1–392.
5. Ascherio A, Willett W. New directions in dietary studies of coronary heart disease. *J Nutr* 1995; 125:647S–655S.
6. Oliver M. It is more important to increase the intake of unsaturated fats than to decrease the intake of saturated fats: evidence from clinical trials relating to ischemic heart disease. *Am J Clin Nutr* 1997:980S–986S.
7. Rimm EB AA, Giovannucci E, Speigelman D, et al. Vegetable, fruit, and cereal fiber intake and risk of coronary heart disease among men. *JAMA* 1996;275:447–451.
8. Hunninghake D, Miller V, LaRosa J, et al. Long-term treatment of hypercholesterolemia with dietary fiber. *Am J Med* 1994;97:504–508.
9. Wynder E, Stellman S, Zang E. High fiber intake. Indicator of a healthy lifestyle. *JAMA* 1996;275: 486–487.
10. Simoes E, Byers T, Coates R, et al. The association between leisure-time physical activity and dietary fat in American adults. *Am J Public Health* 1995; 85:240–244.
11. Anderson K, Castelli W, Levy D. Cholesterol and mortality: 30 years of follow-up from the Framingham Study. *JAMA* 1987;257:2176–2180.
12. Krauss R, Deckelbaum R, Ernst N, et al. Dietary guidelines for healthy American adults. *Circulation* 1996;94:1795–1800.
13. Koop C. *The Surgeon General's report on nutrition and health.* Washington, DC: Department of Health and Human Services, 1988.
14. Goldstein J, Brown M. The LDL receptor and the regulation of cellular cholesterol metabolism. *J Cell Sci Suppl* 1985;3:131–137.
15. Goldstein J, Brown M. Regulation of low-density lipoprotein receptors: implications for pathogenesis and therapy of hypercholesterolemia and atherosclerosis. *Circulation* 1987;76:504–507.
16. Gesquiere L, Loreau N, Minnich A, et al. Oxidative stress leads to cholesterol accumulation in vascular

smooth muscle cells. *Free Radic Biol Med* 1999; 27:134–145.

17. Stein O, Stein Y. Smooth muscle cells and atherosclerosis. *Curr Opin Lipidol* 1995;6:269–274.

18. Plotnick GD, Corrett M, Vogel RA. Effect of antioxidant vitamins on the transient impairment of endothelium-dependent brachial artery vasoactivity following a single high-fat meal. *JAMA* 1997;278:1682–1686.

19. Zilversmit D. Atherogenesis: a postprandial phenomenon. *Circulation* 1979;60:473–485.

20. Lefebvre P, Scheen A. The postprandial state and risk of cardiovascular disease. *Diabetes Med* 1998; 15:S63–S68.

21. Williams M, Sutherland W, McCormick M, et al. Impaired endothelial function following a meal rich in used cooking fat. *J Am Coll Cardiol* 1999; 33:1050–1055.

22. Eaton S, Konner M. Paleolithic nutrition revisited: A twelve-year retrospective on its nature and implications. *Eur J Clin Nutr* 1997;51:207–216.

23. Drewnowski A. Taste preferences and food intake. *Annu Rev Nutr* 1997;17:237–253.

24. Drewnowski A, Schwartz M. Invisible fats: sensory assessment of sugar/fat mixtures. *Appetite* 1990; 14:203–217.

25. Hu F, Stampfer M, Rimm E, et al. A prospective study of egg consumption and risk of cardiovascular disease in men and women. *JAMA* 1999; 281:1387–1394.

26. Temple N, Ascherio A, Willett W. New directions in dietary studies of coronary heart disease. *J Nutr* 1995;125:647s–655s.

27. Leaf A, Kang J, Xiao Y, et al., GISSI-Prevenzione Investigators. Dietary n-3 fatty acids in the prevention of cardiac arrhythmias. *Curr Opin Clin Nutr Metab Care* 1998;1:225–228.

28. Horrocks L, Yeo Y. Health benefits of docosahexaenoic acid. *Pharmacol Res* 1999;40:211–225.

29. Simopoulos A. Essential fatty acids in health and chronic disease. *Am J Clin Nutr* 1999;70:560S–569S.

30. Marckmann P, Gronbaek M. Fish consumption and coronary heart disease mortality. A systematic review of prospective cohort studies. *Eur J Clin Nutr* 1999;53:585–590.

31. Katan M, Grundy S, Willett W. Should a low-fat, high-carbohydrate diet be recommended for everyone? Beyond low-fat diets. *N Engl J Med* 1997;337:563–566.

32. Grundy S. What is the desirable ratio of saturated, polyunsaturated, and monounsaturated fatty acids in the diet? *Am J Clin Nutr* 1997;66:988S–990S.

33. Grundy S. Second International Conference on Fats and Oil Consumption in Health and Disease: how we can optimize dietary composition to combat metabolic complications and decrease obesity. Overview. *Am J Clin Nutr* 1998;67:497S–499S.

34. Grundy S. The optimal ratio of fat-to-carbohydrate in the diet. *Annu Rev Nutr* 1999;19:325–341.

35. Investigators G-P. Dietary supplementation with n-3 polyunsaturated fatty acids and vitamin E after myocardial infarction: results of the GISSI-Prevenzione trial. *Lancet* 1999;354:447–455.

36. Connor W, Connor S. Should a low-fat, high-carbohydrate diet be recommended for everyone? The

37. Kennedy E, Bowman S, Powell R. Dietary-fat intake in the US population. *J Am Coll Nutr* 1999; 18:207–212.

38. Ernst N, Sempos C, Briefel R, et al. Consistency between US dietary fat intake and serum total cholesterol concentrations: the National Health and Nutrition Examination Surveys. *Am J Clin Nutr* 1997;66:965s–972s.

39. Lorgeril MD. Mediterranean diet in the prevention of coronary heart disease. *Nutrition* 1998;14:55–57.

40. Thomsen C, Rasmussen O, Christiansen C, et al. Comparison of the effects of a monounsaturated fat diet and a high carbohydrate diet on cardiovascular risk factors in first degree relatives to type-2 diabetic subjects. *Eur J Clin Nutr* 1999;53:818–823.

41. Kris-Etherton P, Pearson T, Wan Y, et al. High-monounsaturated fatty acid diets lower both plasma cholesterol and triacylglycerol concentrations. *Am J Clin Nutr* 1999;70:1009–1115.

42. Kris-Etherton P. AHA science advisory: monounsaturated fatty acids and risk of cardiovascular disease. *J Nutr* 1999;129:2280–2284.

43. Tsimikas S, Reaven P. The role of dietary fatty acids in lipoprotein oxidation and atherosclerosis. *Curr Opin Lipidol* 1998;9:301–307.

44. Criqui M, Ringel B. Does diet or alcohol explain the French paradox? *Lancet* 1994;344:1719–1723.

45. Singh R, Rastogi S, Verma R, et al. Randomized controlled trial of cardioprotective diet in patients with recent acute myocardial infarction: results of one year follow up. *BMJ* 1992;304:1015–1019.

46. Garg A, Bonamome A, Grundy S, et al. Comparison of a high-carbohydrate diet with a high-monounsaturated-fat diet in patients with non-insulin-dependent diabetes mellitus. *N Engl J Med* 1988; 319:829–843.

47. Garg A, Bantle J, Henry R, et al. Effects of varying carbohydrate content of diet in patients with non-insulin-dependent diabetes mellitus. *JAMA* 1994;271:1421–1428.

48. Grundy S. Hypertriglyceridemia, insulin resistance, and the metabolic syndrome. *Am J Cardiol* 1999;83:25F–29F.

49. Reaven G, Lithell H, Landsberg L. Hypertension and associated metabolic abnormalities—the role of insulin resistance and the sympathoadrenal system. *N Engl J Med* 1996;334:374–381.

50. Lorgeril MD, Salen P, Monjaud I, et al. The "diet heart" hypothesis in secondary prevention of coronary heart disease. *Eur Heart J* 1997;18:13–18.

51. Lorgeril MD, Salen P. What makes a Mediterranean diet cardioprotective? *Cardiol Rev* 1997;14: 15–21.

52. Lorgeril MD, Salen P, Martin J-L, et al. Effect of a Mediterranean type of diet on the rate of cardiovascular complications in patients with coronary artery disease. *J Am Coll Cardiol* 1996; 28:1103–1108.

53. Katan M. High-oil compared with low-fat, high-carbohydrate diets in the prevention of ischemic heart disease. *Am J Clin Nutr* 1997;66[Suppl]:974s–979s.

54. Siscovick D, Raghunathan T, King I, et al. Dietary intake and cell membrane levels of long-chain n-3

polyunsaturated fatty acids and the risk of primary cardiac arrest. *JAMA* 1995;274:1363–1367.

55. Fraser G. Associations between diet and cancer, ischemic heart disease, and all-cause mortality in non-Hispanic white California Seventh-day Adventists. *Am J Clin Nutr* 1999;70:532S–538S.

56. Liu S, Stampfer M, Hu F, et al. Whole-grain consumption and risk of coronary heart disease: results from the Nurses' Health Study. *Am J Clin Nutr* 1999;70:412–419.

57. Slavin J, Martini M, Jacobs DJ, et al. Plausible mechanisms for the protectiveness of whole grains. *Am J Clin Nutr* 1999;70:459S–463S.

58. Kushi L, Meyer K, Jacobs DJ. Cereals, legumes, and chronic disease risk reduction: evidence from epidemiologic studies. *Am J Clin Nutr* 1999;70: 451S–458S.

59. Willett W. Convergence of philosophy and science: the Third International Congress on Vegetarian Nutrition. *Am J Clin Nutr* 1999;70:434S–438S.

60. Chopra M, Thurnham D. Antioxidants and lipoprotein metabolism. *Proc Nutr Soc* 1999;58:663–671:171–180.

60a. Jacob RA, Burri BJ. Oxidative damage and defense. *Am J Clin Nutr* 1996;63:s985–s990.

61. Buring J, Gaziano J. Antioxidant vitamins and cardiovascular disease. In: Bendich A, Deckelbaum RJ, eds. *Preventive nutrition: the comprehensive guide for health professionals.* Totowa, NJ: Humana Press, Inc., 1997:171–180.

62. Tavani A, Vecchia CL. Beta-carotene and risk of coronary heart disease. A review of observational and intervention studies. *Biomed Pharmacother* 1999;53:409–416.

63. Kritchevsky S. Beta-carotene, carotenoids and the prevention of coronary heart disease. *J Nutr* 1999; 129:5–8.

64. Kromhout D. Fatty acids, antioxidants, and coronary heart disease from an epidemiological perspective. *Lipids* 1999;34[Suppl]:s27–s31.

65. Lairon D, Amiot M. Flavonoids in food and natural antioxidants in wine. *Curr Opin Lipidol* 1999;10: 23–28.

66. Vinson J. Flavonoids in foods as *in vitro* and *in vivo* antioxidants. *Adv Exp Med Biol* 1998;439:151–164.

67. Gaziano J, Manson J. Diet and heart disease. The role of fat, alcohol, and antioxidants. *Cardiol Clin North Am* 1996;14:69–83.

68. Hensrud D, Heimburger D. Antioxidant status, fatty acids, and cardiovascular disease. *Nutrition* 1994;10:170–175.

69. Beyer R, Ness A, Powles J, et al. Vitamin C and cardiovascular disease: a systematic review. *J Cardiovasc Risk* 1996;3:513–521.

70. Timimi F, Ting H, Haley E, et al. Vitamin C improves endothelium-dependent vasodilation in patients with insulin-dependent diabetes mellitus. *J Am Coll Cardiol* 1998;31:552–557.

71. Diaz M, Frei B, Vita J, et al. Antioxidants and atherosclerotic heart disease. *N Engl J Med* 1997; 337:408–416.

72. Jha P, Flather M, Lonn E, et al. The antioxidant vitamins and cardiovascular disease. A critical review of epidemiologic and clinical trial data. *Ann Intern Med* 1995;123:860–872.

73. Hodis H, Mack W, LaBree L, et al. Serial coronary angiographic evidence that antioxidant vitamin intake reduces progression of coronary artery atherosclerosis. *JAMA* 1995;273:1849–1854.

74. Rimm E, Stampfer M. The role of antioxidants in preventive cardiology. *Curr Opin Cardiol* 1997; 12:188–194.

75. Gaziano J. Antioxidants in cardiovascular disease: randomized trials. *Nutrition* 1996;12:583–588.

76. Rexrode K, Manson J. Antioxidants and coronary heart disease: observational studies. *J Cardiovasc Risk* 1996;3:363–367.

77. Virtamo J, Rapola J, Rippatti S, et al., GISSI-Prevenzione Investigators. Effect of vitamin E and beta carotene on the incidence of primary nonfatal myocardial infarction and fatal coronary heart disease. *Arch Intern Med* 1998;158:668–675.

78. Stephens N, Parsons A, Schofield P, et al. Randomized controlled trial of vitamin E in patients with coronary disease: Cambridge Heart Antioxidant Study. *Lancet* 1996;347:781–786.

79. The Heart Outcomes Prevention Evaluation Study Investigators. Effects of an angiotensin-converting-enzyme inhibitor, ramipril, on cardiovascular events in high-risk patients. *N Engl J Med* 2000;342:145–153.

80. The Heart Outcomes Prevention Evaluation Study Investigators. Vitamin E supplementation and cardiovascular events in high-risk patients. *N Engl J Med* 2000;342:154–160.

81. Nygard O, Vollset S, Refsum H, et al. Total plasma homocysteine and cardiovascular risk profile. The Hordaland Homocysteine Study. *JAMA* 1995; 274:1526–1533.

82. Mittynen L, Nurminen M, Korpela R, et al. Role of arginine, taurine and homocysteine in cardiovascular diseases. *Ann Med* 1999;31:318–326.

83. Verhoef P, Stampfer M, Buring J, et al. Homocysteine metabolism and risk of myocardial infarction: relation with vitamins B_6, B_{12}, and folate. *Am J Epidemiol* 1996;143:845–859.

84. Rimm E, Willett W, Hu F, et al. Folate and vitamin B6 from diet and supplements in relation to risk of coronary heart disease among women. *JAMA* 1998;279:359–364.

85. Stampfer M, Malinow M. Can lowering homocysteine levels reduce cardiovascular risk? *N Engl J Med* 1995;332:328–329.

86. Rauchova H, Drahota Z, Lenaz G. Function of coenzyme Q in the cell: some biochemical and physiological properties. *Physiol Res* 1995;44: 209–216.

87. Crane F, Sun I, Sun E. The essential functions of coenzyme Q. *Clin Investig* 1993;71:s55–s59.

88. Baggio E, Gandini R, Plancher A, et al. Italian multicenter study on the safety and efficacy of coenzyme Q_{10} as adjunctive therapy in heart failure. *Mol Aspects Med* 1994;15:s287–s294.

89. Langsjoen H, Langsjoen P, Willis R, et al. Usefulness of coenzyme Q_{10} in clinical cardiology: a long-term study. *Mol Aspects Med* 1994;15:s165–s175.

90. Singh R, Wander G, Rastogi A, et al. Randomized, double-blind placebo-controlled trial of coenzyme Q_{10} in patients with acute myocardial infarction. *Cardiovasc Drugs Ther* 1998;12:347–353.

91. Chello M, Mastroroberto P, Romano R, et al. Pro-

tection by coenzyme Q_{10} from myocardial reperfusion injury during coronary artery bypass grafting. *Ann Thorac Surg* 1994;58:1427–1432.

92. Kamikawa T, Kobayashi A, Yamashita T, et al. Effects of coenzyme Q_{10} on exercise tolerance in chronic stable angina pectoris. *Am J Cardiol* 1985; 56:247–251.

93. Langsjoen P, Willis R, Folkers K. Treatment of essential hypertension with coenzyme Q_{10}. *Mol Aspects Med* 1994;15:S265–S272.

94. Singh R, Niaz M, Rastogi S, et al. Effect of hydrosoluble coenzyme Q_{10} on blood pressures and insulin resistance in hypertensive patients with coronary artery disease. *J Human Hypertens* 1999;13: 203–208.

95. Digiesi V, Cantini F, Oradei A, et al. Coenzyme Q_{10} in essential hypertension. *Mol Aspects Med* 1994;15:S257–S262.

96. Thomas S, Neuzil J, Stocker R. Inhibition of LDL oxidation by ubiquinol-10. A protective mechanism for coenzyme Q in atherogenesis? *Mol Aspects Med* 1997;18:S85–S103.

97. Niki E. Mechanisms and dynamics of antioxidant action of ubiquinol. *Mol Aspects Med* 1997;18: S63–S70.

98. Singh R, Niaz M. Serum concentration of lipoprotein(a) decreases on treatment with hydrosoluble coenzyme Q_{10} in patients with coronary artery disease: discovery of a new role. *Int J Cardiol* 1999;68:23–29.

99. Bargossi A, Grossi G, Fiorella P, et al. Exogenous CoQ_{10} supplementation prevents plasma ubiquinone reduction induced by HMG-CoA reductase inhibitors. *Mol Aspects Med* 1994;15:S187–S193.

100. Flegal K, Cauley J. Alcohol consumption and cardiovascular risk factors. *Recent Dev Alcohol* 1985; 3:165–180.

101. Zakhari S, Gordis E. Moderate drinking and cardiovascular health. *Proc Assoc Am Physicians* 1999;111:148–158.

102. Camargo C, Stampfer M, Glynn R, et al. Moderate alcohol consumption and risk for angina pectoris or myocardial infarction in US male physicians. *Ann Intern Med* 1997;126:372–375.

103. Renaud S, Gueguen R, Siest G, et al. Wine, beer, and mortality in middle-aged men from eastern France. *Arch Intern Med* 1999;159:1865–1870.

104. Agewall S, Wright S, Doughty R, et al. Does a glass of red wine improve endothelial function? *Eur Heart J* 2000;21:74–78.

105. Criqui M. Alcohol and coronary heart disease: consistent relationship and public health implications. *Clin Chim Acta* 1996;246:51–57.

106. Kannell W, Ellison R. Alcohol and coronary heart disease: the evidence for a protective effect. *Clin Chim Acta* 1996;246:59–76.

107. Valk BD, Marx J. Iron, atherosclerosis, and ischemic heart disease. *Arch Intern Med* 1999;159: 1542–1548.

108. Ford E. Serum magnesium and ischaemic heart disease: findings from a national sample of US adults. *Int J Epidemiol* 1999;28:645–651.

109. Heber D, Yip I, Ashley J, et al. Cholesterol-lowering effects of a proprietary Chinese red-yeast-rice dietary supplement. *Am J Clin Nutr* 1999; 69:231–236.

110. Fitzpatrick D, Bing B, Rohdewald P. Endothelium-dependent vascular effects of Pycnogenol. *J Cardiovasc Pharmacol* 1998;32:509–515.

111. Lapinleimu H, Viikari J, Jokinen J, et al. Prospective randomized trial in 1062 infants of diet low in saturated fat and cholesterol. *Lancet* 1995;345: 471–476.

112. Writing Group for the DISC collaborative research group. Efficacy and safety of lowering dietary intake of fat and cholesterol in children with elevated low-density lipoprotein cholesterol. The Dietary Intervention Study in Children (DISC). *JAMA* 1995;273:1429–1435.

BIBLIOGRAPHY

See "Sources for All Chapters."

Denke MA. Cholesterol-lowering diets. *Arch Intern Med* 1995;155:17–26.

Dwyer J. Overview: Dietary approaches for reducing cardiovascular disease risks. *J Nutr* 1995;125:656s–665s.

Esrey KL, Joseph L, Grover Sa. Relationship between dietary intake and coronary heart disease mortality: lipid research clinics prevalence follow-up study. *J Clin Epidemiol* 1996;49:211–216.

Gaziano JM, Manson JE. Diet and heart disease. The role of fat, alcohol, and antioxidants. *Cardiology Clin North Am* 1996;14:69–83.

Goldman L, Cook EF. The decline in ischemic heart disease mortality rates. *Annals Int Med* 1984;101: 825–836.

Hensrud DD, Heimburger DC. Antioxidant status, fatty acids, and cardiovascular disease. *Nutrition* 1994;10: 170–175.

Hollman PC, Katan MB. Bioavailability and health effects of dietary falvonols in man. *Arch Toxicol Suppl* 1998;20:237–248.

Jenkins DJA. Optimal diet for reducing the risk of arteriosclerosis. *Can J Cardiol* 1995;11(suppl G):118g–122g.

Kromhout D, Bosschieter EB, Coulander C. The inverse relation between fish consumption and 20-year mortality from coronary heart disease. *N Engl J Med* 1985; 312:1205–1209.

McNamara DJ. Dietary cholesterol and the optimal diet for reducing risk of atherosclerosis. *Clin J Cardiol* 1995;11:123g–126g.

Menotti A. Diet, cholesterol and coronary heart disease. A perspective. *Acta Cardiol* 1999;54:169–172.

Meydani M. Vitamin E. *Lancet* 1995;345:170–175.

Stone NJ, Nicolosi RJ, Kris-Etherton P, Ernst ND, Krauss RM, Winston M. Summary of the scientific conference on the efficacy of hypocholesterolemic dietary interventions. *Circulation* 1996;94:3388–3391.

Tribble DL. AHA Science Advisory. Antioxidant consumption and risk of coronary artery disease: emphasis on vitamin C, vitamin E, and beta-carotene: A statement for healthcare professionals from the American Heart Association. *Circulation* 1999; 99:591–595.

7

Diet and Hypertension

There has long been epidemiologic evidence of variations in blood pressure among diverse populations. Although some of this effect has been attributed to dietary factors, demonstrating causality has been precluded by the multitude of potentially confounding variables. Interest in the role of dietary sodium in the etiology of hypertension has been particularly intense, but the best available evidence suggests that sodium may play a causal role in only a minority of cases of primary, or essential, hypertension. However, data from multiple sources, including the INTERSALT trial, suggest that high intakes of sodium may be shifting population blood pressures means upward (1). There is decisive evidence that dietary interventions are effective in modifying blood pressure. With good patient compliance, diet at times may substitute for pharmacologic management of hypertension. Additionally, there is decisive evidence that weight management often is effective in reducing blood pressure in obese patients. There is suggestive evidence that a variety of micronutrients may modify blood pressure.

OVERVIEW

Diet

Hypertension is unusually prevalent in the United States, with approximately 50 million cases in a population of 265 million. Evidence linking hypertension to diet has been derived in part from transcultural comparisons, demonstrating higher rates of hypertension in the industrialized world. To com-

pensate for the plethora of confounding variables intrinsic to such transcultural comparisons, migration studies have been conducted. Hypertension, like hyperlipidemia, is more prevalent in Asians living in the United States than in their non-emigrating counterparts (2). Similar effects of migration have been reported in other populations (3). Similarly, whereas African-Americans have particularly high rates of hypertension, the rate is low among native Africans living in rural settings and intermediate in Africans exposed to some aspects of the Western lifestyle (4). Among populations in the United States, hypertension is less common among the lean than the overweight, and among vegetarians than among the general population (5). Isolating the direct effects of diet on blood pressure is difficult due to the prevalence of obesity in the United States and the strong association between obesity and hypertension (see Chapters 5 and 10). From a practical perspective, however, patients benefit comparably from dietary interventions that lower blood pressure directly, or indirectly as a result of weight loss. There is decisive evidence that weight loss among obese hypertensives frequently results in blood pressure reduction (6). Even modest weight loss may lower blood pressure in patients who do not reach or even approximate their ideal body weight (6).

In general, diets associated with optimal blood pressure control are similar to diets associated with a variety of other salutary health effects (see Chapter 40). Vegetarianism is associated with lower average blood pressure (see Chapter 37), as is the Mediterranean diet and the low-fat diet typical of the nonindustrialized Far East (5). The association between dietary pattern and blood pressure was confirmed by the results of the DASH study (7), which demonstrated that strict adherence to a diet high in fruit and vegetables, and restricted in total fat, effectively lowered blood pressure among randomized, hypertensive subjects. The DASH diet is apparently particularly beneficial in African-Americans (8). The DISC study suggests that the relationship between diet and blood pressure in children is similar to that in adults (9).

As is the case for the prevention and modification of other cardiovascular risk factors, the optimal diet for management of incipient and established hypertension is not known with certainty. Other avenues of research suggest that restricting total fat may be less beneficial than selectively restricting saturated and trans fat, while liberalizing the intake of monounsaturated fat and particularly n-3 polyunsaturates (10,11). Recommendations for calorie control, abundant intake of fruits and vegetables, and restriction of saturated and trans fat intake may be made with confidence. Of note, such a diet is naturally rich in the micronutrients associated with blood pressure lowering, relatively rich in fiber, and relatively low in sodium. Which of these modifications in dietary behavior is responsible for blood pressure control is important to advance our understanding, but unnecessary to make recommendations likely to benefit patients.

Although stage 1 hypertension has been effectively treated with diet in studies, two caveats should be noted. First, the compliance in a controlled trial is generally greater than is achieved in practice (12). Second, more advanced hypertension has not been shown to respond to dietary management in the absence of pharmacotherapy. One suitable approach in efforts at managing more significant hypertension with lifestyle modification is to initiate pharmacotherapy as indicated, and then taper medications once the blood pressure is well controlled and evidence accrues that the patient is engaged in recommended dietary and lifestyle modifications.

Nutrients and Nutriceuticals

Sodium

Sodium is almost certainly the most extensively studied nutrient influencing blood pressure. Evidence from a variety of sources, including epidemiologic studies as well as intervention trials, suggests that sodium does contribute to blood pressure elevations on a population and individual basis (13,14). Such a conclusion is supported by results of the INTERSALT study, which examined the association between sodium intake and blood pressure in multiple cohorts around the globe (1). Although there is decisive evidence that sodium contributes to blood pressure elevation, the causal role of sodium in hypertension is less well established. Studies suggest that only 10% of hypertensives in the United States are responsive to sodium, demonstrating blood pressure variation with change in sodium intake (15). The efficacy of sodium restriction in the management of hypertension is difficult to demonstrate because it is difficult to achieve patient compliance with low-sodium diets (16), and because such diets almost inevitably introduce other changes as well. Cook and colleagues (17) suggested that the effect of salt restriction on blood pressure has been consistently underestimated.

Despite the uncertainties, recommendations for sodium restriction below prevailing levels in the United States can be made with considerable confidence. Intake in the United States generally exceeds the recommended limit of 3,000 mg per day. Ancestral intake, which may indicate optimal levels, was approximately 700 to 800 mg per day, less than one fourth the average intake today (18). Advocacy of a health-promoting diet will result in sodium restriction by reducing the intake of fast and highly processed foods. Patients should be advised of the importance in reading food labels. The sodium content of many commercial breakfast cereals is comparable to potato chips and pretzels, although the taste of salt in such products is masked by the sugar. In attempting to limit sodium intake, many patients will report not using a salt shaker. However, the salt added to food during preparation is less readily tasted than the salt shaken on just as the food is eaten. Therefore, preparation of low-salt foods and continued, albeit controlled, use of a salt shaker may be a preferred approach. As with other dietary changes, salt restriction becomes less objectionable as it becomes familiar. Whereas the salt content of many processed foods goes unnoticed by most consumers, those acclimated to a lower-sodium diet begin to taste salt more readily and to prefer lower intake levels (19,20). Acclimation to a high-salt diet has the opposite effect (21). So-called "salt substitutes," which replace some of the sodium with potassium or calcium, may serve as a useful aid to patients struggling to acclimate to a salt-restricted diet. However, there is some evidence suggesting that the preferences for dietary salt may vary with factors other than taste perception (22,23).

Potassium

Diets rich in potassium tend to be relatively low in sodium, and vice versa, making the study of isolated dietary potassium difficult. Nonetheless, there is convincing evidence that potassium supplementation has a blood pressure-lowering effect (24). The evidence is decisive that total dietary modification that results in increased potassium intake, and particularly a potassium intake that exceeds sodium intake, lowers blood pressure (7). The average intake of sodium in the United States is approximately 4,000 mg per day, while average daily intake of potassium is approximately 2,500 to 3,400 mg (18). Our prehistoric ancestors are estimated to have consumed approximately 750 to 800 mg per day of sodium and nearly 10,500 mg of potassium (18). As potassium is abundant in a variety of fruits and vegetables, high intake of potassium generally is associated with other dietary changes that may in-

dependently lower blood pressure. In the INTERSALT study, blood pressure rose with age in all populations consuming more sodium than potassium, but not in those consuming more potassium than sodium (1).

Calcium

There is suggestive evidence that high dietary calcium intake contributes to lowering of blood pressure. In the DASH trial, calcium is considered a potentially important mediator of the hypotensive effects of nonfat dairy products (7). A recent (1999) meta-analysis suggests that calcium, either in the diet or as a supplement, has a modest antihypertensive effect (25). However, on the basis of an extensive literature review, the Canadian Hypertension Society has advised against calcium supplementation as a means of either treating or preventing hypertension (26). The isolated effects of calcium supplementation on blood pressure appear to be modest; a dietary pattern providing abundant calcium may be of greater benefit. A particular benefit of calcium in the management and prevention of pregnancy-induced hypertension has been suggested (27). In the aggregate, evidence supports a hypotensive benefit of calcium intake at levels advisable on other grounds (28).

Magnesium

Diets rich in potassium tend to be rich in magnesium, and vice versa (see Chapter 4). Magnesium supplementation may be beneficial in the treatment of hypertension in magnesium-deficient patients, but evidence of treatment benefit is inconclusive (26). Evidence of modest treatment benefit has been reported (29). Although magnesium supplementation is not advocated for the control of hypertension in the United States, a dietary pattern providing abundant magnesium is (30).

Fiber

A potential benefit of dietary fiber in the regulation of blood pressure has been reported both in adults (31,32) and in children (9). However, the isolated effects of dietary fiber on blood pressure remain uncertain (14), as the data available to date are largely from observational studies, and the dietary pattern associated with lowering of blood pressure is naturally high in both soluble and insoluble fiber.

Alcohol

Alcohol contributes to blood pressure elevations when intake exceeds 30 to 45 g of ethanol daily and may contribute at lower intakes in patients with hypertension. Moderate alcohol intake below this level may actually lower blood pressure slightly or may simply have no effect on blood pressure. The cardiovascular benefits of alcohol (see Chapter 6) may help reduce the risk of myocardial infarction in well-controlled hypertensives. When blood pressure is not well controlled, alcohol intake should be discouraged.

Garlic

Garlic is reputed to have antihypertensive effects. Garlic stimulates nitric oxide synthase (33), providing a mechanism by which it might lower blood pressure. Meta-analysis supports a modest antihypertensive effect of garlic, but the evidence is limited (34).

Amino Acids

Arginine and taurine may have antihypertensive properties, but evidence to date is limited (35). Arginine is a precursor in the synthesis of nitric oxide, an endothelium-derived vasodilator; a link between blood pressure and endothelial function is clear, although the direction of causality is not (36,36a). Evidence is insufficient to justify recommendations of amino acid supplementation in efforts to regulate blood pressure.

Coenzyme Q_{10}

An antihypertensive effect of coenzyme Q_{10} is claimed, and it is used in the management of hypertension by alternative medicine practitioners. The evidence for such an effect is limited and not sufficient to justify routine clinical application (37–39).

Caffeine

Caffeine is a pressor and acutely raises blood pressure, generally to a modest degree. The effects of caffeine on blood pressure are apparently greater in hypertensives than in normotensives (40). Evidence is insufficient to warrant population-wide recommendations for caffeine restriction as a means of improving blood pressure. However, caffeine restriction in hypertensives is both reasonable and prudent, even though additional research is needed to provide definitive evidence of benefit.

CLINICAL HIGHLIGHTS

There is decisive evidence that a diet rich in fruits, vegetables, grains, and nonfat dairy products; restricted in saturated and trans fat and their sources; and low in highly processed foods is associated with reductions in blood pressure in hypertensives and preservation of normal blood pressure in normotensives. There is suggestive evidence that such a diet may prevent hypertension on a population basis. The role of sodium in hypertension remains somewhat controversial, but international data now strongly support a consistent and direct relationship between per capita intake of sodium and blood pressure. Therefore, sodium restriction should be encouraged. Most individuals can be expected to acclimate to a salt-reduced diet over a period of weeks, so that preference for higher salt intake abates. Adherence to the dietary patterns advisable both for blood pressure control and health promotion will lead naturally to a salt intake far closer to the recommended 3 g per day than the prevailing level in the United States, which is as much as twice that. Similarly, although there is suggestive evidence of hypotensive effects of potassium, calcium, and magnesium, these nutrients are abundant in the dietary pattern advocated for blood pressure control and, therefore, need not be singled out. Recommendations should be made to all patients to consume such a diet not only for its effects on blood pressure, but for its other health benefits (see Chapter 40).

Hypertensive patients should be advised to read food labels and minimize the intake of processed foods with greater sodium than potassium content. Supplemental calcium, appropriate for the prevention of osteoporosis in many patients (see Chapter 13), may contribute slightly to blood pressure control. Alcohol should be restricted or avoided until blood pressure is normalized. Although there is little evidence that salt substitutes effectively control blood pressure, use of such products as one means of reducing sodium intake is reasonable. Caffeine should be restricted in poorly controlled hypertensives; moderate intake should be advised for all others. Patients with blood pressure in the upper range of normal generally develop hypertension over time (41) and should be encouraged to modify diet in an effort to prevent such progression. Adherence to the recommended dietary pattern can be expected to lower systolic blood pressure by approximately 11 and 6 mm Hg in hypertensives and normotensives, respectively, and diastolic blood pressure by approximately 6 and 3 mm Hg in hypertensives and normotensives, respectively (42).

REFERENCES

1. Stamler J. The INTERSALT Study: background, methods, findings, and implications. *Am J Clin Nutr* 1997;65[2 Suppl]:626S–642S.
2. Imazu M, Sumida K, Yamabe T, et al. A comparison of the prevalence and risk factors of high blood pressure among Japanese living in Japan, Hawaii, and Los Angeles. *Public Health Rep* 1996; 111[Suppl 2]:59.
3. He J, Tell GS, Tang YC, et al. Effect of migration on blood pressure: the Yi People Study. *Epidemiology* 1991;2:88.
4. Grim CE, Robinson M. Blood pressure variation in blacks: genetic factors. *Semin Nephrol* 1996;16:83.
5. Moore TJ, McKnight JA. Dietary factors and blood pressure regulation. *Endocrinol Metab Clin North Am* 1995;24:643.
6. Landsberg L. Weight reduction and obesity. *Clin Exp Hypertens* 1999;21:763.
7. Harsha DW, Lin PH, Obarzanek E, et al. Dietary Approaches to Stop Hypertension: a summary of study results. DASH Collaborative Research Group. *J Am Diet Assoc* 1999;99[8 Suppl]:s35.
8. Tucker K. Dietary patterns and blood pressure in African Americans. *Nutr Rev* 1999;57:356.
9. Simons-Morton DG, Hunsberger SA, Van Horn L, et al. Nutrient intake and blood pressure in the Dietary Intervention Study in Children. *Hypertension* 1997;29:930.
10. Horrocks LA, Yeo YK. Health benefits of docosahexaenoic acid. *Pharmacol Res* 1999;40:211.
11. Grimsgaard S, Bonaa KH, Jacobsen BK, et al. Plasma saturated and linoleic fatty acids are independently associated with blood pressure. *Hypertension* 1999;34:478.
12. Windhauser MM, Ernst DB, Karanja NM, et al. Translating the Dietary Approaches to Stop Hypertension diet from research to practice: dietary and behavior change techniques. DASH Collaborative Research Group. *J Am Diet Assoc* 1999;99 [8 Suppl]:s90.
13. Cutler JA. The effects of reducing sodium and increasing potassium intake for control of hypertension and improving health. *Clin Exp Hypertens* 1999;21:769.
14. He J, Whelton PK. Role of sodium reduction in the treatment and prevention of hypertension. *Curr Opin Cardiol* 1997;12:202.
15. Chrysant GS, Bakir S, Oparil S. Dietary salt reduction in hypertension—what is the evidence and why is it still controversial? *Prog Cardiovasc Dis* 1999; 42:23.
16. Kumanyika S. Behavioral aspects of intervention strategies to reduce dietary sodium. *Hypertension* 1991;17[1 Suppl]:I190.
17. Cook NR, Kumanyika SK, Cutler JA. Effect of change in sodium excretion on change in blood pressure corrected for measurement error. The Trials of Hypertension Prevention, phase I. *Am J Epidemiol* 1998;148:431.
18. Eaton SB, Eaton SB III, Konner MJ. Paleolithic nutrition revisited: a twelve-year retrospective on its nature and implications. *Eur J Clin Nutr* 1997; 51:207.
19. Bertino M, Beauchamp GK, Engelman K. Long-term reduction in dietary sodium alters the taste of salt. *Am J Clin Nutr* 1982;36:1134.
20. Rogers PJ. Eating habits and appetite control: a psychobiological perspective. *Proc Nutr Soc* 1999; 58:59.
21. Bertino M, Beauchamp GK, Engelman K. Increasing dietary salt alters salt taste preference. *Physiol Behav* 1986;38:203.
22. Drewnowski A, Henderson SA, Driscoll A, et al. Salt taste perceptions and preferences are unrelated to sodium consumption in healthy older adults. *J Am Diet Assoc* 1996;96:471.
23. Mattes RD. The taste for salt in humans. *Am J Clin Nutr* 1997;65[Suppl 2]:692s.
24. Whelton PK, He J. Potassium in preventing and treating high blood pressure. *Semin Nephrol* 1999; 19:494.

25. Griffith LE, Guyatt GH, Cook RJ, et al. The influence of dietary and nondietary calcium supplementation on blood pressure: an updated metaanalysis of randomized controlled trials. *Am J Hypertens* 1999;12[1 Pt 1]:84.

26. Burgess E, Lewanczuk R, Bolli P, et al. Lifestyle modifications to prevent and control hypertension. 6. Recommendations on potassium, magnesium and calcium. Canadian Hypertension Society, Canadian Coalition for High Blood Pressure Prevention and Control, Laboratory Centre for Disease Control at Health Canada, Heart and Stroke Foundation of Canada. *CMAJ* 1999;160[9 Suppl]:S35.

27. Yabes-Almirante C. Calcium supplementation in pregnancy to prevent pregnancy induced hypertension (PIH). *J Perinat Med* 1998;26:347.

28. McCarron DA, Reusser ME. Finding consensus in the dietary calcium-blood pressure debate. *J Am Coll Nutr* 1999;18[5 Suppl]:398S.

29. Kawano Y, Matsuoka H, Takishita S, et al. Effects of magnesium supplementation in hypertensive patients: assessment by office, home, and ambulatory blood pressures. *Hypertension* 1998;32:260–265.

30. Appel LJ. Nonpharmacologic therapies that reduce blood pressure: a fresh perspective. *Clin Cardiol* 1999;22[7 Suppl]:III1–III5.

31. Stamler J, Caggiula AW, Grandits GA. Relation of body mass and alcohol, nutrient, fiber, and caffeine intakes to blood pressure in the special intervention and usual care groups in the Multiple Risk Factor Intervention Trial. *Am J Clin Nutr* 1997;65 [1 Suppl]:338S–365S.

32. Ascherio A, Hennekens C, Willett WC, et al. Prospective study of nutritional factors, blood pressure, and hypertension among US women. *Hypertension* 1996;27:1065.

33. Pedraza-Chaverri J, Tapia E, Medina-Campos ON, et al. Garlic prevents hypertension induced by chronic inhibition of nitric oxide synthesis. *Life Sci* 1998;62:PL71–77.

34. Silagy CA, Neil HA. A meta-analysis of the effect of garlic on blood pressure. *J Hypertens* 1994;12:463.

35. Nittynen L, Nurminen ML, Korpela R, et al. Role of arginine, taurine and homocysteine in cardiovascular diseases. *Ann Med* 1999;31:318–326.

36. Hedner T, Sun X. Measures of endothelial function as an endpoint in hypertension? *Blood Press Suppl* 1997;2:58–66.

36a. Panza JA. Endothelial dysfunction in essential hypertension. *Clin Cardiol* 1997;20[11 Suppl 2]:II-26.

37. Langsjoen P, Langsjoen P, Willis R, et al. Treatment of essential hypertension with coenzyme Q_{10}. *Mol Aspects Med* 1994;15:s265–s272.

38. Singh RB, Niaz MA, Rastogi SS, et al. Effect of hydrosoluble coenzyme Q_{10} on blood pressures and insulin resistance in hypertensive patients with coronary artery disease. *J Hum Hypertens* 1999;13: 203–208.

39. Digiesi V, Cantini F, Oradei A, et al. Coenzyme Q_{10} in essential hypertension. *Mol Aspects Med* 1994;15:s257–s262.

40. Nurminen ML, Niittynen L, Korpela R, et al. Coffee, caffeine and blood pressure: a critical review. *Eur J Clin Nutr* 1999;53:831.

41. Sagie A, Larson MG, Levy D. The natural history of borderline isolated systolic hypertension. *N Engl J Med* 1993;329:1912.

42. Kolasa KM. Dietary Approaches to Stop Hypertension (DASH) in clinical practice: a primary care experience. *Clin Cardiol* 1999;22[7 Suppl]:III16.

BIBLIOGRAPHY

See "Sources for All Chapters."

The sixth report of the Joint National Committee on prevention, detection, evaluation, and treatment of high blood pressure. *Arch Intern Med* 1997;157:2413–2446.

Karanja NM, Obarzanek E, Lin PH, et al. Descriptive characteristics of the dietary patterns used in the Dietary Approaches to Stop Hypertension Trial. DASH Collaborative Research Group. *J Am Diet Assoc* 1999;99[8 Suppl]:s19.

8

Diet and Hemostasis

INTRODUCTION

Nutrition plays a vital role in both the manufacture of blood products and in the homeostatic mechanisms governing the function of both cellular and noncellular constituents of blood. Hematopoiesis requires an adequate intake of both energy and an array of micronutrients, including minerals such as iron, vitamins such as folate and B_{12}, and specific amino acids. The manufacture of clotting factors II, VII, IX, and X is dependent on adequate intake of vitamin K.

Provided that both macronutrient and micronutrient intake meets or exceeds recommended levels, diet is unlikely to be a limiting factor in hematopoiesis. However, variations in dietary pattern and in the metabolic responses to such variations appear to play an important and as yet incompletely understood role in modifying hemostasis. Roles for total energy intake, adiposity, alcohol, the quantity and type of dietary fat, and various micronutrients have been tentatively or reliably identified in promoting or inhibiting thrombotic tendencies.

DIET

Excess energy intake leading to obesity appears to be associated with increased thrombotic tendencies. Obesity is associated with increased levels of fibrinogen and plasminogen activator inhibitor (PAI-1) and increased blood viscosity (1). Adiposity, as measured by the waist-to-hip ratio, has been positively correlated with fibrinogen levels (1) and may be particularly associated with a prothrombotic tendency (2). The effects of weight loss on hemostasis are as yet uncertain, but benefits have been reported. Short-term studies have shown variable effects on fibrinogen, apparently mediated by fluctuations in the levels of free fatty acids (1). Rapid weight loss may elevate fibrinogen due to free fatty acid mobilization, whereas more measured weight loss, and the maintenance of such loss, appears to be associated with reduced levels of both fibrinogen and other prothrombotic factors (1,3). Weight loss has been associated with reductions in factor VII coagulant activity (factor VIIc) as well. Physical activity appears to influence hemostasis, reducing levels of fibrinogen and PAI-1 (1); this effect appears particularly robust in diabetics, suggesting that improved insulin sensitivity may reduce thrombotic tendencies.

In a randomized trial of more than 180 adults with impaired glucose tolerance and obesity, Lindahl and colleagues (4) showed that intense behavioral intervention producing significant weight loss also produced significant reductions in PAI-1. Although the intervention subjects also showed declines in tissue plasminogen activator (tPA), these effects were smaller than those on PAI-1, suggesting enhanced fibrinolysis (4). In a randomized trial of physical activity and a low-fat diet with or without daily fish in type II diabetics, Dunstan and colleagues (5) found some prothrombotic and some antithrombotic effects of the interventions.

High dietary fat intake is associated with relatively high levels of factors VIIc and X. Levels of PAI-1 and tPA may rise with increasing fat consumption. Reductions in fat intake have been shown to lower PAI-1 levels, but only if substantial. Elevated serum lipids associated with high dietary fat intake may promote thrombosis both directly and indirectly (1).

The association between vegetarianism and reduced cardiac risk would suggest possible salutary effects on hemostasis; however, evidence to date is inconclusive. In a study of 26 vegetarians and matched omnivorous controls, Mezzano and colleagues (6) found no evidence of reduced thrombotic tendencies in the vegetarians. In general, levels of prothrombotic and fibrinolytic factors were lower in the vegetarians, whereas platelet aggregation was enhanced and plasma homocysteine was relatively elevated (6). A similar study in an African population found vegetarianism to be associated with lower levels of fibrinogen and enhanced fibrinolytic activity (7).

The effects of specific fatty acids on thrombotic tendencies remain controversial. Alterations in the intake of both saturated and monounsaturated fatty acids have yielded inconsistent and conflicting effects on the hemostatic profile, as reviewed by Vorster et al. (1). Even the n-3 polyunsaturated fatty acids, well known to inhibit platelet aggregability, have been associated with reductions in tPA, thus suggesting that fibrinolysis might be impaired by excessive intake. Fish oil may lower fibrinogen levels only when supplemented with vitamin E.

NUTRIENTS AND NUTRICEUTICALS

Alcohol

Alcohol has been shown to increase levels of tPA and to reduce platelet aggregation over time (1). Acute effects of alcohol are just the opposite, inducing a prothrombotic profile in the postprandial state. Alcohol also has been associated with increased levels of PAI-1 in men. Moderate alcohol consumption is associated with reduced levels of fibrinogen, whereas heavier intake is associated with elevated levels. Overall, at a dose of 30 to 40 g per day, alcohol appears to impart greater antithrombotic than prothrombotic effects, accounting for, in whole or in part, its association with reduced risk of atherosclerotic heart disease.

Soluble Fiber

Soluble fiber has been shown to lower fibrinogen levels in diabetics. Raising soluble fiber intake also may improve fibrinolytic activity by increasing levels of tPA. Overall, the evidence is suggestive that dietary soluble fiber should correlate inversely with thrombotic tendency.

n-3 Fatty Acids

The effects of n-3 fatty acid supplementation on the hemostatic profile reported to date are somewhat inconsistent (8,9). Fibrinogen levels are lowered apparently only if vitamin E supplementation is provided. Recent animal data suggest that long-chain n-3 fatty acids reduce platelet aggregation (10). Across the range of typical fish consumption in the United States, no effect on hemostatic factors was seen among young adults in the CARDIA study (11). Similarly, supplementation for 3 months with docosahexaenoic acid did not appreciably alter hemostatic factors in a group of healthy young adults (12). Whereas the serum markers of hemostasis in humans show variable responses, a meta-analysis by Gapinski and colleagues (13) reported promising clinical effects. These investigators reported a nearly 14% reduction in the risk of restenosis at 6 months after coronary angioplasty. The authors recommend use of 4 to 5 g per day of n-3 fatty acids and suggest that seven patients would require treatment for 6 months to prevent restenosis in one. Studies evaluated by Gapinski and colleagues (13), such as that of Dehmer et al. (14), demonstrated a benefit of n-3 fatty acid supplementation in conjunction with use of aspirin. The pertinence of these findings in the context of coronary stenting and use of IIb:IIIa inhibitors is uncertain.

Monounsaturated Fatty Acids

The substitution of monounsaturated fat (oleic acid) for saturated fat has an uncertain effect on thrombotic tendency. *In vitro* data suggest an increase in platelet aggregability (15). Sustained supplementation has been associated with reduced postprandial activation of factor VII (16).

Saturated Fatty Acids

Inconsistent effects of saturated fatty acids on thrombotic tendency have been observed. Tholstrup and colleagues (17) administered meals rich in either stearic or myristic acid to ten healthy men. Although the fats had variable effects on thrombotic factors including PAI-1, factor VIIc, and β-thromboglobulin, both diminished platelet aggregability in the postprandial phase. Temme and colleagues (18) reported increased levels of factor VIIc induced by a high saturated fat diet relative to a high monounsaturated fat diet in women but not in men. Lahoz and colleagues (19) reported increased thromboxane excretion in association with a high saturated fat test diet. Evidence to date does not strongly support assignation of cardiac risk associated with saturated fat intake to effects on hemostasis.

Antioxidant Vitamins

Animal data suggest that both vitamins E and C may inhibit platelet aggregation and delay thrombus formation (20). A study of short-term vitamin E supplementation (400 IU per day) in hypercholesterolemic subjects demonstrated reduced platelet aggregation after 6 weeks (21).

Flavonoids

Flavonoids, such as quercetin, have been shown to inhibit platelet aggregation *in vitro*.

Janssen et al. (22) studied realistic doses of flavonoids from whole-food sources (quercetin from onion; apigenin from parsley) and found no effect on hemostatic variables or platelet aggregation. The authors suggest that cardioprotective effects of flavonoids are unlikely to be related to hemostatic mechanisms.

Arginine

Arginine is a precursor in the manufacture of nitric oxide in the vascular endothelium; nitric oxide levels may influence platelet–endothelium interactions. Animal data have been reported suggesting that L-arginine supplementation reduces levels of thromboxane relative to prostacyclin and inhibits platelet aggregation (23).

CLINICAL HIGHLIGHTS

Hemostatic factors, such as fibrinogen, are strongly associated with the risk of cardiovascular events (24). Evidence from a variety of sources indicates that dietary pattern may play an important role in influencing hemostasis. However, due in part to the wide range of circulating factors involved in hemostatic mechanisms and in part to the difficulties of controlled dietary interventions, little is known with certainty about the effects of specific foods or nutrients on overall thrombotic tendency. Evidence available to date suggests that dietary recommendations to reduce risk of thromboembolic disease are consistent with recommendations to lower risk of cardiovascular disease. Protective factors include the avoidance of excess energy intake and obesity; the avoidance of excess fat consumption; physical activity; abundant dietary fiber, especially soluble fiber; moderate alcohol consumption; and possibly dietary supplementation with n-3 fatty acids and vitamin E. Weight loss in obese patients may be of particular importance. Before definitive dietary recommendations can be offered to modify hemostasis for clinical benefit, observational and ideally interventional studies of diet and clinically important thrombotic events rather than surrogate markers will be needed.

REFERENCES

1. Vorster HH, Cummings JH, Veldman FJ. Diet and haemostasis: time for nutrition science to get more involved. *Br J Nutrition* 1997;77:671–684.
2. Anderssen SA, Holme I, Urdal P, et al. Associations between central obesity and indexes of hemostatic, carbohydrate and lipid metabolism. Results of a 1-year intervention from the Oslo Diet and Exercise Study. *Scand J Med Sci Sports* 1998;8:109–115.
3. Marckmann P, Toubro S, Astrup A. Sustained improvement in blood lipids, coagulation, and fibrinolysis after major weight loss in obese subjects. *Eur J Clin Nutr* 1998;52:329–333.
4. Lindahl B, Nilsson TK, Jansson JH, et al. Improved fibrinolysis by intense lifestyle intervention. A randomized trial in subjects with impaired glucose tolerance. *J Intern Med* 1999;246:105–112.
5. Dunstan DW, Mori TA, Puddey IB, et al. A randomised, controlled study of the effects of aerobic exercise and dietary fish on coagulation and fibrinolytic factors in type 2 diabetics. *Thromb Haemost* 1999;81:367–372.
6. Mezzano D, Munoz X, Martinez C, et al. Vegetarians and cardiovascular risk factors: hemostasis, inflammatory markers and plasma homocysteine. *Thromb Haemost* 1999;81:913–917.
7. Famodu AA, Osilesi O, Makinde YO, et al. The influence of a vegetarian diet on haemostatic risk factors for cardiovascular disease in Africans. *Thromb Res* 1999;95:31–36.
8. Allman-Farinelli MA, Hall D, Kingham K, et al. Comparison of the effects of two low fat diets with different alpha-linolenic:linoleic acid ratios on coagulation and fibrinolysis. *Atherosclerosis* 1999;142:159–168.
9. Sanders TA, Oakley FR, Miller GJ, et al. Influence of n-6 versus n-3 polyunsaturated fatty acids in diets low in saturated fatty acids on plasma lipoproteins and hemostatic factors. *Arterioscler Thromb Vasc Biol* 1997;17:3449–3460.
10. Adan Y, Shibata K, Sato M, et al. Effects of docosahexaenoic and eicosapentaenoic acid on lipid metabolism, eicosanoid production, platelet aggregation and atherosclerosis in hypercholesterolemic rats. *Biosci Biotechnol Biochem* 1999;63:111–119.
11. Archer SL, Green D, Chamberlain M, et al. Association of dietary fish and n-3 fatty acid intake with hemostatic factors in the coronary artery risk development in young adults (CARDIA) study. *Arterioscler Thromb Biol* 1998;18:1119–1123.
12. Nelson GJ, Schmidt PS, Bartolini GL, et al. The effect of dietary docosahexaenoic acid on platelet function, platelet fatty acid composition, and blood coagulation in humans. *Lipids* 1997;32:1129–1136.
13. Gapinski JP, VanRuiswyk JV, Heudebert GR, et al. Preventing restenosis with fish oils following coronary angioplasty. A meta-analysis. *Arch Intern Med* 1993;153:1595–1601.
14. Dehmer GJ, Popma JJ, Van den Berg EK, et al. Reduction in the rate of early restenosis after coronary angioplasty by a diet supplemented with n-3 fatty acids. *N Engl J Med* 1988;319:733–740.
15. Turpeinen AM, Pajari Am, Freese R, et al. Replacement of dietary saturated by unsaturated fatty acids: effects of platelet protein kinase C activity, urinary content of 2,3-dinor-TXB2 and *in vitro* platelet aggregation in healthy man. *Thromb Haemost* 1998;80:649–655.
16. Roche HM, Zampelas A, Knapper JM, et al. Effect of long-term olive oil dietary intervention on postprandial triacylglycerol and factor VII metabolism. *Am J Clin Nutr* 1998;68:552–560.
17. Tholstrup T, Andreasen K, Sandstrom B. Acute effect of high-fat meals rich in either stearic or myristic acid on hemostatic factors in healthy young men. *Am J Clin Nutr* 1996;64:168–176.
18. Temme EH, Mensink RP, Hornstra G. Effects of diets enriched in lauric, palmitic or oleic acids on blood coagulation and fibrinolysis. *Thromb Haemost* 1999;81:259–263.
19. Lahoz C, Alonso R, Ordovas JM, et al. Effects of dietary fat saturation on eicosanoid production, platelet aggregation and blood pressure. *Eur J Clin Invest* 1997;27:780–789.
20. Mehta J, Li D, Mehta JL. Vitamins C and E prolong time to arterial thrombosis in rats. *J Nutr* 1999;129:109–112.
21. Williams JC, Forster LA, Tull SP, et al. Dietary vitamin E supplementation inhibits thrombin-induced platelet aggregation, but not monocyte adhesiveness, in patients with hypercholesterolaemia. *Int J Exp Pathol* 1997;78:259–266.
22. Janssen K, Mensink RP, Cox FJ, et al. Effects of the flavonoids quercetin and apigenin on hemostasis in healthy volunteers: results from an *in vitro* and a dietary supplement study. *Am J Clin Nutr* 1998;67:255–262.
23. Bode-Boger SM, Boger RH, Kienke S, et al. Chronic dietary supplementation with L-arginine inhibits platelet aggregation and thromboxane A2 synthesis in hypercholesterolaemic rabbits *in vivo*. *Cardiovasc Res* 1998;37:756–764.
24. Montalescot G, Collet JP, Choussat R, et al. Fibrinogen as a risk factor for coronary heart disease. *Eur Heart J* 1998;19[Suppl H]:H11–H17.

BIBLIOGRAPHY

See "Sources for All Chapters."

9

Diet and Peripheral and Cerebrovascular Disease

INTRODUCTION

Stroke is the third leading cause of death in the United States, accounting for approximately 150,000 deaths annually. The majority of strokes are the result of thromboembolic events and are associated with atherosclerotic vascular disease. Peripheral vascular disease is the result of systemic atherogenesis and is associated with the same predisposing factors as coronary atherosclerosis. Therefore, dietary recommendations for the prevention and modification of cardiovascular risk generally are pertinent for peripheral vascular disease and stroke risk reduction as well. However, some observational evidence that dietary fat restriction may be associated with increased stroke risk suggests a possible disparity in the optimal dietary interventions for the two conditions. The weight of evidence would still favor fat restriction below levels currently prevailing in the United States. The leading modifiable risk factor for stroke is hypertension, which is amenable to dietary prevention and management, as described in Chapter 7. Approximately 25% of all strokes are cardioembolic, and the prevention of ischemic heart disease might most effectively eliminate events in this category. Less than 10% of all strokes are hemorrhagic. The incidence of hemorrhagic stroke is elevated in Inuit populations with extremely high intake of marine oils rich in n-3 fatty acids, suggesting that the risk of intracranial hemorrhage may be elevated by excessive intake of platelet-inhibiting nutri-

ents. However, thromboembolic stroke risk is reduced by the same practices. The overall evidence that stroke can be prevented by dietary means is convincing, but definitive intervention studies are lacking.

DIET AND STROKE

The risk of stroke is strongly correlated with both systolic and diastolic blood pressure, and advances in the pharmacologic management of hypertension are thought to be the principal explanation for declining stroke incidence and mortality over recent decades. Nonetheless, stroke remains the third leading cause of death and a leading cause of long-term disability among adults in the United States.

Elevated levels of total cholesterol, low-density lipoprotein, triglycerides, and very-low-density lipoprotein, as well as depressed levels of high-density lipoprotein, are linked with atherosclerotic heart disease. Atherosclerosis is known to be a systemic disease, and the same lipid patterns are inferentially linked to cerebrovascular disease. The inference is supported by observational and retrospective studies. Hachinski and colleagues (1) conducted a case-control study enrolling 90 patients with thromboembolic stroke and 90 matched controls. They found total cholesterol, low-density lipoprotein, and triglyceride levels to be significantly higher among the cases and high-density lipoprotein to be significantly lower (1). The inference that dyslipidemia contributes to stroke risk also is supported by secondary analyses of lipid-lowering trials for heart disease prevention that reveal a reduction in stroke risk as well (2,3).

Whereas these trials use pharmacotherapy, namely statin drugs, for lipid reduction, the achievement of lipid reduction by dietary means is thought to confer similar benefit. The possibility that statin-related stroke risk reduction is due to effects other than lipid lowering complicate inferences about diet, serum lipids, and stroke risk (4).

Dietary patterns associated with optimal lipid profiles are described in detail in Chapter 6. In general, dietary fat restriction to approximately 25% of total calories, abundant intake of fruits, vegetables, and whole grains, and moderate intake of lean meats would be indicated. Recommendations for cardiovascular disease include restriction of saturated fat and trans fat, combined, to less than 5% of total calories, with 15% of calories from monounsaturates and the remaining 10% to 15% from polyunsaturates. The ratio of n-3 to n-6 polyunsaturated should be between 1:1 and 1:4 (see Chapters 2, 6, 39, and 40).

Comparable recommendations for cerebrovascular disease are challenged by an observational study by Gillman and colleagues (5). The study followed 832 men in the Framingham cohort over 20 years for incident strokes. Dietary intake was assessed by a single 24-hour recall at baseline. Total intake of fat, saturated fat, and monounsaturated fat was negatively associated with stroke risk. The reliability of dietary intake assessment in this study is suspect, as is the control of confounders. Therefore, the study is provocative and suggests a need for more research, but it does not, on its own, refute the weight of evidence favoring fat restriction for health promotion. Cigarette smoking, a sedentary lifestyle, and obesity are all thought to contribute to stroke risk. A case-control study completed in England suggests that 80% of strokes might potentially be preventable by avoidance of these behavioral risk factors (6).

Hypertension is the single most important modifiable risk factor for stroke, and im-proved detection and treatment of hypertension is thought to be the principal explanation for declining rates of cerebrovascular disease (7). The primary prevention of hypertension often is feasible, with diet playing a major role (see Chapter 7). The prevention of hypertension by dietary means would likely result in the prevention of cerebrovascular events as well.

The hypothesis that antioxidant nutrients may prevent stroke was tested in the Chicago Western Electric Study. A total of 1,843 men contributed to 46,102 person-years of observation, during which 222 incident strokes occurred (8). Although reported intakes of β-carotene and vitamin C were inversely associated with stroke risk, the relationships did not achieve statistical significance. Data from the Honolulu Heart Program were used to assess the association between milk consumption and stroke risk, given an association between dietary calcium and reduced blood pressure (9). A significant inverse association between milk consumption and stroke risk, but not between calcium intake and stroke risk, was reported. The authors suggest that milk consumption might reduce stroke risk or might be associated with other dietary and lifestyle factors contributing to risk reduction.

The importance of adequate micronutrient intake to stroke prevention is supported by data from the Linxian Nutrition Intervention Trial. Subjects from a rural Chinese population with a micronutrient-poor diet had reduced rates of hypertension and stroke when given a multivitamin, multimineral supplement rather than placebo; the effect was more pronounced in men than in women (10).

Population data suggest that fruit and vegetable consumption is associated with reduced stroke risk. Data from the Zutphen study were used to determine the role of specific micronutrients in this association (11). A total of 42 strokes occurred among 552 men followed for 15 years. Dietary histories were obtained at three times, after 5-year intervals. A strong and statistically significant relationship between flavonoid intake, particularly quercetin from black tea, and reduced stroke risk was reported (relative risk = 0.27 by quartile; 95% confidence interval 0.11 to 0.7). A weaker, inverse association with stroke risk was observed for carotenoids. Data extracted from vital statistics in Spain suggest that a marked decline in the incidence of cerebrovascular disease is related to increased fruit and decreased wine consumption (12).

Fish consumption is associated with reduced risk of cardiovascular disease. The association between stroke and fish consumption was assessed in the Chicago Western Electric Study. Among 1,847 men followed for 30 years, stroke incidence was highest among subjects in the highest quartile of fish intake (13) thus failing to suggest any benefit.

In addition to its role in stroke prevention, diet may play a role in recovery. Davalos and colleagues (14) studied 104 acute stroke patients and found that over 25% were malnourished 1 week after the event as measured by both anthropometry and serum markers. Protein-energy malnutrition in this group significantly predicted poor outcome, including death (14).

Although stroke can be prevented by the pharmacologic treatment of hypertension, projections from Framingham and National Health and Nutrition Examination Survey (NHANES) data suggest that a population-based approach would confer additional benefits. Modeling by Cook and colleagues (15) suggests that a reduction of 2 mm Hg in the mean population diastolic blood pressure achieved through lifestyle modification could prevent 67,000 cardiovascular events and 34,000 strokes annually in the 35- to 64-year-old age group.

Alcohol taken in low doses may protect against cerebrovascular disease, whereas higher intakes appear to increase risk. Modest alcohol intake—approximately 30 to 45 g per day of ethanol, or the equivalent of one drink—may independently of other behaviors reduce the risk of atherosclerosis in the carotid arteries (16). Alcohol consumption increases the risk of hemorrhagic stroke in a dose-dependent manner.

Physical activity appears to protect against both incident stroke and the degree of functional disability resulting from stroke (17). Exercise contributes directly to blood pressure control, produces favorable influences on both serum lipids and glucose, and helps control body weight, all of which may influence stroke risk.

Elevated homocysteine levels have been implicated in cardiovascular disease and, to a lesser extent, cerebrovascular disease. A diet rich in B vitamins and folate, or a supplement containing these nutrients, may confer some protection against stroke in vulnerable individuals. Magnesium supplementation, particularly in magnesium-deficient individuals, may mitigate stroke risk by inhibiting spasm of intracranial vessels.

PERIPHERAL VASCULAR DISEASE

Peripheral vascular disease is the result of systemic atherosclerosis and shares risk factors with coronary and cerebrovascular disease. Dietary interventions to modify coronary artery disease risk, described in Chapter 6, should be applied in peripheral arterial disease as well. There is evidence that clinicians tend to modify risk factors less aggressively in peripheral than in coronary arterial disease (18). Peripheral vascular disease is associated with elevated plasma homocysteine and, therefore, may be amenable to intervention with B vitamin and folate supplementation in certain patients (19). As is the case for atherosclerotic disease in general, dietary modification of risk factors should be coupled to other lifestyle interventions, such as smoking cessation and increased physical activity, as well as all indicated pharmacologic interventions (20).

Plasma levels of n-3 fatty acids have been reported to correlate inversely with risk of peripheral vascular disease (21). A strong positive association between smoking and peripheral vascular disease has been consistently reported (22,23). Elevated postprandial insulin levels appear to be an independent risk factor as well, suggesting that dietary intervention to improve glycemic control (see Chapter 10) may play a role in the prevention and control of peripheral vascular disease (24).

NUTRIENTS AND NUTRICEUTICALS

Nutrients and nutriceuticals pertinent to the prevention or management of atherosclerosis and dyslipidemias are discussed in Chapter 6; those related to the control of hypertension in Chapter 7; and those related to control of insulin levels in Chapter 10. Evidence is insufficient to characterize the role of single nutrients in the prevention or amelioration of cerebrovascular or peripheral vascular disease.

CLINICAL HIGHLIGHTS

The predominant risk factor for stroke is hypertension, which can be prevented and modified by dietary interventions. Additional risk may be conferred by low dietary intake of n-3 fatty acids, obesity, hyperinsulinemia, hyperlipidemia, micronutrient deficiencies, and elevated plasma homocysteine. The possibility exists that excessive fat restriction may increase stroke risk, but the data are far from definitive. Certain factors that reduce the risk of thromboembolic stroke, such as platelet-inhibiting nutrients, may increase the risk of hemorrhagic stroke.

Dietary recommendations for prevention of stroke and peripheral vascular disease parallel recommendations for general health promotion. Dietary fat should be restricted to approximately 25% of total calories, with a preponderance from monounsaturated and polyunsaturated fatty acids. Consumption of fish and the use of flaxseed oil to increase the proportion of n-3 fatty acids in the diet appear safe and reasonable in efforts to prevent stroke and peripheral vascular disease, although risk of hemorrhage is raised if consumption is extreme. Vitamin E supplementation in the range of 400 IU per day is reasonable in conjunction with polyunsaturated

fatty acid consumption, although no definitive evidence of stroke or peripheral vascular disease benefit is available. A variety of fruits and vegetables may provide all needed micronutrients, but a multivitamin, multimineral supplement is a reasonable precaution against isolated, subclinical deficiencies, the most pertinent of which are apt to be B vitamins and folate. Dietary sodium restriction and generous intake of potassium, magnesium, and calcium may lower blood pressure. Regular physical activity and smoking cessation are essential elements in lifestyle management of risk for both stroke and peripheral vascular disease. Alcohol intake should not exceed the range consistent with health promotion (i.e., 30 to 45 g per day of ethanol) and at this dose may confer benefit. The value of micronutrient supplements in megadoses for the prevention or modification of either stroke or peripheral vascular disease is unsubstantiated.

REFERENCES

1. Hachinski V, Graffagnino C, Beaudry M, et al. Lipids and stroke: a paradox resolved. *Arch Neurol* 1996;53:303.
2. Crouse JR III, Byington RP, Furberg CD. HMG-CoA reductase inhibitor therapy and stroke risk reduction: an analysis of clinical trials data. *Atherosclerosis* 1998;138:11.
3. Bucher HC, Griffith LE, Guyatt GH. Effect of HMGCoA reductase inhibitors on stroke. A meta-analysis of randomized, controlled trials. *Ann Intern Med* 1998;128:89.
4. Endres M, Laufs U, Huang Z, et al. Stroke protection by 3-hydroxy-3-methylglutaryl (HMG)-CoA reductase inhibitors mediated by endothelial nitric oxide synthase. *Proc Natl Acad Sci USA* 1998; 95:8880.
5. Gillman MW, Cupples LA, Millen BE, et al. Inverse association of dietary fat with development of ischemic stroke in men. *JAMA* 1997;278:2145.
6. Shinton R. Lifelong exposures and the potential for stroke prevention: the contribution of cigarette smoking, exercise, and body fat. *J Epidemiol Community Health* 1997;51:138.
7. He J, Whelton PK. Epidemiology and prevention of hypertension. *Med Clin North Am* 1997;81:1077.
8. Daviglus ML, Orencia AJ, Dyer AR, et al. Dietary vitamin C, beta-carotene and 30-year risk of stroke: results from the Western Electric Study. *Neuroepidemiology* 1997;16:69.
9. Abbott RD, Curb JD, Rodriguez BL, et al. Effect of dietary calcium and milk consumption on risk of

thromboembolic stroke in older middle-aged men. The Honolulu Heart Program. *Stroke* 1996;27:813.

10. Mark SD, Wang W, Fraumeni JF, et al. Lowered risks of hypertension and cerebrovascular disease after vitamin/mineral supplementation: the Linxian Nutrition Intervention Trial. *Am J Epidemiol* 1996; 143:658.

11. Keli SO, Hertog MG, Feskens EJ, et al. Dietary flavonoids, antioxidant vitamins, and incidence of stroke: the Zutphen study. *Arch Intern Med* 1996; 156:637.

12. Rodriguez Artalejo F, Guallar-Castillon P, Banegas JR, et al. Consumption of fruit and wine and the decline in cerebrovascular disease mortality in Spain (1975–1993). *Stroke* 1998;8:1556.

13. Orencia AJ, Daviglus ML, Dyer AR, et al. Fish consumption and stroke in men. 30-year findings of the Chicago Western Electric Study. *Stroke* 1996; 27:204.

14. Davalos A, Ricart W, Gonzalez-Huix F, et al. Effect of malnutrition after acute stroke on clinical outcome. *Stroke* 1996;27:1028.

15. Cook NR, Cohen J, Hebert PR, et al. Implications of small reductions in diastolic blood pressure for primary prevention. *Arch Intern Med* 1995;155:701.

16. Kiechl S, Willeit J, Egger G, et al. Alcohol consumption and carotid atherosclerosis: evidence of dose-dependent atherogenic and antiatherogenic effects. Results from the Bruneck Study. *Stroke* 1994; 25:1593.

17. Fletcher GF. Exercise in the prevention of stroke. *Health Rep* 1994;6:106.

18. McDermott MM, Mehta S, Ahn H, et al. Atherosclerotic risk factors are less intensively treated in patients with peripheral arterial disease than in patients with coronary artery disease. *J Gen Intern Med* 1997;12:209.

19. Cheng SW, Ting AC, Wong J. Fasting total plasma homocysteine and atherosclerotic peripheral vascular disease. *Ann Vasc Surg* 1997;11:217.

20. Cooke JP, Ma AO. Medical therapy of peripheral arterial occlusive disease. *Surg Clin North Am* 1995;75:569.

21. Leng GC, Horrobin DF, Fowkes FG, et al. Plasma essential fatty acids, cigarette smoking, and dietary antioxidants in peripheral arterial disease. A population-based case-control study. *Arterioscler Thromb* 1994;14:471.

22. Fowkes FG, Housley E, Riemersma RA, et al. Smoking, lipids, glucose intolerance, and blood pressure as risk factors for peripheral atherosclerosis compared with ischemic heart disease in the Edinburgh Artery Study. *Am J Epidemiol* 1992;135: 331.

23. Powell JT, Edwards RJ, Worrell PC, et al. Risk factors associated with the development of peripheral arterial disease in smokers: a case-control study. *Atherosclerosis* 1997;129:41.

24. Price JF, Lee AJ, Fowkes FG. Hyperinsulinemia: a risk factor for peripheral arterial disease in the non-diabetic general population. *J Cardiovasc Risk* 1996;3:501.

BIBLIOGRAPHY

See "Sources for All Chapters."

Gillman MW, Cupples LA, Gagnon D, et al. Protective effect of fruits and vegetables on development of stroke in men. *JAMA* 1995;273:1113.

10

Diet, Diabetes Mellitus, and Insulin Resistance

INTRODUCTION

The role of dietary management of both type I and type II diabetes mellitus is conclusively established. Although patients with type I diabetes require exogenous insulin, their glycemic control and the occurrence of diabetes-related complications are related to dietary factors. Most dietary recommendations for diabetes pertain to both types. The one important difference is the need in type I diabetes to maintain a very predictable dietary pattern corresponding to a particular insulin regimen. Of the approximately 15–20 million cases of diabetes in the United States, 90% are type II, and 90% of these patients are overweight (see Chapter 5). Weight control is a fundamental objective in the dietary management of all overweight diabetic patients (see Chapter 5). Whereas traditional approaches to diabetes have focused on the glycemic index of individual foods and on the use of exchange lists, attention is increasingly focused on the effects of foods in combinations and on the overall dietary pattern. The pathogenesis of the insulin resistance syndrome continues to be investigated. There is at least suggestive evidence that obesity is necessary for the insulin resistance syndrome to become clinically discernible (1). Whether an interaction between genetic susceptibility to insulin resistance and particular dietary patterns leads to obesity is uncertain.

OVERVIEW

Pathogenesis of Diabetes Mellitus

Type I Diabetes Mellitus

Type I, or insulin-dependent, diabetes mellitus is due to pancreatic β-cell dysfunction or destruction, generally considered the result of an autoimmune process. Although the inciting event or exposure is not known with certainty, there is some, albeit controversial, evidence that early exposure to bovine milk proteins in predisposed individuals may play a role (2,3). In general, however, there is little to suggest that dietary interventions can be used to prevent type I diabetes.

Insulin Resistance and Type II Diabetes Mellitus

In the United States, there are more than 16 million known diabetics, with a comparable number of undiagnosed cases considered likely (4). More than 90% of the diagnosed cases and virtually all of the undiagnosed cases are type II.

The fundamental distinction between type I and type II diabetes, at times blurred, is the preservation of endogenous insulin production in type II. This distinction results in the susceptibility of type I, but not type II, diabetics to ketoacidosis. Severely uncontrolled hyperglycemia in type II diabetics generally leads instead to nonketotic, hyperosmolar coma, with ketone body production representing the effect of absent insulin-mediated glucose transport.

The development of type II diabetes results from the interplay of genetic susceptibility and environmental factors (5). The responsible genes have not been identified with certainty, although multiple alleles are almost certainly involved, and certain candidate mutations have been under study for some time (6). The clustering of type II diabetes in families is well established. Interest in genetic susceptibility to type II diabetes dates back at least to the early 1960s, when James Neel (7), who went on to head the human genome project, speculated that expression of diabetes was due to the confrontation of a thrifty metabolism designed for dietary subsistence with a world of nutritional abundance. The theory of metabolic thriftiness essentially posits that a brisk insulin release in response to ingestion is advantageous in the utilization and storage of food energy when such energy is only sporadically available. The same brisk response in the context of abundantly available nutrient energy leads to hyperinsulinemia, obesity, insulin resistance, and, ultimately with the advent of β-cell failure, diabetes (7). The thrifty genotype theory, although not universally accepted, is supported by certain lines of evidence and continues to generate considerable interest (8–11).

Factors associated with expression of the disease include excessive nutrient energy intake with resultant obesity, physical inactivity, and advancing age. These factors contribute to the development of insulin resistance at the receptor, a key element in the development of type II diabetes mellitus. Physical activity appears to protect against the advent of type II diabetes mellitus both by preventing and mitigating weight gain and obesity, and independently (12). Insulin resistance generally precedes, by an uncertain and probably variable period of time, the development of diabetes. Diabetes occurs when receptor-mediated resistance is compounded by β-cell dysfunction and reduced insulin secretion.

An association between weight gain and the development of diabetes is supported by prospective cohort studies (13,14), although insulin resistance may contribute to the development of obesity as well, so that causality may be bidirectional (15). Data from such sources suggest that weight loss is protective against the development of diabetes. The currently worsening epidemic of obesity in the United States suggests that the prevalence of diabetes will likely rise and that efforts to combat obesity, if ultimately successful, will translate into reduced rates of diabetes as well.

Under normal circumstances, daily insulin secretion in a healthy adult totals approximately 30 units. In insulin-resistant states, production may rise to more than 100 units per day. This level of insulin production is apparently unsustainable and contributes to the pancreatic endocrine failure that characterizes the transition from insulin resistance to manifest diabetes. Whereas type I diabetes is associated with nearly absent insulin release (0 to 4 units daily), type II diabetes is generally thought to emerge in lean individuals when production falls to approximately 14 units per day.

The development and manifestations of insulin resistance relate to the principal actions of insulin. In liver, insulin inhibits gluconeogenesis, inhibits glycogenolysis, and promotes glycogen production (16). In muscle and adipose tissue, insulin facilities the uptake of glucose, and also its use and storage. Insulin exerts important influence on protein and lipid metabolism as well. The fundamental role of insulin is to coordinate the use and storage of food energy. This requires regulation of both carbohydrate and fat metabolism, as total body glycogen and glucose stores in a healthy adult approximate 300 g. At 4 kcal/g, this represents an energy reserve of 1,200 kcal, enough to support a fast of approximately 12 to 18 hours. Energy stored as triglyceride in adipose tissue in a lean adult totals nearly 120,000 kcal, or 100 times the carbohydrate reserve. Thus, release of energy stores from adipose tissue can protect vital organs during a protracted fast.

In the fed state, the entry of amino acids and monosaccharides into the portal circulation stimulates release of proinsulin from pancreatic β-cells. Insulin is cleaved from the connecting ("C") protein to generate active insulin. Insulin transports both amino acids and glucose into the liver, where it stimulates glycogen synthesis, protein synthesis, and fatty acid synthesis, while suppressing glycogenolysis and gluconeogenesis, as well as proteolysis and lipolysis. Insulin carries both glucose and amino acids into skeletal muscle, and glucose into adipose tissue. Insulin facilitates glycogen synthesis and glycolysis in muscle, and fatty acid synthesis in adipose tissue. Insulin also stimulates the synthesis of lipoprotein lipase in capillaries, facilitating the extraction of fatty acids from circulation, and promotes hepatic very-low-density lipoprotein (VLDL) synthesis.

During a fast, insulin levels decline, as levels of glucagon, a product of the pancreatic α-cells, rise. Falling insulin levels promote glycogenolysis, followed by gluconeogenesis, in the liver. In adipose tissue, low insulin levels stimulate lipolysis, releasing fatty acids for use as fuel; ketones are generated in the process of hepatic fatty acid oxidation. High levels of circulating fatty acids inhibit insulin action. Reduced insulin action at skeletal muscle stimulates proteolysis.

In the insulin-resistant state, insulin levels are high, but receptors, particularly those on skeletal muscle, are relatively insensitive to insulin action. High levels of insulin presumably compensate for receptor-mediated resistance. High insulin levels promote fatty acid synthesis in liver. The accumulation and circulation of free fatty acids and triglycerides packaged in VLDL aggravate insulin resistance, driving insulin levels higher. Thus, the metabolic derangements are self-perpetuating, generating in the process the manifestations of the insulin resistance syndrome associated with cardiovascular risk, until the β-cells fail and diabetes develops.

With β-cell failure, the resultant low levels of circulating insulin mimic conditions during a fast. The metabolic derangements that distinguish diabetes from fasting include pathologically low insulin levels and, of course, high levels of circulating glucose. Hepatic gluconeogenesis compounds the hyperglycemia, with excess glucose leading to tissue damage through glycosylation. Glycosylation of hemoglobin is routinely used as a measure of the extent of prevailing glycemia. High ambient levels of glucose lead to the production of sugar alcohols (e.g., sorbitol, fructose) in many tissues, which in turn can cause cellular distention. The accumulation of such polyols in the lens is causally implicated in the blurred vision that often occurs with poorly controlled diabetes.

In studies of the Pima Indians, a tribe of Native Americans particularly subject to the development of obesity and diabetes mellitus, Lillioja and colleagues (1) showed that insulin resistance is an antecedent of diabetes. During the phase of insulin resistance, serum glucose is normal but insulin levels are abnormally elevated, both in the fasting and postprandial states. The development of obesity appears to be of particular importance in the development of impaired glucose tolerance secondary to insulin resistance. A modest degree of hyperglycemia may occur during the period of insulin resistance, acting as a signal to the endocrine pancreas that insulin action is impaired and stimulating more insulin release (1). Ultimately, both protracted hypersecretion and hyperglycemia may contribute to β-cell dysfunction and overt diabetes (1).

In a longitudinal study of Pima Indians, Lillioja et al. (17) more recently characterized steps in the pathogenesis of type II diabetes. More than 200 nondiabetic subjects were followed for an average of over 5 years, undergoing body composition measures, glucose tolerance testing, and hyperinsulinemic-euglycemic clamp testing to assess insulin action and glucose disposal (17). The single, strongest predictor of the development of diabetes was impaired insulin action, with a relative hazard of over 30; this remained significant after adjustment for body fat (17). Percent body fat and impaired suppression of hepatic gluconeogenesis also were significant predictors of diabetes. The authors concluded that impaired insulin action, or insulin resistance, was the strongest single predictor of impending diabetes (17), while impaired suppression of hepatic gluconeogenesis was likely to be a secondary event. The factors responsible for β-cell failure, possibly including glucose toxicity and/or "fatigue" secondary to hyperfunction over time, are uncertain. The possibility exists, however, that the pathogenesis of type II diabetes is variable in different populations; β-cell failure may occur independently of insulin resistance (18). Noteworthy with regard to the Pima Indians is evidence that restoration of their traditional diet, low in fat and simple sugar and high in fiber from various desert plants, particularly mesquite, ameliorates their tendency toward diabetes and obesity (19). That the habitual nutritional environment should have salutary effects is perhaps supportive of the "thrifty genotype" theory and certainly is supportive of the application of the evolutionary biology model to human nutrition. To what degree this example should be used to guide nutritional management of diabetes in the general population is uncertain.

Reaven and colleagues reported that a substantial proportion of cases of hypertension may be related to insulin resistance (19a). While noting that hypertension may occur independently of insulin resistance, and vice versa, the authors contend that insulin resistance stimulates the sympathetic nervous system. Under normal fasting conditions, low serum glucose and insulin levels stimulate the activity of an inhibitory pathway from the ventromedial hypothalamus to sympathetic centers in the brainstem. With sustained elevations of both glucose and insulin, the inhibitory pathway remains suppressed, with resultant augmentation of sympathetic tone (19a). Invoking this model, the authors suggest that amelioration of insulin resistance, with diet, weight loss, or pharmacotherapy, may be more important to the reduction of cardiovascular risk in certain hypertensive patients than blood pressure control per se (19a).

Thus, the development of type II diabetes often is preceded by a protracted period of insulin resistance manifested as the "metabolic syndrome" of obesity, dyslipidemia, and hypertension (20). Abdominal obesity and hypertriglyceridemia may be particularly early markers of the syndrome and represent a readily detectable indicator of risk for diabetes (20). Interventions during the phase of insulin resistance, particularly supervised weight loss, may both mitigate the cardiovascular risk of the syndrome and prevent its evolution into diabetes.

There is now definitive evidence in type I diabetes (20a) and strongly suggestive evidence in type II diabetes (21) that meticulous control of serum glucose levels to within the physiologic range delays the development of complications. There is consensus that nutritional management is an essential component in efforts to achieve and maintain good glycemic control. Other goals of dietary therapy include regulation of serum lipids, weight control, and targeted management of incipient or advancing complications and concomitants of diabetes, such as hypertension, renal insufficiency, and coronary artery disease.

Although essential to the optimal management of diabetes, nutritional interventions are only rarely sufficient. Judicious combinations of dietary/lifestyle and pharmacologic treatment are generally indicated. Sulfonylureas increase insulin production; α-glucosidase inhibitors such as acarbose delay glucose absorption; biguanides such as metformin reduce hepatic gluconeogenesis; and thiazolidinediones such as troglitazone enhance peripheral insulin receptor sensitivity. Each class of medication, alone and in combination with others as well as insulin, offers distinct advantages and disadvantages.

Excellent reviews of pharmacotherapy are available (22–25).

Diet

The dietary management of diabetes has varied considerably over the course of the past century. The mainstay of treatment in the early decades of this century was carbohydrate restriction. Dietary fat intake was high to compensate for low caloric intake from carbohydrate. The role of carbohydrate restriction entered its modern era with the development of the glycemic index by Jenkins et al. (26). The glycemic index uses a slice of white bread as a reference standard, with a value of 100, and indicates the postprandial rise in serum glucose (and consequently insulin) for fixed portions of specified foods. However, as shown in Table 10.1, the glycemic index does not provide information that is readily translated into clinical advice. Common perceptions about the simple sugar content of foods does not allow one to predict the glycemic response evoked, as exemplified by the relatively low glycemic index of ice cream and the high glycemic index of certain fruits and vegetables. Similarly, variations in the glycemic responses to different polysaccharides are minimal when these sugars are consumed in the context of a meal. Consequently, attention has turned increasingly to overall meal and diet composition.

Foods with a high glycemic index, such as pasta and bread, need not elicit a postprandial spike in glucose and insulin, if such an effect is blunted by other foods consumed concurrently. Foods rich in soluble fiber (see Chapter 1 and Section IIIE) are particularly effective at attenuating such a response. There is some evidence that the distribution of foods may be as important as their glycemic index in the glucose and insulin responses they evoke. Comparing identical diets distributed as either three daily meals or multiple daily snacks, Jenkins and colleagues (27) reported that frequent snacking or "nibbling" resulted in significant reductions in insulin release.

TABLE 10.1. *Glycemic index of common foods*

Food group	Food	Glycemic index
Breads	White bread[a]	100
	Whole wheat bread	99
	Pumpernickel	78
Cereal products	White rice	83
	Spaghetti	66
	Barley	31
	Bulgur wheat	65
	Cornflakes	119
	Shredded wheat	97
	Oatmeal	85
Fruit	Bananas	79
	Apples	53
	Oranges	66
	Grapes	62
	Cherries	32
	Raisins	93
Vegetables	Boiled potato	81
	Baked potato	135
	Corn	87
	Peas	74
	Carrots	133
	Yams	74
	Parsnips	141
Legumes	Lima beans	115
	Baked beans	60
	Chick peas	49
	Red lentils	43
	Peanuts	19
Dairy products	Milk	49
	Yogurt	52
	Ice cream	52
Sugar	Sucrose	86

[a] Reference standard.
Adapted from Jenkins DJA, Jenkins AL. The glycemic index, fiber, and the dietary treatment of hypertriglyceridemia and diabetes. *J Am Coll Nutr* 1987;6:11–17.

The principal goals of nutritional management of diabetes are to maintain a normal or near-normal serum glucose level, to prevent or reverse lipid abnormalities, and to thereby mitigate the potential complications of diabetes. Nutritional management of insulin resistance, if identified as such before the advent of diabetes, is aimed at the prevention of progression to diabetes. Insulin resistance is apt to be detected as the insulin resistance syndrome, alternatively known as the metabolic syndrome, or syndrome X, characterized by obesity (especially central obesity; see Chapter 5), hypertension, and hypertriglyceridemia (28). The combination of elevated serum triglycerides and obesity may be an early indication of insulin resistance (29); postprandial hypertriglyceridemia may be an even earlier indicator.

A mainstay of dietary management of both type II diabetes mellitus in the overweight patient and of insulin resistance is weight loss. Clear clinical benefit of even modest weight loss has been demonstrated (4). There is widespread consensus that restriction of total dietary fat intake is supportive of weight loss efforts, despite the proliferation of fad diets, some high in fat, purported to advance this cause (4).

Dietary guidelines for the management of diabetes have evolved over the twentieth century in light of advances in understanding of nutritional physiology and in an effort to synthesize recommendations for health promotion and disease management apt to pertain simultaneously to individual patients. As of 1986, dietary guidelines for diabetes management were made to resemble the recommendations of the American Heart Association, partly due to the correspondence of heart disease and diabetes in the population. These guidelines have since been modified to accommodate the variable needs and responses of individual patients to nutritional interventions (4).

In general, the protein intake recommended for healthy adults, approximately 0.8 g/kg/day, is appropriate in both insulin-resistant states and in diabetes. Protein restriction may be indicated if renal insufficiency develops (see Chapter 11), but protein restriction to prevent the development of renal insufficiency is not clearly indicated. Excessive protein intake may accelerate the development of renal insufficiency, however. Popular books advocating high-protein diets for weight loss and control of insulin release (30–33) are of dubious merit for healthy individuals and are to be avoided in the management of diabetes.

Although most authorities support maintenance of protein intake in the range from 10% to 20% of energy, opinions vary regarding the optimal distribution of calories between carbohydrate and fat (4). The recent standard recommendation had been to restrict total dietary fat to 30% or less of calories, with saturated fat restricted to less than 10% of calories. Dietary fat restriction in diabetes, resulting in relatively high carbohydrate intake, has been associated with dyslipidemia, specifically hypertriglyceridemia and low high-density lipoprotein (HDL) (4). This experience has led to interest in liberalized fat intake, with attention to the source of fat calories. The substitution of monounsaturated fatty acids for carbohydrate in the diet has been found to improve glycemic control, while lowering triglycerides, raising HDL, and preserving low-density lipoprotein (LDL) levels (34,35). High carbohydrate intake apparently increases serum triglycerides by stimulating increased hepatic synthesis of VLDL particles (36,37) rather than by inhibiting the activity of lipoprotein lipase or hepatic lipase. Elevated triglycerides in turn may exacerbate insulin resistance both by stimulating insulin release and by interfering with insulin action (28,38).

However, studies by Garg and colleagues comparing the effects of diets high in monounsaturated fat to those high in carbohydrate may have biased outcomes in favor of monounsaturated fats by either keeping fiber content the same (34) or equal in proportion to carbohydrate intake (35) between groups. The lipid perturbations seen with high carbohydrate intake may be due, in part or in whole, to ingestion of processed carbohydrate with relatively low fiber content. In a randomized trial, Milne and colleagues (39) found both glycemic and lipid control to be comparably, favorably influenced by either a high-carbohydrate, high-fiber diet, or a diet in which monounsaturated fat was substituted for carbohydrate. Similarly, Luscombe and colleagues (40) found both a high monounsaturated-fat diet and a high-carbohydrate diet with low glycemic index to be superior to a high glycemic index, high-carbohydrate diet with regard to HDL levels; with regard to other outcomes, all three diets were comparable. Of note, subjects in this study all consumed at least 30 g per day of fiber. Heilbronn and colleagues (41) reported data emphasizing the importance of energy restriction in efforts to improve metabolic indices in obese type II diabetics.

In general, when a diabetic patient has elevated LDL, or if weight loss is indicated, restriction of fat below 30% of total energy is appropriate. Priorities for nutritional management will depend in part on whether management of diabetes, other cardiac risk factors, or established cardiovascular disease is the priority. Patients in whom the LDL is normal but who have elevated triglycerides and VLDL generally will benefit from improved glycemic control, which in turn may be produced by weight loss, again suggesting a benefit of fat restriction. If weight loss is achieved in such patients and lipid abnormalities persist, restriction of carbohydrate and liberalized fat intake may be warranted.

The literature on diabetes suggests 10% or less of total energy from saturated fat, approximately 10% from polyunsaturated fat, and up to 20% from monounsaturated fat (4). However, other lines of evidence (see Chapters 5 and 40) suggest that maximal metabolic and cardiovascular benefit may be achieved with restriction of saturated and trans fat in combination to below 10% of energy and preferably below 5%; allocation of between 10% and 15% of calories to polyunsaturated fat, but with a 1:4 or higher ratio of n-3 to n-6 fatty acids; and allocation of approximately 15% of calories to monounsaturated fat. Such a pattern is enhanced further by ensuring that the 50% or more of calories from carbohydrate are derived predominantly from complex carbohydrates with an abundance of fiber, especially soluble fiber. Diets with as much as 50 g per day of fiber have been well tolerated, although they typically require a period of gradual acclimation. Diets high in complex carbohydrate have been shown to elicit metabolic responses that favor efficient glucose utilization and disposal. Thus, high dietary carbohydrate accompanied by high fiber intake may be particularly beneficial. Whereas

high-carbohydrate, low-fiber diets may elevate triglycerides, high-fiber diets generally lower both fasting and postprandial triglycerides. Further research will be required to elucidate the relative advantages and disadvantages, with regard to weight regulation, glycemic control, lipid metabolism, and cardiovascular risk, of diets varying in fat and carbohydrate composition (42).

Exchange lists are a useful, if potentially tedious, tool in dietary management of diabetes. The lists, published at intervals by the American Dietetic Association, generally represent collaborations between the American Dietetic Association and the American Diabetes Association. Foods are grouped by category, with serving sizes that provide comparable amounts of energy and each class of macronutrient indicated. Thus, foods within a category may be substituted or "exchanged" for one another with preservation of a particular nutritional composition for that meal or day. A particular emphasis is generally placed on the quantity and quality of carbohydrate ingested (43). The range of foods included on the lists supports compliance with dietary recommendations over a wide range of dietary options. The general approach to exchange list use calls for estimating the appropriate number of total daily calories; dividing those calories into macronutrient classes; and establishing how many calories from each class of macronutrient should be consumed each day. Pi-Sunyer and colleagues (44) recently reported results of a randomized, multicenter trial in which consistent use of exchange lists was as effective as a prepared meal program in improving a range of pertinent outcome measures in type II diabetic men and women. The most recent iteration of the exchange lists was published in 1995 and can be purchased off the American Dietetic Association web site (www. eatright.org).

The management of diabetes varies to some degree with the circumstances of care for a particular patient. Diabetes management in children must incorporate attention to the maintenance of appropriate growth and invariably should be a collaboration between one or more clinicians (pediatrician or family practitioner and endocrinologist) and a dietitian. Pregnancy induces a sharp decline in insulin requirements during the first trimester, due to glucose uptake by embryo and placenta. Insulin requirements rise markedly in the third trimester, due to high counterregulatory hormone levels. The management of diabetes during pregnancy should best involve obstetrician, endocrinologist, and dietitian. The maintenance of strict glycemic control during pregnancy, both in established and gestational diabetes, is crucial to a good pregnancy outcome and requires intensive and multidisciplinary care. Although complicated by cravings and aversions and increased energy requirements, the principles of nutritional management of diabetes during pregnancy are essentially the same as those applied under other conditions.

Hypoglycemia is a potential complication of tight glycemic control in diabetes. Recent evidence suggests that combination of foods with varying glycemic indices can mitigate the risk of hypoglycemia (45). A nutrition bar, containing sucrose, protein, and cornstarch, results in a "triphasic" glucose release and may be helpful to hypoglycemia-prone diabetics (45).

Glycemic Index

The glycemic index, developed by Jenkins and colleagues (26,46), characterizes the postprandial glucose response to various foods relative to white bread. The area under the postprandial glucose curve for a test food is divided by the area under the curve for white bread with an equal amount of carbohydrate, and multiplied by 100 to establish the glycemic index for the test food. Complex carbohydrate containing starch initially was thought to induce less of a rise in postprandial glucose than simple carbohydrate, but this has been refuted. The glycemic index of foods is unpredictable on the basis of the complexity of their carbohydrate content, as shown in Table 10.1 (47), as it is influenced

by fiber content, processing, and the ratio of amylose to amylopectin (48). Jenkins and Jenkins (47) suggested that dietary fiber may serve as a surrogate measure of the glycemic index of foods, with high fiber content, particularly soluble fiber, lowering the glycemic response. Noteworthy is that sucrose has a lower glycemic index than white bread, carrots, baked potato, and lima beans. Bantle and colleagues (49) studied healthy individuals, as well as type I and type II diabetics, and found virtually no differences in glycemic or insulin responses to test meals containing fixed amounts of total carbohydrate as glucose, fructose, sucrose, potato starch, or wheat starch. The authors interpreted their data to indicate that sucrose consumption in the context of balanced meals need not be restricted in diabetes other than under specific circumstances, such as during intentional weight loss. In general, the weight of evidence indicates that the sucrose content of the diet is not a reliable indicator of glycemic control, and sucrose restriction in diabetes is not specifically indicated to control the serum glucose (50).

A recent study reported by Liljeberg et al. (51) suggests why the glycemic indices of individual foods may be of limited utility in the overall control of glucose metabolism. The investigators found that varying the fiber content of breakfast altered the glucose response to foods with a high glycemic index at lunch in a group of healthy subjects (51).

Nutrients and Nutriceuticals

Fructose

Fructose (see Chapter 1), referred to as fruit sugar, is a monosaccharide that does not require insulin for its metabolism. Fructose intake reduces postprandial glucose relative to other sugars and starches, but it has been associated with increased levels of LDL (52). Fructose restriction in diabetes is not indicated, but substitution of fructose for sucrose does not appear to confer benefit and is not recommended.

Sweeteners

Nutritive sweeteners, including corn syrup, honey, molasses, and fruit juice concentrates, appear to offer no advantage to sucrose in the management of diabetes. Nonnutritive sweeteners (see Chapter 38), such as aspartame and saccharin, confer sweetness without calories and do not raise serum glucose. Such sweeteners may be of some benefit in efforts to control serum glucose and facilitate or maintain weight loss.

Fiber

A daily intake of approximately 30 g of dietary fiber from a variety of food sources is recommended to the general public for health promotion and in the management of diabetes. There is evidence that soluble fiber in particular may be of benefit in controlling both glucose and lipid levels in diabetes (53,53a). However, the levels of fiber intake required to achieve significant improvements in fasting and postprandial glucose levels have been considered too high for practical application. In a study of men with type II diabetes, Anderson and colleagues (54) reported significant improvements in both serum lipids and glucose with twice daily psyllium totaling 10 g, for a period of 8 weeks. Of note, our Paleolithic ancestors were thought to have consumed nearly 100 g of fiber daily, and this pattern persists among rural peoples in the developing world (55). Fruits, oats, barley, and legumes are particularly good sources of soluble fiber (see Section IIIE). Fiber intake of up to 40 g per day is advocated by the American Diabetes Association; average fiber intake by US adults ranges between 12 and 18 g per day.

Ethanol

Ethanol consumption independent of other food intake can result in hypoglycemia by transiently interfering with hepatic gluconeogenesis. Therefore, diabetics, particularly those treated with insulin or sulfonylureas, should be advised to consume alcohol only with food. Excessive alcohol intake may contribute to hypertriglyceridemia and deterioration of glucose control. Moderate alcohol intake in diabetes is generally without known adverse effects. The potential cardiovascular benefits of moderate alcohol consumption are discussed in Chapter 6.

Chromium

Chromium is established as an essential nutrient, with roles in lipid and carbohydrate metabolism. Known to function as an insulin cofactor, chromium may bind to a carrier molecule and thereby activate insulin receptor kinase (56). Chromium may stimulate expression of insulin receptors in skeletal muscle as well (57). Evidence of improved glycemic control with chromium supplementation has been reported (58). Daily supplementation with 200 μg per day (or as much as 8 μg/kg/day) is apparently safe and potentially beneficial.

Vanadium

Vanadium is an ultratrace element. Evidence of a potentially therapeutic role in disorders of glucose metabolism has been reported (59). A recent review of vanadium suggests potential benefit as a cofactor in insulin metabolism in both type I and type II diabetes (60). The therapeutic window for inorganic vanadium is very narrow. Efforts to improve the safety of vanadium are proceeding concurrently with research into its mechanisms of action. Until further progress is made in each of these endeavors, therapeutic applications of vanadium cannot be recommended.

n-3 Fatty Acids (Fish Oil)

Fish oil is used in the treatment of refractory hypertriglyceridemia, typically when treatment with fibric acid derivatives is incompletely effective. A meta-analysis by Friedberg and colleagues (61) indicates that fish oil consistently lowers triglycerides by as much as 30%, with no untoward effects on glucose control in diabetes. The same analysis revealed a modest elevation of LDL in response to fish oil therapy. The authors conclude that fish oil may be an appropriate means of managing the dyslipidemia commonly seen in diabetes. There is some evidence to suggest that n-3 fatty acids stimulate hepatic gluconeogenesis and thereby can degrade glycemic control. Thus, their role in routine diabetes management remains uncertain.

CLINICAL HIGHLIGHTS

The literature guiding management of diabetes is voluminous, complex, and evolving. Placed in the context of nutritional principles pertinent to the management of related conditions, including obesity, cardiovascular disease, hypertension, and renal insufficiency, a cohesive approach to the dietary management of both insulin resistance and diabetes emerges.

For the majority of diabetic patients, weight loss and maintenance are mainstays of clinical management. Complex topics in their own right (see Chapters 5, 39, and 41), weight loss and maintenance are best achieved by restriction of nutrient energy in combination with consistent exercise. Both weight loss and exercise have demonstrated benefit in control of diabetes and its sequelae. Restriction of nutrient energy generally requires restriction of dietary fat due to its energy density. In conjunction with efforts at weight control, diabetes warrants attention to all three classes of macronutrients. Protein intake generally should be maintained at or near 0.8 g/kg/day, with restrictions below this level as required with the advent of renal insufficiency (see Chapter 11). Although controversies persist regarding optimal levels of carbohydrate and fat, the literature on this and other topics supports a carbohydrate intake of approximately 55–60% of calories, with fat comprising 25% to 30%. Carbohydrate should be

complex, and perhaps even more importantly, should provide at least 30 g per day of fiber, preferably more. Sources of soluble fiber, of particular metabolic benefit, include fruits, grains, and legumes. The combination of saturated and trans fat ideally should be restricted to below 5%, and certainly below 10%, of total calories, although the ubiquity of trans fat in processed foods makes this a particular challenge. Although benefits of n-3 fatty acids remain uncertain, other lines of evidence support allocating 10% to 15% of total calories to polyunsaturated fat in a 1:4 ratio of n-3 to n-6. The remaining 10% to 15% of calories should be allocated to monounsaturated fat. Exchange lists, available from the American Dietetic Association, may be of use to both clinician and patient in efforts to translate such guidelines into actual dietary practice. Consultation of a dietitian should be routine in diabetes care and should facilitate the development of meal plans to accommodate clinical recommendations.

Multivitamin/mineral supplementation can be argued on general principles and may be of benefit in diabetes. Additional supplements of vitamins C (500 mg per day) and E (400 IU per day) may be of benefit in the mitigation of sequelae. Chromium is well established as a cofactor in insulin metabolism, and daily supplementation with 200 μg per day (or as much as 8 μg/kg/day) is apparently safe and beneficial.

Weight control, physical activity, and adjustments of both macronutrient and micronutrient intake should be judiciously combined with carefully selected pharmacotherapy to optimize the control and clinical outcomes of diabetes.

REFERENCES

1. Lillioja S, Mott D, Howard B, et al. Impaired glucose tolerance as a disorder of insulin action. *N Engl J Med* 1988;318:1217–1225.
2. Atkinson M, Ellis T. Infants diets and insulin-dependent diabetes: evaluating the "cows' milk hypothesis" and a role for anti-bovine serum albumin immunity. *J Am Coll Nutr* 1997;16:334.
3. Vaarala O, Knip M, Paronen J, et al. Cow's milk formula feeding induces primary immunization to

insulin in infants at genetic risk for type 1 diabetes. *Diabetes* 1999;48:1389–1394.

4. Horton E, Napoli R. Diabetes mellitus. In: Ziegler E, Filer FJ, eds. *Present knowledge in nutrition*, 7th ed. Washington, DC: ILSI Press, 1996:445–455.

5. Lebovitz H. Type 2 diabetes: an overview. *Clin Chem* 1999;45:1339–1345.

6. Moller D, Bjorbek C, Vidal-Puig A. Candidate genes for insulin resistance. *Diabetes Care* 1996; 19:396–400.

7. 7. Neel J. Diabetes mellitus: A "thrifty" genotype rendered detrimental by "progress"? *Am J Human Genet* 1962;14:353–362.

8. Neel J. The "thrifty genotype" in 1998. *Nutr Rev* 1999;57:s2–s9.

9. Joffe B, Zimmet P. The thrifty genotype in type 2 diabetes: an unfinished symphony moving to its finale? *Endocrine* 1998;9:139–141.

10. Fox C, Esparza J, Nicolson M, et al. Is a low leptin concentration, a low resting metabolic rate, or both the expression of the "thrifty genotype"? Results from Mexican Pima Indians. *Am J Clin Nutr* 1998; 68:1053–1057.

11. Sharma A. The thrifty-genotype hypothesis and its implications for the study of complex genetic disorders in man. *J Mol Med* 1998;76:568–571.

12. Spelsberg A, Manson J. Physical activity in the treatment and prevention of diabetes. *Comprehens Ther* 1995;21:559–564.

13. Colditz GA, Willett WC, Rotnitzky A, et al. Weight gain as a risk factor for clinical diabetes mellitus in women [see comments]. *Ann Intern Med* 1995;122: 481–486.

14. Ford E, Williamson D, Liu S. Weight change and diabetes incidence: findings from a national cohort of US adults. *Am J Epidemiol* 1997;146:214.

15. Lazarus R, Sparrow D, Weiss S. Temporal relations between obesity and insulin: longitudinal data from the normative aging study. *Am J Epidemiol* 1998; 147:173–179.

16. Moller D, Flier J. Insulin resistance-mechanisms, syndromes, and implications. *N Engl J Med* 1991; 325:938–948.

17. Lillioja S, Mott D, Spraul M, et al. Insulin resistance and insulin secretory dysfunction as precursors of non-insulin-dependent diabetes mellitus. *N Engl J Med* 1993;329:1988–1992.

18. Pimenta W, Mitrakou A, Jensen T, et al. Insulin secretion and insulin sensitivity in people with impaired glucose tolerance. *Diabet Med* 1996;13: s33–s36.

19. Reaven GM, Lithell H, Landsberg L. Hypertension and associated metabolic abnormalities—the role of insulin resistance and the sympathoadrenal system. *N Engl J Med* 1996;334:374–381.

19a. Cowen R. Seeds of protection. *Sci News* 1990; 137:350–351.

20. Grundy S. Hypertriglyceridemia, insulin resistance, and the metabolic syndrome. *Am J Cardiol* 1999; 83:25F–29F.

20a. The Diabetes Control and Complications Trial Research Group. The effect of intensive treatment of diabetes on the development and progression of long-term complications in insulin-dependent diabetes mellitus. *N Engl J Med* 1993;329:977–986.

21. Clark CM Jr., ed., Adlin V, co-ed. Risks and benefits of intensive management in non-insulin-dependent diabetes mellitus. The Fifth Regenstrief Conference. *Ann Intern Med* 1996;124[1 Pt 2]:81–186.

22. Rao S, Bethel M, Feinglos M. Treatment of diabetes mellitus: implications of the use of oral agents. *Am Heart J* 1999;138:334–337.

23. Bailey C. Insulin resistance and antidiabetic drugs. *Biochem Pharmacol* 1999;58:1511–1520.

24. Ginsberg H, Plutzky J, Sobel B. A review of metabolic and cardiovascular effects of oral antidiabetic agents: beyond glucose-level lowering. *J Cardiovasc Risk* 1999;6:337–346.

25. DeFronzo R. Pharmacologic therapy for type 2 diabetes mellitus. *Ann Intern Med* 1999:281–303.

26. Jenkins D, Wolever T, Taylor R, et al. Glycemic index of foods: a physiological basis for carbohydrate exchange. *Am J Clin Nutr* 1981;34:362–366.

27. Jenkins D, Wolever T, Vuksan V, et al. Nibbling versus gorging: metabolic advantages of increased meal frequency. *N Engl J Med* 1989;321:929–934.

28. DeFronzo R, Prato SD. Insulin resistance and diabetes mellitus. *J Diabetes Complicat* 1996;10:243–245.

29. Zavaroni I, Bonora E, Pagliara M, et al. Risk factors for coronary artery disease in healthy persons with hyperinsulinemia and normal glucose tolerance. *N Engl J Med* 1989;320:702–707.

30. Steward H, Bethea M, Andrews S, et al. *Sugar busters! Cut sugar to trim fat.* New York: Ballantine Books, 1998.

31. Heller R, Heller R. *The carbohydrate addict's lifespan program.* New York: Plume, 1998.

32. Atkins DR. *Atkins' new diet revolution.* New York: M. Evans & Company, Inc., 1999.

33. Sears B, Lawren B. *Enter the zone.* New York: Regan Books, 1995.

34. Garg A, Bonamome A, Grundy S, et al. Comparison of a high-carbohydrate diet with a high-monounsaturated-fat diet in patients with non-insulin-dependent diabetes mellitus. *N Engl J Med* 1988;319: 829–843.

35. Garg A, Bantle J, Henry R, et al. Effects of varying carbohydrate content of diet in patients with non-insulin-dependent diabetes mellitus. *JAMA* 1994; 271:1421–1428.

36. Blades B, Garg A. Mechanisms of increase in plasma triacylglycerol concentrations as a result of high carbohydrate intakes in patients with non-insulin-dependent diabetes mellitus. *Am J Clin Nutr* 1995:996–1002.

37. Lewis G, Steiner G. Acute effects of insulin in the control of VLDL production in humans. *Diabetes Care* 1996;19:390–393.

38. Boden G, Tataranni P, Baier L, et al. Role of lipids in development of noninsulin-dependent diabetes mellitus: lessons learned from Pima Indians. *Lipids* 1996;31:s267–s270.

39. Milne R, Mann J, Chisholm A, et al. Long-term comparison of three dietary prescriptions in the treatment of NIDDM. *Diabetes Care* 1994;17:74–80.

40. Luscombe N, Noakes M, Clifton P. Diets high and low in glycemic index versus high monounsaturated fat diets: effects on glucose and lipid metabolism in NIDDM. *Eur J Clin Nutr* 1999;53:473–478.

41. Heilbronn L, Noakes M, Clifton P. Effect of energy

restriction, weight loss, and diet composition on plasma lipids and glucose in patients with type 2 diabetes. *Diabetes Care* 1999;22:889–895.

42. Roche H. Dietary carbohydrates and triacylglycerol metabolism. *Proc Nutr Soc* 1999;58:201–207.

43. Gillespie S, Kulkarni K, Daly A. Using carbohydrate counting in diabetes clinical practice. *J Am Diet Assoc* 1998;98:897–905.

44. Pi-Sunyer F, Maggio C, McCarron D, et al. Multicenter randomized trial of a comprehensive prepared meal program in type 2 diabetes. *Diabetes Care* 1999;22:191–197.

45. Bell S, Forse R. Nutritional management of hypoglycemia. *Diabetes Educ* 1999;25:41–47.

46. Jenkins D, Wolever T, Jenkins A. Starchy foods and glycemic index. *Diabetes Care* 1988;11:149–159.

47. Jenkins D, Jenkins A. The glycemic index, fiber, and the dietary treatment of hypertriglyceridemia and diabetes. *J Am Coll Nutr* 1987;6:11–17.

48. Morris K, Zemel M. Glycemic index, cardiovascular disease, and obesity. *Nutr Rev* 1999;57:273–276.

49. Bantle J, Laine D, Castle G, et al. Postprandial glucose and insulin responses to meals containing different carbohydrates in normal and diabetic subjects. *N Engl J Med* 1983;309:7–12.

50. American Dietetic Association. Nutrition recommendations and principles for people with diabetes mellitus. *Diabetes Care* 1994;17:519–522.

51. Liljeberg H, Akerberg A, Bjorck I. Effect of the glycemic index and content of indigestible carbohydrates of cereal-based breakfast meals on glucose tolerance at lunch in healthy subjects. *Am J Clin Nutr* 1999;69:647–655.

52. Bantle J, Swanson J, Thomas W, et al. Metabolic effects of dietary fructose in diabetic subjects. *Diabetes Care* 1992;15:1468–1476.

53. Nuttall F. Dietary fiber in the management of diabetes. *Diabetes* 1993;42:503–508.

53a. Chandalia M, Garg A, Lutjohann D, et al. Beneficial effects of high dietary fiber intake in patients with type 2 diabetes mellitus. *N Engl J Med* 2000; 342:1392–1398.

54. Anderson J, Allgood L, Turner J, et al. Effects of psyllium on glucose and serum lipid responses in men with type 2 diabetes and hypercholesterolemia. *Am J Clin Nutr* 1999;70:466–473.

55. Eaton S, Konner M. Paleolithic nutrition revisited: a twelve-year retrospective on its nature and implications. *Eur J Clin Nutr* 1997;51:207–216.

56. Vincent J. Mechanisms of chromium action: low-molecular-weight chromium-binding substance. *J Am Coll Nutr* 1999;18:6–12.

57. McCarty M. Complementary measures for promoting insulin sensitivity in skeletal muscle. *Med Hypotheses* 1998;51:451–464.

58. Anderson R. Chromium, glucose intolerance and diabetes. *J Am Coll Nutr* 1998;17:548–555.

59. Thompson K. Vanadium and diabetes. *Biofactors* 1999:43–51.

60. Badmaev V, Prakash S, Majeed M. Vanadium: a review of its potential role in the fight against diabetes. *J Altern Complement Med* 1999:273–291.

61. Friedberg C, Janssen M, Heine R, et al. Fish oil and glycemic control in diabetes. A meta-analysis. *Diabetes Care* 1998;21:494–500.

BIBLIOGRAPHY

See "Sources for All Chapters."

Anderson JW, Geil PB. Nutritional management of diabetes mellitus. In: Shils ME, Olson JA, Shike M, eds. *Modern nutrition in health and disease,* 8th ed. Philadelphia, PA: Lea & Febiger, 1994.

Henry RR. Glucose control and insulin resistance in non-insulin-dependent diabetes mellitus. *Ann Intern Med* 1996;124:97–103.

Scheen AJ, Lefebvre PJ. Insulin action in man. *Diabetes Metab* 1996;22:105–110.

Cunningham JJ. Micronutrients as nutriceutical interventions in diabetes mellitus. *J Am Coll Nutr* 1998; 17:7–10.

Brand-Miller JC, Colagiuri S. Evolutionary aspects of diet and insulin resistance. *World Rev Nutr Diet* 1999; 84:74–105.

Grundy SM. The optimal ratio of fat-to-carbohydrate in the diet. *Annu Rev Nutr* 1999;19:325–341.

Gilden JL. Nutrition and the older diabetic. *Clin Geriatr Med* 1999;15:371–390.

Rosenbloom Al, Joe JR, Young RS, et al. Emerging epidemic of type 2 diabetes in youth. *Diabetes Care* 1999;22:345–354.

Lipkin E. New strategies for the treatment of type 2 diabetes. *J Am Diet Assoc* 1999;99:329–334.

Hansen BC. Obesity, diabetes, and insulin resistance: implications from molecular biology, epidemiology, and experimental studies in humans and animals. *Diabetes Care* 1995;18:A2–A9.

Lillioja S. Impaired glucose tolerance in Pima Indians. *Diabetic Med* 1996;13:s127–s132.

Feskens EJ, Loeber JG, Kromhout D. Diet and physical activity as determinants of hyperinsulinemia: the Zutphen elderly study. *Am J Epidemiol* 1994;140:350–360.

Wood FC, Bierman EL. Is diet the cornerstone in management of diabetes? *N Engl J Med* 1986;315:1224–1227.

Fernandez-Real J, Ricart W. Insulin resistance and inflammation in an evolutionary perspective: the contribution of cytokine genotype/phenotype to thriftiness. *Diabetologia* 1999;42:1367–1374.

Shulman GI. Cellular mechanisms of insulin resistance in humans. *Am J Cardiol* 1999;84:3J–10J.

Heilbronn LK, Noakes M, Clifton PM. Effect of energy restriction, weight loss, and diet composition on plasma lipids and glucose in patients with type 2 diabetes. *Diabetes Care* 1999;22:889–895.

Mathers JC, Daly ME. Dietary carbohydrates and insulin sensitivity. *Curr Opin Clin Nutr Metab Care* 1998; 1:553–557.

11

Diet and Renal Disease

INTRODUCTION

The development of renal insufficiency often occurs in the context of other chronic conditions, such as hypertension, diabetes, or atherosclerosis, for which dietary management is both essential and of proved benefit. Thus, there is a clear, albeit indirect, role for diet in the prevention of renal insufficiency. With the advent of renal insufficiency of varying severity, diet is of fundamental importance, both in efforts to delay disease progression and to maintain lean body mass. Despite an extensive literature on the role of dietary protein in the development and progression of renal disease, clear support for a single management strategy is lacking. However, evidence that a range of dietary interventions may contribute to the preservation of renal function at varying levels of compromise is increasingly abundant and compelling. The clinician managing patients with, or at risk for, renal insufficiency is obligated to attend to nutrition as well as pharmacotherapy.

Approximately 12% of Americans form renal calculi at some time during their lives. The incidence of stone formation in the urinary tract, and particularly in the upper urinary tract, has been rising over recent decades in westernized countries. The epidemiology of renal calculi is strongly suggestive of an important role for diet. The preponderance of stones contains calcium, and evidence of a link between diet and calcium oxalate stones is convincing.

OVERVIEW

Diet

The two leading causes of renal insufficiency in the United States are diabetes mellitus and hypertension (1–3). There is decisive evidence that diet influences the course of diabetes (see Chapter 10) and accruing evidence that diet may enhance, and at times substitute for, pharmacotherapy in the management of hypertension (see Chapter 7). Both diabetes and hypertension may be preventable by appropriate dietary interventions (see Chapters 7 and 10). Atherosclerosis contributes to the development of renal dysfunction and may be retarded or prevented by dietary management (see Chapter 6). The prevention of risk factors for renal disease may prevent renal insufficiency, although evidence for this is lacking. Lack of evidence cannot be considered the same as negative evidence, however. In the absence of evidence, intuition would suggest that if the course and natural history of the leading causes of renal insufficiency are substantially modifiable by dietary means (see Chapters 7 and 10), then so, too, is the development of renal insufficiency. Consequently, the primary care practitioner may play a role in the prevention of renal insufficiency by optimal dietary management of the principal risk factors.

Evidence for the direct influence of diet, particularly dietary protein, on renal function is less clear. With advanced renal insufficiency, dietary protein restriction is common practice (4) and may serve to slow progressive deterioration of renal function (5–7). However, protein restriction may contribute to nutritional deficiencies, with net adverse effects (7).

The evidence supporting protein restriction in established renal insufficiency is convincing (5). Evidence for the value of protein restriction in the primary prevention of renal insufficiency and the age-related decline in glomerular filtration rate (GFR) is inconclusive (8,9). There is evidence that restriction of phosphorus is beneficial in renal insufficiency, particularly in the prevention of secondary hyperparathyroidism (10,11).

Malnutrition of multifactorial origin often develops in patients with advanced renal insufficiency (12–14), and the primary care provider should play a role in ensuring nutritional adequacy. Just as renal insufficiency may contribute to malnutrition, malnutrition, particularly protein deficiency, tends to lower GFR and impair the concentrating ability of the kidney. These effects are reversible in healthy individuals with the restitution of adequate protein intake.

The complexity of dietary management in advanced renal disease generally requires the input of the primary care provider, a specialized dietitian, and the nephrologist (15). Nutritional management in the setting of acute renal failure may influence prognosis; a benefit of essential amino acid supplementation is suggested in particular (16,17). The diet plan in such a setting should result from a collaborative effort involving, minimally, the nephrologist and nutritionist.

Once symptomatic or clinically overt renal insufficiency has developed, the generalist almost invariably will, and should, be guided by a nephrologist in tailoring both dietary and pharmacotherapy. Such patients are obviously at risk of azotemia (the accumulation of nitrogenous waste) as well as specific micronutrient abnormalities, including phosphorus retention; impaired absorption of calcium and iron; and deficiencies of vitamin B_6, folate, vitamin C, and active vitamin D.

The benefits of protein restriction have been convincingly demonstrated for patients with a GFR below 70 mL/1.73 m^2/min. The standard diet for such patients restricts total protein to approximately 0.55 to 0.60 g/kg/day, with not less than 35 g/kg being of high biologic value (i.e., rich in essential amino acids; see Chapters 3 and 4). For patients with severe renal insufficiency (i.e., GFR below 25), commercial supplements of amino acids, keto acids, and hydroxy acids are available. Patients in this group apparently benefit from protein restriction down to 0.28 g/kg/day. The putative benefits of keto or hydroxy acid supplements is that the amino group, which contributes to the body's nitrogen load, is eliminated. Keto and hydroxy acids can be converted into their respective amino acids endogenously. Although such diets help preserve renal function, they are unpalatable, which makes compliance difficult and increases the risk of nutritional deficiencies (18,19). Whether a delay in the need for dialysis is sufficient cause to implement such dietary therapy will depend on an individual patient's preference.

Although a variety of endocrine abnormalities are associated with renal insufficiency and uremia, most are beyond the scope of this discussion. Most relevant to dietary management is the development of both insulin resistance and elevations of glucagon, which both contribute to impaired glucose metabolism. The dietary approach to impaired glucose metabolism and insulin resistance is discussed in Chapter 10. The basic approaches are unchanged in the setting of renal failure, although medication doses may need adjustment.

Most patients with end-stage renal disease experience some catabolism while on dialysis. Malnutrition, or at least the risk of it, is considered common in this population. Wasting is due both to increased metabolic demand, perhaps due to dialysis, as well as poor intake due to malaise, anorexia, and the unpalatability of a therapeutic diet. Poor nutritional status in dialysis patients appears, not surprisingly, to be a poor prognostic sign.

In a study of 93 subjects, Young et al. (20) found significant elevations in serum leptin levels in malnourished patients with renal failure, suggesting a role for leptin in the malnutrition seen in renal insufficiency.

Patients with chronic renal insufficiency or on dialysis generally require a diet restricted in protein, sodium, and phosphorus, and supplemented with fat-soluble vitamins. The fat intake of uremic patients should be similar to that of nonuremic patients and modified as required to manage comorbid conditions. Carbohydrate intake should represent the majority of calories in these as in other patient groups, with a preponderance of complex carbohydrates rich in fiber.

Nephrolithiasis

The incidence of nephrolithiasis has been increasing sharply over recent decades in affluent populations, and the risk correlates strongly with per capita expenditure on food. Consumption of animal products in particular seems to confer increased susceptibility (21). Observational studies reveal a strong protective effect of vegetarianism, despite a high intake of oxalate in vegetables (21). Dietary protein, generally of animal origin, has a calciuric effect that correlates well with risk of stone formation, although susceptibility to this effect of protein appears to be highly individualized. High dietary protein intake has an acidifying effect, which diminishes urinary citrate excretion; proximal tubular reuptake of citrate is enhanced by acidosis. In the urine, citrate chelates calcium, inhibiting crystallization. The oncotic properties of protein may result in increased GFR, which in turn increases the filtered load of calcium. Protein also increases urinary urate, which is a risk factor for both calcium and uric acid stones (22). Thus, protein intake is presumed to raise the risk of nephrolithiasis by a variety of mechanisms (23). Observational data suggest the relative risk of stone formation associated with high protein intake to be about 1.3 (22). However, negative results of a randomized trial of protein restriction may indicate that increased fluid intake is of greater importance in the prevention of recurrent stones (24).

Mechanisms have been identified by which both dietary fiber and magnesium might protect against stone formation. Insoluble fiber binds calcium in the gastrointestinal tract, potentially reducing urinary calcium. Of greater importance is a positive association between total fiber intake and urinary citrate (25). Magnesium in the urine inhibits the precipitation of calcium oxalate crystals (21). Evidence of clinical benefit specific to fiber or magnesium is lacking at present.

Whereas an increase in total fluid intake appears to be protective, the effects of different fluids may be variable (26,27). Beverages containing caffeine and alcohol may lower risk in particular, as both of these substances oppose antidiuretic hormone (ADH) and result in dilute urine (26). Recent (1998) data suggest that grapefruit juice in particular may increase risk (27). Available data have suggested a positive association between soda intake and stones (27). Solute in urine is diluted as urine volume rises, and hydration is protective against stone formation. Ingestion of not less than 250 mL of fluid every 4 hours, leading to a urine volume not below 1,400 mL per day, is protective (21).

Definitive data to support a benefit of dietary modification from controlled trials are lacking to date, and pharmacotherapy is not much better substantiated. Patients with nephrolithiasis, a high dietary intake of protein, oxalate, and/or salt, and less than optimal fluid intake are likely to benefit from dietary therapy. Therapeutic goals should include restriction of dietary protein intake to not more than 1 g/kg/day and of sodium to not more than 100 mEq per day; avoidance of foods rich in oxalate; and consumption of not less than 2 L per day of fluid (21).

Nutrients and Nutriceuticals

Water

In general, thirst is a reliable indicator of appropriate fluid intake. Adequate intake of water is important in the preservation of renal function over time and in the avoidance of nephrolithiasis. An intake of water equal to urine output plus 500 mL is an appropriate guideline as GFR decreases and thirst becomes a less reliable index.

Protein

Studies in humans indicate that protein restriction slows the progression of renal failure once insufficiency has developed. The ingestion of protein increases renal blood flow and GFR, perhaps through the influence of glucagon. Consequently, the restriction of protein intake reduces glomerular flow and pressures. Protein restriction slows the accumulation of urea, creatinine, and other guanidine compounds in renal insufficiency. Studies have examined the benefits of low-protein, low-phosphorus diets with protein intake of approximately 0.4 to 0.6 g/kg/day, as well as very-low-protein diets with protein intake of approximately 0.28 g/kg/day. The very-low-protein diets are supplemented with essential amino acids or keto acids. Essential amino acids can be manufactured in the body from their keto or hydroxy acid analogues, in which the amino group is replaced. The removal of the amino group results in a smaller nitrogen load to the patient. There is preliminary evidence to date that such diets confer greater benefits than standard protein-restricted diets. There is less convincing evidence that protein restriction can prevent the onset of renal insufficiency in healthy individuals. The average protein intake in the United States exceeds recommendations and may contribute to the age-related decline in GFR. In a recent review of paleolithic nutrition, Eaton and colleagues (28) suggest that our ancestors adapted to high protein intake and that such a diet is unlikely to be harmful in the context of healthy activity levels and overall dietary pattern. However, extrapolation from the prehistoric diet may or may not be appropriate in this instance, given a markedly

shorter life expectancy until, in evolutionary context, quite recently.

In general, it is difficult to demonstrate the efficacy of preventive measures when disease is not common, does not develop rapidly, or lacks good surrogate markers. Perhaps for these reasons, or perhaps because healthy kidneys do not benefit from protein restriction, the benefits of protein restriction have only been convincingly demonstrated for a GFR below 70 mL/1.73 m^2/min.

Dietary Fat

Atherosclerosis affects the renal arteries and is associated with renal insufficiency. The contribution of diabetes and hypertension to atherosclerotic disease of the renal vasculature is one means by which these conditions lead to renal failure. Consequently, dietary interventions to prevent or reverse atherosclerosis may be valuable in preventing or reversing renovascular disease (see Chapter 6). A high intake of dietary fat and cholesterol may contribute to high glomerular pressures. Filtration is impaired by the deposition of foam cells in the glomerular endothelium. Optimal dietary fat intake in the prevention of renal disease is the same as for the prevention of other atherosclerotic conditions. There is evidence that while total, saturated, and trans fat intake should be restricted, intake of polyunsaturated fat, especially n-3 fatty acids, should be liberalized. Through their effects on eicosanoid and prostaglandin metabolism, polyunsaturated fats may indirectly improve glomerular pressures and function.

Phosphorus

Phosphorus restriction, independent of protein restriction, appears to retard the progression of renal insufficiency (10,11). Evidence for the isolated effects of phosphorus restriction in humans is limited, as diets low in phosphorus tend to be low in protein, and vice versa. Calcification of soft tissue is related to the double product (serum levels of phosphorus and calcium, multiplied), and the deposition of calcium in renal tissue is reduced by low phosphorus intake. Serum creatinine rises as the content of calcium in renal tissue rises.

Phosphorus intake should be restricted to 5 to 10 mg/kg/day in patients with a GFR below 25. As renal function declines, phosphate binders may be necessary to control serum levels. In patients with severe renal insufficiency, aluminum toxicity may result from the use of aluminum-containing phosphate binders; this problem can be avoided by using calcium-based binders. The advantages of phosphorus restriction must be weighed against the risks of malnutrition resulting from an unpalatable diet.

A generous intake of dietary phosphate may inhibit the formation of calcium stones by reducing calcium levels in urine (23); however, data from controlled trials are lacking. Further, dietary sources of phosphate and protein tend to correspond, making dietary phosphate supplementation an impractical recommendation for prevention of nephrolithiasis given the prevailing view that dietary protein should be restricted.

Calcium

The restriction of protein and phosphorus in renal insufficiency often requires avoidance of dairy foods, lowering calcium intake, often down to 300 to 400 mg per day. Calcium absorption generally is impaired due to low levels of active vitamin D. Therefore, supplemental calcium often is necessary to raise the intake of uremic patients to the recommended 1,200 to 1,600 mg per day. Patients with renal insufficiency are at risk of osteopathy; chronic ingestion of calcium carbonate may serve to provide needed calcium for skeletal metabolism while compensating for metabolic acidosis. Supplementation of calcium should be deferred if phosphorus levels are elevated, as the double product of calcium and phosphorus correlates with the rate of soft tissue calcification and stone forma-

tion. Vitamin D supplementation is generally indicated as well.

Given that most renal calculi are composed partly or predominantly of calcium, restriction of calcium intake as a means to prevent recurrence has been advocated as an intuitively reasonable precaution. Most of the available evidence now suggests, however, that restriction of dietary calcium results in negative calcium balance, while reducing urinary calcium only slightly and conferring no appreciable protection against stone formation. Calcium in the gastrointestinal tract may complex with oxalate, reducing oxalate absorption and thereby oxalate in the urine. Thus, restriction of dietary calcium may "paradoxically" increase the risk of calcium stone formation and thus is to be discouraged (21). Evidence to date suggests that a high intake of dietary calcium may protect against stone formation, but the implications of this association for calcium in the form of supplements is uncertain (22).

Oxalate

The precipitation of calcium oxalate from urine is much more sensitive to oxalate than to calcium. Although oxalate levels are influenced by dietary intake, the preponderance of urinary oxalate is derived from metabolism. The metabolism of several amino acids contributes to oxalate levels in blood and urine; therefore, oxaluria correlates directly with protein intake. Ascorbate can be converted to oxalate. Although this generally contributes minimally to oxalate levels, ingestion of megadoses of vitamin C can lead to hyperoxaluria in susceptible individuals (21). Pyridoxine serves as a cofactor in glycine metabolism, and its deficiency leads to excess oxalate production. Patients with a tendency to produce calcium oxalate stones may benefit from restriction of dietary oxalate in the context of other generally advisable dietary modifications. Among foods known to be high in oxalate are chocolate, peanuts, and spinach (22). Limited data on the bioavailability of oxalate from various dietary sources complicate assessment of the role of dietary oxalate on the risk of nephrolithiasis (22).

Ascorbate

The metabolic conversion of ascorbate to oxalate suggests that high levels of vitamin C intake might increase the risk of stone formation. Urinary oxalate has been shown to increase with high ascorbate intake, but the effects on actual stone formation have not been confirmed. Thus, the risk of nephrolithiasis with an intake of vitamin C above 5 g per day may be increased, and this should be considered by those favoring megadosing of this nutrient. No change in the risk of nephrolithiasis attributable to vitamin C was seen in the Health Professionals Follow-up Study (29).

Pyridoxine

Vitamin B_6 is a cofactor in the metabolism of glyoxalic acid. High levels of B_6 intake reduce the production of oxalate by shifting the pathway toward the production of glycine. Pyridoxine has been used to treat oxalate stones with anecdotal success. A dose of 100 mg per day has been recommended, although further study is indicated (30). In the Health Professionals Follow-up Study, variation in pyridoxine intake did not emerge as a predictor of risk of nephrolithiasis (29).

Uric Acid

Uric acid excretion in urine rises with the intake of dietary protein. The solubility of urate is reduced in an acid environment, and ingestion of amino acids acidifies the urine. Thus, purine ingestion both increases urinary urate and reduces its solubility. Hyperuricosuria contributes to the development of calcium oxalate stones by saturating urine and reducing the threshold for solute precipitation. Thus, relative protein restriction may protect against urate and calcium oxalate stone formation by reducing urinary urate.

Magnesium

Magnesium tends to accumulate in renal failure, and intake should generally not exceed 200 mg per day. The restriction of protein and phosphorus generally serves to restrict magnesium intake as well, so that it need not be selectively targeted.

Sodium

Sodium filtration and reabsorption are both reduced with renal insufficiency; therefore, restriction of sodium intake in renal insufficiency generally is not necessary. As renal insufficiency becomes more severe, sodium restriction to between 1,000 and 3,000 mg per day is appropriate. The role of sodium restriction in the primary prevention of renal disease is unclear, although sodium restriction may play a role in the control of blood pressure (see Chapter 7).

Dietary sodium is related to urinary sodium levels, and calcium excretion in urine tends to parallel that of sodium. High salt intake is associated with calciuria and an increased risk for calcium oxalate stone formation (21). Stone formation may result in part from enhanced susceptibility to a calciuric effect of dietary sodium (22).

Potassium

Tubular secretion of potassium tends to rise as GFR falls, preserving the ability to excrete potassium in the urine. When urine output falls below 1,000 mL per day, potassium accumulation becomes a threat. In such patients, the restriction of potassium intake to approximately 70 mEq per day is recommended.

Potassium intake appears to be protective against stone formation. Foods rich in potassium, specifically fruits and vegetables, tend to be alkaline and naturally low in sodium. Alkalinity increases urinary citrate, reducing the risk of stone formation. The degree to which potassium provides specific protection versus the degree to which it is simply a marker of a low-protein, low-sodium diet is uncertain (22).

Iron

Iron deficiency is relatively common in chronic renal insufficiency and generally is multifactorial. Iron supplementation is appropriate. A multivitamin designed for use in renal insufficiency usually is adequate. Provision of adequate iron is necessary for exogenous erythropoietin to be effective.

Zinc

There is increasing evidence of widespread zinc deficiency in the US population. In renal insufficiency, zinc absorption may be impaired and deficiency is likely to be more significant. Zinc supplementation in renal insufficiency is appropriate. A multivitamin designed for use in renal insufficiency generally is adequate.

Aluminum

Patients with renal insufficiency are at risk of aluminum toxicity if aluminum-based products are used to bind phosphate. Calcium-based phosphate binders are recommended for this reason.

Vitamin D

Renal insufficiency is associated with decreased activation of 25-hydroxycholecalciferol to 1,25-dihydroxycholecalciferol in the kidney. Vitamin D supplementation is generally indicated; a preparation that does not depend on activation by renal hydroxylation is essential.

Water-soluble Vitamins

Dietary restrictions and anorexia place patients with chronic renal insufficiency at risk for deficiencies of B vitamins, folate, and vitamin C. Ascorbate can be metabolized to oxalate, and this conversion is accelerated by renal insufficiency. Therefore, excessive ascorbate ingestion in renal failure can lead

to stone formation; an intake of 60 mg per day should generally not be exceeded. A multivitamin providing the RDA/DRI (Recommended Dietary Allowance/Dietary Reference Intake) of other water-soluble vitamins is appropriate.

Carnitine

Carnitine is a nitrogenous compound abundant in meat and dairy products. Carnitine serves as a cofactor in the mitochondrial oxidation of long-chain fatty acids and buffers the pool of coenzyme A by accepting an acyl group in transfer (31). Carnitine requirements are met by carnitine ingestion and by carnitine biosynthesis, which occurs in the liver and kidneys. Renal insufficiency may lead to carnitine deficiency by several mechanisms, including reductions in both intake and manufacture. Hypertriglyceridemia is common in renal failure and may be due in part to impairments in fatty acid oxidation resulting from carnitine deficiency. There is suggestive evidence that carnitine supplementation may be effective in the treatment of hypertriglyceridemia associated with renal insufficiency (31). To date, reliable data characterizing carnitine balance in uremic and dialysis patients are lacking (31). Carnitine has been used in attempts to lower triglycerides; ameliorate muscle cramps and other symptoms associated with dialysis; improve exercise tolerance; enhance responsiveness to erythropoietin; and improve cardiac function (31). The current evidence is inconclusive for any of the outcomes. Doses and routes of administration have varied in studies; an oral dose of 2 g per day is reasonable (31). Use of carnitine should be considered experimental until additional evidence becomes available.

Fiber

Dietary fiber confers comparable benefits in renal failure patients as in other patients (see Chapter 3). In addition, insoluble fiber may lower serum nitrogen by enhancing fecal nitrogen excretion. High-fiber foods often contain protein of low biologic value, as well as potassium and phosphorus, which may be poorly tolerated by patients with advanced renal insufficiency.

Sucrose

Sucrose and other simple sugars in the diet impede tubular reabsorption of calcium and thereby increase calciuria. Although this provides a mechanism for a contribution of dietary sugar to stone formation, this association has not been demonstrated in studies controlling for other aspects of diet (22).

L-Arginine

There is animal evidence that dietary supplementation with L-arginine prevents age-related decline in renal function (33). The mechanism for this effect is unclear and may be independent of nitric oxide (33). Implications for humans are as yet uncertain.

TOPICS OF SPECIAL INTEREST

Nephrotic Syndrome

Evidence suggests that the combination of dietary protein restriction and angiotensin-converting enzyme inhibitor therapy reduces protein loss in urine without contributing to declines in serum albumin levels. In general, restriction of total protein intake to 0.7 g/kg/day is recommended, with 1.0 g of high-biologic value protein each day for each gram of protein lost in the urine. Nephrotic patients generally require vitamin and mineral supplementation, as they are subject to vitamin D and trace element deficiencies. Hypoalbuminemia results from albumin losses in urine in the nephrotic syndrome, increased albumin catabolism in chronic ambulatory peritoneal dialysis, and reduced synthetic capacity in hemodialysis (33).

Acute Renal Failure

The dietary management of acute renal failure is not well delineated in the literature and depends in part on the etiology. When acute renal failure occurs in the context of shock, parenteral nutrition may be necessary. The composition of parenteral nutrition formulas should be developed with the input of a nephrologist and hospital-based dietitian. Excellent references on total parenteral nutrition in general and renal failure in particular are available (see Chapter 24). Enteral feeding should be maintained whenever possible (see Chapter 24).

Acute renal failure is characterized by a state of accelerated protein breakdown that is not suppressed by provision of exogenous protein. The causes of excessive protein catabolism are diverse, including uremic toxins, insulin resistance, metabolic acidosis, inflammatory mediators, and dialysis-related losses of nutrients, as well as declines in the multiple metabolic and endocrine functions of the kidney (34). Patient requirements for dietary protein vary and are influenced more by the illness causing renal failure and by the extent of hypercatabolism, as well as by the type and frequency of renal replacement therapy, than by the renal insufficiency (34). Intake of 1 g per kilogram of body weight per day is appropriate for noncatabolic patients. Hypercatabolic patients undergoing continuous renal replacement therapy may require up to 1.5 g amino acids per kilogram of body weight per day to maintain nitrogen balance (36). A dietitian should be involved in the management of all patients with acute renal failure that persists for more than several days.

Dialysis

Patients on dialysis tend to lose protein and would benefit from protein intake in the range from 1.0 to 1.2 g/kg/day. In peritoneal dialysis, protein losses are particularly high, and intakes of 1.2 to 1.3 g/kg/day are encouraged. In all dialysis patients, 50% of ingested protein should be of high biologic value (see Chapter 3). To maintain lean body mass, nonobese patients with renal insufficiency, whether or not on dialysis, generally should receive an energy intake of approximately 35 kcal/kg/day.

Peritoneal dialysis is conducive to weight gain and obesity in patients receiving adequate nutrition, due to the delivery of 400 to 700 kcal per day in dialysate glucose. Obesity may contribute to the development and progression of renal insufficiency and should be avoided due to its other associated hazards as well (see Chapter 5). Obesity in renal failure is managed as for other patients.

Hyperlipidemia

Elevations of both low-density lipoprotein and very-low-density lipoprotein occur commonly in renal disease. Management is as described in Chapter 6.

CLINICAL HIGHLIGHTS

There is no conclusive evidence that diet can prevent renal insufficiency. However, the established role of diet in the prevention and management of hypertension, diabetes, atherosclerosis, and obesity suggests that successful primary prevention of renal disease may be achieved by limiting the size of the at-risk population. In renal insufficiency, judicious and tailored restriction of protein and phosphorus is indicated, along with supplementation of vitamins and trace elements. Other aspects of the optimal renal diet are similar to the diet recommended for general health promotion (see Chapter 40). The dietary management of patients with severe renal insufficiency should be a collaborative effort involving the patient and the patient's family, the primary care provider, the nephrologist, and a dietitian with expertise in renal disease. An effort to delay dialysis in a patient with advanced renal insufficiency may involve complex dietary management, including the use of keto or hydroxy acids to minimize nitrogen load while preserving adequate nutriture.

The contribution of dietary pattern to the risk of renal stone formation is uncertain, but it appears to be considerable. The difference in rates of stone formation between developed and developing countries suggests that nephrolithiasis may be largely preventable through dietary modification. A diet rich in fruits and vegetables and restricted in animal protein and sodium is indicated. Fluid intake leading to a urine output of not less than 2 L per day is likely protective. Relative restriction of dietary oxalate and purines is a prudent precaution in patients with a history of stone formation. A generous intake of magnesium, potassium, and fiber may be beneficial and is indicated for purposes of health promotion (see Chapter 40). Dietary calcium should not be restricted and actually may be protective. Dietary measures to prevent renal calculi are largely consistent with recommendations for health promotion and may be advocated to patients both with and without a history of nephrolithiasis. Grapefruit juice should be avoided on the basis of available evidence. Patients with recurrent stone disease despite prudent dietary interventions are candidates for pharmacotherapy and/or more tailored nutritional therapies. Potassium citrate has shown promise in the management of recurrent calcium stones. Thiazide diuretics are indicated for hypercalciuria and allopurinol for hyperuricosuria (27) associated with stone formation. The use of high-dose pyridoxine for oxalate stones may be effective and apparently is safe.

REFERENCES

1. Brazy PC. Epidemiology and prevention of renal disease. *Curr Opin Nephrol Hypertens* 1993;2:211.
2. Mogensen CE. Preventing end-stage renal disease. *Diabet Med* 1998;15[Suppl 4]:S51–S56.
3. Valderrabano F, Gomez-Campdera F, Jones EH. Hypertension as cause of end-stage renal disease: lessons from international registries. *Kidney Int Suppl* 1998;68:S60.
4. Maroni BJ, Mitch WE. Role of nutrition in prevention of the progression of renal disease. *Annu Rev Nutr* 1997;17:435.
5. Levey AS, Adler S, Caggiula AW, et al. Effects of dietary protein restriction on the progression of advanced renal disease in the Modification of Diet in Renal Disease Study. *Am J Kid Dis* 1996;27:652.
6. Holm EA, Solling K. Dietary protein restriction and the progression of chronic renal insufficiency: a review of the literature. *J Intern Med* 1996;239:99.
7. Burgess E. Conservative treatment to slow

deterioration of renal function: evidence-based recommendations. *Kidney Int Suppl* 1999;70:S17–S25.

8. Brandle E, Sieberth HG, Hautmann RE. Effect of chronic dietary protein intake on the renal function in healthy subjects. *Eur J Clin Nutr* 1996;50:734.

9. Kimmel PL, Lew SQ, Bosch JP. Nutrition, ageing and GFR: is age-associated decline inevitable? *Nephrol Dial Transplant* 1996;11[Suppl 9]:85–88.

10. Martinez I, Saracho R, Montenegro J, et al. The importance of dietary calcium and phosphorus in the secondary hyperparathyroidism of patients with early renal failure. *Am J Kidney Dis* 1997;29: 496–502.

11. Hsu CH. Are we mismanaging calcium and phosphate metabolism in renal failure? *Am J Kidney Dis* 1997;29:641–649.

12. Lusvarghi E, Fantuzzi AL, Medici G, et al. Natural history of nutrition in chronic renal failure. *Nephrol Dial Transplant* 1996;11[Suppl 9]:75.

13. Dobell E, Chan M, Williams P, et al. Food preferences and food habits of patients with chronic renal failure undergoing dialysis. *J Am Diet Assoc* 1993; 93:1129.

14. Oldrizzi L, Rugiu C, Maschio G. Nutrition and the kidney: how to manage patients with renal failure. *Nutr Clin Pract* 1994;9:3–10.

15. Beto JA. Which diet for which renal failure: making sense of the options. *J Am Diet Assoc* 1995;95:898–903.

16. Alvestrand A. Nutritional aspects in patients with acute renal failure/multiorgan failure. *Blood Purif* 1996;14:109.

17. Kopple JD. The nutrition management of the patient with acute renal failure. *J Parenteral Enteral Nutr* 1996;20:3–12.

18. Mitch WE. Dietary protein restriction in chronic renal failure: nutritional efficacy, compliance, and progression of renal insufficiency. *J Am Soc Nephrol* 1991;2:823–831.

19. Kopple JD, Levey AS, Greene T, et al. Effect of dietary protein restriction on nutritional status in the Modification of Diet in Renal Disease Study. *Kidney Int* 1997;52:778.

20. Young GA, Woodrow G, Kendall S, et al. Increased plasma leptin/fat ratio in patients with chronic renal failure: a cause of malnutrition? *Nephrol Dial Transplant* 1997;12:2318–2323.

21. Goldfarb S. Diet and nephrolithiasis. *Annu Rev Med* 1994;45:235.

22. Curhan GC, Curhan SG. Dietary factors and kidney stone formation. *Comprehens Ther* 1994;20:485–489.

23. Parivar F, Low RK, Stoller ML. The influence of diet on urinary stone disease. *J Urol* 1996;155:432.

24. Hiatt RA, Ettinger B, Caan B, et al. Randomized controlled trial of a low animal protein, high fiber diet in the prevention of recurrent calcium oxalate kidney stones. *Am J Epidemiol* 1996;144:25.

25. Jaeger P. Prevention of recurrent calcium stones: diet versus drugs. *Miner Electrolyte Metab* 1994;20: 410.

26. Curhan GC, Willett WC, Rimm EB, et al. Prospective study of beverage use and the risk of kidney stones. *Am J Epidemiol* 1996;143:240.

27. Curhan GC, Willett WC, Speizer FE, et al. Beverage use and risk for kidney stones in women. *Ann Intern Med* 1998;128:534.

28. Eaton SB, Eaton SB III, Konner MJ. Paleolithic nutrition revisited. A twelve-year retrospective on its nature and implications. *Eur J Clin Nutr* 1997; 51:207.

29. Curhan GC, Willett WC, Rimm EB, et al. A prospective study of the intake of vitamins C and B$_6$, and the risk of kidney stones in men. *J Urol* 1996; 155:1847.

30. Goldenberg RM, Girone JAC. Oral pyridoxine in the prevention of oxalate kidney stones [Letter]. *Am J Nephrol* 1996;16:552–553.

31. Brass EP. Carnitine in renal failure. In: Kopple JD, Massry AG, eds. *Nutritional management of renal disease.* Baltimore: Williams & Wilkins, 1997.

32. Reckelhoff JF, Kellum JA Jr., Racusen LC, et al. Long-term dietary supplementation with L-arginine prevents age-related reduction in renal function. *Am J Physiol* 1997;272[6 Pt 2]:R1768.

33. Kaysen GA. Albumin turnover in renal disease. *Miner Electrolyte Metab* 1998;24:55.

34. Druml W. Protein metabolism in acute renal failure. *Miner Electrolyte Metab* 1998;24:47.

BIBLIOGRAPHY

See "Sources for All Chapters."

Broquist HP. Carnitine. In: Shils ME, Olson JA, Shike M, eds. *Modern nutrition in health and disease*, 8th ed. Philadelphia: Lea & Febiger, 1994.

Kopple JD, Massry AG, eds. *Nutritional management of renal disease.* Baltimore: Williams & Wilkins, 1997.

Kopple JD. Nutrition, diet, and the kidney. In: Shils ME, Olson JA, Shike M, eds. *Modern nutrition in health and disease*, 8th ed. Philadelphia: Lea & Febiger, 1994.

Klahr S. Renal disease. In: Ziegler EE, Filer LJ, eds. *Present knowledge in nutrition*, 7th ed. Washington, DC: ILSI Press, 1996.

12

Diet and Cancer

INTRODUCTION

The link between diet and cancer, supported by *in vitro,* animal, and epidemiologic studies, is convincing. Decisive intervention trials are lacking, however, because of the protracted time course of carcinogenesis and a lack of reliable surrogate markers in most cases. Most reviews of diet and cancer cite the work of Doll and Peto (1) and suggest that a third or more of all cancer is related to nutritional factors and potentially preventable by nutritional means. Dietary factors may influence cancer initiation, promotion, and progression.

As is the case for atherogenesis, the process of carcinogenesis may be affected both favorably and unfavorably by micronutrients and macronutrients. Initiation is linked to mutagenic micronutrients, whereas cancer promotion and progression appear to be more meaningfully associated with macronutrient intake. Procarcinogens in the diet include heterocyclic amines and polycyclic aromatic hydrocarbons that result from pyrolysis (i.e., charring); nitrosamines used or produced in the curing of meats; naturally occurring contaminants, such as aflatoxin B-1; naturally occurring chemicals in plants; and chemicals added to the food supply as a result of agricultural practices and food handling.

Whereas mutagenicity has been demonstrated for most of these factors, there are of course no intervention trials demonstrating carcinogenicity directly in humans. Epidemiologic studies support an association between excess dietary fat intake and cancer incidence at a variety of sites. Diet may lead indirectly to cancer by contributing to obesity. Associations with cancer incidence have been suggested for both dietary protein and simple sugars.

The most convincing evidence for the cancer-fighting potential of diet supports a high total intake of fruits and vegetables. Less extensive evidence suggests that energy restriction may reduce cancer risk, either directly or indirectly through effects on body fat. Dietary fiber and a variety of micronutrients to be discussed are thought to reduce cancer risk. Nutrients with antioxidant properties are thought to be particularly important in cancer prevention by neutralizing the carcinogenic potential of free radicals ingested or generated by metabolism and radiation exposure.

In clinical practice, dietary recommendations may be made based on available evidence to reduce both aggregate cancer risk and the risk of certain specific cancers. Similar recommendations are indicated for secondary prevention. In general, dietary recommendations for cancer prevention are entirely consistent with recommendations for health promotion. As clinically overt cancer is invariably a catabolic process, nutritional support is important in the management and tertiary prevention of cancer.

OVERVIEW

Diet

Cancer as a pathologic category is diverse and complex, as is the literature associating carcinogenesis with diet. Numerous attempts have been made to review and summarize the pertinent literature (1–9), but none is truly comprehensive. The lack of readily measurable and modifiable risk factors for cancer renders the study of human carcinogenesis extremely difficult. Prospective interventions must rely on actual cancer or precancerous dysplasia as endpoints. Of necessity, such interventions are lengthy and large, and often prohibitively expensive. Further complicating the relationship between diet and cancer is the prevailing view that cancer is a nonthreshold risk. Therefore, establishing a dose–response relationship between any isolated dietary factor and cancer may prove daunting.

Despite the complexity of both cancer and nutritional epidemiology, there is considerable uniformity in published recommendations for prevention of cancer by dietary means (2,3). As summarized by the American Cancer Society in 1996, current guidelines for the dietary prevention of cancer include consumption of five or more servings of vegetables and fruits each day, along with a relative abundance of other plant-based foods such as cereals and grains; limitation of dietary fat intake, particularly saturated fat from animal sources; maintenance of weight within a "healthy" range; maintenance of physical activity; and limitation of alcohol intake (9).

Evidence in support of these recommendations derives principally from observational and retrospective studies, and is of varying strength with regard to specific cancers and specific aspects of diet (2). A mechanistic understanding of nutrients in the prevention of cancer is developing and should guide future studies and recommendations (10,11).

Diet and Specific Neoplasms

Colon Cancer

A link between diet and colon cancer risk would seem virtually intuitive, and indeed diet is thought to be one of the, if not the, most important modifiable risk factors (12).

Evidence of an inverse association between dietary fiber intake and the risk of colorectal cancer has been consistent overall and convincing (9). High intake of fruits and vegetables is associated with reduced risk, but the extent to which this is due to fiber or other nutrients is uncertain. A positive association has been reported for high intake of dietary fat and red meat, although these, too, tend to covary. Physical inactivity and obesity may increase risk.

Prospective data from the Nurses' Health Study demonstrate an association between animal fat consumption and colon cancer risk (13). The same study revealed no association between low-fat meats, specifically fish and skinless poultry, and colon cancer risk. A case-control study conducted by Neugut et al. (14) using patients with colorectal adenomatous polyps as cases demonstrated an increased risk of colon cancer among those in the highest quartile of saturated fat intake, red meat consumption, and total dietary fat. High consumption of fiber showed a strong protective effect (14). Fiber has been shown to prevent the induction of colon cancer in rats fed a "high-risk" diet (15).

Results of the Health Professionals Follow-up Study suggest an inverse association between physical activity and colon cancer risk, and an independent association between body mass index (BMI) and colon cancer risk. The association was even stronger for the waist-to-hip ratio than for BMI, suggesting that adiposity and fat distribution may influence colon cancer development (16). The hypothesis that calcium and dairy products rich in calcium reduce colon cancer risk was not supported by data from either the Health Professionals Follow-up Study or the Nurses' Health Study (17).

Data from the Iowa Women's Health Study, obtained prospectively over a 5-year period, demonstrated an inverse association between vegetable and fiber intake and colon cancer risk, although the associations were not statistically significant. A protective effect of garlic was reported in this study, but has not since been convincingly replicated (18).

Diet is thought to be one of the most potent determinants of colon cancer risk (12). High dietary fat intake is thought to influence colon cancer development through effects on bile acid production and bacterial flora (12). High fiber intake lowers risk by any of several possible mechanisms, including dilution of mutagens, reduction of gastrointestinal transit time, and alteration of pH.

In an innovative application of factor analysis, Slattery and colleagues (19) studied nearly 2,000 cases of colon cancer in comparison to 2,400 controls. They found that a "western"-style diet (with high intake of fat, cholesterol, and protein and a high BMI) was associated with significantly increased risk compared to other dietary patterns.

Recommendations supported by the weight of available evidence include a diet rich in vegetables and other plant-based foods, with a high intake of insoluble fiber. Consumption of red meat should be moderate, although there is no evidence implicating fish or poultry. Alcohol intake should be kept at moderate levels. To date, no convincing evidence supports micronutrient supplements as a specific strategy for preventing colon cancer (20,21).

Breast Cancer

Evidence linking dietary factors to breast cancer risk is based predominantly on a combination of animal studies, ecologic studies between and among populations, and retrospective studies within populations. Although some of the findings are consistent, they are best described as suggestive at this time. Prospective studies are on-going, including primary and secondary prevention studies (22).

The American Cancer Society recommends avoidance or limitation of alcohol intake, avoidance of obesity, maintenance of physical activity, and abundant intake of vegetables and fruits as means to lower breast cancer risk (9). The evidence is stronger for alcohol and obesity than for other aspects of diet. Most reviews over recent years offer similar advice, albeit with variable degrees of enthusiasm for the quality of evidence gathered to date (23–25).

In an effort to quantify the relationship between micronutrient intake and breast cancer risk, Kushi et al. (26) assessed the association between breast cancer incidence and intake of vitamins A, C, and E, retinol, and carotenoids among more than 34,000 women in the Iowa Women's Health Study. No protective effect was found for women with high intake of any of these nutrients. Some protective effect was noted for megadose supplements of vitamins C and A, but the associations did not reach significance (26). Similar results were reported from the Nurses' Health Study, where intake of vitamins C and E showed no association with breast cancer risk; vitamin A intake was inversely associated with risk in this study (27). The effectiveness of vitamin A supplementation is currently under evaluation in a prospective, randomized trial with prevention of a second primary breast cancer the outcome of interest (28).

Herbert and Rosen (29), comparing breast cancer incidence among 66 countries, used food intake and socioeconomic status (SES) data to develop predictive multivariable models. The strongest predictors of breast cancer risk in their study were total calories, total dietary fat, red meat, dairy, and alcohol. Fish and cereal products showed protective effects (29). The strength of association for dietary factors was commensurate with that for fertility; SES factors dropped out in multivariable models due to covariance with dietary and fertility factors. The biologic plausibility for a relationship between dietary fat intake and breast cancer is supported by prior literature (30–34).

Dorgan et al. (35) compared serum levels of carotenoids, retinol, selenium and α-tocopherol between 105 breast cancer cases and matched controls. Only lycopene emerged as significantly protective, whereas the trend for β-cryptoxanthin was favorable but did not reach statistical significance (35). Lycopene is found principally in tomatoes, whereas β-cryptoxanthin is found in tangerines, nectarines, oranges, peaches, papaya, and mango.

Evidence linking alcohol consumption to breast cancer risk has been fairly consistent, as recently reported in a meta-analysis by Smith-Warner et al. (36), Schatzkin et al. (37), and van den Brandt et al. (38). The pooled data suggest a relative risk of approximately 1.4 among moderate drinkers (30 to 60 g of ethanol per day; two to five drinks) compared with nondrinkers.

In a recent analysis of data from a large case-control study in Italy, Mezzetti et al. (39) suggest that modification of dietary antioxidant intake, body weight, alcohol consumption, and physical activity level could eliminate up to one third of breast cancers in the population studied.

The association between dietary fat intake and breast cancer risk is both controversial and complex. Animal studies and cross-cultural comparisons in humans suggest that total fat, saturated fatty acids, and ω-6 polyunsaturated fatty acids may increase breast cancer risk, whereas ω-3 polyunsaturated fatty acids and possibly monounsaturates decrease risk (23,40,41).

Data from recent case-control and observational cohort studies, however, have largely failed to corroborate such associations (42–45). Similar doubts have been cast on the relationship between adiposity and breast cancer risk (46). A recent case-control study found no significant effect of dietary fat intake during adolescence on subsequent risk of breast cancer (47).

A case-control study in Italy found an inverse association between intake of unsaturated fat and breast cancer, and a positive association for starch, although fat and vegetable intake were highly correlated (41). Thus, the dietary contributors to breast cancer risk may vary with population characteristics and prevailing dietary patterns. Complications in establishing a definitive link between dietary fat and breast cancer have been described (25).

Given the inconsistencies in evidence gathered to date, few definitive recommendations can be offered to women attempting to reduce breast cancer risk (48,49). The results from on-going and future prospective studies should be informative. In particular, results of the Women's Health Initiative, a randomized trial of dietary modification, including fat restriction, as primary prevention, and of the Women's Intervention Nutrition Study, a randomized trial of fat restriction in the prevention of breast cancer recurrence in women with resected, localized cancers (25), should prove important. A diet rich in fruits, vegetables, and grains, modest to no alcohol intake, and avoidance of excess meat, fat, calories, and obesity are consistent with recommendations for health promotion. Such recommendations may serve to reduce breast cancer risk as well (24,50).

Lung Cancer

As is widely known, tobacco is by far the most important modifiable risk factor for lung cancer. However, as only a minority of smokers develop cancer, there are likely to be other important exposures, as well as variability in genetic susceptibility (51). There has long been evidence of a protective effect of fruit and vegetable intake. The association of reduced risk with consumption of green and yellow vegetables has suggested a protective effect of β-carotene (51).

The results of randomized clinical trials to date have largely refuted the efficacy of β-carotene in cancer prevention. Specifically with regard to lung cancer, two negative trials are noteworthy. In the CARET trial, current smokers and asbestos-exposed workers had a statistically significant increase in risk of both incident lung cancer and lung cancer mortality when taking supplemental β-carotene as opposed to placebo (52). Similarly, β-carotene supplementation was associated with a higher incidence of lung cancer than placebo in the Alpha-Tocopherol, Beta-Carotene Cancer Prevention Study (53–55).

In a case-control study of lung cancer among nonsmoking women, Alavanja and colleagues (56) reported increased risk in association with red meat and dairy intake, and particularly total and saturated fat intake; a protective effect of vegetables was not seen. A case-control study among men in Sweden identified low vegetable intake and high milk consumption as lung cancer risk factors in a mixed group of smokers and nonsmokers (57). In a review of studies of lung cancer risk factors among nonsmoking women in China, the dietary factors reported to be most consistently associated with increased risk were low intake of vegetables and fruits, particularly vegetables and fruits rich in carotene and vitamin C (58).

A separate case-control study in Chinese women identified frequent consumption of fried food as a risk factor and frequent carrot consumption as protective (59). At least one case-control study in China demonstrated a decreased risk of lung cancer with increasing intake of meat as well as vegetables among men in a mining town (60). The discrepant findings with regard to red meat are likely due to variable population characteristics; red meat may be protective when diet is marginal and harmful when diet tends to be excessive. Alternatively, as yet unspecified confounders may account for the observed associations between meat consumption and lung cancer.

The results of a large cohort study conducted in Finland suggest that flavonoids, particularly quercetin, confer protection against cancer in general and lung cancer in particular. The primary source of flavonoids in the study population was apples (61). The results of this study were relatively unaffected by adjusting for intake of vitamins C and E and β-carotene.

The sum of available evidence supports recommendations to consume an abundance of fruits and vegetables. Recommendations to avoid meat or dairy, or to consume any particular micronutrient, cannot be made with confidence (9). However, restriction of meat and fat intake is indicated for general health promotion and may confer some benefit with regard to lung cancer as well (62).

Prostate Cancer

There is considerable interest in dietary and lifestyle risk factors for prostate cancer, but there is little definitive evidence to date. Ecologic and migrant studies suggest that the dietary patterns of industrialized countries, associated with high saturated fat and protein intake and relatively low intake of fruits and vegetables, contribute to increased risk (63). There is evidence of an increased risk in association with high intake of saturated fat from animal and dairy sources (64–66). However, fat intake was not predictive of risk in a recent case-control study in England, thought to be due in part to a high mean fat intake and a relatively narrow range (67). Based on the results of a case-control study in Sweden, Andersson and colleagues (68) suggest that the association between prostate cancer risk and dietary fat is eliminated by controlling for total energy intake. The discrepancies in the available literature may be interpreted as suggesting that intake of dietary fat or total energy, which is highly correlated with fat consumption, is among the factors contributing to population risk for prostate cancer, but that other important factors remain to be identified to further the risk among members of a population with high or low mean fat and energy intake.

A variety of micronutrients have been suggested to protect against prostate cancer, although for most the evidence is limited. However, as virtually all of the putatively protective nutrients are found in fruits and vegetables, the evidence is more convincing that fruit and vegetable intake may be protective (66). The evidence in support of a specific protective effect of tomatoes and/or their lycopene content raises the possibility that high fruit and vegetable intake is a marker of high tomato intake (63). Of note, whereas the incidence of clinically apparent prostate cancer varies markedly among populations, the incidence of latent cancer appears to be fairly consistent among diverse populations (69,70). This observation suggests that the role of dietary factors may be to inhibit or stimulate the promotion of microscopic tumor foci. Such inhibitory effects have been observed for fat-restricted and soy-supplemented diets in animals (69).

Preliminary evidence has suggested protective effects of vitamins D and E, but further study is required before a basis for recommendations is established (64). Recent data from the ATBC trial suggest that α-tocopherol may inhibit the transformation of clinically latent to clinically active prostate cancer. The same study showed a decrease in prostate cancer risk in nonalcohol drinkers receiving β-carotene, but an increased risk in drinkers (71,72). Like lycopene, β-carotene is concentrated in the prostate (73).

An inverse association between retinoid intake and prostate cancer risk has been reported fairly consistently. In contrast, intake of retinol has been positively associated with risk in several studies (64). Data from the Health Professionals Follow-up Study suggested an inverse association between prostate cancer risk and intake of lycopene, but not other carotenoids (74); a positive association between retinol and cancer risk was not seen. Recent studies suggesting a protective effect of lycopene have generated considerable interest (73). An association with lycopene was not seen in recent case-control studies (67,75). Further study of this nutrient in prospective studies is needed to provide more definitive evidence of benefit. As tomatoes are the highly predominant source of dietary lycopene, associations observed between lycopene intake and prostate cancer risk may pertain to some other nutrient in tomatoes (74).

Uncertainties about dietary factors in the etiology of prostate cancer are highlighted by a recent case-control study conducted in the United Kingdom, which revealed essentially no association with either fat or carotenoid intake (67). On-going trials, both case-control and cohort, should advance our understanding in the near future (70).

The difference in rates of clinically manifest prostate cancer in the United States and Japan has generated interest in the potential promotional effects of ω-6 fatty acids and inhibitory effects of ω-3 fatty acids. An *in vitro* study designed to test this hypothesis had negative results, demonstrating promotional effects of all fats (76).

Other Cancers

The principal risk factor for cancer of the esophagus appears to be tobacco exposure, but the effect is apparently promoted by alcohol (77). Fruit and vegetable intake is inversely associated with risk for esophageal cancer. An association with obesity has been suggested.

The link between alcohol consumption and gastric cancer risk is less clear. Epidemiologic studies suggest that risk is increased by high intake of salted, cured, smoked, and pickled foods (77), with salt apparently the dominant factor (78). High fruit and vegetable intake has been consistently associated with reduced risk of gastric cancer (77).

An ecologic study of populations in twenty-four European countries suggests that when total fat intake is high, fish and fish oil confer protection against both colorectal and breast cancers (79). The etiology of childhood cancers is poorly understood at present. An association between maternal consumption of cured meats containing *N*-nitroso compounds and brain tumor risk has been suggested (80). Recommendations to avoid such products are consistent with general dietary guidelines. Other specific recommendations to reduce the risk of childhood cancer cannot be made on the basis of available evidence.

Data from the Iowa Women's Health Study suggest that fat from animal sources, and a diet high in meat, may increase risk of non-Hodgkin's lymphoma (81); fruit consumption appeared to be protective.

A case-control study in Japan, where the incidence of pancreatic cancer is rising concurrently with lifestyle changes, suggests that a predominantly plant-based diet is protective, whereas meat consumption increases risk (82). The prevailing consensus is that fruits and vegetables are protective, whereas high intake of meat, fat, or both increases risk (83). Obesity is associated with increased risk (84). Obesity and adiposity have been associated with several tumors of hormonal tissues, including ovary, uterus, breast, and prostate. Obesity is thought to promote tumorigenesis by raising estrogen levels (9,84). Obesity also has been linked to renal cell cancer, particularly in women (85). In a case-control study, Davies and colleagues (86) found an association between the risk of testicular cancer and milk consumption, compatible with prior work suggesting an association with fat intake. A case-control study in Washington state suggests that fried food consumption may increase bladder cancer risk, whereas fruit, vitamin C from both diet and supplements, and multivitamin use may decrease risk (87).

Animal and *in vitro* studies implicate nitrates, nitrites, and *N*-nitroso compounds, but no definitive evidence is available in humans (88). In a concise summary of current evidence, Willett (2) made the following observations: cancer of the oral cavity is inversely associated with fruit and possibly vegetable intake, and positively associated with alcohol intake; esophageal cancer is inversely associated with fruit and vegetable intake, and positively associated with alcohol and hot drink consumption; gastric cancer is inversely associated with fruit and vegetable intake, is positively associated with salt intake, and may be positively associated with egg and total carbohydrate intake; pancreatic cancer risk may be reduced by fruit, vegetable and fiber intake, and increased by intake of alcohol, meat, protein, and carbohydrate; both endometrial and renal cancer are convincingly associated with obesity; and fruit and vegetable consumption appears to be at least weakly protective against most cancers studied. Summary recommendations of most agencies attempting to prevent cancer are consistent with these associations and include reduced fat intake; increased fruit, vegetable, and fiber intake; maintenance of body weight near ideal; and minimizing consumption of salt-cured, pickled and smoked foods, and alcohol (3).

NUTRIENTS AND NUTRICEUTICALS

The natural reductionist tendencies of western science are perhaps nowhere more evident, for good or for bad, than in efforts to elucidate the relationships between dietary constituents and cancer risk. As stated earlier, the weight of evidence clearly favors a diet rich in fruits and vegetables. Whether or not isolated nutrients found in plant foods can provide the benefits of a prudent dietary pattern is far from established. Nonetheless, a variety of nutrients and nutrient categories have received considerable attention in both the professional literature and lay press, and they are addressed briefly here.

Vitamin C

Despite long-standing interest in the potential for vitamin C to prevent cancer by virtue of its antioxidant properties, to date there is no convincing evidence that supplementation effectively prevents or treats cancer. High dietary intake of vitamin C is consistently associated with reduced cancer risk, but such intake invariably is associated with high fruit and vegetable consumption (89). The evidence regarding vitamin C supplementation is summarized in a Nutrient Reference Table in Section III.

Carotenoids

There are more than 600 carotenoids in nature, most of which are widespread in plants, lending pigment that functions in photoprotection and photosynthesis (90). Approximately 50 carotenoids are retinoids, moieties with varying vitamin A activity (91). The hypothesis that carotenoids in general may prevent cancer is based on associations between cancer risk and dietary intake patterns (92) and on a mechanistic rationale (93).

β-Carotene

Abundant in dark green, yellow, and orange fruits and vegetables, β-carotene is the most extensively studied of the carotenoids

Interest in the cancer-fighting properties of the nutrient derived from observational and ecologic studies. Intervention trials to date report consistently negative results, however, with β-carotene in supplement form increasing cancer risk in smokers in both CARET (52) and the ATBC trial (53). β-carotene has failed to reduce the development of colorectal adenomas in an intervention trial (94) and showed no benefit in a prospective study of prostate cancer (95). Results from these and other studies resulted in recommendations to avoid supplemental β-carotene, particularly in smokers, and have shifted interest to other carotenoids, alone or in combination with each other and unrelated antioxidants. The evidence regarding β-carotene supplementation is summarized in a Nutrient Reference Table in Section III.

Lycopene

Lycopene is the carotenoid responsible for the bright red color of tomatoes. It differs from other carotenoids in several respects. Lycopene lacks a ring structure; therefore, it cannot be converted to vitamin A. Because of its 11-carbon chain of conjugated double bonds, lycopene has exceptional antioxidant capacity. Lycopene may be protective against prostate cancer in particular, but no intervention trials have been conducted to date (96). The evidence regarding lycopene supplementation is summarized in a Nutrient Reference Table in Section III.

Vitamin E

Vitamin E, or α-tocopherol, is a lipid-soluble antioxidant. Like β-carotene, it has been studied in cancer prevention with largely disappointing results. The ATBC and CARET studies both included vitamin E and showed no significant benefit (52,53). In contrast to β-carotene, vitamin E appeared innocuous in these studies. There is currently interest in the role of vitamin E in combination with water-soluble antioxidants such as vitamin C in cancer prevention. Evidence supporting a role for vitamin E in cancer prevention is in

the aggregate unconvincing at present, but preliminary (97). The evidence regarding vitamin E supplementation is summarized in a Nutrient Reference Table in Section III.

Selenium

Selenium is an essential mineral with antioxidant properties. Studies in China, where soil is generally selenium poor, and the United States, where selenium deficiency is rare, suggest a possible role in cancer prevention (98). The evidence regarding selenium supplementation is summarized in a Nutrient Reference Table in Section III.

Fiber

Dietary fiber, a diverse group of indigestible components of plant cell walls, is thought to mediate cancer risk by several mechanisms (99). By increasing fecal bulk and reducing intestinal transit time, insoluble fibers may reduce the risk of colon cancer. Dietary fiber has shown inverse associations with colon cancer risk in both retrospective (100,101) and prospective studies (102). Wheat bran fiber has been shown to reduce bile acid excretion in patients with resected colon adenomas, suggesting an additional mechanism by which colon cancer risk may be reduced (103). However, recent data from the Health Professionals Follow-up Study failed to demonstrate an association between fiber intake and colon cancer risk (104). As the overall evidence on the effects of fiber supplementation rather than fiber from dietary sources is mixed at best, use of supplemental fiber to reduce colon cancer risk has been discouraged (105). A protective effect of soluble fibers and cellulose in breast cancer has been reported from a large case-control study (106). The weight of evidence favors a diet rich in both soluble and insoluble fibers found in fruits, vegetables, and whole grains. Evidence is insufficient to support supplementation as a means of reducing cancer risk (99). Soluble and insoluble fiber are discussed in Nutrient Reference Tables in Section III.

Other Nutrients

To date, no other micronutrients have been studied adequately to permit definitive recommendations regarding a role in cancer prevention in humans. However, a variety of substances are biologically plausible inhibitors of cancer and are supported in this role by preliminary evidence.

Allyl compounds, found in garlic, onion, chives, and leeks, demonstrate inhibition of tumor induction *in vitro* and are associated with reduced rates of cancer, particularly gastric cancer, in epidemiologic studies. Isothiocyanates, organic compounds distributed widely in plants and particularly abundant in cruciferous vegetables, appear to suppress carcinogen activation by the cytochrome P-450 system. Indole compounds, also abundant in cruciferous vegetables, demonstrate inhibition of carcinogenesis in mammary cell lines, possibly mediated by effects on estrogen. Flavonoids, organic antioxidants widely distributed in plants, may have cancer-fighting properties. This class of compounds includes flavones, flavonols, and isoflavones. Flavones found in citrus fruit have been shown to inhibit growth of malignant cells in tissue culture. Of the flavonols, quercetin has been most extensively studied and has been shown to inhibit growth of neoplastic cells.

Tea leaves used to prepare green, black, and oolong tea contain polyphenols, including catechins and flavonols. Quinones are produced when the tea is oxidized. The constituents of such tea have been shown to inhibit nitrosamine formation *in vitro*. Tea consumption has been associated with reduced cancer risk in observational studies (107,108).

Soybeans are a rich source of isoflavones, which are converted by intestinal bacteria to substances with weak estrogen activity and the capacity to function as estrogen antagonists in certain tissues. These substances appear to inhibit the growth of mammary cell tumors, as well as tumor-induced angiogenesis.

Terpenes, lipid-soluble compounds found in a variety of herbs, have demonstrated a variety of anticancer properties, including suppression of cellular proliferation and induction of apoptosis (109,110).

TOPICS OF INTEREST

Calorie Restriction

Energy restriction has been shown to have tumor-inhibiting properties in animal studies (111). No long-term studies of calorie restriction have been conducted in humans, nor do such studies seem probable. Several cancers, including breast, prostate, ovarian, endometrial, and renal, may be promoted by either high calorie intake or the resultant high BMI. Further study of calorie restriction in cancer prevention is warranted and may be most effectively approached in the context of secondary prevention studies (i.e., prevention of cancer recurrence following successful treatment).

Diet and Cancer Management

By a variety of mechanisms, cancer tends to induce malnutrition (112). Although there is theoretical concern that nutritional support might stimulate tumor growth, there is no evidence of such an effect in humans (113). While in part the result of cancer and treatment factors that may reduce nutrient intake, cancer cachexia differs from starvation in that basal energy expenditure, lipolysis, and protein turnover are increased rather than decreased (112).

Learned Food Aversions

Foods associated circumstantially with the unpleasant effects of cancer treatments may result in aversions. Nearly 50% of untreated cancer patients have such aversions, and new ones develop with treatment in more than 50% of all patients. Although several approaches have been tried to prevent learned food aversions from developing, the most promising approach to date is the administration of nutritionally unimportant foods near treatment times, so that learned food aversions are directed toward such foods rather than those with important nutritional value (114).

CLINICAL HIGHLIGHTS

Inconsistent and conflicting literature on the relative effectiveness of specific nutrients in preventing cancer of various tissues may be seen as a hopeless quagmire from which no meaningful message can be extracted. If one looks at dietary pattern rather than nutrient consumption, however, the literature is remarkably consistent. The risk for virtually all cancers influenced by diet can be reduced by a diet rich in fruits and vegetables. Avoidance of excess dietary fat and the sources of that fat, typically red meat and dairy products, also has strong support. Both obesity and high total energy intake, correlated with one another, appear to increase risk of several cancers. When fat intake is relatively high, the greater the proportion of fat that is n-3 polyunsaturated, such as that found in fish, the less the cancer risk; no such benefit is seen when fat intake is low. Similarly, a variety of micronutrients that show benefit in populations with marginal diets show no such benefits in populations with abundant diets.

Patients wishing to minimize cancer risk should be encouraged to eat a diet rich in fruits and vegetables and relatively low in total fat. Meat should be predominantly poultry and fish, and dairy products should be reduced fat. Alcohol consumption should be moderate. Ideal body weight should be maintained by prudent energy intake and regular physical activity. A daily multivitamin/multimineral supplement seems prudent and is free of known harmful effects. High doses of any single micronutrient cannot be recommended based on currently available evidence.

REFERENCES

1. Doll R, Peto R. The causes of cancer: quantitative estimates of avoidable risks of cancer in the United States today. *JNCI* 1981;66:1191.
2. Willett WC. Nutrition and cancer: a summary of the evidence. *Cancer Causes Control* 1996;7:178–180.
3. Greenwald P. The potential of dietary modification to prevent cancer. *Prev Med* 1996;25:41.
4. Fraser D. Nutrition and cancer: epidemiological aspects. *Public Health Rev* 1996;24:113.
5. Prasad KN, Cole W, Hovland P. Cancer prevention studies: past, present, and future directions. *Nutrition* 1998;14:197–210.
6. Laviano A, Meguid MM. Nutritional issues in cancer management. *Nutrition* 1996;12:358–371.
7. Butrum RR, Clifford CK, Lanza E. NCI dietary guidelines: rationale. *Am J Clin Nutr* 1988;48:888.
8. Lindsay DG. Dietary contribution to genotoxic risk and its control. *Food Chem Toxicol* 1996; 34:423.
9. The American Cancer Society 1996 Advisory Committee on Diet, Nutrition, and Cancer Prevention. Guidelines on diet, nutrition, and cancer prevention: reducing the risk of cancer with healthy food choices and physical activity. *CA Cancer J Clin* 1996;46:325.
10. Rose DP. The mechanistic rationale in support of dietary cancer prevention. *Prev Med* 1996;25:34.
11. Birt DF, Pelling JC, Nair S, et al. Diet intervention for modifying cancer risk. In: *Genetics and cancer susceptibility: implications for risk assessment.* New York: Wiley-Liss, 1994:223–234.
12. Peipins LA, Sandler RS. Epidemiology of colorectal adenomas. *Epidemiol Rev* 1994;16:273.
13. Willett WC, Stampfer MJ, Colditz GA, et al. Relation of meat, fat, and fiber intake to the risk of colon cancer in a prospective study among women. *N Engl J Med* 1990;323:1664.
14. Neugut AI, Garbowski GC, Lee WC, et al. Dietary risk factors for the incidence and recurrence of colorectal adenomatous polyps. A case-control study. *Ann Intern Med* 1993;118:91.
15. Alabaster O, Tang Z, Shivapurkar N. Dietary fiber and the chemopreventive modulation of colon carcinogenesis. *Mutat Res* 1996;350:185.
16. Giovannucci E, Ascherio A, Rimm EB, et al. Physical activity, obesity, and risk for colon cancer and adenoma in men. *Ann Intern Med* 1995;122:327.
17. Kampman E, Giovannucci E, van't Veer P, et al. Calcium, vitamin D, dairy foods, and the occurrence of colorectal adenomas among men and women in two prospective studies. *Am J Epidemiol* 1994;139:16.
18. Steinmetz KA, Kushi LH, Bostik RM, et al. Vegetables, fruit, and colon cancer in Iowa Women's Health Study. *Am J Epidemiol* 1994;139:1.
19. Slattery ML, Boucher KM, Caan BJ, et al. Eating patterns and risk of colon cancer. *Am J Epidemiol* 1998;148:4.
20. Bostik RM. Diet and nutrition in the etiology and primary prevention of colon cancer. In: Bendich A, Deckelbaum RJ, eds. *Preventive nutrition. The comprehensive guide for health professionals.* Totowa, NJ: Humana Press, 1997;57–96.
21. Goldin-Lang P, Kreuser ED, Zunft HJF. Basis and consequences of primary and secondary prevention of gastrointestinal tumors. *Recent Results Cancer Res* 1996;142:163.
22. Noguchi M, Rose DP, Miyazaki I. Breast cancer chemoprevention: clinical trials and research. *Oncology* 1996;53:175.

23. Hulka BS, Stark AT. Breast cancer: cause and prevention. *Lancet* 1995;346:883–887.
24. Hunter DJ, Willet WC. Nutrition and breast cancer. *Cancer Causes Control* 1996;7:56.
25. Greenwald P, Sherwood K, McDonald SS. Fat, caloric intake, and obesity: lifestyle risk factors for breast cancer. *J Am Diet Assoc* 1997;97:s24.
26. Kushi LH, Fee RM, Sellers TA, et al. Intake of vitamins A, C, E and postmenopausal breast cancer. *Am J Epidemiol* 1996;144:165.
27. Hunter DJ, Manson JE, Olditz GA, et al. A prospective study of the intake of vitamins C, E, and A and the risk of breast cancer. *N Engl J Med* 1993;329:234.
28. Costa A, Formelli F, Chiesa F, et al. Prospects of chemoprevention of human cancers with synthetic retinoid fenretinide. *Cancer Res* 1994;54:2032s.
29. Hebert JR, Rosen A. Nutritional, socioeconomic, and reproductive factors in relation to female breast cancer mortality: findings from a cross-national study. *Cancer Detect Prev* 1996;20:234.
30. Hershcoppf RJ, Bradlow HL. Obesity, diet, endogenous estrogens and the risk of hormone-sensitive cancer. *Am J Clin Nutr* 1987;45[Suppl]:283.
31. Gregario DI, Emrich LJ, Graham S, et al. Dietary fat consumption and survival among women with breast cancer. *JNCI* 1985;75:37.
32. Zumoff B. Hormonal profiles in women with breast cancer. *Anticancer Res* 1988;8:627.
33. Johnston PV. Dietary fat, eicosanoids, and immunity. *Adv Lipid Res* 1985;21:103.
34. Hebert JR, Augustine A, Barone J, et al. Weight, height and body mass in the prognosis of breast cancer: early results of a prospective study. *Int J Cancer* 1988;42:315.
35. Dorgan JF, Sowell A, Swanson CA, et al. Relationships of serum carotenoids, retinol, α-tocopherol, and selenium with breast cancer risk: results from a prospective study in Columbia, Missouri (United States). *Cancer Causes Control* 1998;9:89.
36. Smith-Warner SA, Spiegelman D, Yaun SS, et al. Alcohol and breast cancer in women: a pooled analysis of cohort studies. *JAMA* 1998;279:535.
37. Schatzkin A, Jones Y, Hoover RN, et al. Alcohol consumption and breast cancer in the epidemiologic follow-up study of the first National Health and Nutrition Examination Survey. *N Engl J Med* 1987;316:1169.
38. van den Brandt PA, Goldbohm A, van't Veer P. Alcohol and breast cancer: results from the Netherlands cohort study. *Am J Epidemiol* 1995;141:907.
39. Mezzetti M, La Vecchia C, Decarli A, et al. Population attributable risk for breast cancer: diet, nutrition, and physical exercise. *J Natl Cancer Inst* 1998;90:389.
40. Schatzkin A, Greenwald P, Byar DP, et al. The dietary fat-breast cancer hypothesis is alive. *JAMA* 1989;261:3284.
41. Franceschi S, Favero A, Decarli A, et al. Intake of macronutrients and risk of breast cancer. *Lancet* 1996;347:1351.
42. Willett WC, Hunter DJ, Stampfer MJ, et al. Dietary fat and fiber in relation to risk of breast cancer. An 8-year follow-up. *JAMA* 1992;268:2037.
43. Willett WC, Stampfer MJ, Colditz GA, et al. Dietary fat and the risk of breast cancer. *N Engl J Med* 1987;316:22.
44. Holmberg L, Ohlander EM, Byers T, et al. Diet and breast cancer risk. Results from a population-based, case-control study in Sweden. *Arch Intern Med* 1994;154:1805.
45. Hunter DJ, Spiegelman D, Adami H-O, et al. Cohort studies of fat intake and the risk of breast cancer—a pooled analysis. *N Engl J Med* 1996;334:356.
46. Petrek JA, Peters M, Cirrincione C, et al. Is body fat topography a risk factor for breast cancer? *Ann Intern Med* 1993;118:356.
47. Potischman N, Weiss HA, Swanson CA, et al. Diet during adolescence and risk of breast cancer among young women. *J Natl Cancer Inst* 1998;90:226.
48. Clinton SK. Diet, anthropometry and breast cancer: integration of experimental and epidemiologic approaches. *J Nutr* 1997;127:916s.
49. Kohlmeier L, Mendez M. Controversies surrounding diet and breast cancer. *Proc Nutr Soc* 1997;56:369.
50. Howe GR. Nutrition and breast cancer. In: Bendich A, Deckelbaum RJ, eds. *Preventive nutrition. The comprehensive guide for health professionals.* Totowa, NJ: Humana Press, 1997.
51. Colditz GA, Stampfer MJ, Willett WC. Diet and lung cancer. A review of the epidemiologic evidence in humans. *Arch Intern Med* 1987;147:157.
52. Omenn GS, Goodman GE, Thornquist MD, et al. Risk factors for lung cancer and for intervention effects in CARET, the Beta-Carotene and Retinol Efficacy Trial. *J Natl Cancer Inst* 1996;88:1550.
53. The Alpha-Tocopherol, Beta-Carotene Cancer Prevention Study Group. The effect of vitamin E and beta carotene on the incidence of lung cancer and other cancers in male smokers. *N Engl J Med* 1994;330:1029.
54. Albanes D, Heinonen OP, Taylor PR, et al. α-Tocopherol and β-carotene supplements and lung cancer incidence in the Alpha-Tocopherol, Beta-Carotene Cancer Prevention Study: effects of baseline characteristics and study compliance. *J Natl Cancer Inst* 1996;88:1560.
55. Omenn GS, and CARET, et al. Re: Risk factors for lung cancer and for intervention effects in CARET, the Beta-Carotene and Retinol Efficacy Trial [Letter]. *J Natl Cancer Inst* 1997;89:326.
56. Alavanja MCR, Brownson RC, Benichou J. Estimating the effect of dietary fat on the risk of lung cancer in nonsmoking women. *Lung Cancer* 1996;14:s63.
57. Rylander R, Axelsson G, Andersson L, et al. Lung cancer, smoking and diet among Swedish men. *Lung Cancer* 1996;14:s75.
58. Gao Y. Risk factors for lung cancer among nonsmokers with emphasis on lifestyle factors. *Lung Cancer* 1996;14:s39.
59. Dai X, Lin C, Sun X, et al. The etiology of lung cancer in nonsmoking females in Harbin, China. *Lung Cancer* 1996;14:s85.
60. Sanson CA, Mao BL, Li JY, et al. Dietary determinants of lung cancer risk: results from a case-control study in Hunan Province. *Int J Cancer* 1992;50:876.

61. Knekt P, Jarvinen R, Seppanen R, et al. Dietary flavonoids and the risk of lung cancer and other malignant neoplasms. *Am J Epidemiol* 1997;146: 223–230.

62. Comstock GW, Helzlsouer KJ. Preventive nutrition and lung cancer. In: Bendich A, Deckelbaum RJ, eds. *Preventive nutrition. The comprehensive guide for health professionals.* Totowa, NJ: Humana Press, 1997.

63. Giovannucci E, Clinton SK. Tomatoes, lycopene, and prostate cancer. *Proc Soc Exp Biol Med* 1998;218:129–139.

64. Giovannucci E. How is individual risk for prostate cancer assessed? *Hematol Oncol Clin North Am* 1996;10:537.

65. Kolonel LN. Nutrition and prostate cancer. *Cancer Causes Control* 1996;7:83–94.

66. Pienta KJ, Esper PS. Risk factors for prostate cancer. *Ann Intern Med* 1993;118:793–803.

67. Key TJA, Silcocks PB, Davey GK, et al. A case-control study of diet and prostate cancer. *Br J Cancer* 1997;76:678.

68. Andersson S, Wolk A, Bergstrom R, et al. Energy, nutrient intake and prostate cancer risk: a population-based case-control study in Sweden. *Int J Cancer* 1996;68:716.

69. Fair WR, Fleshner NE, Heston W. Cancer of the prostate: a nutritional disease? *Urology* 1997;50: 840.

70. Giles G, Ireland P. Diet, nutrition, and prostate cancer. *Int J Cancer* 1997;10:s13.

71. Heinonen OP, Albanes D, Virtamo J, et al. Prostate cancer and supplementation with α-tocopherol and β-carotene: incidence and mortality in a controlled trial. *J Natl Cancer Inst* 1998;90:440.

72. Olson KB, Pienta KJ. Vitamins A and E: further clues for prostate cancer prevention. *J Natl Cancer Inst* 1998;90:414.

73. Clinton SK, Emenhiser C, Schwartz SJ, et al. Cis-trans Lycopene isomers, carotenoids, and retinol in the human prostate. *Cancer Epidemiol Biomarkers Prev* 1996;5:823.

74. Giovannucci E, Ascherio A, Rimm EB, et al. Intake of carotenoids and retinol in relation to risk of prostate cancer. *J Natl Cancer Inst* 1995;87:1767.

75. Nomura AM, Stemmermann GN, Lee J, et al. Serum micronutrients and prostate cancer in Japanese Americans in Hawaii. *Cancer Epidemiol Biomarkers Prev* 1997;6:487.

76. Pandalai PK, Pilat MJ, Yamazaki K, et al. The effects of omega-3 and omega-6 fatty acids on *in vitro* prostate cancer growth. *Anticancer Res* 1996; 16:815.

77. Fontham ETH. Prevention of upper gastrointestinal tract cancers. In: Bendich A, Deckelbaum RJ, eds. *Preventive nutrition. The comprehensive guide for health professionals.* Totowa, NJ: Humana Press, 1997.

78. Joosens JV, Hill MJ, Elliott P, et al. Dietary salt, nitrate and stomach cancer mortality in 24 countries. *Int J Epidemiol* 1996;25:494.

79. Caygill CPJ, Charlett A, Hill MJ. Fat, fish, fish oil, and cancer. *Br J Cancer* 1996;74:159.

80. Bunin GR, Cary JM. Diet and childhood cancer. In: Bendich A, Deckelbaum RJ, eds. *Preventive nutrition. The comprehensive guide for health professionals.* Totowa, NJ: Humana Press, 1997.

81. Chiu BC-H, Cerhan JR, Folsom AR, et al. Diet and risk of non-Hodgkin lymphoma in older women. *JAMA* 1996;275:1315.

82. Ohba S, Nishi M, Miyake H. Eating habits and pancreas cancer. *Int J Pancreatol* 1996;20:37.

83. Warshaw AL, Fernandez-Del Castillo C. Pancreatic carcinoma. *N Engl J Med* 1992;326:455.

84. Rao GN. Influence of diet on tumors of hormonal tissues. In: Huff J, Boyd J, Barrett JC, eds. *Cellular and molecular mechanisms of hormonal carcinogenesis: environmental influences.* New York: Wiley-Liss, 1996.

85. Chow W-H, McLaughlin JK, Mandel JS, et al. Obesity and risk of renal cell cancer. *Cancer Epidemiol Biomarkers Prev* 1996;5:17.

86. Davies TW, Palmer CR, Ruja E, et al. Adolescent milk, dairy product and fruit consumption and testicular cancer. *Br J Cancer* 1996;74:657.

87. Bruemmer B, White E, Vaughan TL, et al. Nutrient intake in relation to bladder cancer among middle-aged men and women. *Am J Epidemiol* 1996; 144:485.

88. Eichholzer M, Gutzwiller F. Dietary nitrates, nitrites, and N-nitroso compounds and cancer risk: a review of the epidemiologic evidence. *Nutr Rev* 1998;56:95.

89. Weber P, Bendich A, Schalch W. Vitamin C and human health—a review of recent data relevant to human requirements. *Int J Vit Nutr Res* 1996;66:19.

90. Mayne ST. Beta-carotene, carotenoids, and disease prevention in humans. *FASEB J* 1996;10:690.

91. Lotan R. Retinoids in cancer chemoprevention. *FASEB J* 1996;10:1031.

92. Ziegler RG. A review of epidemiologic evidence that carotenoids reduce the risk of cancer. *J Nutr* 1989;119:116.

93. Edge R, McGarvey DJ, Truscott TG. The carotenoids as anti-oxidants—a review. *J Photochem Photobiol* 1997;41:189.

94. Greenberg ER, Baron JA, Tosteson TD, et al. A clinical trial of antioxidant vitamins to prevent colorectal adenoma. *N Engl J Med* 1994;331:141.

95. Daviglus ML, Dyer AR, Persky V, et al. Dietary beta-carotene, vitamin C, and the risk of prostate cancer: results from the Western Electric Study. *Epidemiology* 1996;7:472.

96. Clinton SK. Lycopene: chemistry, biology, and implications for human health and disease. *Nutr Rev* 1998;56:35.

97. Meydani M. Vitamin E. *Lancet* 1995;345:170.

98. Blot WJ. Vitamin/mineral supplementation and cancer risk: international chemoprevention trials. *Proc Soc Exp Biol Med* 1997;216:291.

99. Gallaher DD, Schneeman BO. Dietary fiber. In: Ziegler EE, Filer LJ Jr., eds. *Present knowledge in nutrition,* 7th ed. Washington, DC: ILSI Press, 1996.

100. Martinez ME, McPherson RS, Annegers JF, et al. Association of diet and colorectal adenomatous polyps: dietary fiber, calcium, and total fat. *Epidemiology* 1996;7:264.

101. Le Marchand L, Hankin JH, Wilkens LR, et al.

Dietary fiber and colorectal cancer risk. *Epidemiology* 1997;8:658.

102. Giovannucci E, Stampfer MJ, Colditz G, et al. Relationship of diet to risk of colorectal adenoma in men. *J Natl Cancer Inst* 1992;84:91.

103. Alberts DS, Ritenbaugh C, Story JA, et al. Randomized, double-blind, placebo-controlled study of effect of wheat bran fiber and calcium on fecal bile acids in patients with resected adenomatous colon polyps. *J Natl Cancer Inst* 1996;88:81.

104. Giovannucci E, Rimm EB, Stampfer MJ, et al. Intake of fat, meat, and fiber in relation to risk of colon cancer in men. *Cancer Res* 1994;54:2390.

105. Wasan HS, Goodlad RA. Fibre-supplemented foods may damage your health. *Lancet* 1996; 348:319.

106. LaVecchia C, Ferraroni M, Franceschi S, et al. Fibers and breast cancer risk. *Nutr Cancer* 1997; 28:264.

107. Zheng W, Doyle TJ, Kushi LH, et al. Tea consumption and cancer incidence in a prospective cohort study of postmenopausal women. *Am J Epidemiol* 1996;144:175.

108. Gao YT, McLaughlin JK, Blot WJ, et al. Reduced risk of esophageal cancer associated with green tea consumption. *J Natl Cancer Inst* 1994;86:855.

109. Milner JA. Nonnutritive components in foods as modifiers of the cancer process. In: Bendich A, Deckelbaum RJ, eds. *Preventive nutrition. The comprehensive guide for health professionals.* Totowa, NJ: Humana Press, 1997.

110. Murray MT. *Encyclopedia of nutritional supplements.* Rocklin, CA: Prima Publishing, 1996.

111. Kolaja KL, Bunting KA, Klauning JE. Inhibition of tumor promotion and heptocellular growth by dietary restriction in mice. *Carcinogenesis* 1996; 17:1657.

112. Rivadeneira DE, Evoy D, Fahey, TJ III, et al. Nutritional support of the cancer patient. *CA Cancer J Clin* 1998;48:69.

113. Copeland EM III. Historical perspective on nutritional support of cancer patients. *CA Cancer J Clin* 1998;48:67.

114. Mattes. In: Shils.

BIBLIOGRAPHY

See "Sources for All Chapters."

National Research Council. *Carcinogens and anticarcinogens in the human diet.* Washington, DC: National Academy Press, 1996.

National Research Council. *Recommended dietary allowances,* 10th ed. Washington, DC: National Academy Press, 1989.

Margen S. *The wellness nutrition counter.* New York: Health Letter Associates, 1997.

Murray MT. *Encyclopedia of nutritional supplements.* Rocklin, CA: Prima Publishing, 1996.

Shils ME, Olson JA, Shike M, eds. *Modern nutrition in health and disease,* 8th ed. Philadelphia: Lea & Febiger, 1994.

Ziegler EE, Filer LJ Jr., eds. *Present knowledge in nutrition,* 7th ed. Washington, DC: ILSI Press, 1996.

Ensminger AH, Ensminger ME, Konlande JE, et al. *The concise encyclopedia of foods and nutrition.* Boca Raton: CRC Press, 1995.

United States Department of Agriculture. *USDA nutrient database for standard reference.* Release 11-1, 1997.

Bendich A, Deckelbaum RJ, eds. *Preventive nutrition. The comprehensive guide for health professionals.* Totowa, NJ: Humana Press, 1997.

Institute of Medicine (U.S.). *Improving America's diet and health: from recommendations to action.* Thomas PR, ed. Washington, DC: National Academy Press, 1991.

Thomas B. *Nutrition in primary care.* Oxford, England: Blackwell Science, 1996.

Schottenfeld D, Fraumeni JF, eds. *Cancer epidemiology and prevention,* 2nd ed. New York: Oxford University Press, 1996.

World Cancer Research Fund in Association with American Institute for Cancer Research. *Food, nutrition and the prevention of cancer: a global perspective.* Washington, DC: American Institute for Cancer Research, 1997.

Committee on Diet and Health, Food and Nutrition Board, Commission on Life Sciences, National Research Council. *Diet and health. Implications for reducing chronic disease burden.* Washington, DC: National Academy Press, 1989.

13

Diet and Osteoporosis

INTRODUCTION

The hydroxyapatite crystals of bone are made up predominantly of calcium and phosphorus. Osteoporosis is the demineralization of bone due to a net movement of calcium from bone to serum, mediated by a predominance of osteoclast over osteoblast activity. Osteoporosis is to be distinguished from osteomalacia, a different pattern of demineralization resulting from vitamin D deficiency.

Osteoporosis affects more than 20 million adults in the United States. Risk factors include gender (female), early menopause, ethnicity (white or Asian), thin bone structure, low body mass index, smoking, heavy consumption of alcohol, sedentary lifestyle, and family history.

Dietary pattern, use of supplements, physical activity, and sunlight exposure at various periods of life have the potential to affect peak bone density, the rate of bone mineral losses, and the propensity to bone injuries such as traumatic and pathologic fractures. The principal dietary consideration in the prevention and management of osteoporosis is lifetime calcium intake. In addition to lifestyle interventions, various pharmacologic interventions may be indicated in efforts to prevent disability from skeletal demineralization.

OVERVIEW

Diet

Bone metabolism is influenced by a variety of hormone actions. The serum calcium level is a stimulus to both parathyroid hormone (PTH) and calcitonin. Parathyroid hormone varies inversely, and calcitonin directly, with circulating calcium; PTH mobilizes calcium from bone, whereas calcitonin enhances skeletal deposition of calcium. Parathyroid hormone also increases activation of vitamin D, enhancing intestinal calcium absorption, and reduces urinary calcium excretion.

Peak bone mass is reached in the third to fourth decade of life, with gradual demineralization thereafter. Relatively rapid bone loss occurs in women during the 5 years following cessation of menses, with spine density diminished by 3% to 6% annually. Bone loss in men apparently occurs at a fairly constant rate of 0.5% to 2% annually, depending on site, after peak bone mass is achieved. The clinical sequelae of osteoporosis result from fracture, most commonly at the wrist, hip, and spine. More than 50% of women past the age of 80 have experienced compression fracture of the spine.

Definitive evidence that increasing dietary intake of calcium increases peak bone density is lacking. However, suggestive evidence is available. A National Institutes of Health (NIH) consensus panel convened in 1994 concluded that average calcium intake in the United States is too low to support optimal bone health, and it revised recommended intake ranges upward (1). The basis for the NIH-recommended intake levels is the evidence of threshold doses above which further incorporation of calcium into bone does not occur. Optimal calcium intake over time is the level that allows bone density to reach the maximum genetically "encoded" for a given individual. Paleolithic intake of calcium is estimated in the range of 2 g per day for adults (2) (see Nutrient Reference Data Table in Section III). Relative inefficiency in the absorption of ingested calcium is protection against calcium excess under the conditions prevailing during our evolutionary history.

Calcium requirements are lower when sodium and protein intake is low, as both of these increase urinary losses of calcium. The reduced calcium requirements associated with nonwestern diets may partly explain the inability to demonstrate a transcultural dietary calcium gradient that corresponds with osteoporosis or fracture risk. Vegetarianism (see Chapter 37) need not, therefore, have adverse effects on calcium nutriture. There is longitudinal evidence from the Framingham cohort that diets high in alkaline-producing components, specifically fruits, vegetables, potassium, and magnesium, are associated with preservation of bone mass in both men and women (3). A strictly vegetarian diet that excludes dairy products and is high in sodium would likely have an adverse effect on the skeleton.

Dietary factors thought to influence the incorporation of calcium into bone include vitamin D, copper, zinc, manganese, fluorine, silicon, and boron. The predominant effects of protein and phosphorus on bone metabolism are mediated by the fractional reabsorption of calcium in the renal tubule. Protein decreases, and phosphorus increases, calcium reabsorption. The concomitant ingestion of protein and phosphorus in meat and dairy products has little net effect on calcium losses.

On the basis of the available epidemiologic evidence, recommended calcium intake for adolescents has been raised to 1,200 mg daily. More conclusive evidence from prospective trials is available that higher calcium intake, about 1,500 mg daily, reduces the rate of spinal bone loss in premenopausal women. Supplemental calcium appears to be less effective at reducing the rate of bone loss during the immediate postmenopausal period during which rapid bone loss occurs. More than 5 years after menopause, when the rate of bone loss slows, responsiveness to supplementation increases, particularly in women with relatively low dietary intake. With high dietary intake, the benefit of supplementation in this age group is less discernible. Calcium supplementation in men with adequate dietary intake (more than 1,000 mg per day) has not been shown to influence the rate of bone demineralization; the effects of supplementation in men with low dietary intake are not known. Epidemiologic data suggest that hip fracture rates are lower in populations with high habitual intake of dietary calcium.

The recommended intakes of calcium at different stages of life (see Nutrient Reference Data Table, Section III) are based on what is known about obligate daily calcium losses in stool and urine (200 to 250 mg per day in adults), an absorption rate of 30% to 40%, and the rate of calcium incorporation into bone during the growth phase (from 140 to 500 mg per day during various stages). Finally, recent recommendations have been revised up to account for the rate of bone loss in older adults, as well as reduced intestinal absorption.

Although supplements may be useful in achieving the recommended 800 to 1,500 mg per day of calcium, food sources offer the benefits of other nutrients known or thought to confer benefits on the skeleton, including vitamin D and trace minerals. A diet rich in nonfat dairy products and a variety of vegetables and grains will provide all of the nutrients thought to optimize bone health and may be recommended on other grounds as well. Calcium intake up to 2,500 mg per day is generally safe, although extreme intake may contribute to the formation of renal calculi (see Chapter 11) and interfere with the absorption of iron, zinc, and other minerals. Physical activity, particularly repetitive weight-bearing activities and resistance training, confer benefit to bone mass and strength in addition to that attainable by nutritional means. In addition, fitness reduces the risk of injurious falls (4).

Calcium needs in adolescence have been studied by examining variation in dietary intake and associated variation in bone density in populations, by calcium balance studies, and by the provision of supplements in controlled trials. Bone density in adolescence is consistently influenced by age, weight, height, and pubertal status. Evidence indicating a role for dietary calcium intake is less consistent. To some degree, inconsistency in the results with dietary supplementation may be due to limited sample sizes, variation in the calcium preparations used, habitual calcium intake, or the predominant effects of physical activity, weight, and hormonal status. Despite the inconsistency in research findings to date, the possible benefits and lack of potential harm in raising calcium intake during adolescence have resulted in recommendations from the NIH to increase the recommended calcium intake for adolescents to 1,200 to 1,500 mg per day.

Pregnancy (see Chapter 25) is associated with the diversion of approximately 30 g of calcium from the maternal circulation to the fetal skeleton. The effects of this process on the maternal skeleton remain uncertain. Were maternal calcium absorption or ingestion not to increase or excretion not to decrease, the formation of the fetal skeleton would consume 3% of maternal bone calcium. However, the increased levels of estrogen in pregnancy, resulting from placental estradiol production, favor osteoblast action and calcium deposition in bone.

Studies of multiparity are inconsistent; some demonstrate increased bone mass and others show no change. The same uncertainty exists for fractures in later life. If multiparity contributes to increased bone mass, the extent to which it is due to pregnancy versus increased weight is uncertain. Pregnancy is associated with increased levels of circulating active vitamin D (1,25-dihydroxy vitamin D) and consequently with enhanced intestinal absorption of calcium. The effects of adolescent pregnancy on bone mass are uncertain. There is concern that the need for both fetal and maternal bone mineralization

might exceed compensatory mechanisms. The fetal calcium demands in total approximately 3% of the maternal skeletal depot. Without compensatory mechanisms, each pregnancy might reduce maternal bone mass by this amount.

Lactation (see Chapter 25) is associated with an initial loss of bone mineral, with subsequent compensation when menses is restored. Approximately 150 to 200 mg per day of calcium is diverted to breast milk at 3 months post partum, and nearly 300 mg at 6 months. A total of 6 months of breast-feeding would require 4% to 6% of the maternal skeletal calcium without compensation.

High levels of prolactin and reduced levels of estrogen are associated with reductions in bone mass. Net loss of maternal bone apparently does not occur at detectable levels if breast-feeding is sustained for less than 6 months. Loss of calcium from bone apparently occurs with breast-feeding beyond 6 months even with optimal dietary intake (5). With restoration of menses, bone density is restored provided that dietary intake is adequate. As with pregnancy, the effects of lactation on bone density in adolescents are less certain and of potentially greater concern. The net effect of lactation on the skeleton when vitamin D or calcium intake is deficient has not been adequately addressed.

Senescence (see Chapter 29), in both men and women, is associated with progressive demineralization of bone and increasing fracture risk. Although the focus in the elderly had until recently been on calcium intake, interest has shifted somewhat to stores of vitamin D. Vitamin D levels in the elderly are generally lower than in younger adults, with actual deficiency not uncommon in institutionalized elderly not exposed to natural light. Because of reduced sunlight exposure among the elderly in general, dietary intake of vitamin D appears to be an important determinant of circulating levels. The principal source of dietary vitamin D is fortified milk. There is some evidence that vitamin D supplementation given either intramuscularly or orally to elderly men and women can increase bone density and decrease the fracture rate relative to untreated controls.

The rapid phase of bone demineralization following menopause results in the loss of approximately 15% of skeletal calcium before a new steady state is reached. This loss is approximately equal to one standard deviation of bone density; thus, greater than average bone density during the premenopause can result in ostensibly "normal" bone density even after rapid postmenopausal bone loss. Conversely, failure to optimize bone density before menopause renders a woman much more susceptible to clinical sequelae of the bone loss induced by menopause.

Whereas the rapid phase of postmenopausal bone loss is highly dependent on estrogen, the maintenance or loss of bone calcium thereafter apparently is quite responsive to dietary calcium. Although evidence has been gathered demonstrating a reduction in the fracture rate with calcium supplementation, particularly when combined with vitamin D, the benefit would likely be much greater were calcium intake to be adequate throughout life. Thus, it is probable that the fracture rates in the treatment groups of even the most successful trials are higher than they would have to be if lifelong calcium intake were optimized.

There is some evidence that calcium supplementation may retard bone loss in postmenopausal women with habitually low calcium intake (less than 400 mg per day). The efficacy of calcium supplementation when dietary intake is greater than 400 mg daily is unclear (5), although there is some evidence of slowed bone loss even in women with high-to-normal habitual intake (750 mg per day). Particular benefits have been demonstrated when calcium supplementation has been combined with vitamin D supplementation; increased bone density and reduced fracture rate in elderly women has been reported. Based on currently available evidence, a total daily intake of 1,500 mg of calcium is appropriate for both elderly men and women, with supplementation indicated to compensate for lesser dietary intake. Vita-

min D supplementation also is reasonable; the 400 IU contained in a typical multivitamin is sufficient.

Vitamin D intake among adults in the United States is generally about 100 IU per day; the most recent recommended dietary allowance (RDA) is 200 IU per day. Circulating levels of vitamin D tend to be lower during the winter in higher latitudes; effects on bone metabolism have not been established with certainty. Epidemiologic data support an association between low serum vitamin D, and lower rates of intestinal calcium absorption, and osteoporosis. Vitamin D supplementation as an isolated intervention has not shown consistent utility in preventing fractures in osteoporotic or healthy postmenopausal women. The potential benefits of vitamin D supplementation are most likely to be realized in subjects with low habitual vitamin D intake or limited sun exposure, and if coadministered with supplemental calcium.

Phosphorus, the other main mineral in bone, is abundantly available in the diet. Excess intake of phosphorus suppresses activation of vitamin D, with resultant reduction in intestinal absorption of calcium. Parathyroid hormone levels rise when phosphorus intake is high. However, high dietary phosphorus is associated with reduced urinary calcium losses, so no net effect on bone has been demonstrated. Sodas contain phosphorus. Diets high in processed foods with phosphate additives, meat, and soda may contain an excess of phosphorus that is detrimental to bone. If calcium and phosphorus in the diet remain proportional, high phosphorus intake does not appear to be harmful.

Protein, and therefore nitrogen, intake results in increased urinary calcium losses. The mobilization of mineral from bone induced by protein intake is thought to be due to the buffering of acid generated during protein metabolism. Most dietary sources of protein also are sources of phosphorus, which, as noted, reduces urinary calcium. Thus, there appears to be little net effect of protein intake on bone density. To the extent that protein ingestion does contribute to calcium loss in urine, it is the result of the sulfur load imposed and consequent acidification of serum and urine. As vegetable protein imposes less of a sulfur load than animal protein, protein from vegetable sources may be less likely to contribute to urinary loss of calcium.

Controversy persists regarding the significance to bone mass of protein intake. In a prospective study of postmenopausal women in Iowa, increasing protein intake was actually found to be protective against hip fracture (6). Protein may be beneficial to bone when habitual intake is low or in the context of malnutrition (7). There is preliminary evidence from animal research that a diet high in saturated fat may have deleterious effects on the mineral content of cancellous bone (8).

Once osteoporosis has developed, dietary manipulations are relatively, if not completely, ineffective at restoring bone density. Pharmacotherapy is required for this effect. The principal intervention for postmenopausal women is estrogen replacement. The topic of hormone replacement is complex and was reviewed recently (9). Estrogen directly stimulates osteoblasts and enhances production of active vitamin D. Estrogen supplementation prevents the rapid bone loss that occurs at menopause, but rapid bone loss ensues if estrogen administration is later discontinued. The selective estrogen receptor modulators, such as raloxifene, appear to have comparable effects on bone.

Supplemental calcium may reduce the dose of estrogen necessary to preserve bone density. Salmon calcitonin is available as a nasal spray. It reduces osteoclast activity and bone resorption. Finally, biphosphonates, such as alendronate, inhibit osteoclast activity. Marketed as Fosamax, alendronate has been shown to increase bone density in osteoporosis and to reduce the fracture rate (10). Similar results have been reported for other biphosphonates (11). The role of pharmacotherapeutics warrants mention in defining the limitations of dietary management of osteoporosis. Malnutrition contributes importantly to adverse outcomes following hospitalization of elderly patients for hip fracture. Sequelae are partly preventable with a vigorous program of nutritional support, which should be a part of the management plan for every such patient (see Chapter 24).

Nutrients and Nutriceuticals

Calcium

Calcium intake is essential to bone health and the prevention of osteoporosis, as discussed earlier. More detail regarding calcium intake is provided in the Nutrient Reference Data Table in Section III. Good sources include dairy products, mustard greens, almonds, tofu, and sardines. Other seafood is a moderately good source. High oxalate vegetables, such as spinach, provide little calcium that is bioavailable.

A variety of calcium preparations are available, and most are well absorbed. Calcium carbonate predominates in the United States. Its absorption is enhanced if the tablet is chewed or disintegrates readily. Calcium citrate and phosphate are widely available, and they are well absorbed. Split dosing enhances absorption, as only a portion of calcium ingested at any time is absorbed. Although some controversy exists regarding the optimal dose of calcium for prevention of osteoporosis, a teleologic view would favor fairly high intake. Our paleolithic ancestors apparently consumed considerably more calcium than we do (2,12).

Magnesium

Although magnesium is essential for the secretion and action of PTH, supplementation of magnesium has not been shown to benefit bone metabolism, even though the average intake in the United States is below the RDA (13). Magnesium supplementation concurrent with calcium may limit calcium absorption.

Approximately half of the body's magnesium stores are in bone: one third on the bone surface and two thirds incorporated into hydroxyapatite. Under conditions of calcium deficiency, magnesium may displace calcium in bone mineral. The exact influences of magnesium nutriture on osteoporosis or fracture risk are uncertain (17).

Vitamin K

Vitamin K functions in the gamma carboxylation of glutamic acid, contributing to the production of a variety of physiologically important proteins. The most prominent products of vitamin K metabolism participate in coagulation (see Chapters 4 and 8). Several protein products dependent on vitamin K are incorporated in bone. One such product, osteocalcin, can be measured in serum as a marker of bone turnover. Circulating osteocalcin is low in low vitamin K states, such as use of warfarin (Coumadin). Further, signs of impaired vitamin K metabolism are common in patients with osteoporosis. To date, however, a specific role for vitamin K nutriture in the prevention or amelioration of osteoporosis has not been defined (13). Data from the Nurses' Health Study suggest that low intake of vitamin K may increase risk for hip fracture; women in the lowest quintile of intake had significantly higher hip fracture risk than other women in the cohort (14).

Iron

Calcium in a meal or supplement ingested with iron will interfere with iron absorption.

Phosphorus

Phosphorus is stored in bone at a ratio of 1:2 with calcium based on mass. Although 85% of body phosphorus is stored in the skeleton, it contributes to a wide range of physiologic functions, including the storage and generation of energy in the phosphate bonds of ATP. Phosphorus is widely distributed in the diet; a typical American diet provides approximately 1 g per day for adult women and 1.5 g for adult men. The major sources are dairy, meat, poultry, and fish; cereals contribute approximately 12% of the total. Phosphorus is abundant in food additives; a highly processed diet may provide as much as 30% of intake in the form of additives. Of note, the ratio of calcium to phosphorus in human milk is nearly twice as high as that in bovine milk. Phosphorus deficiency does not occur under normal dietary conditions. It may be induced by protracted use of aluminum-based antacids, which bind phosphorus. Bone loss results when phosphorus deficiency occurs. Recommended intake of phosphorus is based on the maintenance of a 1:1 ratio with calcium.

Vitamin D

Vitamin D is essential in the intestinal absorption of calcium and may be derived from food sources or synthesized in skin with exposure to sunlight. The RDA for vitamin D in adults is 200 IU, 5 μg of cholecalciferol activity. When exposure to sunlight is consistent, there is no dietary requirement. Although the evidence base is limited, an intake of 400 IU per day is recommended for children older than 6 months, as well as for pregnant or lactating women. The principal dietary source of vitamin D in the United States is fortified milk, which contains 400 IU per quart. The vitamin is stable with regard to processing, storage, and cooking.

Phytoestrogens

Although there is considerable interest in the potential of phytoestrogens to ameliorate the impact of ovarian endocrine failure at menopause on bone density, to date there is no definitive evidence of any effect (15). Isoflavones, a group of phytoestrogens, are particularly abundant in soy; diets rich in soy products have been associated with low rates of osteoporotic fracture (16).

Boron

Boron appears to influence calcium balance, reducing urinary losses. The mechanisms of boron's action on calcium metabolism are uncertain. Postulated effects include hydroxylation of vitamin D and stimulation of increased estradiol production. Boron may enhance the effects of estrogen on bone. Excess from diet is unlikely, and doses up to 10 mg per day are nontoxic. Doses exceeding 50 mg per day in the form of supplements have induced gastrointestinal discomfort and possibly seizures. Estimated intake in the United States ranges from 0.5 to just over 3 mg per day; 1 mg per day is believed to be sufficient. Boron is found in beans, beer, nuts, legumes, wine, and green leafy vegetables (see Section IIIE).

Fluoride

Fluoride is nearly ubiquitous in soil and water, but in small and variable amounts. The incorporation of fluoride into bone is proportional to intake. Food sources of fluoride in the United States contribute an estimated 0.3 to 0.6 mg per day, with the distribution of foods obscuring differences in the regional fluoride contents of soil.

The principal determinant of variation in fluoride intake is water and beverages. An intake of 1.5 to 4.0 mg per day is recommended for adults; average intake is in this range. Intake of 0.1 to 1 mg daily during the first year of life, and up to 1.5 mg for the next 2 years, is recommended. Mottling of teeth occurs in children with a fluoride intake above 2 mg per day. Chronic intake of more than 20 mg per day induces toxicity in adults, leading to disruption of bone architecture and adverse effects on kidney, muscle, and nerve. High-dose fluoride (50 mg per day) has been shown to increase bone density in osteoporosis and to reduce the rate of vertebral fracture [18]. For benefit to occur with fluoride supplementation, sufficient calcium must be provided concomitantly; fluoride induces osteogenesis and especially consequent "bone hunger" in the spine. If calcium is unavailable from the diet, it may be leached from other skeletal sites [19].

A recently reported randomized trial again demonstrated increased bone density and reduced fractures with fluoride, but demonstrated that a low-dose regimen (approximately 11.2 mg per day) was more effective at preventing fractures, even though it raised bone density less than a higher-dose (20 mg per day) regimen [20].

Variation in doses and regimens used in clinical trials have perpetuated controversy regarding the role of fluoride in the treatment and prevention of osteoporosis [21-25].

Fluoride is incorporated into hydroxyapatite and stimulates the action of osteoblasts. Fluoride increases bone density and strength, but, because of reduced elasticity, the resistance of bone to fracture is not necessarily enhanced by fluoride supplementation. Most controlled trials of fluoride supplementation have demonstrated increased bone density, but no benefit with regard to the rate of fracture.

Caffeine

Caffeine apparently reduces active transport of calcium in the intestine, thereby reducing absorption. The effect is modest and completely compensated by the addition of milk to coffee.

Sodium

Sodium and calcium share a transport system in the kidney, and filtered sodium is accompanied by calcium. For every 2.3 g of sodium excreted in urine, 20 to 60 mg of calcium is lost [13,26].

Other Nutrient Effects

Phytate and oxalate in food complex with calcium. They are abundant in cruciferous vegetables and limit the bioavailability of calcium from such sources. Although phytate and oxalate levels are high in beans, calcium from beans is relatively bioavailable. Fiber can interfere with calcium absorption, and wheat bran seems to have a particularly strong influence.

Unlike phytate and oxalate, the effects of concomitantly ingested fiber generalize to calcium from other foods. In the average US diet, the effects of fiber intake on calcium absorption are negligible (13).

A role for zinc, manganese, and copper as cofactors in enzymatic processes germane to bone metabolism has stimulated interest in the influence dietary levels of these trace minerals may have on bone. To date, there is no more than preliminary evidence in humans that these trace minerals exacerbate osteoporosis when intake is low or ameliorate it when intake is raised.

Elevated serum homocysteine levels have been associated with osteoporosis, as well as vascular disease, raising the possibility that vitamins B_{12}, B_6 and folate may affect bone metabolism (27). In particular, these nutrients tend to be deficient in the diets of elderly people. Evidence that B vitamin supplementation may play a role in the prevention of osteoporosis is not available.

A prospective study suggests that relatively high intake of vitamin C or E, or both, may protect against the adverse effects smoking has on bone. The investigators postulate that oxidation plays a role in the acceleration of osteoporosis seen in smokers (28).

CLINICAL HIGHLIGHTS

Dietary management is fundamental to the primary and secondary prevention of osteoporosis, and it plays an important role in tertiary prevention. The origins of osteoporosis are in childhood and adolescence, during which time adequate physical activity and dietary calcium are particularly important. Peak bone density is reached by around the end of the third decade. Calcium intake of about 1,500 mg per day is advisable during adolescence. To achieve this amount and to optimize bone metabolism, the diet should be rich in nonfat dairy products and a variety of vegetables, fruits, and grains. Moderation in protein and sodium intake is advisable.

These recommendations are compatible with the dietary pattern advisable on other grounds (see Chapter 40). For women with apparent osteoporosis risk factors, hormone replacement therapy (of some variety) should be given serious consideration (9). If estrogen replacement is not an option for whatever reason, the use of calcium and fluoride supplementation, calcitonin, or alendronate might be considered. These options have not been studied for primary prevention, but evidence supports consideration of their use for secondary prevention.

In older adults, vitamin D supplementation to achieve an intake of at least 400 IU per day is indicated; such an intake can be achieved with use of a multivitamin. As calorie intake declines, the need to supplement calcium to achieve recommended intake levels is more probable. Calcium carbonate is readily available and inexpensive. Any calcium preparation should be given in divided doses to optimize absorption.

A diet in compliance with overall recommendations for fruit, vegetable, grain, meat, and dairy intake will provide various nutrients—including magnesium, zinc, boron, and vitamin K—in amounts adequate to contribute to the health of bone. Brief recommendations in office practice should focus on diversity in the diet, consumption of nonfat dairy products, avoiding or quitting smoking, limiting alcohol intake, and engaging in consistent weight-bearing physical activity, at least some of which should be outdoors in sunlight.

REFERENCES

1. NIH Consensus Conference. Optimal calcium intake. NIH Consensus Development Panel on Optimal Calcium Intake. *JAMA* 1994;272:1942.
2. Eaton SB, Eaton SB III, Konner MJ. Paleolithic nutrition revisited: a twelve-year retrospective on its nature and implications. *Eur J Clin Nutr* 1997; 51:207.

3. Tucker KL, Hannan MT, Chen H, et al. Potassium, magnesium, and fruit and vegetable intakes are associated with greater bone mineral density in elderly men and women. *Am J Clin Nutr* 1999;69:727.

4. Lewis RD, Modlesky CM. Nutrition, physical activity, and bone health in women. *Int J Sport Nutr* 1998;8:250.

5. Ziegler EE, Filer LJ Jr., eds. *Present knowledge in nutrition,* 7th ed. Washington, DC: ILSI Press, 1996.

6. Munger RG, Cerhan JR, Chiu BC. Prospective study of dietary protein intake and risk of hip fracture in postmenopausal women. *Am J Clin Nutr* 1999;69:147.

7. Bonjour JP, Schurch MA, Rizzoli R. Nutritional aspects of hip fractures. *Bone* 1996;18:139s.

8. Wohl GR, Loehrke L, Watkins BA, et al. Effects of high-fat diet on mature bone mineral content, structure, and mechanical properties. *Calcif Tissue Int* 1998;63:74.

9. Nawaz H, Katz DL. American College of Preventive Medicine position statement on post-menopausal hormone replacement therapy. *Am J Prev Med* 1999;17(3):250–254.

10. Liberman UA, Weiss SR, Broll J, et al. Effect of oral alendronate on bone mineral density and the incidence of fractures in postmenopausal osteoporosis. *N Engl J Med* 1995;333:1437.

11. Watts NB, Harris ST, Genant HK, et al. Intermittent cyclical etidronate treatment of postmenopausal osteoporosis. *N Engl J Med* 1990;323:73.

12. Patrick L. Comparative absorption of calcium sources and calcium citrate malate for the prevention of osteoporosis. *Altern Med Rev* 1999;4:74.

13. Heaney HP. Osteoporosis: vitamins, minerals, and other micronutrients. Bendich A, Deckelbaum RJ, eds. *Preventive nutrition. The comprehensive guide for health professionals.* Totowa, NJ: Humana Press, 1997.

14. Feskanich D, Weber P, Willett WC, et al. Vitamin K intake and hip fractures in women: a prospective study. *Am J Clin Nutr* 1999;69:74.

15. Strauss L, Santii R, Saarinen N, et al. Dietary phytoestrogens and their role in hormonally dependent disease. *Toxicol Lett* 1998;102–103:349.

16. Tham DM, Gardner CD, Haskell WL. Clinical review 97: potential health benefits of dietary phytoestrogens: a review of the clinical, epidemiological, and mechanistic evidence. *J Clin Endocrinol Metab* 1998;83:2223.

17. Shils.

18. Pak CYC, Sakhaee K, Piziak V, et al. Slow-release sodium fluoride in the management of postmenopausal osteoporosis. A randomized, controlled trial. *Ann Intern Med* 1994;120:625.

19. Ringe JD, Kipshoven C, Coster A, et al. Therapy of established postmenopausal osteoporosis with monofluorophosphate plus calcium: dose-related effects on bone density and fracture rate. *Osteoporosis Int* 1999;9:171.

20. Heaney RP. 1994; Meunier PJ. Evidence based medicine and osteoporosis: a comparison of fracture risk reduction data from osteoporosis randomised clinical trials. *Int J Clin Pract* 1999;53:122.

21. Heaney RP. Fluoride and osteoporosis. *Ann Intern Med* 1994;120:689.

22. Meunier PJ. Evidence-based medicine and osteoporosis: a comparison of fracture risk reduction data from osteoporosis randomised clinical trials. Int J Clin Pract. 1999;53:122–129.

23. Fluoride and bone: a second look. No use in osteoporosis. *Prescrire Int* 1998;7:110.

24. Meunier PJ, Sebert JL, Reginster JY, et al. Fluoride salts are no better at preventing new vertebral fractures than calcium-vitamin D in postmenopausal osteoporosis: the FAVO study. *Osteoporosis Int* 1998;8:4.

25. Kleerekoper M. The role of fluoride in the prevention of osteoporosis. *Endocrinol Metab Clin North Am* 1998;27:441.

26. Devine A, Criddle RA, Dick IM, et al. A longitudinal study of the effect of sodium and calcium intakes on regional bone density in postmenopausal women. *Am J Clin Nutr* 1995;62:740–745.

27. Bunker VW. The role of nutrition in osteoporosis. *Br J Biomed Sci* 1994;51:228.

28. Melhus H, Michalsson K, Holmberg L, et al. Smoking, antioxidant vitamins, and the risk of hip fracture. *J Bone Miner Res* 1999;14:129.

BIBLIOGRAPHY

See "Sources for All Chapters."

Standing Committee on the Scientific Evaluation of Dietary Reference Intakes, Food and Nutrition Board, Institute of Medicine. *Dietary reference intakes for calcium, phosphorus, magnesium, vitamin D, and fluoride.* Washington, DC: National Academy Press, 1997.

Sowers MF. Nutritional advances in osteoporosis and osteomalacia. In: Ziegler.

Krall EA, Dawson-Hughes B. Osteoporosis. In: Shils.

Nordin BE, Need AG, Steurer T, et al. Nutrition, osteoporosis, and aging. *Ann NY Acad Sci* 1998;20:336–351.

Lau EM, Woo J. Nutrition and osteoporosis. *Curr Opin Rheumatol* 1998;10:368.

Nordin BE. Calcium and osteoporosis. *Nutrition* 1997;13:664.

14

Diet and Obstructive Airway Disease

INTRODUCTION

Nutritional and respiratory status are related in a variety of ways. Malnutrition, either in isolation or as the result of acute or chronic illness, impairs respiratory function directly by weakening diaphragmatic contractions (see Chapter 24). Malnutrition impacts the respiratory system indirectly by causing relative immunosuppression (see Chapter 15). As pneumonia is a leading cause of hospitalization due to infectious disease and is a leading nosocomial infection, the relationship among nutritional status, immune function, and the respiratory system is of particular importance.

The link between diet and the pulmonary system is especially clear in patients with limited respiratory reserve and CO_2 retention. The respiratory quotient (see later) of carbohydrate is higher than that of either fat or protein, justifying the restriction of carbohydrate in certain patients. Evidence that manipulation of diet to reduce the respiratory quotient will modify long-term outcomes in patients with chronic obstructive pulmonary disease (COPD) is lacking, although the practice is supported by short-term studies. Dietary triggers of asthma and exacerbations of COPD are under active investigation. Dietary intake may influence the production of surfactant. Whereas conclusive evidence supports a role for adequate nutritional status in obstructive pulmonary disease, evidence for a protective or provocative role of specific micronutrients is mostly preliminary to date. The antiinflammatory properties of n-3 fatty acids described in other chapters

pertain to airway inflammation as well and may prove to be of benefit in obstructive disease such as asthma and chronic bronchitis.

OVERVIEW

Diet

Malnutrition has been shown to be common among patients with clinically significant obstructive airway disease, ranging from 20% to 25% in published series (1). Mortality rates among patients with COPD rise substantially with the advent of malnutrition. Airway obstruction increases the metabolic costs of breathing, as does the need for higher respiratory rates to compensate for a reduction in the proportion of tidal volume effective in gas exchange.

Macronutrient intake patterns may directly influence the adequacy of gas exchange by leading to variable CO_2 production. Every molecule of carbohydrate ingested results in a molecule of CO_2 produced; therefore, the respiratory quotient of carbohydrate has a value of 1. The respiratory quotient of protein is 0.8, whereas that of fat is 0.7. Protein supplementation may increase oxygen consumption due to its relatively high thermic effect. Protein consumption also tends to increase ventilation, potentially leading to dyspnea in patients with limited reserve. Thus, on the basis of metabolic effects, a relatively high-fat, carbohydrate-restricted diet is indicated for patients with CO_2 retention. The capacity of such diets to reduce CO_2 production has been shown, whereas the capacity of such diets to modify clinical outcomes has not been demonstrated to date.

Weight loss in chronic pulmonary disease, such as COPD, and cystic fibrosis has been attributed to an increased resting energy expenditure, although evidence in support of this is inconsistent. An increased work of breathing may contribute to an elevation of resting energy consumption, but inefficiency in oxygen metabolism with exertion may contribute more. Cytokines associated with the disease state may contribute to catabolism and attenuate appetite. Negative energy balance during acute exacerbations of COPD apparently is due to both reduced energy intake relative to baseline and an increase in resting energy expenditure (2). Elevated levels of tumor necrosis factor α, and other acute-phase-reactant proteins, have been reported in patients with COPD and weight loss, although causality has not been adequately studied to date (2).

A review of nutritional support for severe pulmonary disease of diverse etiologies suggests that weight loss, particularly loss of fat-free mass, is a poor prognostic sign. However, evidence of benefit for aggressive nutritional support is lacking (3). Further investigation of effective means of suppressing inflammatory mediator activity and preferentially restoring lean body mass is indicated.

In COPD, energy intake of 1.4 to 1.6 times the resting energy expenditure is indicated during periods when lean body mass is being recovered; energy then should be maintained at 1 to 1.2 times resting energy expenditure to avoid increased CO_2 generation (4). A high intake of protein and fat relative to carbohydrate is indicated, although this is more based on theoretical grounds than outcome evidence (4).

Protein supplementation at approximately 1.5 g/kg/day is advocated by some in the aftermath of COPD exacerbation to facilitate the reconstitution of lean body mass (2). Ingestion and postprandial gastric distension may impair gas exchange slightly, leading to reduced calorie consumption as a means to avoid dyspnea. Although nutritional support with high-fat rather than high-carbohydrate preparations offers the theoretical advantage of a lower respiratory quotient, in most cases the actual clinical significance appears to be small. COPD patients receiving calorie supplementation in combination with exercise have shown improvement, although not all those studied responded.

Reduction in the mass and contractility of the diaphragm has been observed in both animals and humans subject to malnutrition. Nutritional support may reverse this effect (5). Growth hormone and anabolic steroids have been used with some success, but their roles in clinical management are uncertain (6). Muscle wasting is characteristic during exacerbations of COPD and is compounded by the administration of corticosteroids. Dietary supplementation has been shown to attenuate, but not reverse, this tendency (7).

The energy requirements of patients with COPD and malnutrition are estimated at 45 kcal/kg/day, approximately 80% to 90% higher than predicted resting energy expenditure (see Nutrition Formulas in Section III) (8). In such patients, expert opinion favors a diet relatively high in total fat (45% to 55% of total calories), with low intake of saturated fat to avoid cardiovascular sequelae (8).

Difficulty in achieving measurable improvements in anthropometry or pulmonary function with energy-supplemented diets has been reported (9). Therefore, current interest has largely shifted from isolated dietary intervention to diet combined with exercise and/or anabolic agents.

Benefits of n-3 fatty acid supplementation in asthma have been reported (10). Population-based survey data suggest an inverse association between dietary fish intake and the development of smoking-related COPD (11).

The generation of lactic acid, and resultant cellular acidosis, is thought to contribute to muscle fatigue by a variety of mechanisms, including interference with calcium release, glycolytic enzyme activity, and neural impulse propagation (12). The retention of CO_2

and the resultant systemic acidosis impose a respiratory workload on patients with COPD, limiting exercise capacity. Sodium bicarbonate has been studied as an ergogenic aid in healthy subjects with mixed results; approximately half of the published trials show benefit (see Chapter 30). In a small study, Coppoolse and colleagues (12) demonstrated no increase in exercise capacity in COPD subjects given an acute oral bicarbonate load. Potential benefits of chronic bicarbonate supplementation remain speculative.

Data from the Nurses' Health Study suggest that vitamin E intake may be inversely associated with the risk of asthma development, although the association was relatively weak; other antioxidants did not reveal significant effects (13). Evidence that a variety of dietary antioxidants, especially vitamin C, vitamin E, and n-3 fatty acids, may protect against COPD is preliminary but provocative (14). The evidence and biologic plausibility of antioxidant benefits in asthma are less robust, although vitamin E, vitamin C, and selenium appear protective based on available evidence. A recent review emphasizes the apparent benefit of vitamin C, as well as the need for further study of diet and asthma given the preliminary evidence suggesting important associations (15). Folklore has long suggested that dairy product consumption increases the production of respiratory tract mucus and exacerbates asthma. A recently completed double-blind, placebo-controlled crossover trial in 20 subjects showed no effect of acute milk consumption on symptoms or pulmonary function (16).

In a recent survey of readers of a peer-reviewed journal of alternative and complementary medical practices, nutritional therapy for asthma was the most frequently cited practice among MD and non-MD providers, testifying to widespread interest in the topic (17). Use of nutrition and other alternative medical practices also was reported by 55% of 51 consecutive asthmatic children seen at a conventional medical clinic in south Australia (18).

Nutrients and Nutriceuticals

Phosphorus

Hypophosphatemia is known to impair diaphragmatic contractility and exacerbate CO_2 retention. Phosphorus depletion commonly occurs due to intracellular shifts following the correction of respiratory acidosis (19).

Impaired skeletal muscle function, attributable to loss of lean body mass, is associated with functional deterioration in COPD (20). Weight loss generally correlates with loss of respiratory muscle strength, which in turn is predictive of CO_2 retention. Nonetheless, patients not demonstrably underweight may be impaired due to losses of fat-free mass.

Monosodium Glutamate

The perception among asthma sufferers that the condition is exacerbated by food additives is widespread (see Chapter 17). Monosodium glutamate (MSG) is the substance most commonly implicated. In a recent double-blind, placebo-controlled crossover trial of 12 subjects who reported MSG sensitivity, no effect of MSG was demonstrated (21).

Antioxidants

Inverse associations between dietary antioxidants and both asthma and COPD have been reported. A recent case-control study noted inverse associations with zinc, magnesium, and manganese, as well as vitamin C (22). Theoretical support is strongest for vitamin C, which is found abundantly in pulmonary secretions (23).

Magnesium

Magnesium relaxes bronchial and vascular smooth muscle. It has been studied for the treatment of acute, reversible bronchoconstriction, but there have been mixed results. A recent double-blind, placebo-controlled crossover trial of 17 stable asthmatic patients showed improvement in symptoms, but not objective measures of pulmonary function, when taking supplemental magnesium compared to placebo (24). The study may have lacked power to detect clinically meaningful improvements in pulmonary function.

n-3 Fatty Acids

There is considerable interest in the potential benefits of n-3 fatty acid supplementation on inflammatory conditions in general and pulmonary diseases in particular. Evidence in support of this interest is limited to date, but appears promising. A recent double-blind, randomized trial of fish oil in asthmatic children showed a decrease in tumor necrosis factor α in the intervention group, but over the 6-month study period there was no difference in disease activity (25).

CLINICAL HIGHLIGHTS

Inflammation is important in the pathogenesis of chronic airway diseases. The inflammatory process leads to oxidative cell injury, implicating oxidation in chronic airway disease as well. Therefore, a theoretical basis exists for optimizing intake of antiinflammatory and antioxidant nutrients. Although definitive evidence of benefit in airway disease has been reported for neither, both are supported by other lines of evidence and may be recommended on general principles (see Chapter 40). Minimally, a diet rich in fruits, vegetables, whole grains, and fish is advisable. Supplementation with vitamin C 500 mg per day, vitamin E 400 to 800 IU per day, and flaxseed oil, one tablespoon per day, would appear reasonable components of an overall plan to ameliorate the course of chronic airway disease despite the lack of conclusive outcome data. On general principles, a daily multivitamin/mineral supplement is appropriate for all patients with chronic airway disease.

Patients with more advanced airway disease are at risk of malnutrition and should be monitored closely for signs thereof. Nutritional consultation is indicated at the earliest emergence of such signs and, not unreasonably, even before. Increased energy expenditure and decreased intake both may contribute to catabolism, and the diet should be tailored to compensate. Relative restriction of carbohydrate may be indicated to limit CO_2 production in retainers, but conclusive evidence of benefit for this practice is lacking. More convincing is evidence of benefit of maintaining nutritional adequacy, with relatively high protein intake, in combination with a program of conditioning exercise.

REFERENCES

1. Chin R Jr., Haponik EF. Nutrition, respiratory function, and disease. In: Shils.
2. Vermeeren MAP, Schols AMWJ, Wouters EFM. Effects of an acute exacerbation on nutritional and metabolic profile of patients with COPD. *Eur Respir J* 1997;10:2264.
3. Donahoe MP. Nutrition in end-stage pulmonary disease. *Monaldi Arch Chest Dis* 1995;50:47.
4. Pezza M, Iermano C, Tufano R. Nutritional support for the patient with chronic obstructive pulmonary disease. *Monaldi Arch Chest Dis* 1994;49[Suppl 1]: 33.
5. Dureuil B, Matuszczak Y. Alteration in nutritional status and diaphragm muscle function. *J Reprod Nutr Dev* 1998;38:175.
6. Schols AMWJ. Nutrition and outcome in chronic respiratory disease. *Nutrition* 1997;13:161.
7. Saudny-Unterberger H, Martin JG, Gray-Donald K. Impact of nutritional support on functional status during an acute exacerbation of chronic obstructive pulmonary disease. *Am J Respir Crit Care Med* 1997;156:794.
8. Goldstein-Shapses SA. Nutritional treatment in chronic respiratory failure: the effect of macronutrients on metabolism and ventilation. *Monaldi Arch Chest Dis* 1993;48:535.
9. Sridhar MK, Galloway A, Lean MEJ, et al. An outpatient nutritional supplementation programme in COPD patients. *Eur Respir J* 1994;7:720.
10. Vincent D. Relationship of dietary fish intake to level of pulmonary function. *Eur J Respir* 1995;8: 507.
11. Silverman EK, Speizer FE. Risk factors for the development of chronic obstructive pulmonary disease. *Med Clin North Am* 1996;80:501.
12. Coppoolse R, Barstow TJ, Stringer WW, et al. Effect of acute bicarbonate administration on exercise responses of COPD patients. *Med Sci Sports Exerc* 1997;29:725.
13. Troisi RJ, Willett WC, Weiss ST, et al. A prospective study of diet and adult-onset asthma. *Am J Respir Crit Care Med* 1995;151:1401.
14. Burney P. The origins of obstructive airways disease. A role for diet? *Am J Respir Crit Care Med* 1995; 151:1292.
15. Weiss ST. Diet as a risk factor for asthma. In: *The*

rising trends in asthma. Ciba Foundation Symposium 206. Chichester: Wiley, 1997:244.
16. Woods RK, Weiner JM, Abramson M, et al. Do dairy products induce bronchoconstriction in adults with asthma? *J Allergy Clin Immunol* 1998;101:45.
17. David PA, Gold EB, Hackman RM, et al. The use of complementary/alternative medicine for the treatment of asthma in the United States. *Invest Allergol Clin Immunol* 1998;8:73.
18. Andrews L, Lokuge S, Sawyer M, et al. The use of alternative therapies by children with asthma: a brief report. *J Paediatr Child Health* 1998;34:131.
19. Chin, Haponik. In: Shils.
20. Schols AMWJ. Nutrition and outcome in chronic respiratory disease. *Nutrition* 1997;13:161.
21. Woods RK, Weiner JM, Thien F, et al. The effects of monosodium glutamate in adults with asthma who perceive themselves to be monosodium glutamate-intolerant. *J Allergy Clin Immunol* 1998;101[6 Pt 1]:762.
22. Soutar A, Seaton A, Brown K. Bronchial reactivity and dietary antioxidants. *Thorax* 1997;52:166.
23. Hatch GE. Asthma, inhaled oxidants, and dietary antioxidants. *Am J Clin Nutr* 1995;61[Suppl]:625s.
24. Hill J, Micklewright A, Lewis S, et al. Investigation of the effect of short-term change in dietary magnesium intake in asthma. *Eur Respir J* 1997;10:2225.
25. Hodge L, Salome CM, Hughes JM, et al. Effect of dietary intake of omega-3 and omega-6 fatty acids on severity of asthma in children. *Eur Respir J* 1998;11:361.

BIBLIOGRAPHY

See "Sources for All Chapters."
Feldman EB. Nutrition and diet in the management of hyperlipidemia and atherosclerosis. In: Shils ME, Olson JA, Shike M, eds. *Modern nutrition in health and disease,* 8th ed. Philadelphia: Lea & Febiger, 1994.
McNamar DJ. Cardiovascular disease. In: Shils ME, Olson JA, Shike M, eds. *Modern nutrition in health and disease,* 8th ed. Philadelphia: Lea & Febiger, 1994.
Margen S, ed. *The wellness nutrition counter.* New York: Rebus, 1997.

15

Diet and Immunity

INTRODUCTION

Immune function refers broadly to the actions of both the humoral and cell-mediated systems in defense of the body against microbial and toxic invasions. The humoral immune system comprises the five immunoglobulin classes, IgA, D, E, G, and M, produced by B lymphocytes. Immunoglobulins are glycoproteins and therefore are dependent on adequate protein nutriture, as well as on the enzymes and cofactors essential to protein metabolism. The cell-mediated system includes T lymphocytes and various granulocytes, both phagocytic and nonphagocytic. Normal immune function is dependent as well on cytokines and complement, chemical messengers orchestrating the response of immune cells. The entire immune system is subject to neuroendocrine regulation, which in turn is influenced by nutritional status. The bone marrow is one of the largest and most metabolically active tissues in the body, producing billions of blood cells daily. Hematopoiesis is dependent on the availability of adequate substrate for cell formation. Intake of nutrients likely to be rate limiting in the production of immune system components offers the possibility of modifying immunocompetence by dietary manipulation.

OVERVIEW

Diet

Antibody formation is impaired by deficiencies in total protein and/or B-complex vitamins. Natural conditions make the study of single-nutrient deficiencies on immune function difficult, as nutrient deficiency is typically the result of generalized malnutrition. Environmental circumstances conducive to malnutrition tend to favor the transmission of infectious disease as well (e.g., poverty, poor sanitation, displacement), further complicating interpretation of naturally occurring states of nutritional immunosuppression in humans. Therefore, the effects of isolated nutrient deficiencies on immune function have been investigated predominantly by use of animal models.

Protein-energy malnutrition in humans is associated with impairment of both humoral and cell-mediated immunity; T-helper cells are suppressed, whereas T-suppressor cells are spared or even generated at an increased rate. Production of, and response to, interleukin 1 appears to be diminished by protein malnutrition.

Of the B complex, pyridoxine, pantothenic acid, riboflavin, folate, and B_{12} have the greatest impact on immune function. B_{12} repletion in patients with pernicious anemia has been shown to reverse anergy on skin testing.

Malnutrition during gestation apparently can result in prolonged immunocompromise even if the diet is adequate during the neonatal period. Low birth weight is associated with impaired development of the spleen and thymus and possibly impaired placental transfer of maternal immunoglobulin G.

Overnutrition may interfere with immunity, although data are limited. The relationship between obesity and immunocompetence is uncertain, although obese infants appear to experience more lower respiratory infections than lean counterparts. Excess intake of dietary fat may interfere with reticuloendothelial system function. Phagocyte function is impaired by hyperglycemia in diabetes; the role of dietary sugar in nondiabetics is less clear. In general, the rate of infection in states of extreme malnutrition is lower than the immune system disruption would suggest. Some authorities have speculated that malnutrition might result in some enhancement of immune function or merely render the body less accommodating to microbial pathogens.

Epidemiologic data reveal the total leukocyte count to be a potent predictor of various morbidities and all-cause mortality. Leukocyte activity generates reactive oxygen moieties, a possible mechanism for adverse effects (1). Reactive oxidant species such as H_2O_2 and HOCl exert an inhibitory influence on both T and B lymphocytes and natural killer cells. Dietary intake levels and serum levels of several antioxidant nutrients, including vitamin C, vitamin E, and β-carotene, are inversely correlated with neutrophil and total leukocyte counts (1). Thus, the white blood cell count may emerge as a convenient gauge of the adequacy of antioxidant intake (1). These findings are preliminary and require further study before routine clinical application is indicated.

The health benefits of a diet with relatively high fruit and vegetable intake are thought to include enhanced immunity. Although the nutrient complexity of whole foods makes nutrient-specific causality difficult to establish, potential benefits of dietary antioxidants (2), plant sterols (3), and flavonoids (4) have been proposed.

Gradual attenuation of immune function with aging is well established and may be an important contributor to functional deterioration with age (5). Reduced T-cell function may be the earliest harbinger of age-related immunocompromise and may be related to thymic involution (5). Although a decline in immune function with age has been deemed normal, recent evidence suggests that age-related immune dysfunction may be due, at least in part, to nutritional deficiencies (6). The regulation of T-cell function tends to deteriorate with age, whereas immunoglobulin levels tend to rise. Specific antibody responses diminish. Protein and zinc deficiencies appear to be particularly prevalent and important contributors to dysregulation of immune function in elderly individuals. Limited evidence suggests that supplementation can confer clinical benefit (6). There is some evidence, reviewed by Bogden and Louria (5), that a daily multivitamin/mineral supplement for 6 to 12 months in older adults improves measures of cell-mediated immunity. Data on the benefits of multivitamin supplementation much beyond 1 year are lacking (5). Given that deficiencies of one or more micronutrients are found in up to one third of all free-living elderly, a multivitamin/mineral supplement for all individuals over age 50 is likely to be both appropriate and cost effective (7).

Human Immunodeficiency Virus Infection

Energy expenditure rises with human immunodeficiency virus (HIV) infection, and depletion of vitamin B_{12}, folate, zinc, and selenium has been reported as the CD4 count falls below 500 (8). The acquired immunodeficiency syndrome (AIDS) is associated with wasting; the wasting syndrome seen in HIV infection is an AIDS-defining condition (9). Loss of 10% or more of baseline body weight generally is associated with diminished functional capacity.

In addition to appropriate antiretroviral therapy, nutritional supplementation and appetite stimulation are important adjuvants in this syndrome. An imbalance between caloric intake and the metabolic demands imposed by the primary HIV infection as well as any secondary opportunistic infections is thought to be the principal antecedent of wasting, but effects of specific inflammatory cytokines have been suggested (9). A recent review (9) addresses the role of pharmacologic support with megestrol acetate, dronabinol, and/or testosterone analogues, as well as that of growth hormone (10). Nutritional supplementation should focus on adequate total energy to prevent on-going weight loss, as well as balanced intake of macronutrients and micronutrients. Nutrition counseling apparently is more effective when combined with an appropriate oral supplement than when given alone (11). Glutamine supplementation has been studied with limited evidence of benefit. The role, if any, of potentially immune-enhancing nutrients, such as zinc, arginine, or n-3 fatty acids, in HIV in general, and the AIDS wasting syndrome specifically, is unknown.

Nutrients and Nutriceuticals

Zinc

Zinc deficiency is considered one of the most prevalent nutritional deficiencies worldwide, due both to limited dietary intake and the presence in the food supply of phytic acid, a zinc chelator. Zinc is an essential cofactor in more than 90 metalloenzyme systems; its deficiency interferes with cellular replication. Zinc deficiency in particular appears to arrest T-cell maturation. Studies in mice have shown that moderate-to-severe zinc deficiency leads to bone marrow depletion of B lymphocytes and to peripheral lymphopenia.

These studies suggest that zinc deficiency leads to chronic elevation of glucocorticoid levels, which in turn suppress immunity. The combination of zinc deficiency and elevated cortisol is thought to augment apoptosis of prelymphocytes in the bone marrow. The same conditions that lead to lymphopenia apparently spare, at least relatively, granulocyte precursors. The possibility exists that granulocytosis and lymphopenia in response to zinc deficiency represent a form of homeostatic prioritization in the face of resource shortages. Phagocytic cells, representing a first line of defense, may be favored over lymphocytes during periods of malnutrition. Zinc repletion appears to restore normal immunity in zinc-deficient organisms

within as little as 2 weeks. Excessive zinc supplementation may adversely effect immune function (5).

Iron

Iron deficiency is associated with impaired cell-mediated immunity. If iron deficiency occurs in the context of general malnutrition, protein deficiency will suppress levels of transferrin. Under such circumstances, repleted iron is readily available to microorganisms; therefore, iron repletion before protein repletion might be harmful, promoting bacterial replication. Iron excess is associated with impaired immunity and susceptibility to tumorigenesis.

Essential Amino Acids/Arginine

Deficiency of any of the essential amino acids appears to suppress humoral immunity, whereas intake of nonessential amino acids appears not to be limiting given adequate total protein intake. Animal studies suggest that imbalances of protein intake can impair immunity even in the absence of overt deficiency; excessive dietary leucine has been shown to reduce antibody responses in animals. Sulfur-containing amino acids involved in the synthesis of glutathione may be in particular demand during infection/inflammation due to the increased oxidative stresses, suggesting that supplementation might be beneficial (12).

Arginine is a conditionally essential amino acid (see Chapter 3). Studies in animals and *in vitro* suggest that supplemental L-arginine may be immunostimulatory (13). The use of L-arginine in states of human immunodeficiency has been proposed. Reduced hospital stay following surgery has been observed in supplemented patients. Arginine is an essential nitrogen donor in nitric oxide synthesis. The effects of nitric oxide on the vasculature are potentially an important component of the response to severe infection (14). Immune enhancement has been ascribed to both glutamine (15) and taurine (16).

randomized controlled trial evaluating nutrition counseling with or without oral supplementation in malnourished HIV-infected patients. *J Am Diet Assoc* 1998;98:434–438.

12. Grimble RF, Grimble GK. Immunonutrition: role of sulfur amino acids, related amino acids, and polyamines. *Nutrition* 1998;14:605–610.
13. Evoy D, Lieberman MD, Fahey TJ 3rd, et al. Immunonutrition: the role of arginine. *Nutrition* 1998;14: 611–617.
14. Kelly E, Morris SM Jr., Billiar TR. Nitric oxide, sepsis, and arginine metabolism. *J Parenteral Enteral Nutr* 1995;19:234–238.
15. Wilmore DW, Shabert JK. Role of glutamine in immunologic responses. *Nutrition* 1998;14:618–626.
16. Redmond HP, Stapleton PP, Neary P, et al. Immunonutrition: the role of taurine. *Nutrition* 1998;14: 599.
17. Friis H, Ndhlovu P, Kaondera K, et al. Serum concentration of micronutrients in relation to schistosomiasis and indicators of infection: a cross-sectional study among rural Zimbabwean schoolchildren. *Eur J Clin Nutr* 1996;50:386.
18. Das BS, Thurnham DI, Bas DB. Plasma α-tocopherol, retinol, and carotenoids in children with falciparum malaria. *Am J Clin Nutr* 1996;64:94.
19. Semba RD. Impact of vitamin A on immunity and infection in developing countries. In: Bendich A, Deckelbaum RJ, eds. *Preventive nutrition: the comprehensive guide for health professionals.* Totowa, NJ: Humana Press, 1997.
20. Beharka A, Redican S, Leka L, et al. Vitamin E status and immune function. *Methods Enzymol* 1997;282:247–263.
21. Meydani SN, Meydani M, Blumberg JB, et al. Vitamin E supplementation and *in vivo* immune response in healthy elderly subjects. A randomized controlled trial. *JAMA* 1997;277:1380–1386.
22. Wu D, Maydani M, Leka LS, et al. Effect of dietary supplementation with black currant seed oil on the immune response of healthy elderly subjects. *Am J Clin Nutr* 1999;70:536.
23. Wu D, Maydani SN. N-3 polyunsaturated fatty acids and immune function. *Proc Nutr Soc* 1998;57: 503–509.

BIBLIOGRAPHY

See "Sources for All Chapters."

Beisel WR, Edelman R, Nauss K, et al. Single-nutrient effects on immunologic functions. Report of a workshop sponsored by the department of Food and Nutrition and its Nutrition Advisory Group of the American Medical Association. *JAMA* 1981;245:53–58.

Levy J. Immunonutrition: the pediatric experience. *Nutrition* 1998;14:641.

Beaumier L, Castillo L, Yu YM, et al. Arginine: new and exciting developments for an "old" amino acid. *Biomed Environ Sci* 1996;9:296.

Mainous MR, Deitch EA. Nutrition and infection. *Surg Clin North Am* 1994;74:659.

Calder PC. N-3 polyunsaturated fatty acids and cytokine production in health and disease. *Ann Nutr Metab* 1997;41:203.

Scrimshaw NS, SanGiovanni JP. Synergism of nutrition, infection, and immunity: an overview. *Am J Clin Nutr* 1997;66:464s.

16

Diet and Wound Healing

INTRODUCTION

Overall nutritional status influences the response of the body to metabolic stress. Wound healing requires sufficient nutritional substrate to support the formation of granulation tissue. Adequate intake of energy, protein, and various micronutrients, before, during, and after either surgical or traumatic injury can influence the speed and vitality of tissue repair. Nutritional assessment and management strategies for the promotion of optimal wound healing have been elaborated, although evidence for certain interventions remains preliminary.

OVERVIEW

A patient's nutritional status is of vital importance to tissue repair in the advent of injury. The adequacy of various micronutrients, total protein, and total energy influence wound healing. Metabolic demand is increased during wound healing, increasing the likelihood of negative nitrogen balance and catabolism. Energy, protein, and micronutrient deficiencies are among the more common impediments to optimal wound healing (1).

Evaluation of all patients' nutritional status should be performed before elective surgery. In patients with no clinical evidence of compromised nutritional status, no laboratory testing is indicated. Patients with recent weight loss or those who are chronically underweight require a more extensive evaluation (see Chapter 24 and Nutrition Formulas in Section III). Dietary consultation in such cases is indicated. Preoperative nutritional support may be important to postoperative healing. Total parenteral nutrition (TPN; see Chapter 24) is an intervention of last resort; it has been shown to reduce noninfectious complications of surgery in select patients while increasing infectious complications.

In general, preoperative nutrition support is indicated in patients unfed for a period of 7 days or more as well as patients expected not to eat for 10 days or more and patients with loss of more than 10% of lean body mass. Such patients should receive enteral nutrition support unless contraindicated by intolerance or gastrointestinal tract dysfunction; only in such circumstances should TPN be used. In patients with evidence of poor nutritional status before elective surgery, enteral supplementation preoperatively may shorten recovery time (2). In patients who are well nourished before surgery, a 5% dextrose infusion for up to 1 week postoperatively has not been shown to impair recovery.

Because elderly patients have reduced appetite possibly compounded by impaired sensorium or functional status, they are highly subject to protein-calorie malnutrition and involuntary weight loss during wound healing (3). Nutritional status is correlated with the rate of wound healing (3). If compromised nutritional status results in losses of lean body mass, wound healing is delayed; therefore, nutritional support during wound healing should begin early, even when there is no evidence of nutritional impairment (3). Children, particularly neonates, are susceptible to loss of lean body mass during wound healing because their tissue reserves are limited (4).

The effects of specific nutrient deficiencies, and isolated nutrient supplements, on wound healing have been studied predominantly in animals. There is some evidence that pantothenic acid (vitamin B_5) supplementation can increase the tensile strength of aponeuroses and dermal scars. Thiamine is essential to normal collagen synthesis and metabolism, and animal studies have demonstrated impaired wound healing with deficiency.

Animal studies have demonstrated enhanced scar-tissue strength with vitamin A or provitamin A carotenoid supplementation, and impaired healing with deficiency. Vitamin C, which is essential to the metabolism of both collagen and elastin, has been studied in humans to a limited extent. Studies summarized by Werbach (5) suggest that vitamin C supplementation at a dose of 500 mg per day can accelerate the healing of surgical wounds and pressure sores. Supplementation with vitamin E 800 IU per day is supported by anecdotal evidence in humans, as well as by animal research.

Evidence regarding zinc to date suggests that its nutriture is essential to healing, but that supplementation is of importance only when zinc stores are deficient. Animal evidence suggests that zinc is concentrated at the site of wound healing, with impaired tensile strength of skin resulting when zinc is deficient (6). Recent epidemiologic data suggest that incipient zinc deficiency may be relatively widespread in the United States, particularly among the elderly. Thus, studies demonstrating accelerated wound healing with zinc supplementation may be of generalized relevance.

In a case-control study of chronic lower-extremity ulcers, Rojas and Phillips (7) found patients to have lower serum levels of vitamin A and carotenes, vitamin E, and zinc. These nutrients are generally thought to influence wound healing capacity (8). Supplements of the amino acids glutamine and argi-nine, and n-3 fatty acids, have shown promise in accelerating a patient's recovery from burns (9).

Wound infection has the potential to disrupt the healing process, while placing further metabolic demands on the patient. The adequacy of nutrition during wound healing will have systemic effects on immune function, thereby influencing susceptibility to wound infection (10).

Among the metabolic derangements associated with trauma is accelerated gluconeogenesis, which contributes to a state of catabolism (11). Protein requirements rise during recovery from trauma, and supplemental protein should be provided during periods of wound healing.

In addition to adequate nutritional support, pain control, conditioning exercises, and anabolic agents may contribute to preservation of lean body mass and to wound healing (11). In a study of eight patients with nonhealing wounds, Demling and De Santi (11) found that all subjects had lost at least 10% of body weight. Nutritional support alone failed to restore the lost weight or influence wound closure. The addition of oxandrolone, an oral anabolic agent, in combination with nutritional support led to weight gain and wound healing, with complete or partial wound closure in all subjects over 12 weeks. The authors noted a high correlation between restoration of lean body mass and wound healing (12).

CLINICAL HIGHLIGHTS

Evidence in the aggregate is conclusive that overall nutritional status influences the pace and quality of wound healing. Evidence for specific nutritional manipulations to enhance wound healing capacity is generally less definitive. Patients scheduled for elective surgery should routinely be assessed for the adequacy of their diets, recent weight loss history, and preservation of lean body mass. Preoperative nutrition supplementation in marginally malnourished patients may be of benefit and is of clear benefit when malnutrition is advanced.

Energy and protein needs are increased in patients recovering from surgical trauma as well as during healing of traumatic wounds. Multivitamin and mineral supplements are advisable in older adults on general principles and may be of particular benefit to wound healing. Additional supplementation with vitamin C 500 mg per day and vitamin E 800 IU per day may be of benefit and are unlikely to be of any harm. Topical vitamin A and E ointment may confer additional benefit. Zinc supplementation is beneficial over time in zinc-deficient patients. Supplementation with glutamine and arginine may be of benefit, but this is uncertain. A beneficial role of n-3 fatty acids has been suggested.

Dietary consultation to optimize nutrition is prudent in patients with nonhealing wounds, as case reports of rapid recovery following nutritional adjustments have been published. In general, the nutritional guidelines to promote wound healing are consistent with those that can be advocated on general principles.

REFERENCES

1. Stadelmann WK, Digenis AG, Tobin GR. Impediments to wound healing. *Am J Surg* 1988;176[2A Suppl]:39s–47s.
2. McClave SA, Snider HL, Spain DA. Preoperative issues in clinical nutrition. *Chest* 1999;115[5 Suppl]:64s–70s.
3. Himes D. Protein-calorie malnutrition and involuntary weight loss: the role of aggressive nutritional intervention in wound healing. *Ostomy Wound Manage* 1999;45:46–51, 54–55.
4. Shew SB, Jaksic T. The metabolic needs of critically ill children and neonates. *Semin Pediatr Surg* 1999; 8:131–139.
5. Werbach MR. *Nutritional influences on illness*. New Canaan, CT: Keats Publishing, 1988.
6. Nezu R, Takagi Y, Ito T, et al. The importance of total parenteral nutrition-associated tissue zinc distribution in wound healing. *Surg Today* 1999;29: 34–41.
7. Rojas AI, Phillips TJ. Patients with chronic leg ulcers show diminished levels of vitamins A and E, carotenes, and zinc. *Dermatol Surg* 1999;25:601–604.
8. Thomas DR. Specific nutritional factors in wound healing. *Adv Wound Care* 1997;10:40–43.
9. De-Souza DA, Greene LJ. Pharmacological nutrition after burn injury. *J Nutr* 1998;128:797–803.
10. Thornton FJ, Schaffer MR, Barbul A. Wound healing in sepsis and trauma. *Shock* 1997;8:391–401.
11. Demling RH, De Santi L. Involuntary weight loss and the nonhealing wound: the role of anabolic agents. *Adv Wound Care* 1999;12[1 Suppl]:1–14.
12. Demling R, De Santi L. Closure of the "non-healing wound" corresponds with correction of weight loss using the anabolic agent oxandrolone. *Ostomy Wound Manage* 1998;44:58–62, 64, 66.

BIBLIOGRAPHY

See "Sources for All Chapters."

Hunt TK, Hopf HW. Wound healing and wound infection. What surgeons and anesthesiologists can do. *Surg Clin North Am* 1997;77:587.

Souba WW Jr., Wilmore DW. Diet and nutrition in the care of the patient with surgery, trauma, and sepsis. In: Shils.

Thomas DR. Nutritional factors affecting wound healing. *Ostomy Wound Manage* 1996;42:40–42, 44–46, 48, 49.

Thomas DR. The role of nutrition in prevention and healing of pressure ulcers. *Clin Geriatr Med* 1997; 13:497.

Whitney JD, Heitkemper MM. Modifying perfusion, nutrition, and stress to promote wound healing in patients with acute wounds. *Heart Lung* 1999;28:123.

17

Food Allergy and Intolerance

INTRODUCTION

Adverse reactions to food include intolerance, a nonimmune-mediated abnormal physiologic response, and true food allergy, an immunologic reaction to ingested antigens. Intolerance may be mediated by metabolic processes (e.g., lactose intolerance), contaminants (e.g., bacteria or toxins), or pharmacologic effects of ingested food chemicals (e.g., alcohol, caffeine). Other adverse reactions are idiosyncratic. Although there is considerable uncertainty about the epidemiology of food allergy, the best available data suggest a prevalence in the range of 2%.

Generally, the predominant antibody reaction to ingested antigen is mediated by immunoglobulin A (IgA). Systemic hypersensitivity reactions to food are predominantly mediated by immunoglobulin E (IgE). Ingested antigens must traverse the intestinal mucosa and enter the circulation to elicit a hypersensitivity response; thus, food antigens are stable, water-soluble proteins of predictable size. The foods most commonly responsible for hypersensitivity reactions include eggs, peanuts, other nuts, milk, soy, wheat, fish, and shellfish. Bovine milk allergy is common in infancy.

OVERVIEW

Diet

The prevalence of true food allergy is estimated at approximately 2%, although in most surveys more than ten times that proportion of the population believe themselves to have food allergy. A random-digit-dial telephone survey in the United States of more than 4,000 households found the prevalence of peanut or tree nut allergy to approximate 1% of the general population (1). Intolerance to food additives is quite uncommon, estimated to be one per 10,000 population. There is some preliminary evidence associating food allergy in childhood with *Helicobacter pylori* infection; disruption of the gastrointestinal barrier by ingested antigens is the presumed mechanism (2).

With the exception of hypersensitivity to peanuts, nuts, fish, and shellfish, most food allergies occur in infancy and are outgrown by early childhood. Overall, approximately 40% of food allergies in children subside by age 5. Once a food allergen is identified and excluded from the diet, rechallenge after 1 to 2 years is appropriate, as most allergies abate with time. Allergies to nuts, peanuts, and seafood are particularly persistent, and rechallenge at 4- to 8-year intervals is more appropriate when these foods are implicated.

Exposure to food antigens in early infancy may be particularly likely to lead to hypersensitivity in susceptible individuals because of low levels of secretory IgA. Limited binding of antigen in the gastrointestinal tract leads to greater absorption and more IgE generation. The risk of food allergy appears to be reduced by delaying the introduction of solid foods to an infant until after 6 months of age and by maternal avoidance of such common allergens as bovine milk, eggs, peanuts, and fish during pregnancy and lactation. Infants born to atopic parents are at increased risk of atopy and may particularly benefit from delayed weaning and exclusions from the maternal diet during gestation. There is no evidence that the substitution of soy-based formulas for milk-based formulas attenuates the risk of atopy. Hypoallergenic formulas are available (Alimentum, Nutramigen, Pregestimil) (3) and are preferred, at least for high-risk infants weaned before 6 months. The avoidance of milk, egg, peanuts, peanut butter, and fish for the first 2 to 3 years of life may reduce the risk of food allergy in highly susceptible children. To effect such exclusions is challenging and of uncertain efficacy; therefore, these recommendations are appropriate only when the child is deemed at high risk and the family is highly motivated to use prophylactic measures of possible value.

The most common manifestation of true food allergy is cutaneous, ranging from urticaria and angioedema to atopic dermatitis; the link between food allergy and atopic dermatitis is particularly important. The spectrum of cutaneous manifestations of food allergy has been reviewed (4). Gastrointestinal reactions, including nausea, vomiting, pain, and blood in the stool, are relatively common and typically occur within 1 hour of ingestion. A condition known as Heiner's syndrome is a form of pulmonary hemosiderosis associated with hypersensitivity to bovine milk or, less commonly, egg or pork. Symptoms resolve with avoidance of the implicated food.

Contact hypersensitivity of the oropharynx (oral allergy syndrome) typically is associated with fresh fruits and raw vegetables. Specifically, the syndrome is induced in individuals with respiratory allergy to birch pollen, potatoes, carrots, celery, hazelnuts, and apples; in individuals with respiratory allergy to ragweed pollen, melons and bananas are implicated. The putative mechanism is antigenic cross-reactivity, although the responsible antigens have, for the most part, not been identified.

Among the varieties of food intolerance distinct from allergy is pseudoallergy, in which symptoms are related to the release

of histamine. The histamine release appears to be related to chemical rather than immunologic mechanisms, and it requires a large exposure. Dietary chemicals with pharmacologic properties often produce intolerance. Caffeine may be poorly tolerated, as may vasoactive amines such as histamine in fermented deli meats (sausage) and sauerkraut, and tyramine in cheese, chocolate, and red wine. Monosodium glutamate, typically associated with Chinese food, may lead to flushing and palpitations. Sulfites added to wine may be poorly tolerated, as may strong spices and capsaicin.

An association between "colic" in infants and the presence of bovine milk immunoglobulin G in maternal breast milk has been established, suggesting that hypersensitivity may account for some cases of colic (10% to 15%). Chronic constipation in young children may be a manifestation of allergy to bovine milk proteins (5). Although respiratory manifestations of food allergy are relatively less common, rhinitis and exacerbations of asthma have been convincingly associated with foods in blinded challenges.

Food-mediated anaphylaxis does occur, as does a variant, in which both food hypersensitivity and exercise are required in combination to induce the anaphylactic response. Eosinophilic gastroenteritis may be induced by milk protein hypersensitivity in infants and may require 12 weeks to resolve after removal of the offending antigen from the diet; short-term corticosteroid therapy may be indicated for both eosinophilic gastroenteritis and food-induced enterocolitis. Food allergy has been implicated in some cases of migraine headache. Although there is interest in the possible role of food allergy in inflammatory arthritis, inflammatory bowel disease, dysmenorrhea, chronic fatigue, and a variety of other constitutional symptoms, there currently is no convincing evidence.

The diagnosis of food allergy is facilitated by a history that establishes a temporal link between ingestion and the manifestations of hypersensitivity. Food allergy is much more likely when a family history of atopy is present. A diet diary is useful in identifying potential allergens.

Skin testing is reliable in excluding IgE-mediated food allergy, as the test is highly sensitive; it performs less well as a rule-in test because of limited specificity (6). Radioallergosorbent tests (RAST) are conducted *in vitro,* identifying IgE antibody responses to specific antigens; the performance characteristics of RAST are similar to those of skin testing.

Recent data suggest that skin prick tests may be of variable utility depending on the allergen; such tests perform poorly for soy allergy in particular (7). No laboratory tests are available for the detection of non–IgE-mediated food allergies. Elimination diets are useful both diagnostically and therapeutically, requiring that the correct food antigen be entirely eliminated from the diet for a period of 1 to 2 weeks. Software to facilitate the detection of food allergens and safe foods in food diaries is under development (8). The most definitive diagnostic method is double-blind, placebo-controlled challenge with the suspected antigen; such testing is potentially hazardous and should only be done when truly necessary, and then only under carefully controlled circumstances. The diagnostic approach to food allergy has been reviewed (9–11).

Treatment of food allergy depends on elimination of the implicated antigen(s) from the diet. The antigenic proteins should be identified, rather than the whole food most likely to contain them, as the proteins may be present in other foods. The milk proteins responsible for hypersensitivity, casein and whey, for example, may be included on ingredient lists independent of milk. Lecithin often is derived from either soy or egg, but the source frequently will not be included on ingredient labels.

Because food allergens tend to be widely distributed in the food supply, elimination requires expert dietary advice both to achieve full elimination and to avoid nutrient deficiencies. Modification of foods and manipulation of the gut microflora may provide alter-natives to elimination in the future, but their use remains experimental to date (12,13).

The most common food allergies in adults are to fish, shellfish, nuts, and peanuts; in children, the most common reactions are to milk, eggs, peanuts, soy, and wheat. Peanuts are in the legume family and, therefore, have antigens that do not generally cross-react with those of other nuts. There is little evidence implicating food additives in hypersensitivity reactions. Celiac disease is the result of hypersensitivity to gluten present in wheat, oat, rye, and barley.

Nutrients and Nutriceuticals

Lactose

Intolerance to lactose, a milk sugar, results from deficiency of the enzyme lactase. Deficiency actually is considered the normal condition for adult mammals, with preservation of enzyme activity into adulthood the result of a genetic mutation. Lactase deficiency is considered the most common enzyme deficiency; more than half of all adults are affected. Deficiency is especially common in individuals of African, Asian, Mediterranean, or Native-American origin; lactose tolerance is highly prevalent in northern Europeans.

Lactose intolerance is distinct from allergy to milk proteins. For individuals allergic to bovine milk protein, alternative milks may be substituted. However, all milks (cow, goat, sheep) contain lactose. Milk products such as cheese and butter contain milk protein, so they cannot be eaten by individuals with true allergy, but they contain trivial amounts of lactose. Most individuals with lactose intolerance of genetic origin can tolerate at least 5 g of lactose (contained in 100 mL of milk) with no symptoms. In a randomized, double-blind crossover trial, Suarez and colleagues (14) demonstrated that adults self-reporting severe lactose intolerance could tolerate up to 15 g of lactose in 250 mL of milk.

In a separate study, Suarez et al. (15) demonstrated that lactose intolerance is unlikely to interfere meaningfully with a dietary pattern providing the recommended 1,500 mg of daily calcium in adult women. The gastrointestinal symptoms attributed by many individuals to lactose intolerance may represent a form of irritable bowel syndrome of as yet uncertain etiology (16–19). To the extent that symptoms are induced by lactose in maldigesters, there is no appreciable difference between whole-fat and fat-free milk; recommendations to such individuals to use whole-fat dairy products to reduce symptoms are unfounded (20). For lactose-intolerant patients consuming more than 15 g per day of lactose, a variety of lactose-free or hydrolyzed-lactose products are available (see Section III).

Gluten

Gluten is a protein found in many cereal grains, but it is especially abundant in wheat. Intolerance to gluten causes villous atrophy, the hallmark of celiac sprue. Dermatitis herpetiformis is associated with gluten intolerance as well. Antibody testing to endomysial tissue indicates gluten sensitivity is more prevalent than the number of clinically overt cases would suggest; thus, mild cases may go clinically undetected (21). The prevalence of gluten intolerance is estimated to be one in 300 for individuals of European origin. Gluten intolerance is lifelong, and exclusion of gluten from the diet is the only known treatment to date (22). Lymphoma risk rises with celiac disease, but is mitigated by adherence to a gluten-free diet. As gluten is virtually ubiquitous in the diet, expert dietary advice is essential. (Registries of gluten-free foods are available on-line; see Section III.) Most gluten-free diets traditionally exclude oats, but this may prove to be unnecessary, at least for some patients (see Chapter 22) (23).

CLINICAL HIGHLIGHTS

Food allergy is sufficiently common that most clinicians are likely to encounter it. The manifestations span a wide spectrum, although the more common manifestations are fairly prototypical. The prevalence of true food allergy is higher in children than adults, and many children can be expected to outgrow their allergies. Diagnosis can be confirmed only with elimination diets and double-blind challenges, but skin testing often is helpful. The most common food allergies in adults are to fish, shellfish, nuts and peanuts; in children, the most common reactions are to milk, eggs, peanuts, soy, and wheat. If food allergy is confirmed, a dietitian should be consulted to help the patient (or their parents) develop a nutritionally complete diet completely free of the offending antigen. Allergy to gluten produces celiac disease and requires complete and permanent elimination of gluten from the diet (see Chapter 22).

Food intolerance, as opposed to allergy, is not immune mediated. Lactose intolerance is perhaps the most common and best-known example. Although patients with lactose intolerance may report an inability to tolerate any milk, randomized double-blind trials are consistent in demonstrating that most individuals can tolerate up to 15 g per day of lactose, and that adequate calcium intake from dairy sources remains feasible. Breastfeeding up to the age of 6 months may reduce the risk of food allergy, although more extreme measures, such as maternal dietary exclusions to prevent the presence of food antigens in breast milk, may be unrealistic for most patients. The role of food allergy in a host of conditions and constitutional symptoms remains speculative at present. Advances in the modification of food antigenicity and intestinal microflora show promise in offering new alternatives for the prevention and management of food allergy.

REFERENCES

1. Sicherer SH, Munoz-Furlong A, Burks AW, et al. Prevalence of peanut and tree nut allergy in the US determined by a random digit dial telephone survey. *J Allergy Clin Immunol* 1999;103:559–562.
2. Corrado G, Luzzi I, Lucarelli S, et al. Positive association between Helicobacter pylori infection and

food allergy in children. *Scand J Gastroenterol* 1998;33:1135–1139.

3. Host A, Koletzko B, Dreborg S, et al. Dietary products used in infants for treatment and prevention of food allergy. Joint statement of the European society for paediatric allergology and clinical immunology (ESPACI) committee on hypoallergenic formulas and the European society for paediatric gastroenterology, hepatology and nutrition (ESPGHAN) committee on nutrition. *Arch Dis Child* 1999;81:80–84.

4. Wuthrich B. Food-induced cutaneous adverse reactions. *Allergy* 1998;53[Suppl]:131–135.

5. Iacono G, Cavataio F, Montalto G, et al. Intolerance of cow's milk and chronic constipation in children. *N Engl J Med* 1998;339:1100–1104.

6. Majamaa H, Moiso P, Holm K, et al. Wheat allergy: diagnostic accuracy of skin prick and patch test and specific IgE. *Allergy* 1999;54:851–856.

7. Eigenmann PA, Sampson HA. Interpreting skin prick tests in the evaluation of food allergy in children. *Pediatr Allergy Immunol* 1998;9:186–191.

8. Kueper T, Martinelli D, Konetzki W, et al. Identification of problem foods using food and symptom diaries. *Otolaryngol Head Neck Surg* 1995;112:415–420.

9. Terho EO, Savolainen J. Diagnosis and food hypersensitivity. *Eur J Clin Nutr* 1996;50:1–5.

10. Sampson HA. Food allergy. Part 1: immunopathogenesis and clinical disorders. *J Allergy Clin Immunol* 1999;103:717–728.

11. Sampson HA. Food allergy. Part 2: diagnosis and management. *J Allergy Clin Immunol* 1999;103:981–989.

12. Isolauri E, Salminen S, Mattila-Sandholm T. New functional foods in the treatment of food allergy. *Ann Med* 1999;31:299–302.

13. Kirjavainen PV, Gibson GR. Healthy gut microflora and allergy: factors influencing development of the microbiota. *Ann Med* 1999;31:288–292.

14. Suarez FL, Savaiano DA, Levitt MD. A comparison of symptoms after the consumption of milk or lactose-hydrolyzed milk by people with self-reported severe lactose intolerance. *N Engl J Med* 1995; 333:1–4.

15. Suarez FL, Adshead J, Furne JK, et al. Lactose maldigestion is not an impediment to the intake of 1500 mg calcium as dairy products. *Am J Clin Nutr* 1998;68:1118–1122.

16. Vesa TH, Korpela RA, Sahi T. Tolerance to small amounts of lactose in lactose maldigesters. *Am J Clin Nutr* 1996;64:197–201.

17. Suarez F, Levitt MD. Abdominal symptoms and lactose: the discrepancy between patients' claims and the results of blinded trials. *Am J Clin Nutr* 1996;64:251–252.

18. Mascolo R, Saltzman JR. Lactose intolerance and irritable bowel syndrome. *Nutr Rev* 1998;56:306–308.

19. Vesa TH, Seppo LM, Marteau PR, et al. Role of irritable bowel syndrome in subjective lactose intolerance. *Am J Clin Nutr* 1998;67:710–715.

20. Vesa TH, Lember M, Korpela R. Milk fat does not affect the symptoms of lactose intolerance. *Eur J Clin Nutr* 1997;51:633–636.

21. Parnell ND, Ciclitira PJ. Review article: coeliac disease and its management. *Aliment Pharmacol Ther* 1999;13:1–13.

22. Murray JA. The widening spectrum of celiac disease. *Am J Clin Nutr* 1999;69:354–365.

23. Thompson T. Do oats belong in a gluten-free diet? *J Am Diet Assoc* 1997;97:1413–1416.

BIBLIOGRAPHY

See "Sources for All Chapters."

Malagelada J-R. Lactose intolerance. *N Engl J Med* 1995;333:53–54.

Rance F, Kanny G, Dutau G, et al. Food hypersensitivity in children: clinical aspects and distribution of allergens. *Pediatr Allergy Immunol* 1999;10:3–38.

18

Diet and Rheumatologic Disease

INTRODUCTION

Interest among patients in dietary management of various inflammatory diseases of soft tissue and joints generally exceeds the availability of rigorously obtained scientific evidence. Much of the evidence in support of nutritional therapies for rheumatologic conditions is anecdotal; little of the evidence is better than suggestive. There are, however, clear links between diet and the natural history of certain arthritides. Further, there is a biologically plausible link between dietary patterns and inflammatory activity in general.

Preliminary evidence of the beneficial effects of n-3 fatty acids in rheumatoid arthritis (RA) is fortified by the clearly established role of polyunsaturated fats in the manufacture of inflammatory and antiinflammatory cytokines. The impact of diet on weight may indirectly have important effects on the degree to which arthritis of any etiology translates into functional limitations and on its rate of progression. Rheumatologic diseases arising from errors in intermediate metabolism, such as gout, are decisively influenced by diet. There is sufficient evidence of possible benefit, and sufficiently limited evidence of likely toxicity, to support consideration of nutritional interventions for osteoarthritis (OA), RA, and gout.

Evidence for nutritional therapies in other conditions is less interpretable. In general, the magnitude of benefit from nutritional interventions appears insufficient to replace conventional treatments; nutritional and pharmacologic interventions should be considered potentially complementary. Diet and nutriceuticals are most important in patients intolerant of, or unresponsive to, conventional treatments. Finally, the dissemination of unsubstantiated claims for nutrients with healing properties in diverse rheumatologic conditions does a disservice to patients by cultivating misapprehensions, and perhaps even more so to physicians, among whom this trend may cultivate inattention to the actual potential benefits of nutritional therapies.

OVERVIEW

Diet

Overall dietary pattern may influence the risk of rheumatologic disease, as well as the risk of functional limitations in the advent of such disease. Mechanisms for these associations are both direct and indirect. Directly, there is a link between dietary pattern and immune function, mediated by a variety of micronutrients including antioxidant substances and zinc (Chapter 15), as well as the pattern of fatty acid intake. Indirectly, diet will influence the impact of arthritic conditions on function by contributing to overall health status and the extent of comorbidities, including vascular disease.

Most of the claims for an effect of general dietary pattern on the development and progression of rheumatologic conditions are consistent with dietary recommendations for general health maintenance. Excess body weight secondary to caloric excess increases joint stress, and particularly may exacerbate size generally has been small (11). The available evidence is preliminary, but other lines of argument support increased n-3 fatty acid intake (see Chapter 40). Studies combining n-6 fatty acid restriction, n-3 supplementation, and antiinflammatory drug use are indicated.

Glucosamine Sulfate

Glucosamine is found in the body as a precursor of glycosaminoglycans, which are used by chondrocytes in the manufacture of proteoglycans incorporated into articular cartilage. The body's manufacture of glucosamine declines with age at variable rates, apparently leaving some people vulnerable to deficiency. The use of supplemental glucosamine is promoted as a means of compensating for a decline in endogenous production, thereby reconstituting worn articular surfaces.

Although glucosamine is available in various forms, its use as a sulfate salt is most convincingly supported by available evidence, perhaps because sulfur is another integral component of cartilage. Glucosamine available as a nutriceutical agent is derived from the exoskeletons of shrimps, lobsters, and crabs.

Data from a number of methodologically rigorous studies, including double-blind, randomized trials, demonstrate the efficacy of glucosamine in OA (12). Glucosamine works slowly by reconstituting cartilage and has no known direct analgesic properties. Antiinflammatory effects have been reported (13); therefore, pain relief is faster with nonsteroidal antiinflammatory drugs (NSAIDs).

One double-blind trial demonstrated superior pain relief with ibuprofen at 2 weeks, but a superior effect of glucosamine at 4 weeks (14). There is evidence that NSAIDs, while alleviating symptoms, may actually accelerate the degeneration of articular cartilage (15,16). There is no known toxicity of glucosamine sulfate. Doses up to 500 mg three times daily are generally recommended; higher doses may be required in obese patients or those on diuretics.

Recent literature reviews highlight important gaps in the evidence supporting use of glucosamine. Trials conducted to date have been small and short term. No controlled trials conducted in the United States have been reported (17). Thus, even though the available evidence is provocative, it can be considered only suggestive (18). Clearly further study of glucosamine is indicated.

Cartilage Extracts and Chondroitin Sulfate

Alternative medicine publications support the use of various cartilage extracts, including shark cartilage, sea cucumber, chondroitin sulfate, and green-lipped mussel for chronic, degenerative arthroses. These products either contain glycosaminoglycans or, in the case of chondroitin, are glycosaminoglycans, and putatively function by incorporation into joints (19). However, absorption apparently is very poor, with rates between 0% and 8% (12). In contrast, absorption of glucosamine, a much smaller molecule, is estimated to be about 98%.

The available evidence, and the established pharmacokinetics, support the use of glucosamine over these products. The combination of chondroitin sulfate and glucosamine sulfate has become popular, but there is no evidence that the combination is any more effective than glucosamine monotherapy (20).

Nightshade Vegetables

The nightshade family of plants, known scientifically as the *Solanaceae*, has been implicated in the alternative medicine literature as a cause of arthritis. The literature is poorly substantiated, and the type of arthritis rarely specified.

The family *Solanaceae* is diverse and includes the potato, tomato, red pepper, eggplant, tobacco, paprika, pimento, cayenne pepper, and chili pepper. There is little evidence to support elimination of one or more of these foods from the diet to manage any particular type of arthritis. Elimination diets, however, are occasionally helpful in RA, and the elimination of nightshades might be considered in that context in an effort to manage refractory disease.

CLINICAL HIGHLIGHTS

There is sufficient evidence to justify offering tailored dietary advice to patients suffering from various forms of arthritis. Avoidance of obesity should be encouraged. A balanced diet conforming to recommendations for health promotion (see Chapter 40) is advisable on general principles. Abundant calcium intake may be beneficial, particularly in OA, and should be derived from either diet or supplements.

Daily use of a multivitamin/multimineral supplement seems a prudent addition to, but not substitute for, a diet conforming to recommendations. A vegetarian diet may be advantageous in RA and, providing all nutrient needs are met (see Chapter 37), is conducive to health promotion goals. Alcohol intake should be restricted or avoided. Regular consumption of fish or soybeans and regular use of flaxseed oil as a means of increasing n-3 fatty acid intake are advisable both for arthritis management and on general principles (see Chapter 40). In progressive RA, use of fish oil capsules may be indicated.

The use of glucosamine sulfate is supported by studies of reasonable quality and apparently is safe. While further study is desirable, a trial of glucosamine sulfate 500 mg three times daily for patients with chronic joint pain seems appropriate, and even more so in patients intolerant of NSAIDs. Fasting and elimination diets may offer at least temporary relief to a minority of patients with RA. The avoidance of nightshade vegetables does not appear to offer any consistent benefit, although the practice is supported by anecdotal reports.

REFERENCES

1. Sperling RI. Eicosanoids in rheumatoid arthritis. *Rheum Dis Clin North Am* 1995;21:741.
2. Cleland LG, Hill CL, James MJ. Diet and arthritis. *Bailleres Clin Rheumatol* 1995;9:771.
3. McAlindon T, Felson DT. Nutrition: risk factors for osteoarthritis. *Ann Rheum Dis* 1997;56:397.
4. Adam O. Anti-inflammatory diet in rheumatic disease. *Eur J Clin Nutr* 1995;49:703.
5. Martin RH. The role of nutrition and diet in rheumatoid arthritis. *Proc Nutr Soc* 1998;57:231.
6. Schrander JJP, Marcelis C, De Vries MP, et al. Does food intolerance play a role in juvenile chronic arthritis? *Br J Rheumatol* 1997;36:905.
7. Stone J, Doube A, Dudson D, et al. Inadequate calcium, folic acid, vitamin E, zinc, and selenium intake in rheumatoid arthritis patients: results of a dietary survey. *Semin Arthritis Rheum* 1997;27:180–185.
8. Ebringer A, Wilson C. The use of a low-starch diet in the treatment of patients suffering from ankylosing spondylitis. *Clin Rheumatol* 1996;15:62.
9. Eaton SB, Eaton SB, Konner MJ. Paleolithic nutrition revisited: a twelve-year retrospective on its nature and implications. *Eur J Clin Nutr* 1997;51:207.
10. Calder PC. N-3 polyunsaturated fatty acids and cytokine production in health and disease. *Ann Nutr Metab* 1997;41:203.
11. James MJ, Cleland LG. Dietary n-3 fatty acids and therapy for rheumatoid arthritis. *Semin Arthritis Rheum* 1997;27:85.
12. Murray MT. *Encyclopedia of nutritional supplements.* Rocklin, CA: Prima Publishing, 1996.
13. Gottlieb MS. Conservative management of spinal osteoarthritis with glucosamine sulfate and chiropractic treatment. *J Manipulat Physiol Ther* 1997;20:400.
14. Vaz AL. Double-blind clinical evaluation of the relative efficacy of ibuprofen and glucosamine sulfate in the management of osteoarthrosis of the knee in out-patients. *Curr Med Res Opin* 1982;8:145.
15. Newman NM, Ling RSM. Acetabular bone destruction related to non-steroidal anti-inflammatory drugs. *Lancet* 1985;ii:11.
16. Brandt KD. Effects of nonsteroidal anti-inflammatory drugs on chondrocyte metabolism *in vitro* and *in vivo*. *Am J Med* 1987;83[Suppl 5a]:29.
17. da Camara CC, Dowless GV. Glucosamine sulfate for osteoarthritis. *Ann Pharmacother* 1998;32:580.
18. Barclay TS, Tsourounis C, McGart GM. Glucosamine. *Ann Pharmacother* 1998;32:574.
19. Pipitone VR. Chondroprotection with chondroitin sulfate. *Drugs Exp Clin Res* 1991;17:3.
20. Kelly GS. The role of glucosamine sulfate and chondroitin sulfates in the treatment of degenerative joint diseases. *Altern Med Rev* 1998;31:27.

See "Sources for All Chapters."

disability, including cerebrovascular disease (see Chapter 9) and Parkinson's disease (17) are associated with a risk of malnutrition. Nutritional assessment at regular intervals is indicated in all such patients, with nutritional support as required to maintain muscle mass and metabolic balance (18) (see Chapter 24).

Neuropathy

Vitamin B_6 (pyridoxine) is routinely administered in conjunction with isoniazid for prevention of peripheral neuropathy. It has been studied for the treatment of neuropathy, especially carpal tunnel syndrome, with mixed results (19). Some randomized, controlled trials have shown a benefit of B_6 at a dose of 50 mg two to three times daily for a period of weeks, whereas others have shown no benefit.

Nutrients and Nutriceuticals

Manganese

Manganese is widely distributed in grains, cereals, and nuts, and is present in lower levels in fruits and vegetables. As a result, overt deficiency is extremely rare. However, low levels have been associated with epilepsy, and optimal intake is uncertain. Paleolithic intake of manganese has not yet been estimated in a published report, but given the characteristics of our ancestral diet, intake was likely to have been greater than it is today. Any benefit of manganese supplementation in reducing the severity or frequency of seizures in some patients with epilepsy remains to be shown.

Thiamine

Thiamine deficiency in the context of alcoholism may result in Wernicke's encephalopathy or Korsakoff psychosis. The latter may cause unconsciousness or coma; thus, parenteral thiamine supplementation (generally 1 mg) is an established component in the early response to coma of uncertain etiology.

It is important in such situations to administer thiamine prior to glucose, as carbohydrate induces thiamine metabolism. Thiamine supplementation has been shown to enhance cognition in epileptic patients on long-term phenytoin (Dilantin) therapy (20).

Pyridoxine (Vitamin B_6)

Seizures resulting from pyridoxine deficiency have been reported in infants, and they respond when pyridoxine is given in doses approximating the recommended dietary allowance. Other infantile seizures of uncertain etiology have been characterized as pyridoxine dependent and occur despite ostensibly adequate pyridoxine intake. These seizures reportedly respond to high-dose supplementation, in the range from 25 to 50 mg per day (21). There is some suggestion that pyridoxine-dependent seizures, thought to be due to an inborn derangement of γ-aminobutyric acid synthesis (22), may represent only the extreme form of a syndrome with various neurocognitive deficits (23). A potential role for pharmacologic dosing of pyridoxine (50 mg b.i.d. to t.i.d.) in the treatment of carpal tunnel syndrome remains controversial, as noted earlier.

Selenium

Brain cells are apparently guarded against oxidative injury, at least in part, by two enzymes that require selenium, glutathione peroxidase and phospholipid hydroperoxide glutathione peroxidase. In other tissues, catalase inactivates hydrogen peroxide, but the central nervous system is catalase deficient (24). At least one report suggests that selenium deficiency should be considered when intractable seizures develop in children (24). The value of routine selenium supplementation as adjuvant therapy in epilepsy has not been established.

CLINICAL HIGHLIGHTS

The specific role for nutritional management of neurologic conditions as defined by outcome data is limited but nonetheless important. Malnutrition is a common sequela of chronic, disabling neurologic conditions and can be prevented by continual monitoring and early intervention. Diet may play a role in the precipitation of headaches in some patients, although this appears not to be a predominant factor on a population basis. The use of dietary interventions for the management of seizures, alone or in combination with pharmacotherapy, is well established. The therapeutic efficacy of the ketogenic diet is supported by definitive evidence, but the circumstances under which it should be applied remain controversial. Pyridoxine is of well-defined benefit in certain cases of pediatric seizure disorder; its role in the treatment of peripheral neuropathies remains controversial.

Although direct evidence of specific neurologic benefit is lacking, a balanced diet rich in the sources of micronutrients and with a judicious distribution of macronutrients (see Chapter 40) could be expected to be supportive of optimal neurologic health on theoretical grounds. The dietary pattern advocated for health promotion offers benefit with regard to immune function (see Chapter 15), susceptibility to inflammation (see Chapter 18), cognitive function (see Chapter 33), brain development (see Chapter 27), and susceptibility to cerebrovascular disease (see Chapter 9). Thus, although largely indirect, the evidence linking dietary practices to neurologic health is substantial in the aggregate.

REFERENCES

1. Peatfield RC. Relationship between food, wine, and beer-precipitated migrainous headaches. *Headache* 1995;35:355.
2. Marcus DA, Scharff L, Turk D, et al. A double-blind provocative study of chocolate as a trigger of headache. *Cephalalgia* 1997;17:855.
3. Jarisch R, Wantke F. Wine and headache. *Int Arch Allergy Immunol* 1996;110:7.
4. Mosek A, Korczyn AD. Yom Kippur headache. *Neurology* 1995;45:1953.
5. Barzideh O, Burright RG, Donovick PJ. Dietary iron and exposure to lead influence susceptibility to seizures. *Psychol Rep* 1995;76:971.
6. Ramaekers VT, Calomme M, Vanden Berghe D, et al. Selenium deficiency triggering intractable seizures. *Neuropediatrics* 1994;25:217.
7. Tallian KB, Nahata MC, Tsao CY. Role of the ketogenic diet in children with intractable seizures. *Ann Pharmacother* 1998;32:349.
8. Nordli DR, De Vivo C. The ketogenic diet revisited: back to the future. *Epilepsia* 1997;38:743.
9. Carroll J, Koenigsberger D. The ketogenic diet: a practical guide for caregivers. *J Am Diet Assoc* 1998;98:316.
10. Berryman MS. The ketogenic diet revisited. *J Am Diet Assoc* 1997;97:s192–s194.
11. Swink TD, Vining EP, Freeman JM. The ketogenic diet: 1997. *Adv Pediatr* 1997;44:297.
12. Ballaban-Gil K, Callahan C, O'Dell C, et al. Complications of the ketogenic diet. *Epilepsia* 1998;39:744.
13. Bazil CW, Pedley TA. Advances in the medical treatment of epilepsy. *Annu Rev Med* 1998;49:135.
14. Arnold ST, Dodson WE. Epilepsy in children. *Bailleres Clin Neurol* 1996;5:783.
15. Prasad AN, Stafstrom CF, Holmes GL. Alternative epilepsy therapies: the ketogenic diet, immunoglobulins, and steroids. *Epilepsia* 1996;37:s81.
16. Ghadirian P, Jain M, Ducic S, et al. Nutritional factors in the aetiology of multiple sclerosis: a case-control study in Montreal, Canada. *Int J Epidemiol* 1998;27:845.
17. Beyer PL, Palarino MY, Michalek D, et al. Weight change and body composition in patients with Parkinson's disease. *J Am Diet Assoc* 1995;95:979.
18. Britton JER, Lipscomb G, Mohr PD, et al. The use of percutaneous endoscopic gastrostomy (PEG) feeding tubes in patients with neurological disease. *J Neurol* 1997;244:431.
19. Bender DA. Non-nutritional uses of vitamin B$_6$. *Br J Nutr* 1999;81:7.
20. Botez MI, et al. Thiamine and folate treatment of chronic epileptic patients: a controlled study with the Wechsler IQ scale. *Epilepsy Res* 1993;16:157.
21. Jiao FY, Gao DY, Takuma Y, et al. Randomized, controlled trial of high-dose intravenous pyridoxine in the treatment of recurrent seizures in children. *Pediatr Neurol* 1997;17:54.
22. Gospe SM Jr., Hecht ST. Longitudinal MRI findings in pyridoxine-dependent seizures. *Neurology* 1998;51:74.
23. Baxter P, Griffiths P, Kelly T, et al. Pyridoxine-dependent seizures: demographic, clinical, MRI and psychometric features and effect of dose on intelligence quotient. *Dev Med Child Neurol* 1996;38:998.
24. Ramaekers VT, Calomme M, Vanden Berghe D, et al. Selenium deficiency triggering intractable seizures. *Neuropediatrics* 1994;25:217.

See "Sources for All Chapters."

spicy food. The belief that capsaicin contributes to dyspepsia or symptoms of heartburn associated with GERD is widespread. Evidence in the medical literature of such an effect, however, is quite limited. A recent (2000) small blinded, controlled trial demonstrated a reduction in time to peak symptoms of heartburn when capsaicin was provided along with a test meal (17).

CLINICAL HIGHLIGHTS

Despite the prevailing and intuitive view that certain foods irritate the GI tract directly or indirectly by effects on motility, gastroesophageal sphincter tone, or acid production, evidence linking diet or nutrients with peptic ulcer disease, GERD, or dyspepsia is very limited. What evidence there is suggests that a diet high in fiber is likely to be of benefit. Data supporting the protective effects of fermented milk products and detrimental effects of unfermented milk are preliminary and of uncertain significance. On the basis of available evidence, no strong argument can be made for significant adjustment of dietary pattern, including alterations in intake of alcohol or caffeine, specifically to address symptoms of dyspepsia.

Dietary practices consistent with health promotion (see Chapter 40) appear to be appropriate for purposes of preventing or managing dyspepsia or peptic ulcer disease. A diet rich in fiber should receive emphasis, as is true on general principles. Despite the lack of compelling evidence in the literature, interventions supported by judgment and physiologic mechanism, such as restriction in alcohol or caffeine intake, are reasonable on a trial basis in individual patients. Advances in the pharmacotherapy of dyspeptic syndromes, including treatment of *H. pylori* and the use of proton pump inhibitors, are such that most patients need not impose dietary restrictions.

REFERENCES

1. Aldoori WH, Giovannucci EI, Stampfer MJ, et al. Prospective study of diet and the risk of duodenal ulcer in men. *Am J Epidemiol* 1997;145:42.
2. Aldoori WH, Giovannucci EI, Stampfer MJ, et al. A prospective study of alcohol, smoking, caffeine, and the risk of duodenal ulcer in men. *Epidemiology* 1997;8:420.
3. Kato K, Nomura AMY, Stemmerman GN, et al. A prospective study of gastric and duodenal ulcer and its relation to smoking, alcohol, and diet. *Am J Epidemiol* 1992;135:521.
4. Katschinski BD, Logan RFA, Edmond M, et al. Duodenal ulcer and refined carbohydrate intake: a case-control study assessing dietary fiber and refined sugar intake. *Gut* 1990;31:993.
5. Grant HW, Palmer KR, Riermesma RR, et al. Duodenal ulcer is associated with low dietary linoleic acid intake. *Gut* 1990;31:997.
6. Elmstahl S, Svensson U, Berglund G. Fermented milk products are associated to ulcer disease. Results from a cross-sectional population study. *Eur J Clin Nutr* 1998;52:668.
7. Johnsen R, Forde OH, Straume B, et al. Aetiology of peptic ulcer: a prospective population study in Norway. *J Epidemiol Community Health* 1994;48:156.
8. Scolapio JS, Camilleri M. Nonulcer dyspepsia. *Gastroenterologist* 1996;4:13.
9. Colin-Jones DG, Bloom B, Bodemar G, et al. Management of dyspepsia: report of a working party. *Lancet* 1988;I:576.
10. Barbara L, Camilleri M, Corinaldesi R, et al. Definitions and investigation of dyspepsia, consensus of an international ad hoc working party. *Dig Dis Sci* 1989;34:1272.
11. Heading RC. Definitions of dyspepsia. *Scand J Gastroenterol* 1991;26[Suppl 82]:1.
12. Talley NJ, Phillips SF. Non-ulcer dyspepsia: potential causes and pathophysiology. *Ann Intern Med* 1988;108:865.
13. Talley NJ, McNeil D, Piper DW. Environmental factors and chronic unexplained dyspepsia: association with acetaminophen but no other analgesics, alcohol, coffee, tea or smoking. *Dig Dis Sci* 1988;33:641.
14. Cuperus P, Keeling PWN, Gibney MJ. Eating patterns in functional dyspepsia: a case control study. *Eur J Clin Nutr* 1996;50:520.
15. Mullan A, Kavanagh P, O'Mahony P, et al. Food and nutrient intakes and eating patterns in functional and organic dyspepsia. *Eur J Clin Nutr* 1994;48:97.
16. Chyou P-H, Nomura AMY, Hankin JH, et al. A case-control study of diet and stomach cancer. *Cancer Res* 1990;50:7501.
17. Rodriguez-Stanley S, Collings KL, Robinson M, et al. The effects of capsaicin on reflux, gastric emptying and dyspepsia. *Aliment Pharmacol Ther* 2000;14:129.

See "Sources for All Chapters."

21

Diet and Liver Disease

INTRODUCTION

The importance of the liver in the metabolism of ingested nutrients and drugs suggests that hepatic function can be influenced by dietary manipulations. Less obvious is the potential role of specific nutrients in ameliorating the natural history of various chronic liver diseases or toxic exposures. Preliminary evidence supports the use of several nutriceutical agents in the treatment of liver diseases for which conventional therapies are limited.

OVERVIEW

Diet in compensated chronic liver disease need not differ from that recommended for general health promotion (1). In uncompensated liver disease, malnutrition is a common sequela (2). The increased energy demands in chronic liver disease are at least comparable to those in dialysis patients (3). Malnutrition in patients with chronic liver disease may develop despite near-normal dietary intake (4).

Liver disease directly influences the biomarkers of nutrient energy deficiency, such as albumin, prealbumin, transferrin, and retinol-binding protein, rendering nutritional assessment difficult (5,6). Upper body anthropometry, such as triceps skin-fold thickness, may be necessary to assess body fat reserves in a patient with ascites. For bedside assessment, clinical parameters such as weight change, functional status, and visible muscle wasting are reliable indexes of nutritional status, particularly when used in com-

bination (5). Given the frequency of protein energy malnutrition in patients with advanced liver disease and the complexity of evaluating the nutritional status of such patients, a dietary consultation is generally indicated for inpatients and outpatients alike.

Maintenance of adequate nutritional status should be a priority in patients with chronic liver disease and hepatic insufficiency. Ascites is associated with anorexia and has been shown to increase energy expenditure (5). Nausea, which frequently accompanies liver disease, further reduces dietary intake. Malabsorption and poor dietary intake associated with alcoholism are other common reasons for malnutrition in chronic liver disease.

Although protein restriction is indicated for patients with hepatic encephalopathy, the restoration of normal protein intake once the encephalopathy is controlled generally is indicated. A goal of managing the cirrhotic patient over time should be to provide the maximal level of protein tolerated without inducing encephalopathy (5). Lactulose may be used to facilitate clearance of nitrogenous waste, while permitting protein intake adequate for metabolic needs.

An unpalatable diet may exacerbate the tendency toward malnutrition common to patients with advanced liver disease and, therefore, may be harmful even if the dietary restriction imposed would otherwise be judicious. In such situations, there is a tradeoff between control of specific nutrients and ensuring the adequacy of energy intake.

Adequate energy intake generally should be a priority (7). The recommended energy improve hepatic encephalopathy in alcoholic patients (16).

Vitamins

Use of a multivitamin supplement is advocated for all patients with chronic liver disease (16). Thiamine supplementation is indicated in all alcoholic patients.

CLINICAL HIGHLIGHTS

Liver disease, whether cholestatic or noncholestatic, of alcoholic, viral, or other origin, imposes significant nutritional demands. Once severe, liver disease increases energy demands considerably. The sequelae of liver disease make malnutrition common.

Nutritional management should be directed toward preventing protein-energy malnutrition. Protein intake should be unrestricted unless encephalopathy is present. In patients intolerant of standard protein, branched-chain amino acids or ketoacids should be considered, although their benefit and particularly their cost-effectiveness are as yet uncertain. All patients should receive vitamin and mineral supplements.

Patients with ascites should consume a salt-restricted and, if necessary, water-restricted diet. In the setting of malabsorption, MCTs may be advantageous. The possible benefits of silymarin and other nutriceuticals in the amelioration of hepatocyte function once cirrhosis has developed are intriguing, but such benefits are as yet inadequately demonstrated.

REFERENCES

1. Corish C. Nutrition and liver disease. *Nutr Rev* 1997;55:17.
2. Cabre E, Gassull MA. Nutritional therapy in liver disease. *Acta Gastroenterol Belg* 1994;57:1.
3. Cano N, Leverve XM. Influence of chronic liver disease and chronic renal failure on nutrient metabolism and undernutrition. *Nutrition* 1997;13:381.
4. Levine JA, Morgan MY. Weighed dietary intakes in patients with chronic liver disease. *Nutrition* 1996;12:430.
5. Munoz SJ. Nutritional therapies in liver disease. *Semin Liver Dis* 1991;11:278.
6. Crawford DHG, Cuneo RC, Shepherd RW. Pathogenesis and assessment of malnutrition in liver disease. *J Gastroenterol Hepatol* 1993;8:89.
7. Siriboonkoom W, Gramlich L. Nutrition and chronic liver disease. *Can J Gastroenterol* 1998; 12:201.
8. Novy MA, Schwarz KB. Nutritional consideration and management of the child with liver disease. *Nutrition* 1997;13:177.
9. Utrilla MP. Natural products with hepatoprotective action. *Meth Find Exp Clin Pharmacol* 1996; 18[Suppl]:11.
10. Pares A, Planas R, Torres M, et al. Effects of silymarin in alcoholic patients with cirrhosis of the liver: results of a controlled, double-blind, randomized and multicenter trial. *J Hepatol* 1998;28:615.
11. Velussi M, Cernigoli AM, De Monte A, et al. Long-term (12 months) treatment with an anti-oxidant drug (silymarin) is effective on hyperinsulinemia, exogenous insulin need and malondialdehyde levels in cirrhotic diabetic patients. *J Hepatol* 1997;26:871.
12. Miguez M, Anundi I, Sainz-Pardo LA, et al. Hepatoprotective mechanism of silymarin: no evidence for involvement of cytochrome P450 2EI. *Chem Biol Interact* 1994;91:51.
13. Boigk G, Stroedter L, Herbst H, et al. Silymarin retards collagen accumulation in early and advanced biliary fibrosis secondary to complete bile duct obliteration in rats. *Hepatology* 1997;26:643.
14. Flora K, Hahn M, Rosen H, et al. Milk thistle (*Silybum marianum*) for the therapy of liver disease. *Am J Gastroenterol* 1998;93:139.
15. Loguercio C, De Girolamo V, Federico A, et al. Trace elements and chronic liver diseases. *J Trace Elem Med Biol* 1997;11:158.
16. Levinson MJ. A practical approach to nutritional support in liver disease. *Gastroenterologist* 1995; 3:234.

See "Sources for All Chapters."

22

Diet and Common
Gastrointestinal Disorders

INTRODUCTION

Normal functioning of the gastrointestinal tract is essential to normal digestion, nutrient absorption, and egestion. Gastrointestinal pathology can impair nutritional status in a variety of ways, depending on the site, nature, and extent of disease or injury. Conversely, nutritional status and specific exposures to ingested substances can significantly affect the health of the gastrointestinal tract via both direct and systemic influences. Gastrointestinal diseases often can be prevented or managed, in whole or in part, by dietary means.

CONSTIPATION

Constipation refers to infrequent bowel movements associated with abdominal discomfort and straining. The frequency of bowel movement is quite variable, and there is an insufficient basis for defining a pathologic state. Constipation is associated with hemorrhoids, diverticulosis, and appendicitis. Prolonged gastrointestinal transit time is thought to increase the risk of colon cancer, and constipation and colon cancer share some risk factors (see Chapter 12). Constipation should be managed with diet whenever possible, as laxatives generally fail to address the problem at its source and may cause worsening of bowel function over time.

Dietary management consists principally of increasing fiber intake, with an emphasis on cereal fibers, and on maintaining good hydration. Whole grain breads and cereals are excellent sources of insoluble fiber, and patients should be encouraged to eat them. Fruits and vegetables provide soluble and insoluble fiber in combination, and their consumption should be encouraged, both for the prevention or management of constipation and on general principles. Use of bran supplements may be injudicious, as it poses a threat of obstruction and may interfere with micronutrient absorption. Bran in whole grains is safer and generally effective. However, used appropriately and in conjunction with adequate fluid intake, wheat bran added to food can help prevent constipation, as 2 tablespoons of wheat bran contains 3 g of fiber. Dried fruits are an excellent source of fiber and should be incorporated into the diet in efforts to prevent constipation and on general principles, as they are nutrient dense. Although other dried fruits provide more fiber, prunes also provide phenolphthalein, which is used in commercial laxatives. Therefore, regular consumption of prunes may be particularly helpful.

Constipation in children is likely to be related to dietary fiber intake. A case-control study of more than 100 Brazilian children found low intake of fiber, particularly insoluble fiber, to be a risk factor for constipation (1). Similar results were obtained from a larger case-control study in Greece (2).

Even with adequate fiber intake (30 g per day is recommended), hard stools and constipation are likely if hydration status is poor. Fiber increases stool bulk by absorbing water. A glass of water with every meal (and in between) should be encouraged. Anti and colleagues (3) reported results of a randomized trial in adults that demonstrated a significant benefit in the treatment of constipation of fiber intake and 1.5 to 2.0 L of fluid per day. Physical activity may stimulate gastrointestinal peristalsis and contribute to the prevention of constipation; it is advisable on general principles as well.

PEDIATRIC COLIC

"Colic" refers to periods of nearly inconsolable crying in infants between the ages of 2 weeks and 4 months, apparently induced by abdominal distention and pain. The etiology of the condition and its pathophysiology are uncertain. Colic occurs more commonly in bottle-fed than breast-fed infants. Breast-fed infants with colic may benefit from modification of maternal diet, with avoidance of bovine milk, peanuts, eggs, seafood, or wheat, or several of these items. Temporary elimination of bovine milk protein from the diet of a colicky infant with appropriate substitution of soy protein is reasonable, although not certain to alleviate the condition. Bovine milk may be reintroduced after resolution of symptoms; it is then generally well tolerated.

Nucleotides, such as nucleic acids and nucleosides, are present in human milk in much greater quantities than in cow's milk or infant formula. There is increasing evidence that dietary nucleotides enhance both immune and gastrointestinal function in the infant and may account for some of the functional benefit associated with breast-feeding (4).

DIARRHEA

Diarrhea generally is due to a specific perturbation of gastrointestinal homeostasis, often infectious, and treatment should be directed at the underlying cause as indicated. Viral gastroenteritis is among the more common conditions affecting healthy children. The mainstay of management is repletion of lost fluid and electrolytes. Children under the age of 2 should be given a commercially prepared solution with balanced electrolytes (see Section III). Older children may replenish fluid and electrolyte loss with clear liquids, broth, or commercial drinks. Highly sweetened drinks of any kind may worsen diarrhea and should be avoided.

Gastroenteritis in children may result in a state of temporary lactose intolerance. During and immediately after (up to 1 week) an acute diarrheal illness, milk and milk products should be avoided if there is evidence of lactose intolerance; lactose-free or lactose-reduced products may be substituted. A meta-analysis suggests that most children continue to tolerate nonhuman milk during the period of acute diarrheal illness (5). Although lactose intolerance can be problematic in children with significant dehydration.

There is evidence of some benefit of lactose-free or lactose-reduced refeeding after rehydration in underweight infants (6). In a population of Indian children with persistent diarrhea, Bhatnagar and colleagues (7) demonstrated that moderate milk consumption was well tolerated, producing no meaningful outcome differences as compared to a milk-free diet. The consensus supporting oral rehydration and continuous feeding of staples, including lactose, is well established.

Breast-fed infants should continue to be breast-fed, and older children generally should continue to receive their normal diet whenever possible (8). The so-called BRAT diet (bananas, rice, apples, toast) is no longer recommended, although these foods may be included as part of a more balanced diet during the illness. Other foods rich in soluble fiber, such as oatmeal, have a binding effect and can be helpful. Foods high in insoluble fiber, such as wheat bran, should be avoided during the illness. Excessive fruit juice consumption in toddlers can induce an osmotic diarrhea; fruit juice intake is best limited to 2 to 3 ounces per day until after age 2.

APPENDICITIS

Specific dietary precipitants of appendicitis are generally unknown. Population studies link the disease to relatively low intake of dietary fiber. A diet rich in cereal grains, fruits, and vegetables is thought to be protective. Epidemiologic data suggest that improved sanitation and reduced exposure to food-borne pathogens in early life may increase the incidence of childhood appendicitis by fostering a more extreme hyperplasia of appendiceal lymphoid tissue when viral exposure does occur. Uncertainties about the etiology of appendicitis limit the security with which targeted dietary recommendations can be made. A lower than average risk has been associated with vegetarianism (9).

Conventional clinical wisdom holds that particulate matter in the diet, such as small seeds, may contribute to episodes of acute appendicitis or diverticulitis by luminal occlusion; however, evidence in support of this perception is lacking in the peer-reviewed literature.

DIVERTICULOSIS/DIVERTICULITIS

Diverticula develop as a direct consequence of high intraluminal pressure in the bowel. Outpouchings typically occur in the sigmoid colon, as pressures increase with solidification of the stool. Long gastrointestinal transit time and increased pressure are associated with low dietary fiber, thought to be a strong determinant of diverticulosis in both populations and individuals. Diverticulitis occurs when bacteria are trapped within a diverticulum, leading to infection. Dietary interventions to prevent diverticulosis are aimed at preventing constipation and the attendant elevations of intraluminal pressure (see "Constipation" discussed earlier). The principal strategy is to achieve and maintain a high intake of dietary fiber, indicated on general principles of health promotion as well. Vegetarianism is associated with reduced risk for diverticulosis (9). Data from the Health Professionals Follow-up Study suggest that physical activity, particularly vigorous activity, may be protective against diverticular disease in men (10).

PANCREATITIS

The only aspect of diet reliably known to cause pancreatitis is excessive alcohol intake. Diet may contribute indirectly to the development of pancreatitis by leading to cholelithiasis (discussed later). Bowel rest is standard care in acute pancreatitis, with the goal of eliminating stimulation of pancreatic enzyme release. Resumption of oral intake, preferably of low-fat foods, can generally take place within 5 days of the onset of symptoms.

When pancreatitis is more severe and protracted, enteral nutritional support should be considered. Total parenteral nutrition is one option; enteral nutrition with tube placement in the jejunum is the other. The more distally a tube is placed in the small bowel, the less pancreatic stimulation occurs. Placement of a jejunostomy tube beyond the ligament of Treitz, coupled with slow continuous infusion of an enteral formula, results in almost no pancreatic stimulation and offers considerable advantages over total parenteral nutrition (see Chapter 24).

Among the symptoms of chronic pancreatitis, associated with exocrine failure of the pancreas, is fat malabsorption. Treatment strategies include moderate restriction of dietary fat (advisable on general principles, but potentially ill-advised in a malnourished patient); use of commercial pancreatic enzyme supplements; and supplementation with medium-chain triglycerides. The dietary management of a patient with chronic loss of exocrine pancreatic function should involve both a gastroenterologist and a dietitian.

CHOLESTASIS/CHOLELITHIASIS

Definitive associations between diet and cholelithiasis have not been established.

Epidemiologic data suggest associations with high intake of dietary fat, excess body weight, rapid weight loss, and low dietary fiber. A case-control study in southern Italy found physical inactivity and consumption of animal fats and refined sugars to increase risk, whereas physical activity, monounsaturated fats, and dietary fiber appeared to be protective (11). A comparable study in France had similar findings and suggested that moderate alcohol consumption (20 to 40 g per day of ethanol) is protective (12). Results of a large population survey in Italy are somewhat less clear, reporting differing associations by gender (13). Rapid weight loss seems to lead to cholelithiasis over a range of dietary fat content (14), but risk may vary when the manipulation of dietary fat content is more extreme (15).

The level of calorie restriction achievable with over-the-counter meal replacements may be sufficient to raise substantially the risk of gallstone formation (16). There is evidence, however, that energy restriction to 1,200 kcal per day by use of regular food rather than liquid diet does not increase the risk of cholelithiasis (17).

Recommendations for reducing the risk of cholelithiasis consistent with general dietary guidelines include consuming a diet rich in fiber, particularly soluble fiber; restricting dietary fat to 30% or less of total calories; avoiding excess body weight; avoiding "crash" diets with less than 1,000 to 1,200 kcal daily; avoiding rapid swings in weight; avoiding extended fasts followed by binges; and, possibly, increasing n-3 fatty acid intake by consuming fish or plant sources (flaxseeds, linseeds) regularly (18). The n-3 fatty acids may reduce crystallization from bile. Vegetarianism is associated with a lower risk of gallstone formation (9).

GASTROESOPHAGEAL REFLUX DISEASE

Gastroesophageal reflux disease (GERD) is the preferred term for acid reflux into the esophagus associated with pain typically referred to as heartburn. Symptoms of GERD typically occur postprandially. Dietary precipitants are thought to include large meals, fatty meals, coffee, and alcohol. Dietary interventions to control GERD include eating small, regularly spaced meals and/or snacks; avoiding food within several hours of sleep; avoiding meals with high fat content; avoiding carbonated beverages and excess caffeine; and weight control (see Chapter 25). Dietary interventions are complementary to pharmacotherapy with histamine (H_2) receptor antagonists or proton pump inhibitors.

GASTRECTOMY

Dietary interventions in the advent of surgical gastrectomy are aimed at mitigating the symptoms of the dumping syndrome. The syndrome, as a result of rapid entry of a nutrient load into the jejunum, is characterized by tachycardia, nausea, and even hypotension. Rapid insulin release can result in hypoglycemia. Dietary interventions include small, evenly spaced meals; avoidance of meals with a high content of sugar or processed carbohydrate; use of nutrient-dense foods or supplements to prevent malnutrition due to early satiety; iron supplementation as indicated; and parenteral B_{12} due to loss of intrinsic factor.

SHORT BOWEL SYNDROME

Short Bowel syndrome, in which resection or loss of major lengths of the small bowel for any reason leads to impaired nutrient absorption, is associated with diarrhea, weight loss, and malnutrition. Resection of the small bowel impairs absorption of salt, water, various nutrients, and bile salts. Loss of bile salts in stool in the short bowel syndrome is associated with impaired fat absorption. Delivery of salt, water, and bile salts to the large bowel induces an osmotic diarrhea. Malabsorption tends to occur when more than 75% of the total small bowel length is lost; parenteral nutrition support generally is required. With lesser degrees of resection, oral intake can be maintained. Vitamin B_{12} generally needs to be supplemented parenterally, and oral calcium supplementation is indicated.

Short bowel syndrome generally is consequent to severe Crohn's disease, radiation enteritis, neoplastic disease, infarction, or trauma. The condition occurs in infants due to congenital malformations or necrotizing enterocolitis. When bowel resections occur at specific sites, there is some adaptation over remaining lengths of bowel to develop compensatory absorptive capacity. Nonetheless, some degree of site specificity persists, so that nutrient deficiencies are characteristic to sites of resection. The colon principally resorbs water and electrolytes.

The duodenum absorbs iron, folate, and calcium preferentially. Water-soluble vitamins, proteins, electrolytes, and minerals (particularly trace elements) are well absorbed in the jejunum and ileum. Glucose uptake is coupled to active sodium absorption in the jejunum. Reduced secretion of cholecystokinin-pancreozymin after jejunal resection is associated with cholestasis and cholelithiasis, whereas loss of various hormones from the jejunum can lead to gastric hypersecretion as a result of unregulated release of gastrin. The distal ileum absorbs fat-soluble vitamins and vitamin B_{12}. Loss of the ileum results in bile salt malabsorption, bile acid delivery to the colon, and diarrhea accompanied by loss of fat-soluble nutrients. Loss of the ileocecal valve can allow colonic bacteria to migrate into the small bowel.

Bacterial metabolism in the small bowel can generate nonmetabolizable D-lactic acid, resulting in acidosis. The condition may manifest with slurred speech and ataxia, mimicking intoxication with ethanol. Treatment of acidosis may require supplemental base, such as bicarbonate or citrate, and reduced carbohydrate to limit the generation of acid. Bile salt malabsorption results in binding of calcium to fatty acids in the gut, which in turn leads to absorption of free oxalate, normally bound by calcium. Oxalate excretion in urine can lead to formation of oxalate stones. Reduction of dietary oxalate may be indicated when significant portions of the ileum are missing. Also of use in preventing formation of renal oxalate stones is the binding of bile salts with cholestyramine, increased calcium intake, increased fluid intake, and alkalinization of urine with citrate to prevent crystallization.

Villous height and crypt depth both increase in response to small bowel resections, facilitating nutritional support with enteral preparations. Adaptation apparently can be expected to continue as long as 2 years after surgery. Enteral feeding stimulates continued adaptation, whereas exclusive parenteral nutrition induces atrophy. Immediately after small bowel resection, total parenteral nutrition is required; careful monitoring of electrolytes is necessary during this period. Enteral feeding should be initiated as soon as feasible (see Chapter 24). Pharmacotherapy likely will be needed to slow motility and reduce gastric acid secretion. Cholestyramine may help control diarrhea induced by malabsorption of bile acids. A period of overlapping enteral and parenteral nutrition is commonly indicated.

Energy requirements are increased by malabsorption and in the short bowel syndrome may be twice normal. Supplements of folate, iron, and fat-soluble vitamins generally are indicated; B_{12} injection is indicated after loss of the terminal ileum. Preliminary evidence and data from animal studies suggest that glutamine and pectin may stimulate enhanced intestinal adaptation.

Specific nutritional strategies may be tailored to the site and extent of small bowel resection. When only the jejunum has been resected, a near-normal diet can be maintained. When less than 100 cm of ileum is resected, cholestyramine and parenteral B_{12} generally are indicated. When more than 100 cm of ileum is resected, parenteral B_{12} is required, cholestyramine is not indicated (due to depletion of bile salts), and fat restriction is necessary to limit steatorrhea. Massive bowel resection (less than 60 cm of intact small bowel) requires home parenteral nutrition, although even in this group gut adaptation may permit restoration of at least partial enteral nutrition in time. Nutritional management of the short bowel syndrome has been reviewed (19).

Studies of enteral solutions in malabsorption and the short bowel syndrome have largely failed to demonstrate the superiority of hydrolyzed protein or free amino acids, apparently because of the absorptive capacity of the intestine even when impaired. The higher costs of solutions containing free amino acids or peptides suggest they be used only when absorption is severely impaired and other solutions are not tolerated.

GLUTEN ENTEROPATHY (CELIAC SPRUE)

Gluten enteropathy (see Chapter 17), is a cell-mediated hypersensitivity reaction to gluten, a protein found predominantly in wheat, but also in barley, rye, and oats. When severe, gluten enteropathy can lead to nearly complete villous atrophy and malabsorption. Secondary pancreatic insufficiency may occur because of impaired release of cholecystokinin-pancreozymin and secretin.

Although clearly familial, gluten enteropathy requires environmental triggers, possibly adenovirus infection. Breast-fed babies and those with delayed exposure to wheat have reduced risk of the condition.

Gluten enteropathy is associated with various systemic diseases and particularly autoimmune conditions. Diagnosis is made definitively by small bowel biopsy; antigliadin and antiendomysial antibodies are strongly suggestive. A gluten-free diet is therapeutic, but difficult to follow. Print and on-line information is available to assist a patient in efforts to adhere to a gluten-free diet (see Section III). Consultation with a dietitian is always indicated.

IRRITABLE BOWEL SYNDROME

Irritable bowel syndrome affects up to 25% of the population and is responsible for up to 50% of referrals to gastroenterologists. Of unknown etiology, the syndrome is characterized by crampy, abdominal pain and diarrhea, constipation, or cycles of both. Gradual increases in dietary fiber generally are recommended, helping most when constipation predominates. The use of diet to attenuate stress may be helpful, as stress and anxiety are linked with exacerbations (see Chapter 32). Irritable bowel syndrome, and other functional gastrointestinal disturbances, may be associated with dieting practices in young women (20). The role of intolerance of specific foods in irritable bowel syndrome remains unclear (21). Individualization of therapy within a range of general guidelines is most appropriate (22,23). Randomized trials of peppermint oil have been conducted and summarized by meta-analysis (24). The data are promising but inconclusive to date.

LACTOSE INTOLERANCE

Lactose intolerance is discussed in Chapter 17. The symptom complex of lactose intolerance is very similar to that of irritable bowel syndrome, with the important difference that the etiology and optimal management of the latter are ill defined (25). Definitive diagnosis of lactose intolerance requires dietary challenge and elimination.

INFLAMMATORY BOWEL DISEASE

Both ulcerative colitis and Crohn's disease can lead to malabsorption and malnutrition. In adults, weight loss is common; in children, growth failure occurs. The adequacy of the diet is threatened not only by malabsorption due to mucosal injury or surgery, but also by anorexia, diarrhea, increased metabolic demand, and medication effects. Inflammatory bowel disease (IBD) is more common in industrialized than developing nations, and dietary factors are thought to influence the natural history of the disease. Nutritional management principles of the two variants overlap, but are in some ways distinct, as discussed later. Highlights of nutritional management have been summarized (26).

ULCERATIVE COLITIS

Because ulcerative colitis involves only the large bowel, it is potentially curable with total colectomy. After colectomy, dietary interventions pertain to the avoidance of dehydration and electrolyte imbalance, and the management of an ileostomy (see later). Other than the dietary interventions indicated with colectomy, to date there is little to suggest that diet influences the course of ulcerative colitis. Dietary consultation is indicated to support efforts to maintain a diet adequate in energy and all essential nutrients.

CROHN'S DISEASE

In general, a balanced diet should be maintained during periods of remission in Crohn's disease. Dietary consultation is indicated to help ensure the adequacy of energy and nutrient intake. Avoidance of excessive fiber generally is indicated to prevent the dilution of nutrient energy and to reduce the risk of obstruction. Restriction of lactose or use of supplemental lactase often is indicated. Restriction of dietary fat intake is useful in the prevention of steatorrhea.

Evidence derived from studies subject to methodologic limitations suggests a possible role for corn, wheat, eggs, potatoes, tea, coffee, apples, mushrooms, oats, chocolate, dairy products, and yeast in the induction of flares of Crohn's disease. Evidence is stronger that elemental diets based on oligopeptides or amino acids are of potential benefit. Overall, the evidence to date is considered insufficient to justify widespread use of elimination or restricted diets. Such diets pose the threat of worsening nutrient deficiencies if they are found to be unpalatable by patients often already experiencing anorexia.

Nutritional deficiencies common in IBD include protein/energy; zinc, magnesium, and selenium; and vitamins A, E, B_6, thiamine, riboflavin, and niacin (27). Zinc deficiency impairs wound healing (see Chapter 16) as well as taste sensation, potentially compounding anorexia. The most reliable measure of zinc status is 24-hour urinary zinc excretion. Magnesium deficiency can similarly impair wound healing and is best gauged by 24-hour urine collection. Serum levels of magnesium and zinc may be altered by globulin status and, therefore, are potentially unreliable in states of generalized malnutrition. Selenium deficiency can be assessed by measurement of serum level, erythrocyte level, or erythrocyte glutathione peroxidase. Routine selenium supplementation in IBD apparently is warranted.

Nutritional therapy can be used to influence the course of IBD. Parenteral nutrition and bowel rest are indicated during acute flares and can contribute to induction of remission while preventing malnutrition. However, as enteral feeding often can accomplish the same end with lower cost and risk, it is preferred unless clearly contraindicated (see Chapter 24). Elemental diets have been shown to induce remission in up to two thirds of patients, but they are costly and generally unpalatable. Use of enteral nutrition formulas may induce remissions of Crohn's disease, although they are less effective than steroids. The best formula is unknown as yet (28).

Meta-analysis indicates that polymeric enteral feeds are as effective as elemental diets at lower cost and with improved palatability (29). Steroids are more effective at inducing remission than enteral formulae of either variety. The nutritional risk index, based on serum albumin and weight loss, can be used to gauge the need for, and urgency of, nutritional support (28). Guidelines for the use of enteral formula feeding in the management of Crohn's disease have been published (30).

Current interest in dietary therapy for IBD focuses on the use of n-3 fatty acids to suppress leukotriene production. Preliminary studies show evidence of benefit (29).

OSTOMIES

Ileostomies are associated with the passage of rather liquid stool, raising the risk of dehydration and electrolyte imbalance. Patients should be advised to remain well hydrated at all times and to keep handy oral rehydration formula (see Section III). Diarrhea may be associated with consumption of raw fruit and vegetables, beer, and spicy foods. These reactions are somewhat idiosyncratic, and diet should be adjusted individually as indicated. Fiber intake should be moderate, as very high fiber intake may lead to stomal blockage.

Colostomies are associated with a risk of constipation, and high dietary fiber intake along with good hydration generally is indicated. Flatus may be a problem and is associated particularly with onions, leeks, and garlic; cruciferous vegetables; beans; resistant starches; cucumbers; and yeast. Again, dietary adjustment should be guided by general principles but individualized.

General recommendations in stomal management include chewing food well and maintaining good hydration status at all times. Stomal blockage is associated with very fibrous vegetables such as celery and asparagus; citrus fruits; nuts; cabbage; and the skins of apples, tomatoes, and potatoes. Individual, empirical dietary adjustments are indicated rather than blanket dietary exclusions. Foods particularly associated with stool odor include fish, eggs, cabbage, onion, garlic, and leeks. Stool odor may be reduced in some individuals by consumption of parsley or yogurt. Diarrhea may be induced by raw fruit, highly fibrous vegetables, and beer.

PROBIOTICS AND INTESTINAL MICROFLORA

To date there is suggestive and rapidly proliferating evidence that manipulation of the intestinal microflora can influence health and alter outcomes of clinical importance (31,32). Probiotics refer generically to commensal organisms associated with putative health benefits, but in particular connote *Lactobacillus acidophilus* and *Bifidobacterium bifidum* (33). Both organisms colonize the intestinal tract after birth; *L. acidophilus* is introduced from foods, whereas *B. bifidum* is introduced by breast-feeding. The concentration of lactobacilli in the gastrointestinal tract can be increased by ingestion of fermented dairy products, such as yogurt, or certain nondigestible substances, such as oligofructose or other short-chain polysaccharides (34).

Yogurt may be made with other bacteria, such as *L. bulgaricus* and *Streptococcus thermophilus*; therefore, cannot be assumed to be a source of acidophilus. Yogurts made with acidophilus generally are explicit on their labels. Commercial preparations of variable quality are available. Short-chain polysaccharides preferentially nourish probiotic bacteria and are widely marketed in other countries, especially Japan. Fructooligosaccharides are found naturally in onions, garlic, asparagus, and artichokes.

The intestinal flora are involved in nutrient metabolism, immune function, and cholesterol metabolism. They influence the susceptibility of colonic epithelial cells to mutations. Claims made for the probiotics include defense against pathogenic bacteria in the gastrointestinal tract by a variety of mechanisms, including elaboration of lactic acid, hydrogen peroxide, and bacteriocidal proteins known as bacteriocins. Thus, probiotics are thought to reduce the risk of gastroenteritis (35). Probiotic supplementation has been advocated after, or during, use of broadspectrum antibiotics for reconstitution of flora (36). In a randomized trial of nearly 200 children, Vanderhoof et al. (37) demonstrated a significant reduction in diarrhea associated with antibiotic use for common infections with probiotic supplementation.

Vaginal douching as well as oral *L. acidophilus* may help prevent recurrences of candida vaginitis and gram-negative urinary tract infection. There is early evidence that vaginal colonization with lactobacilli may offer some protection against sexually transmitted disease, including human immunodeficiency virus (38). Preliminary data suggest reduced cancer risk (39), particularly but not necessarily limited to cancers of the gastrointestinal tract, with high habitual intake or supplementation of *L. acidophilus.* A variety of mechanisms by which probiotics and prebiotics may serve as anticarcinogens are under investigation (40). There may be beneficial effects on gastrointestinal function after radiation therapy. Intestinal flora influence lipid metabolism, and salutary effects of probiotics and prebiotics on serum lipids have been reported (41).

Lactobacilli in foods and commercial supplements generally are categorized as GRAS ("generally recognized as safe") by the Food and Drug Administration (42). The potential participation of such organisms in the transmission of antibiotic resistance is a lingering concern. The incorporation of nutrients such as oligosaccharides in the diet may alter more sustainably intestinal flora than the ingestion of probiotic organisms *per se*; such substances have been characterized as prebiotics (43). A consensus panel convened by the European Commission highlighted the potential health benefits of prebiotics and characterized the need for further research (44).

CLINICAL HIGHLIGHTS

That impaired gastrointestinal function would adversely affect nutritional status, and that nutrition would influence gastrointestinal function and health, are rather self-evident. Thus, nutritional management and dietary pattern are of considerable importance in gastrointestinal disorders. The details of management vary with the specific effort to prevent or ameliorate a particular disorder.

Breast-feeding may offer some protection against infantile colic, which in any event is a self-limited disorder. Diarrhea is best managed with vigorous oral hydration and, generally, maintenance of a varied diet. Constipation is best managed by increasing dietary fiber in combination with adequate hy-

dration and physical activity; the folklore regarding prunes is valid. Abrupt and extreme weight loss raise the risk of cholelithiasis, possibly compounded when dietary fat intake is severely restricted. The best preventive measure is to avoid excessive weight gain in the first place. Diverticular disease and appendicitis may be related in part to deficient dietary fiber.

States of malabsorption related to resection or inflammation of the small or large bowel require meticulous attention to nutritional status; collaboration with a dietitian or other nutritionist in all such cases is indicated. Supplements of vitamins and minerals generally are warranted. A growing body of evidence emphasizes the preferability of enteral to parenteral nutrition support unless truly precluded by obstruction or intolerance. Advances in understanding of the immunomodulation of gastrointestinal tract function by altering the composition of dietary fat or using probiotics or prebiotics offer promise for health promotion and disease prevention.

On general principles, an effort to include n-3 fatty acids in the diet appears warranted. In the aggregate, gastrointestinal health can be promoted, and gastrointestinal disorders prevented, by adherence to a dietary pattern indicated on general principles. They include moderate intake of total calories with maintenance of nearly ideal weight; restriction of dietary fat to less than 30% of calories, distributed appropriately among polyunsaturated (n-6, n-3, and nonessential), monounsaturated, and saturated fats with avoidance of animal fat in particular; abundant and consistent consumption of cereal grains, vegetables, and fruits, with approximately 30 g (or more) of fiber intake per day; moderate intake of refined carbohydrate; moderate alcohol intake; adequate hydration; and regular physical activity.

REFERENCES

1. Morais MB, Vitolo MR, Aguirre AN, et al. Measurement of low dietary fiber intake as a risk factor

for chronic constipation in children. *J Pediatr Gastroenterol Nutr* 1999;29:132.

2. Roma E, Adamidis D, Nikolara R, et al. Diet and chronic constipation in children: the role of fiber. *J Pediatr Gastroenterol Nutr* 1999;28:169.

3. Anti M, Pignataro G, Armuzzi A, et al. Water supplementation enhances the effect of high-fiber diet on stool frequency and laxative consumption in adult patients with functional constipation. *Hepatogastreoenterology* 1998;45:727.

4. Carver JD. Dietary nucleotides: effects on the immune and gastrointestinal systems. *Acta Paediatr Suppl* 1999;88:83.

5. Brown KH, Peerson JM, Fontaine O. Use of nonhuman milks in the dietary management of young children with acute diarrhea: a meta-analysis of clinical trials. *Pediatrics* 1994;93:17.

6. Wall CR, Webster J, Quirk P, et al. The nutritional management of acute diarrhea in young infants: effect of carbohydrate ingested. *J Pediatr Gastroenterol Nutr* 1994;19:170.

7. Bhatnagar S, Bhan MK, Singh KD, et al. Efficacy of milk-based diets in persistent diarrhea: a randomized, controlled trial. *Pediatrics* 1996;98:1122.

8. Brown KH. Dietary management of acute diarrheal disease: contemporary scientific issues. *J Nutr* 1994; 124[8 Suppl]:1455s.

9. Key TJ, Davey GK, Appleby PN. Health benefits of a vegetarian diet. *Proc Nutr Soc* 1999;58:271.

10. Aldoori WH, Giovannucci EL, Rimm EB, et al. Prospective study of physical activity and the risk of symptomatic diverticular disease in men. *Gut* 1995;36:276.

11. Misciagna G, Centonze S, Leoci C, et al. Diet, physical activity, and gallstones—a population-based, case-control study in southern Italy. *Am J Clin Nutr* 1999;69:120.

12. Caroli-Bose FX, Deveau C, Peten EP, et al. Cholelithiasis and dietary risk factors: an epidemiologic investigation in Vidauban, Southeast France. *Dig Dis Sci* 1998;43:2131.

13. Attili AF, Scafato E, Marchioli R, et al. Diet and gallstones in Italy: the cross-sectional MICOL results. *Hepatology* 1998;27:1492.

14. Vezina WC, Grace DM, Hutton LC, et al. Similarity in gallstone formation from 900 kcal/day diets containing 16 vs. 30 g of daily fat: evidence that fat restriction is not the main culprit of cholelithiasis during rapid weight reduction. *Dig Dis Sci* 1998; 43:554.

15. Gebhard RL, Prigge WF, Ansel HJ, et al. The role of gallbladder emptying in gallstone formation during diet-induced rapid weight loss. *Hepatology* 1996; 24:544.

16. Spirt BA, Graves LW, Weinstock R, et al. Gallstone formation in obese women treated by a low-calorie diet. *Int J Obes Relat Metabol Disord* 1995;19:593.

17. Heshka S, Spitz A, Nunez C, et al. Obesity and risk of gallstone development on a 1200 kcal/d (5025 Kj/d) regular food diet. *Int J Obes Relat Metab Disord* 1996;20:450.

18. Tseng M, Everhart JE, Sandler RS. Dietary intake and gallbladder disease: a review. *Public Health Nutr* 1999;2:161.

19. Nightingale JM. Management of patients with a short bowel. *Nutrition* 1999;15:633.

20. Krahn D, Kurth C, Nairn K, et al. Dieting severity and gastrointestinal symptoms in college women. *J Am Coll Health* 1996;45:67.

21. Niec Am, Frankum B, Talley NJ. Are adverse food reactions linked to irritable bowel syndrome? *Am J Gastroenterol* 1998;93:2184.

22. Bonis PA, Norton RA. The challenge of irritable bowel syndrome. *Am Fam Physician* 1996;53:1229.

23. Paterson WG, Thompson WG, Vanner SJ, et al. Recommendations for the management of irritable bowel syndrome in family practice. *IBS Consensus Conference Participants CMAJ* 1999;161:154.

24. Pittler MH, Ernst E. Peppermint oil for irritable bowel syndrome: a critical review and metaanalysis. *Am J Gastroenterol* 1998;93:1131.

25. Shaw AD, Davies GJ. Lactose intolerance: problems in diagnosis and treatment. *J Clin Gastroenterol* 1999;28:208.

26. Dieleman LA, Heizer WD. Nutritional issues in inflammatory bowel disease. *Gastroenterol Clin North Am* 1998;27:435.

27. Geerling BJ, Badart-Smook A, Stockbrugger RW, et al. Comprehensive nutritional status in patients with long-standing Crohn disease currently in remission. *Am J Clin Nutr* 1998;67:919.

28. Duerksen DR, Nehra V, Bistrian BR, et al. Appropriate nutritional support in acute and complicated Crohn's disease. *Nutrition* 1998;14:462.

29. Griffiths AM. Inflammatory bowel disease. *Nutrition* 1998;14:788.

30. Ferguson A, Glen M, Ghosh S. Crohn's disease: nutrition and nutritional management. *Baillieres Clin Gastroenterol* 1998;12:93.

31. Salminen S, Bouly C, Boutron-Ruault MC, et al. Functional food science and gastrointestinal physiology and function. *Br J Nutr* 1998;80[Suppl 1]: s147.

32. Goldin BR. Health benefits of probiotics. *Br J Nutr* 1998;80:s203.

33. Von Wright A, Salminen S. Probiotics: established effects and open questions. *Eur J Gastroenterol Hepatol* 1999;11:1195.

34. Kasper H. Protection against gastrointestinal diseases—present facts and future developments. *Int J Food Microbiol* 1998;41:127.

35. Salminen S, Isolauri E, Onnela T. Gut flora in normal and disordered states. *Chemotherapy* 1995; 41[Suppl 1]:5.

36. Gismondo MR, Drago L, Lombardi A. Review of probiotics available to modify gastrointestinal flora. *Int J Antimicrob Agents* 1999;12:287.

37. Vanderhoof JA, Whitney DB, Antonson DL, et al. Lactobacillus GG in the prevention of antibiotic-associated diarrhea in children. *J Pediatr* 1999; 135:564.

38. Martin HL, Richardson BA, Nyange PM, et al. Vaginal Lactobacilli, microbial flora, and risk of human immunodeficiency virus type 1 and sexually transmitted disease acquisition. *J Infect Dis* 1999; 180:1863.

39. Hirayma K, Rafter J. The role of lactic acid bacteria in colon cancer prevention: mechanistic considerations. *Antonie van Leeuwenhoek* 1999;76:391.

40. Reddy BS. Possible mechanisms by which pro- and prebiotics influence colon carcinogenesis and tumor growth. *J Nutr* 1999;129[7 Suppl]:1478s.
41. Taylor GR, Williams CM. Effects of probiotics and prebiotics on blood lipids. *Br J Nutr* 1998; 80:s225.
42. Salminen S, von Wright A, Morelli L, et al. Demonstration of safety of probiotics—a review. *Int J Food Microbiol* 1998;44:93.
43. Gibson GR, Roberfroid MB. Dietary modulation of the human colonic microbiota: introducing the concept of prebiotics. *J Nutr* 1995;125:1401.
44. Van Loo J, Cummings J, Delzenne N, et al. Functional food properties of non-digestible oligosaccharides: a consensus report from the ENDP project (DGXII AIRII-CT94-1095). *Br J Nutr* 1999; 81:121.

BIBLIOGRAPHY

See "Sources for All Chapters."

Abyad A, Mourad F. Constipation: common-sense care of the older patient. *Geriatrics* 1996;51:28.

Camilleri M. Review article: clinical evidence to support current therapies of irritable bowel syndrome. *Aliment Pharmacol Ther* 1999;13[Suppl 2]:48.

Collins MD, Gibson GR. Probiotics, prebiotics, and synbiotics: approaches for modulating the microbial ecology of the gut. *Am J Clin Nutr* 1999;69:1052s.

Drossman DA. Review article: an integrated approach to the irritable bowel syndrome. *Aliment Pharmacol Ther* 1999;13[Suppl 2]:3.

Dunne C, Murphy L, Flynn S, et al. Probiotics: from myth to reality. Demonstration of functionality in animal models of disease and in human clinical trials. *Antonie Van Leeuwenhoek* 1999;76:279.

Gibson GR. Dietary modulation of the human gut microflora using the prebiotics oligofructose and insulin. *J Nutr* 1999;129[7 Suppl]:1438s.

Han PD, Burke A, Bladassano RN, et al. Nutrition and inflammatory bowel disease. *Gastroenterol Clin North Am* 1999;28:423.

Hove H, Norgaard H, Mortensen PB. Lactic acid bacteria and the human gastrointestinal tract. *Eur J Clin Nutr* 1999;53:339.

Husain A, Korzenik JR. Nutritional issues and therapy in inflammatory bowel disease. *Semin Gastrointest Dis* 1998;9:21.

Hyams JS. Functional gastrointestinal disorders. *Curr Opin Pediatr* 1999;11:375.

Joachim G. The relationship between habits of food consumption and reported reactions to food in people with inflammatory bowel disease—testing the limits. *Nutr Health* 1999;13:69.

Lifschitz CH. Treatment of acute diarrhea in children. *Curr Opin Pediatr* 1997;9:498.

Meyers A. Modern management of acute diarrhea and dehydration in children. *Am Fam Physician* 1995; 51:1103.

Rhoads M. Management of acute diarrhea in infants. *J Parenteral Enteral Nutr* 1999;23[5 Suppl]:s18.

Sferra TJ, Heitlinger LA. Gastrointestinal gas formation and infantile colic. *Pediatr Clin North Am* 1996;43:489.

Sullivan PB. Nutritional management of acute diarrhea. *Nutrition* 1998;14:758.

23

Eating Disorders

INTRODUCTION

Eating disorders refer to aberrant eating behavior, with or without discernible physical consequences. The prototypical conditions are anorexia nervosa and bulimia nervosa. A more recent addition is binge-eating disorder.

As obesity is a state of imbalance between energy needs and energy intake, it, too, may be considered a disorder of eating, although it generally is categorized and managed differently, partly because of its prevalence. Disorder or not, obesity and overweight now afflict more than half of the adult population in the United States. By virtue of prevalence alone it cannot be considered "aberrant." Extreme degrees of obesity represent aberrancy and as such share characteristics with the other eating disorders. In these cases, elements of management borrowed from the other disorders may be helpful.

Occasional or mildly disordered eating, related to cravings, aversions, and dissatisfaction with body image, is very prevalent, if not universal. Bona fide eating disorders are considered principally psychopathologies, and management relies heavily on psychotherapy. Nonetheless, the disorders are expressed in interactions with food, requiring that dietary management be addressed.

OVERVIEW

The prevalence and public health importance of eating disorders has risen steeply since the 1970s, concurrent with a rapid rise in the prevalence of obesity. At the same time, societal concepts of beauty have increasingly prioritized thinness. Thus, although previously considered a consequence of family dysfunction and psychopathology, the link between eating disorders and prevailing imbalance between dietary goals and dietary practices seems self-evident.

Dieting appears to increase susceptibility to disordered eating (1). A population-based survey in Spain suggests that eating disorders occur against a backdrop of highly prevalent, less extreme, unhealthy eating practices (2).

Eating disorders are perceived as conditions that overwhelmingly affect young women. There is increasing evidence that the disorders occur in men as well, but tend to go unreported in this group. Nonetheless, the clinical experience to date and epidemiologic data currently available pertain to women in particular.

The age distribution of the conditions also may be changing, with more cases coming to attention in the third and fourth decades. In all eating disorders, a family history of either affective disorder or substance abuse is common. A personal history of obesity or perceived obesity is commonly reported as well, particularly in bulimia. Individuals encouraged to be preoccupied with weight control, such as models, actresses, and athletes, appear to be at increased risk.

Eating disorders share features with depression and obsessive-compulsive disorder, but they are distinguished by the preoccupation with body weight. Familial clustering and twin studies in particular suggest genetic susceptibility is contributory. Diagnostic criteria for eating disorders have been codified in the *Diagnostic and Statistical Manual of Mental Disorders* (DSM) and the *International Classification of Diseases* (ICD).

Anorexia Nervosa

Fundamentally, anorexia nervosa is a morbid fear of becoming fat, an inability to gauge correctly the degree of thinness, and consequent self-starvation (3). *DSM-IV* criteria include refusal to maintain a minimally normal weight; intense fear of weight gain; distorted perception of body image; and attendant metabolic disturbance, such as amenorrhea. Diet usually is strictly controlled in anorexia, and the patient is apt to deny and genuinely not recognize that a problem exists. However, in some variants, bingeing and purging occur, with the distinction from bulimia resting on the degree of underweight.

Anorexia nervosa typically develops between the ages of 14 and 18. The prototypical family dynamic is one of close-knit, even "enmeshed" relationships, with a characteristic rigidity.

Medical complications of anorexia are those of starvation. Basal metabolism is slowed, with potential hypotension and bradycardia. Amenorrhea due to reduced production of follicle-stimulating hormone and luteinizing hormone and reduced estrogen levels is common and may be one of the earliest indicators. Skin discoloration due to hypercarotenemia may occur, related to either dietary habits or metabolic dysfunction.

Characteristic features of hypothyroidism often develop. Potentially irreversible bone loss may occur at a rate of up to 15% per year during periods of cachexia and amenorrhea. With protracted and severe starvation, visceral protein loss has the potential to become life threatening. Myocardial protein loss renders the anorexic susceptible to sudden cardiac death. The mortality rate in untreated anorexia nervosa approaches 20%.

Bulimia Nervosa

Bulimia is more common and more difficult to "cure" than anorexia. In bulimia, as in anorexia, there is preoccupation with body weight and fear of weight gain. *DSM-IV* criteria include recurrent binges characterized by excessive calorie consumption and loss of control; recurrent purges; and undue preoccupation with body habitus. The distinguishing features tend to be the degree of dietary control, which is strict in anorexia but poor in bulimia, and the related degree of thinness (3).

Bulimics tend to binge eat, then "purge" by self-induced vomiting, use of laxatives, use of diuretics, calorie restriction, bouts of exercise, or some combination of these actions. Unlike anorexics, who appear unwell to any objective observer but tend to be unaware of a problem, bulimics generally appear well (unless the condition is advanced or decompensated) but tend to know their dietary behavior is pathologic. Nonetheless, bulimics often are reluctant to disclose the condition to even close friends.

Most bulimics had the condition for up to 5 years before seeking treatment, and often then only because of some acute disruption. Survey data suggest that more than two thirds of the bulimics who have a primary care physician conceal the condition. Limited data suggest that impaired metabolism of cholecystokinin may contribute to lack of normal satiety signals.

Bulimia generally manifests between the ages of 18 and 22. The family situation often is characterized by conflict and instability. Medical complications result from trauma to the gastrointestinal tract and electrolyte imbalance. Bingeing can lead to gastric rupture. Pancreatitis may occur following a binge. Enlargement of the parotid glands may be induced by a binge.

Purging can result in esophagitis and esophageal tear or rupture. Ipecac taken in high doses is cardiotoxic, potentially leading to myocarditis and dysrhythmia. Repeated bouts of emesis erode dental enamel and can lead to tooth loss. Loss of gastric acid can lead to hypochloremic alkalosis and hypokalemia, potentially inducing shock. Laxatives can lead to renal tubular damage and can chronically impair gastrointestinal motility. Bruised knuckles as a result of self-inflicted vomiting may be an early clue to the diagnosis.

Binge-eating Disorder

Binge-eating disorder is similar to bulimia in the commonly reported loss of impulse control that leads to a binge. The distinction is that, in binge-eating disorder, extreme forms of purging such as self-induced vomiting, are not applied. Binges tend to take place in private, with normal, or even subnormal, food intake in public. Recurrent binges contribute to the development of obesity over time.

Atypical Eating Disorders

States of aberrant eating behavior that do not meet criteria for anorexia, bulimia, or binge eating exist, but receive limited attention in the medical literature. Such conditions include psychogenic loss of appetite, pica, and psychogenic overeating (4). Recognition of such disorders may be particularly important in sensitizing the primary care community to the prevalence and clinical impact of disordered eating.

Management

The management of eating disorders is multidisciplinary and relies heavily on expert psychiatric or psychological care. There is some evidence of benefit from use of selective serotonin reuptake inhibitors. In addition to the primary care provider, the management team generally should involve a mental health specialist, dietitian, and social worker. Excellent and extensive literature is available on the various theories and approaches to the counseling of eating-disordered patients (see Bibliography). Dietary management per se is an important but limited aspect of the care plan.

Diet

Severe anorexia may require hospitalization and enteral nutrition support, with meticulous management of electrolytes. A body mass index below 13, severe electrolyte imbalance, or suicidality is an indication for hospitalization. Refeeding should be gradual to avoid the refeeding syndrome, characterized by congestive heart failure, hypophosphatemia, or both. Inpatient care should be supervised by a dietitian or other nutrition consultant.

Ambulatory care calls for close follow-up. The principles of dietary counseling discussed in Chapter 41 are applicable. Nutritional management should begin with a dietary history (5). The history should include not only a description of current and past dietary behaviors, but the beliefs and motivations underlying them.

Weekly visits are appropriate until a consistent therapeutic response has been achieved. Weight monitoring should be routine. The patients should maintain a food diary, which should be reviewed at office visits. Because preoccupation with weight is predominant, patient education regarding healthy weight and dietary practices conducive to weight maintenance is essential.

Because the pathology is related to a very restrictive diet in anorexia, emphasis should be placed on a prudent but balanced and unrestricted diet. A similar goal is pertinent in the management of bulimia, with a need to emphasize that the disordered eating typically is a result of overly restrictive attitudes about food rather than overeating (5,6). Establishment of a consistent, moderate dietary pattern is helpful in resolving the tendencies to binge and purge.

If weight gain is indicated in anorexia, it should be gradual. The addition of approximately 500 kcal per day beyond what is required for maintenance will result in a weight gain of 1 lb per week. Involvement of a dietitian in the development of meal plans to facilitate weight gain or maintenance is indicated. In anorexia, the suppression of basal metabolism is such that seemingly modest intake of food energy may be sufficient to support weight maintenance or gradual weight gain. Rapid weight gain should be avoided, as much for its adverse psychological effects as for its physiologic effects.

A dietitian should determine the basal metabolic rate as a means of estimating caloric needs. The diet should be advanced gradually to allay the patient's anxieties about excessive weight gain. In bulimia, stabilization of the dietary pattern and weight should be addressed initially. An effort should be made to identify foods associated with binges so that they can be avoided or their intake strictly controlled. If indicated, a diet for measured weight loss may be developed once the eating pattern has reliably stabilized. Dietary counseling (see Chapter 41) should be coupled to cognitive-behavioral therapy to ameliorate perceptions of body image and establish a sustainable dietary pattern that supports weight control efforts.

An additional challenge to the physician is the concurrence of an eating disorder and a metabolic disease, such as diabetes mellitus. Rydall and colleagues (7) reported that disordered eating in young women with insulin-dependent diabetes mellitus accelerates the development of retinopathy. Given the prevalence of both diabetes and eating disorders, the authors encourage consideration of concurrence whenever diabetes proves difficult to manage, especially in a young woman.

CLINICAL HIGHLIGHTS

A pervasive struggle with weight control, epidemic obesity, and fascination with thinness characterize modern society. A rising prevalence of eating disorders may be attributable to both individual susceptibility and environmental conditions. Increased awareness among clinicians with enhanced detection may also be contributory. The environmental contribution is such that every patient may reasonably be considered at some degree of risk for some degree of disordered eating. The incorporation of nutrition education and limited dietary counseling into primary care practice may support efforts at primary prevention of eating disorders, particularly by revealing the dietary habits imparted by parents to their children.

Eating disorders generally require a care team including a mental health specialist and dietitian. However, a therapeutic alliance between the patient and a primary care provider with a good working knowledge of nutrition is conducive to early detection and optimal management. Patients need education regarding healthy weight and dietary practices, and the adverse effects of disordered eating. A balanced but not overly restricted diet is conducive to overcoming eating disorders and to preventing excessive weight gain, which may precipitate recurrences of disordered eating.

A dietary pattern consistent with principles of health promotion and weight control (see Chapters 5 and 40) should be encouraged. Frequent follow-up, with monitoring of weight and dietary pattern, is essential until a therapeutic response is achieved and sustained.

REFERENCES

1. Howard CE, Porzelius LK. The role of dieting in binge eating disorder: etiology and treatment implications. *Clin Psychol Rev* 1999;19:25–44.
2. Martin AR, Nieto JM, Jimenez MA, et al. Unhealthy eating behaviour in adolescents. *Eur J Epidemiol* 1999;15:643–648.
3. Garfinkel PE. Classification and diagnosis of eating disorders. In: Brownell DK, Fairburn CG, eds. *Eating disorders and obesity. A comprehensive handbook.* New York: Guilford Press, 1995.
4. Fairburn CG, Walsh BT. Atypical eating disorders. In: Brownell DK, Fairburn CG, eds. *Eating disorders and obesity. A comprehensive handbook.* New York: Guilford Press, 1995.
5. Beumont PJV, Touyz SW. The nutritional management of anorexia and bulimia nervosa. In: Brownell DK, Fairburn CG, eds. *Eating disorders and obesity. A comprehensive handbook.* New York: Guilford Press, 1995.
6. Steiger H, Lehoux PM, Gauvin L. Impulsivity, dietary control and the urge to binge in bulimic syndromes. *Int J Eat Disord* 1999;26:261.
7. Rydall AC, Rodin GM, Olmsted P, et al. Disordered eating behavior and microvascular complications in young women with insulin-dependent diabetes mellitus. *N Engl J Med* 1997;336:1849.

BIBLIOGRAPHY

See "Sources for All Chapters."

American Psychiatric Association. *Diagnostic and statistical manual of mental disorders,* 4th ed. Washington, DC: American Psychiatric Association, 1994.

Becker AE, Grinspoon SK, Klibanski A, et al. Eating disorders. *N Engl J Med* 1999;340:1092–1098.

Brownell DK, Fairburn CG, eds. *Eating disorders and obesity. A comprehensive handbook.* New York: Guilford Press, 1995, in particular the following chapters:

> Andersen AE. Eating disorders in males.
>
> Beumont PJV. The clinical presentation of anorexia and bulimia nervosa.
>
> Cooper Z. The development and maintenance of eating disorders.
>
> Fairburn CG. The prevention of eating disorders.
>
> Halmi KA. Hunger and satiety in clinical eating disorders.
>
> Hsu LKG. Outcome of bulimia nervosa.

Steinhausaen H-C. The course and outcome of anorexia nervosa.

Kaye WH, Gendall K, Kye C. The role of the central nervous system in the psychoneuroendocrine disturbances of anorexia and bulimia nervosa. *Psychiatr Clin North Am* 1998;21:381–396.

Mizes JS. Neglected topics in eating disorders: guidelines for clinicians and researchers. *Clin Psychol Rev* 1998;18:387–390.

Schebendach J, Nussbaum MP. Nutrition management in adolescents with eating disorders. *Adolesc Med* 1992;3:541.

Stunkard A. Eating disorders: the last 25 years. *Appetite* 1997;29:181.

Walsh BT, Devlin MJ. Eating disorders: progress and problems. *Science* 1998;29:1387.

World Health Organization. *International classification of diseases (ICD) 10. Classification of mental and behavioral disorders.* Geneva, Switzerland: World Health Organization, 1992.

24

Malnutrition and Cachexia

INTRODUCTION

Impaired functional status and anorexia of various etiologies may result in nutrient and energy intake inadequate for metabolic demand. Similarly, physiologic stresses including acute illness or injury may raise metabolic demand to a level not easily accommodated by a conventional diet. Often, impaired nutrient intake and increased metabolic demand are concurrent, as is the case in cancer, acquired immunodeficiency syndrome (AIDS), burns, or other acute and chronic disease states. Although there is little evidence to suggest that nutrient deficiency under such conditions strongly influences the course of illness or recovery over the first several days, nutritional status is fundamental to convalescence and health maintenance over time. Nutritional status influences immune function (see Chapter 15) and wound healing (see Chapter 16), both vital to recovery from acute and chronic illness.

To achieve adequate nutriture in the context of disease or disability, nutritional support may be indicated. Whenever possible, that support should be enteral, either by mouth or feeding tube. Parenteral nutrition can meet all metabolic need, but at the cost of gastrointestinal (GI) atrophy and a risk of line sepsis. Adjuvant therapies, such as megestrol acetate or growth hormone, have been used with variable success to enhance appetite and promote preferential restitution of lean body mass. Increasingly, nutritional formulas tailored to a patient's particular condition and nutrient needs are available. The selection and modification of nutrition

support formulas generally should be overseen by a dietitian or other nutritionist; such consultation typically is readily available in the inpatient setting.

OVERVIEW

Decisions about nutritional support are based on the nutritional status of the patient as well as the clinical context. Nutritional status is evaluated by use of body weight, particularly in comparison with baseline weight. The measure "percent usual body weight," actual body weight divided by usual body weight times 100, often is used in anthropometric assessment. Height can be measured along with weight to obtain body mass index in adults (weight in kilograms divided by height in meters squared). Length and head circumference are useful in young children.

Calipers (typically, Lange skin-fold calipers) can be used to measure skin-fold thickness and provide a measure of subcutaneous fat as compared with a reference standard; triceps skin-fold is used most often because the site is easy to reach and there is usually no edema. In men, a triceps skin-fold thickness less than 12.5 mm indicates malnutrition, whereas a thickness above 20 mm indicates overnutrition. The comparable values in women are 16.5 and 25 mm, respectively. Measures of body composition including bioelectrical impedance and transaxial computed tomography are useful in research settings, but rarely applied clinically.

TABLE 24.1. *Cutoff values for visceral and somatic protein assays in clinical use*

Level	Albumin (g/dL)	Transferrin (mg/dL)	Prealbumin (mg/dL)	Retinol-binding protein (mg/dL)	Urinary creatinine (% of reference value)
Normal	3.5–5.5	250–300	15.7–29.6	2.6–7.6	>90
Mild depletion	2.8–3.5	150–250	10–15	N/A	80–90
Moderate depletion	2.1–2.7	100–150	5–10	N/A	60–80
Severe depletion	<2.1	<100	<5	N/A	<60

Biochemical indexes of nutritional status include both somatic and visceral proteins (Table 24.1). The visceral proteins include albumin, transferrin, prealbumin, and retinol-binding protein. Albumin is used most commonly; its level varies consistently with the adequacy of protein stores. Albumin has a half-life of approximately 20 days and, therefore, cannot be used to measure acute states of malnutrition. Conversely, albumin levels tend to drop precipitously in septic states independent of nutritional status. An albumin level from 3.5 to 5.5 g/dL is considered normal; 2.8 to 3.5 g/dL is considered mild depletion; 2.1 to 2.7 g/dL is moderate depletion; and levels below 2.1 g/dL indicate severe depletion of visceral protein.

Transferrin, with a half-life of 8 to 10 days, can be used instead of albumin when acute nutritional perturbations are under evaluation. The half-life of prealbumin is approximately 2 days; like the level of albumin, the prealbumin level is acutely depressed by severe physiologic stress. The half-life of retinol-binding protein is approximately 10 hours, but its sensitivity to even minor stress limits the clinical utility of its measurement.

Somatic proteins are those that indicate the state of skeletal muscle mass. The most commonly used index is 24-hour urinary creatinine excretion. The index is expressed as (milligram of urinary creatinine in 24 hours for the patient per milligram of urinary creatinine in 24 hours by a normal subject of the same height and sex) times 100.

Functional testing, of muscle strength, for example, has advantages over biochemical and anthropometric assessments, but is not used consistently. Other indicators of malnutrition include leukopenia and lymphopenia and skin-test anergy. Essential fatty acid deficiency can be detected as a plasma triene to tetraene ratio greater than 0.4.

Malnutrition results from deficient nutrient intake, impaired metabolism, excessive losses, or some combination of these factors. Clinical evaluation for malnutrition should include not only examination for signs of wasting (e.g., at the temples or in the hands), but also examination of hair for thinning or poor attachment, the skin for xerosis, and the mouth for inflammation, all indicative of macronutrient or micronutrient deficiencies (Table 24.2).

Hospitalized patients are subject to marasmus (a term derived from the Greek meaning "to waste"), a state of both protein and total energy malnutrition. Marasmus is

TABLE 24.2. *Physical findings associated with common nutrient deficiencies*

Physical finding	Responsible nutrient deficiency
Muscle wasting (temples, hands)	Protein; energy
Hair: thinning, poor attachment, pigment changes	Protein; energy
Skin: xerosis, scaling, bruising	Protein; energy; vitamins A, C, K
Mouth: glossitis, swelling	B vitamins

distinguished from kwashiorkor, a Bantu word meaning "displaced child," which describes the state of protein deficiency despite adequate energy intake. Kwashiorkor occurs in babies weaned from the breast in many developing countries with subsistence diets. Kwashiorkor can be associated with a serum albumin as low as 1 g/dL as compared with the fourfold higher normal value, resulting in very low oncotic pressure and characteristic edema.

Approximately 25% of the body's protein reserves can be consumed to generate energy during starvation, sparing vital functions for a period as long as 50 days. In a well-nourished adult, nearly 3 kg of protein can be turned over to generate 12,000 kcal of energy.

Energy requirements in hospitalized patients can be estimated by application of the Harris-Benedict equation (see Section IIIA) or, when available, by use of indirect calorimetry. No clinical outcome data indicate the superiority of measurement versus estimation of energy requirements. Protein requirements rise with metabolic stress. Baseline protein needs of approximately 0.8 g/kg/day nearly triple after a significant burn and rise to lesser degrees with all disease states.

NUTRITION SUPPORT

Dietary Supplements

Anorexia, or simply small appetite, may occur in patients with current nutritional deficiencies or patients at risk of developing them. Simple strategies to combat a persistently small appetite include frequent spacing of small meals and the prioritization of energy-dense (usually high-fat) foods.

When efforts to modify the diet fail to provide adequate nutrition, powdered (for reconstitution) or liquid supplements may be indicated. A wide variety of commercial products is available; selection often is best based on the recommendations of an experienced dietitian and patient preference. Some of the available supplements are nutritionally complete and can be used as needed as the sole source of nutrients and energy.

Enteral Nutrition Support

Enteral nutrition support involves the administration of nutrient formulas into the GI tract through a tube. The weight of evidence clearly favors enteral over parenteral nutrition support whenever either is an option, leading to the axiom that the gut should be used whenever it works. When nutrients are not administered via the GI tract, mucosal atrophy occurs, as does dysfunction of the pancreatic/biliary system. Options in enteral nutrition have been enhanced over recent years by the development of low-risk procedures for tube insertion and by the development of a variety of commercial preparations tailored to differing clinical situations. For the most part, enteral feeding formulas are classified according to energy density, protein content, intended administration route, and molecular complexity.

Feeding Tubes

There are two types of feeding tubes: those that enter the GI tract through the nose and those that enter through the abdominal wall. Nasogastric tubes are used for short-duration feeding and when the risk of aspiration is low. Nasoduodenal and nasojejunal tubes are preferable for longer-term feeding and when the risk of aspiration is higher. The risk of aspiration falls the more distally the tube is placed.

Tubes placed through the abdominal wall are more appropriate in general for long-term supplementation. Such tubes are less likely to kink or occlude, and they reduce the risk of aspiration. Gastrostomy and jejunostomy tubes can be inserted endoscopically or surgically. The percutaneous endoscopic gastrostomy (PEG) tube is increasingly popular. Insertion requires an endoscopy laboratory and local anesthesia with sedation, and is routinely done on an outpatient basis. Jejunostomy tubes, placed endoscopically or surgically, may be indicated when the risk of aspiration is considered particularly high. The technical difficulty is greater for jejunostomy tubes, and the complication rate is higher. Recent advances in technique permit endoscopic tube placement in most circumstances, except when anatomy is distorted by surgery or pathology (1). A button gastrostomy is an option in particularly active patients for whom a tube gastrostomy is inconvenient or embarrassing.

Enteral Formulas

Conventional enteric formulas are polymeric, containing oligosaccharides, intact protein, and triglycerides. Commercial preparations are lactose free and can provide approximately 2,000 kcal per day. The energy density varies from 1 to 2 kcal/mL, with high-energy-density preparations indicated when fluid restriction is required. Formula proteins are derived from egg albumin, milk protein, or both. The fat is of vegetable origin. Such formulas can be delivered directly into the stomach, duodenum, or jejunum. Added fiber often is used to prevent osmotic diarrhea and to even out serum glucose responses.

Monomeric formulas contain partially hydrolyzed protein and monosaccharides and disaccharides. These formulas are available at higher cost and in general are not known to offer appreciable advantages over polymeric preparations. Theoretically, such solutions should be advantageous in states of impaired absorption, such as pancreatic insufficiency.

Targeted formulas are intended for use in particular disease states. Tailored formulations for many conditions lack evidence of benefit compared with conventional preparations. Use of formulas tailored for hepatic dysfunction, containing a high ratio of branched-chain to aromatic amino acids, is supported by available evidence. Solutions based on essential amino acids have been developed for renal failure.

Formulas tailored for pulmonary disease exploit the lower respiratory quotient (RQ) of fat and protein relative to carbohydrate. The RQ refers specifically to the molar ratio of carbon dioxide produced per oxygen consumed. The RQ is 1 for carbohydrate, 0.7 for fat, and approximately 0.8 for protein. Thus, fat and protein can be used to generate energy with less CO_2 production, of particular value in states of CO_2 retention (see Chapter 14).

Formulas specifically tailored for inborn errors of metabolism are of clear value in defined circumstances. There is some evidence that solutions using ketoacids rather than amino acids can slow progression of chronic renal failure (2). Glycemic control can be improved with formulas tailored for diabetes (3). One solution, Impact, was designed to enhance immune function by supplementing n-3 fatty acids, RNA, and arginine. Results of a randomized trial using such a solution in patients undergoing cancer surgery indicate benefits with regard to postoperative infections and length of hospitalization (4). There is increasing interest in the addition of glutamine to enteral solutions, as it is the preferred energy substrate of the GI tract. Preliminary studies of its use are encouraging, but as it is the preferred energy source for GI tumors as well, its use in cancer patients remains controversial (5). The inclusion of fiber in enteral solutions, often in the form of soy polysaccharide, has become common practice.

Modular solutions are available to supplement commercial preparations so that nutrient composition can be tailored to the individual patient's need. There are more than 100 commercially available enteral feeding solutions. Selection is best based, other than for the nutrition specialist, on the advice of a consulting dietitian; inpatient use will be constrained by the hospital formulary.

Enteral solutions can be delivered as bolus feeds or continuous infusions; bolus feeding is feasible only when the tube is in the stomach. Bolus feeds are more convenient, with infusions typically requiring a pump.

Infusions into the small bowel generally can be tolerated at a rate up to 150 mL per hour.

Aspiration is the principal risk of enteral feeding. Risk is reduced by feeding with the torso at a 30- to 45-degree angle of inclination rather than supine. When the gag reflex is absent or impaired or gastric emptying is delayed, feeding into the jejunum is preferred. Diarrhea occurs not uncommonly, especially in patients taking antibiotics concomitantly. The risk generally is reduced by the use of isoosmolar solutions.

Parenteral Nutrition Support

The delivery of nutrition directly into the bloodstream poses risks enteral feeding does not and should be avoided when possible. Indications for parenteral feeding include states of severe malabsorption; such states occur in extensive bowel resection, radiation enteritis, severe inflammatory bowel disease; disordered intestinal motility, obstruction, or persistent vomiting; premature birth; or states of extreme catabolism, such as extensive burns, for which enteral feeding may not be adequate.

Whereas enteral solutions are approved as foods, parenteral solutions must be approved by the Food and Drug Administration as drugs. Intravenous nutrient infusions are intended to meet energy and nutrient requirements completely (total parenteral nutrition; TPN) or incompletely (peripheral parenteral nutrition; PPN). The PPN solutions generally can be delivered through a peripheral or central vein, but TPN requires central venous access. Near-complete nutrition support via peripheral access may be achievable in patients who can tolerate a high volume of isotonic solution. To meet energy needs while limiting the proportion of calories from fat, hypertonic carbohydrate solutions must be used, thus requiring TPN and central access.

Access for TPN generally is via the subclavian or jugular veins. Peripheral placement of long catheters threaded into the superior vena cava and creation of an arteriovenous fistula as in dialysis are alternatives. Surgical insertions are used to tunnel the catheter under the skin to reduce the risk of infection. Other vascular approaches are used less frequently. The risk of line sepsis is reduced by strict adherence to aseptic technique and infection control guidelines. Dedicated TPN lines can be maintained for months, if not years. Indwelling central venous catheters pose a risk not only of sepsis but also of thrombosis.

Various plastics are used for TPN delivery. There is some absorption of insulin by commonly used plastics, so the glucose levels of patients with diabetes should be monitored carefully, with adjustments in infused insulin made accordingly.

Parenteral nutrition generally is indicated only when intestinal absorption is impaired. Benefit is convincingly established only in the short bowel syndrome. Studies to date in surgical and oncology patients have yielded equivocal results at best, with some studies showing clear advantage for controls over those receiving TPN. Lipid emulsions generally are provided as adjuvants to TPN formula. Micronutrient doses in TPN formulas are standardized, but they may need to be tailored in certain conditions. Glutamine-supplemented formulas may enhance outcomes, but the data are preliminary (5). Glutamine is the preferred fuel of the gut.

There are clear disadvantages to overnutrition beyond those related to weight gain (6). In normal states, adults can oxidize glucose at a rate of up to approximately 14 mg/kg/min. This rate is reduced to as low as 5 mg/kg/min in burn patients. Glucose infused beyond this capacity is converted to fat, with elevation of the RQ to above 1 and loss of available energy due to metabolic demand and waste. Fatty liver may result over time from excessive hepatic synthesis of triglycerides.

Lipid emulsions administered with TPN become coated with apolipoproteins in circulation, much the same way as do endogenously produced lipoprotein particles. Because infused lipid particles differ from chylomicrons, they are metabolized differently, eliciting the formation of a novel lipoprotein (lipoprotein X). Emulsified lipid droplets are acted on by endothelial lipoprotein lipase and undergo metabolism much the way as does ingested fat (see Chapter 2).

Because lipid solutions are highly susceptible to microbial growth, infusion times of less than 12 hours are recommended. Lipid mixed with the other components of TPN, known as total nutrient admixture, can allow lipid infusions over 24-hour periods, but have disadvantages as well, among them catheter occlusions. Total nutrient admixture may be particularly useful in premature neonates, who may not tolerate standard lipid infusions.

Lipid infusions increase the risk of bacteremia and rarely can result in the fat overload syndrome, which is characterized by fever, hepatosplenomegaly, and coagulopathy due to fat sludging. Impaired pulmonary function and interference with immune function by occupation of the reticuloendothelial system also occur. Lipid emulsions containing balanced mixtures of medium-chain triglycerides (MCTs) and long-chain triglycerides (LCTs) apparently mitigate most of these complications (7).

The use of TPN in children is associated with metabolic bone disease (8). The etiology of the condition is not completely understood, with calcium and phosphate deficiencies only partially accountable (8).

Use of TPN is associated with gallstone formation, due to stasis in the gallbladder (9). Protracted use of TPN warrants periodic evaluation of the gallbladder by ultrasound, with consideration of elective cholecystectomy if stones develop. Use of ursodeoxycholic acid and S-adenosyl-L-methionine have shown promise in preventing TPN-induced cholelithiasis (10). Both cholelithiasis (10) and immune dysfunction (11) associated with TPN may be reduced by "gut stimulation" with limited enteral feeds. Meta-analysis indicates there is no net mortality benefit associated with use of TPN in surgical or critical care patients (12).

As is the case for enteral solutions, a variety of commercial parenteral formulas are available. The selection and constitution of parenteral solutions should be overseen by a dietitian or nutrition consult service.

Other

The progestational agent megestrol acetate (Megace) has been studied as an appetite stimulant in cancer and AIDS patients, with generally promising results (13–16). Although effective in stimulating appetite and supporting an increase in body mass, megestrol is associated with an increased risk of deep venous thrombosis.

Growth hormone has been shown to increase lean body mass in human immunodeficiency virus wasting syndrome, but at the cost of hypertriglyceridemia and hyperglycemia. Data are available only from short-term interventions. MCTs in either enteral or parenteral preparations may be useful in states of malabsorption. MCTs are more readily oxidized, whereas LCTs are needed to provide the essential fatty acid linoleic acid. Balanced mixtures of MCT/LCT may be particularly advantageous.

Use of both enteral and parenteral feeding may fail to suppress appetite completely, because of the dependence of satiety in part on the sensations elicited during ingestion (17).

Preoperative enteral nutrition support has proven benefit in patients with even moderate nutritional impairment (18), whereas parenteral nutrition preoperatively has no proven benefit and should be reserved for severely impaired patients in whom enteral nutrition is precluded. Postoperative TPN should be considered only if the period of needed support is likely to exceed 1 week (19). In a retrospective chart review, Pettignano and colleagues (20) reported the superiority of enteral to parenteral nutrition in pediatric patients requiring extracorporeal membrane oxygenation.

In 23 patients with AIDS and malabsorption, an oral semielemental diet was as effective at controlling weight loss and wasting as TPN, while performing better with regard to physical functioning (21).

A study in 16 children with cystic fibrosis comparing a semielemental formula to a nonelemental formula supplemented with pancreatic enzymes demonstrated that the enzyme-supplemented formula performed as well (22).

CLINICAL HIGHLIGHTS

Clinical assessment for malnutrition can and should be routinely incorporated into the history and physical examination of both inpatients and outpatients. For chronically malnourished patients able to eat, dietary adjustments or supplements may permit restoration of nutritional adequacy. When eating is precluded by illness, enteral nutrition support is preferred to parenteral nutrition whenever the GI tract is functioning. Enteral formulas increasingly can be tailored to the condition and metabolic state of individual patients; dietary consultation is indicated to facilitate optimal choices.

Parenteral nutrition support is riskier and costlier than enteral support, but is indicated when the GI tract is nonfunctioning. Improvements in the composition of formulas and the techniques for vascular access offer the promise of TPN with lower rates of complication. Nutrition service consultation is always indicated when TPN is to be used.

REFERENCES

1. Campos AC, Marchesini JB. Recent advances in the placement of tubes for enteral nutrition. *Curr Opin Clin Nutr Metab Care* 1999;2:265.
2. Koretz RL. Does nutritional intervention in protein-energy malnutrition improve morbidity or mortality? *J Ren Nutr* 1999;9:119–121.
3. Coulston AM. Clinical experience with modified enteral formulas for patients with diabetes. *Clin Nutr* 1998;17[Suppl 2]:46–56.
4. Braga M, Gianotti L, Radaelli G, et al. Perioperative immunonutrition in patients undergoing cancer surgery: results of a randomized double-blind phase 3 trial. *Arch Surg* 1999;134:428–433.
5. Sacks GS. Glutamine supplementation in catabolic patients. *Ann Pharmacother* 1999;33:348–354.
6. Klein CJ, Stanek GS, Wiles CE 3rd. Overfeeding macronutrients to critically ill adults: metabolic complications. *J Am Diet Assoc* 1998;98:795–806.
7. Adolph M. Lipid emulsions in parenteral nutrition. *Ann Nutr Metab* 1999;43:1–13.
8. Klein GL. Metabolic bone disease of total parenteral nutrition. *Nutrition* 1998;14:149–152.
9. Moss RL, Amii LA. New approaches to understanding the etiology and treatment of total parenteral nutrition-associated cholestasis. *Semin Pediatr Surg* 1999;8:140–147.
10. Amii LA, Moss RL. Nutritional support of the pediatric surgical patient. *Curr Opin Pediatr* 1999; 11:237–240.
11. DeWitt RC, Kudsk KA. The gut's role in metabolism, mucosal barrier function, and gut immunology. *Infect Dis Clin North Am* 1999;13:465–481.
12. Heyland DK, MacDonald S, Keefe L, et al. Total parenteral nutrition in the critically ill patient: a meta-analysis. *JAMA* 1998;280:2013–2019.
13. Loprinzi CL, Kugler JW, Sloan JA, et al. Randomized comparison of megestrol acetate versus dexamethasone versus fluoxymesterone for the treatment of cancer anorexia/cachexia. *J Clin Oncol* 1999;17:3299.
14. Tchekmedyian NS, Hickman M, Heber D. Treatment of anorexia and weight loss with megestrol acetate in patients with cancer or acquired immunodeficiency syndrome. *Semin Oncol* 1991;18 [1 Suppl 2]:35.
15. De Conno F, Martini C, Zecca E, et al. Megestrol acetate for anorexia in patients with far-advanced cancer: a double-blind controlled clinical trial. *Eur J Cancer* 1998;34:1705.
16. Corcoran C, Grinspoon S. Treatments for wasting in patients with the acquired immunodeficiency syndrome. *N Engl J Med* 1999:340:1740.
17. Stratton RJ, Elia M. The effects of enteral tube feeding and parenteral nutrition on appetite sensations and food intake in health and disease. *Clin Nutr* 1999;18:63–70.
18. McClave SA, Snider HL, Spain DA. Preoperative issues in clinical nutrition. *Chest* 1999;115[5 Suppl]: 64s–70s.
19. Waitzberg DL, Plopper C, Terra RM. Postoperative total parenteral nutrition. *World J Surg* 1999; 23:560–564.
20. Pettignano R, Heard M, Davis R, et al. Total enteral nutrition versus total parenteral nutrition during pediatric extracorporeal membrane oxygenation. *Crit Care Med* 1998;26:358–363.
21. Kotler DP, Fogleman L, Tierney AR. Comparison of total parenteral nutrition and an oral, semielemental diet on body composition, physical function, and nutrition-related costs in patients with malabsorption due to acquired immunodeficiency syndrome. *J Parenteral Enteral Nutr* 1998;22:120–126.
22. Erskine JM, Lingard CD, Sontag MK, et al. Enteral

nutrition for patients with cystic fibrosis: comparison of a semi-elemental and nonelemental formula. *J Pediatr* 1998;132:265–269.

BIBLIOGRAPHY

See "Sources for All Chapters."
Bozzetti F, Gavazzi C, Mariani L, et al. Artificial nutrition in cancer patients: which route, what composition? *World J Surg* 1999;23:577–583.

Chan S, McCowen KC, Blackburn GL. Nutrition management in the ICU. *Chest* 1999;115[5 Suppl]:145s–148s.

Jolliet P, Pichard C, Biolo G, et al. Enteral nutrition in intensive care patients: a practical approach. *Clin Nutr* 1999;18:47–56.

Varella LD, Young RJ. New options for pumps and tubes: progress in enteral feeding techniques and devices. *Curr Opin Clin Nutr Metab Care* 1999;2:271–275.

Special Topics in Clinical Nutrition

25

Diet, Pregnancy, and Lactation

INTRODUCTION

Optimal maternal nutrition during pregnancy and lactation is vitally important to the health of mother and infant. Nutritional needs rise during pregnancy (Table 25.1) in response to the metabolic demand of the developing embryo as well as to changes in maternal physiology.

There is definitive evidence that periconceptual folate supplementation decreases the incidence of neural tube defects. The maternal diet often is deficient in calcium, iron, and other micronutrients, and supplementation with a prenatal vitamin throughout pregnancy is indicated. Vitamin A at doses of about 10,000 IU per day is teratogenic and to be avoided during pregnancy. Carotenoids with vitamin A activity are safe. Caloric needs rise in pregnancy, but excessive weight gain is potentially disadvantageous to mother and fetus.

Under most circumstances, breast-feeding is the preferred nutritional source for neonates. The composition of human milk changes in response to maternal diet. A generous intake of dietary calcium and continued use of prenatal vitamins are indicated throughout the period of lactation. The pattern of macronutrient intake indicated for general health promotion is appropriate during pregnancy and lactation as well. Biologic maturity occurs on average 5 years after menarche. Before this time, a woman may still be growing herself, creating metabolic demands in conflict with the needs of pregnancy.

OVERVIEW

Diet

Maternal weight should be nearly ideal at the start of pregnancy to prevent complications that may arise from either maternal obesity or underweight. Underweight in the mother is associated with low birth weight, whereas maternal overweight is associated with increased risks of gestational hypertension, diabetes, and toxemia.

Maternal hemoglobin at sea level during pregnancy should consistently be higher than 11 g/dL to ensure adequate oxygen delivery to the fetus. Nutritional causes of anemia should be considered if the hemoglobin level falls below this value and another explanation is not evident. A microcytic anemia suggests iron deficiency, whereas a macrocytic anemia suggests folate or B_{12} deficiency; the former is the more common.

Maternal weight gain during pregnancy should occur predominantly during the second and third trimesters. Weight gain of more than 1 kg per week at any time generally is excessive, whereas weight loss or weight gain of less than 1 kg per month generally indicates inadequate nutrition.

Plasma volume expands nearly 50% during pregnancy. Total mass of red blood cells increases 20% over prepregnancy levels. These

TABLE 25.1. *Recommended nutrient intake changes associated with pregnancy and lactation*

Nutrient	Recommended intake by subject category				Average US dietary intake in adult women	Content of representative prenatal vitamin[b]
	Female (19–24 yr)	Female (25–50 yr)	Pregnancy	Lactation (initial 6 mo)		
Calcium (mg)	1,200	800	1,200[d]	1,200[d]	530	250
Folate[a] (μg)	180	180	400[d]	280[d]	280–300	1,000
Iodine (μg)	150	150	175	200[c]	170	150
Iron (mg)	15	15	30[d]	15	10.7	60
Magnesium (mg)	280	280	300[d]	355[c]	207	25
Niacin (mg NE)	15	15	17	20[c]	16	20
Phosphorus (mg)	1,200	800	1,200[d]	1,200[d]	1,000	—
Protein (g)	46	50	60[c]	65[d]	70	—
Riboflavin (mg)	1.3	1.3	1.6[c]	1.8[c]	1.34	3.4
Selenium (μg)	55	55	65[c]	75[c]	108	—
Thiamine (mg)	1.1	1.1	1.6[c]	1.6[c]	1.05	3
Vitamin A (μg RE)	800	800	800	1,300[d]	1,170	1,500
Vitamin B_2 (μg)	2.0	2.0	2.2	2.6[c]	4.85	12
Vitamin B_6 (mg)	1.6	1.6	2.2[c]	2.1[c]	1.16	10
Vitamin C (mg)	60	60	70	95[d]	77	100
Vitamin D (μg)	10	5	10[d]	10[d]	1.5	10
Vitamin E (mg TE)	8	8	10[c]	12[d]	7.1	22.2
Vitamin K (μg)	60	65	65	65	300–500	—
Zinc (mg)	12	12	15[c]	19[d]	10–15	25

[a] Intake of folate 400 μg per day is now recommended for all women of child-bearing age to ensure adequate stores at the time of conception.

[b] Maternal prenatal vitamins, Lederle Laboratories, 1997.

[c] Nutrient intake levels represent a 20% or more increase over recommendations for nonpregnant adult women.

[d] Nutrient intake levels represent a 50% or more increase over recommendations for nonpregnant adult women.

NE, niacin equivalent equal 1 mg of dietary niacin or 60 mg of dietary tryptophan; RE, retinol equivalent; TE, α-tocopherol equivalent.

Adopted from the National Research Council. *Recommended dietary allowances,* 10th ed. Washington, DC: National Academy Press, 1989, with permission.

changes require increased intake of energy, nutrients, and fluid. The greater increase in plasma volume than red cell mass will cause the hematocrit to fall during pregnancy; however, the mean corpuscular hemoglobin concentration (MCHC) should remain fairly constant, barring a concurrent anemia. The tendency of serum lipids to rise during pregnancy is due largely to the effects of progesterone.

Requirements for folate, calcium, iron, and zinc rise disproportionately during pregnancy. In general, intestinal nutrient absorption is enhanced during pregnancy as an adaptation to increased metabolic demands.

Whereas electrolytes, fatty acids, and fat-soluble vitamins cross the placenta by simple diffusion, sugars are carried to the fetus by facilitated diffusion so that glucose levels tend to be higher in fetal than in maternal blood. Amino acids, water-soluble vitamins, sodium, calcium, and iron are actively transported across the placenta to the fetal circulation.

In general, pregnancy requires a calorie increase over baseline of approximately 300 kcal per day, and lactation requires 500 kcal per day. Nutrients for which the recommended dietary allowance is specifically raised in pregnancy include total protein, total energy, magnesium, iodine, zinc, selenium, vitamin E, vitamin C, thiamine, niacin, iron, calcium, and folate. Lactation requires additional increases in protein, zinc, vitamin A, vitamin E, vitamin C, and niacin; requirements for iron and folate decline (see Table 25.1).

A total weight gain of 12.5 kg (approximately 27.5 lb) is appropriate during pregnancy, although weight gain will vary with maternal and fetal size. Pregnancy is thought to require an increase in energy consumption of 45,000 to 110,000 kcal over the level required for weight maintenance in the nonpregnant state; an 80,000-kcal increase is the standard estimate. Inadequate weight gain during pregnancy is associated with low birth weight, whereas excessive weight gain is associated with macrosomia, fetopelvic disproportion, and attendant complications of labor and delivery.

The Women, Infants, and Children (WIC) program is designed to meet the nutritional needs of women and infants. The program assists nearly one million women annually in meeting nutritional needs during pregnancy. Because WIC supplements tend to be shared with family members, the nutrient intake of pregnant women in this population often is suboptimal and requires close scrutiny to ensure optimal pregnancy outcomes.

Weight gain recommendations for pregnancy vary with prepregnant weight. For women with a baseline body mass index (BMI) below 20 kg/m², weight gain of 1.1 lb (0.5 kg) per week during the second and third trimesters is indicated. For women with a BMI greater than 26, weight gain of 0.7 lb (just under one third of a kilogram) per week during the same period is recommended. Obligatory weight gain during pregnancy, attributable to fetal growth, placental growth, amniotic fluid production, uterine and breast enlargement, and expansion of the blood volume, accounts for approximately 16.5 lb (7.5 kg) on average. Weight gain in excess of this amount represents weight the woman will need to lose through a combination of calorie restriction and increased energy expenditure, following pregnancy, to return to prepregnant weight. Available evidence suggests that biologically immature women, i.e., those less than 5 years after beginning menarche, require on average an additional 150 kcal per day, and an additional 3-kg weight gain, to avoid low birth weight.

Weight gain targets can be tailored to the particular situation. A woman who is over-weight before pregnancy (BMI greater than 25) should gain as little over the obligatory 7.5 kg as possible; the rate of weight gain should be approximately 300 g per week. A woman with BMI below 25 who does not plan on breast-feeding should gain approximately 10 kg at a rate of 350 g per week. A woman with BMI less than 25 and above 20 and planning to breast-feed should gain approximately 12 kg at a rate of 400 g per week. Underweight (BMI less than 20) and biologically immature women should gain 14 to 15 kg at a rate of 500 g per week. Women bearing twins generally should gain at least 18 kg at a rate of 650 g per week (1). For women in the United States, each pregnancy adds an average of approximately 2.5 kg (5.5 lb) of permanent weight.

Physical activity during pregnancy offers benefits to the mother at no cost to the fetus, provided maternal tolerance is not taxed. Extreme exertion will result in elevated fetal temperature. Maintenance of moderate exercise during pregnancy is appropriate unless precluded by complications. Exercise with potential high impact, such as skiing, or at altitude is to be avoided during pregnancy. Postpartum exercise facilitates desired weight loss.

A total of approximately 925 g of protein is incorporated into the developing fetus and other products of conception. Peak requirements during pregnancy add a need for 8.5 g of protein to basal requirements. Protein intake by women in the United States is typically about 70 g per day, a figure well in excess of minimal requirements for all stages of pregnancy. Therefore, no particular effort to raise protein intake during pregnancy is indicated unless the diet is atypical. The fetus gains approximately 30 g per day during the third trimester. Interventions to ensure term delivery are essential in maintaining this rate of development. Intensive care of premature babies can rarely sustain more than 20 g of growth per day.

Overall, the increased micronutrient requirements of pregnancy exceed the increased energy requirements. Therefore, vitamin supplementation during pregnancy is universally indicated, and the nutrient density of foods assumes increased importance.

The teratogenicity of vitamin A in high doses was revealed through the use of the vitamin A analogue isotretinoin for acne. Ingestion of 20,000 IU or more of vitamin A per day is thought to be potentially teratogenic as well. Carotenoid precursors of vitamin A provide adequate retinol while avoiding any known toxicity. Therefore, prenatal vitamin supplements typically provide vitamin A at well below the toxic threshold, and precursor, generally in the form of β-carotene.

Successful pregnancy outcomes depend heavily on maternal health and lifestyle, but of course are mediated as well by the condition of the fertilizing sperm. Preliminary evidence suggests that vitamin C, which is concentrated in semen, and vitamin E, which is not, may play important roles in protecting the integrity of DNA in sperm from oxidative injury (2). There also is preliminary evidence that folate and zinc, which are highly concentrated in seminal fluid, may influence spermatogenesis.

Immediately following a birth for a period of approximately 3 to 5 days, the mother's mammary glands produce colostrum, a fluid rich in sodium, chloride, and immunoglobulins that confer passive immunity to the newborn. Colostrum is replaced by milk, which is rich in lactose and protein, and comparatively low in sodium and chloride. Milk volume consumed by the neonate is 50 mL per day at birth, 500 mL by day 5, and 750 mL at 3 months.

Milk production is maintained by infant suckling, which suppresses hypothalamic dopamine production, thereby disinhibiting prolactin release. The first 4 months of lactation consume, and convey to the infant, an amount of energy comparable to that of the entire gestational period. Human milk is appropriate as the sole source of infant nutrition for up to 6 months. There is uncertainty whether milk meets all of the infant's nutritional needs beyond this point (see Chapter 27).

The fatty acid composition of human milk varies with maternal dietary intake. With the exception of iodine and selenium, there is little evidence that the levels of minerals and trace elements in milk vary with maternal diet. In contrast, vitamin levels in milk are responsive to dietary intake, with the strength of the relationship varying by nutrient. The levels of both fat- and water-soluble vitamins in milk vary in proportion to maternal intake. Calcium and folate, and possibly other nutrients, are preserved in milk at the expense of maternal stores when maternal intake is less than daily requirements.

Breast milk contains more than 100 different oligosaccharides. There is current interest in the influence these carbohydrates have on intestinal flora of the infant and their capacity to play a role in the prevention of infection (3).

As noted above, maternal diet strongly influences the fatty acid and vitamin composition of breast milk, but generally exerts a modest influence on minerals (4,5). Iodine and selenium are exceptions, varying substantially in response to maternal intake (6). Vitamins D and K generally are present at low levels in breast milk, and supplementation is recommended (7); however, a recent study suggests that low vitamin D intake in breast-fed neonates may not adversely affect bone metabolism (8).

Breast-feeding has been associated with a decline in maternal bone density, and this association was not influenced by maternal calcium intake (9). A recent study of 52 lactating women in the United States suggests that intake of calcium, zinc, folate, vitamin E, vitamin D, and pyridoxine may tend to be deficient in this group (10). A recent study demonstrates that the transfer of fatty acids to breast milk occurs within several hours of ingestion, with the maximum effect varying with the particular fat source (11).

Breast milk and infant formulas differ substantially in a variety of nutrients (12). The significance of all of the differences has yet to be established. The prevailing view is that breast milk favors optimal brain development, and breast-feeding is associated with greater intelligence, at least during childhood (13) (see Chapter 27).

Energy requirements to sustain lactation are based on the caloric density of human milk (approximately 70 kcal per 100 mL), the metabolic cost of milk production, and total milk volume. The consensus view that lactation requires 500 kcal per day above the energy required to maintain maternal weight assumes that approximately 200 kcal per day of milk production energy will derive from pregnancy-related fat stores. Loss of 0.5 to 1 kg per month is common during lactation, whereas loss in excess of 2 kg per month implies inadequate nutrition. Weight maintenance and weight gain during lactation are not uncommon.

Weight loss of up to 2 kg per month appears to be safe during lactation, with preservation of energy transfer to breast milk. The safety of more rapid weight loss is uncertain. Prolactin levels tend to rise in response to maternal energy restriction during lactation, perhaps serving to preserve energy delivery to the neonate (14). A recent study suggests that energy restriction beginning 1 month post partum can facilitate maternal weight loss without adverse effects on milk production or infant growth (15). An accompanying editorial, however, urges caution in the application of energy-restricted diets during lactation, encouraging instead judicious management of diet and weight throughout the gestational and postpartum periods (16).

Exercise during lactation, independent of energy restriction, is not known to pose any threat to mother or infant, and it offers a range of benefits. Lactation does not specifically aid in weight loss, despite the suggestion in folklore that it does. Women do tend to lose weight while breast-feeding (17), as is to be expected in the postpartum period. Generally, however, nonlactating women lose weight more readily than do their breast-feeding counterparts.

There is interest in the role breast-feeding may play in preventing the development of atopy, but the data are preliminary (18)

(see Chapter 17). Evidence is convincing that breast-feeding confers protection against infections, although the mechanisms by which breast milk influences infant immunity remain under study (19,20). Erythropoietin in breast milk apparently is resistant to degradation in the infant gastrointestinal tract and may stimulate the newborn's marrow (21).

The amino acid pattern of breast milk is species specific, suggesting another way in which human milk might make unique contributions to early development (22). Maternal diet influences the flavor of breast milk and thereby serves as a means of introducing the neonate to a variety of taste experiences (23,24).

Strong flavors, and the familiarity or novelty of such flavors, may influence the feeding behaviors of infants. Ingestion of garlic by the mother has been shown to lengthen feeding at first, but shortens feeding when exposure is recurrent (25). Alcohol ingested by a breast-feeding woman is conveyed to breast milk and generally results in reduced feeding by the infant. Research by Mennella (26) and Mennella and Beauchamp (27) suggests that this effect is not due to the taste of alcohol per se, but some other effect of alcohol on the feeding experience. Contrary to folklore, maternal alcohol ingestion may actually decrease the sleep of a breast-feeding infant (28).

A study of more than 170,000 women demonstrated that weight gain during pregnancy in ranges recommended by the Institute of Medicine decreased the incidence of low-birth-weight babies for lean white and Hispanic women. The data were less consistent with regard to black women. Low birth weight was uncommon among obese or high BMI white and Hispanic women, and the benefit of recommended weight gain in these groups was unclear (29). Nutritional support of malnourished women during pregnancy is beyond the scope of this discussion, but in general is approached as is malnutrition under other circumstances (see Chapter 24). The topic has been reviewed (30).

Nutrients and Nutriceuticals

Folate

Supplementation with approximately 400 μg of folic acid per day beginning before conception markedly reduces the risk of neural tube defects, including anencephaly and spina bifida. Evidence for this association has been extensively reviewed and is considered definitive (31,32). Ingestion of more than 1 mg per day of folate is generally not recommended. However, in women with prior pregnancies leading to neural tube defects, the ingestion of up to 4 mg per day of folate may confer additional benefit.

Fluoride

Breast milk does not provide optimal fluoride levels to term infants, and supplementation generally is recommended (33).

Iron

Anemia is the most common nutrient-related abnormality of pregnancy and is attributable to iron deficiency nearly 90% of the time, with the remainder due primarily to folate deficiency. Because of the cessation of menses, iron requirements drop during the first trimester. Demands increase over baseline in the second trimester and peak in the third trimester at 4.0 mg per day.

Pregnancy consumes approximately 1,040 mg of iron in total, of which 200 mg is recaptured after pregnancy from the expanded red cell mass and 840 mg is permanently lost. The iron is lost to the fetus (300 mg), the placenta (50 to 75 mg), expanded red cell mass (450 mg), and blood loss at parturition (200 mg). Only about 10% of ingested iron is absorbed in the nonpregnant state, but pregnancy may enhance absorption by as much as 30%. Therefore, an intake between 13 and 40 mg per day is required during the third trimester. Vitamin/mineral supplements generally contain 30 mg of iron, and the diet provides an additional 15 mg, easily

meeting the needs of most women without anemia.

Women with iron deficiency anemia during pregnancy require increased intake to replenish bone marrow stores and still provide for the metabolic needs of the fetus. In this situation, daily iron intake between 120 and 150 mg typically is required. Iron supplementation before conception will facilitate meeting the iron needs of pregnancy and lactation, which together result in a net loss between 420 and 1,030 mg of elemental iron. Iron supplementation should continue post partum, both to provide iron for breast milk and to replenish losses due to bleeding at delivery.

Calcium

The need for calcium supplementation was discussed earlier. There is preliminary evidence that calcium supplementation may reduce the risk of pregnancy-induced hypertension and preterm delivery (34).

Magnesium

The evidence that magnesium supplementation may prevent preeclampsia is mixed. Alternative medicine sources recommend supplements of about 500 mg per day, which appears to be safe. Conventional prenatal vitamins provide only 25 mg per day; as a result, intake often is below recommended levels.

Selenium

Based on reported association between selenium deficiency and sudden infant death syndrome, as well as low birth weight, selenium supplementation of 200 μg/day is advocated in the complementary and alternative medicine literature (35). The benefits of selenium may be limited to individuals from areas with selenium-deficient soil. Selenium deficiency in the United States, where soil levels are high, is not generally considered a problem. Selenium in breast milk is very responsive to maternal intake, which distinguishes it from most other minerals (36).

Zinc

Studies of zinc nutriture in relation to pregnancy outcome have shown mixed results. There is some evidence that zinc supplementation may extend pregnancy to term among women with low levels of serum zinc. Zinc supplementation may directly contribute to normal birth weight through its effects on protein metabolism, or the influence may be indirect as a result of extended gestation (34). Zinc levels in breast milk are not thought to vary readily with dietary intake. However, a cohort study in Spain suggests that low dietary zinc intake during the third trimester predicts relatively low levels in breast milk (37). Relative zinc deficiency among US adults has been reported.

Caffeine

Available evidence indicates that caffeine intake of up to 300 mg per day, the equivalent of up to five or six cups of coffee, is not harmful to mother or fetus. Caffeine is particularly concentrated in brewed coffee, which contains on average 125 mg of caffeine per 8 oz.

Alcohol

Heavy alcohol ingestion during pregnancy is associated with the fetal alcohol syndrome, a condition of fetal developmental delay and cognitive deficits. The incidence of fetal alcohol syndrome in the United States among offspring of women consuming 1.5 to 8 drinks per week is approximately 10%. A "drink" contains on average 17 g of ethanol. An occasional alcoholic drink during pregnancy is not known to be harmful, but recommendations in the United States favor abstinence.

n-3 Fatty Acids

Preliminary evidence suggests that high consumption of marine oils is associated with longer gestation, and that dietary supplementation with n-3 polyunsaturated oils may increase the proportion of term births in diverse populations (34). There is evidence that n-3 fatty acids are important in the normal development of eye and brain function (13). The n-3 content of breast milk is mediated by maternal intake. The impact of n-3 supplementation during pregnancy or lactation remains to be elucidated.

A case-control study in Greece supports the hypothesis that n-3 fatty acids may be especially important in fetal brain development, and that low maternal fish consumption may elevate risk of cerebral palsy (38). Increased consumption of n-3 fatty acids may confer health benefits to mother and baby. Relative to the prehistoric dietary pattern, the modern diet is deficient in n-3 fatty acids (39), lending the support of an evolutionary context to the hypothesis that increased intake may be beneficial.

Vitamin B_6

Other than its role in metabolism, supplemental B_6 is recommended for treatment of pregnancy-induced nausea based on the results of small randomized, double-blind trials (35). A dose range from 50 to 100 mg per day is advised, and this level exceeds the content of diet and prenatal vitamins combined.

Gingerroot

Ground gingerroot, at a dose of 250 mg four times daily, has been shown effective in the treatment of hyperemesis gravidarum (40). The combination of ginger and vitamin B_6 may be more effective than either used alone (35).

Vitamin C

The naturopathic literature suggests that vitamin C supplementation of about 500 mg per day may play a role in the prevention of preeclampsia and premature rupture of membranes. Evidence in support of either claim is minimal at present. This dose apparently is safe. Third-trimester maternal intake of ascorbic acid has been shown to influence the level of ascorbate in breast milk (37).

SPECIAL CONSIDERATIONS
Diabetes/Gestational Diabetes

Diabetes during pregnancy should be controlled so that blood sugar is consistently in the normal range to prevent macrosomia and sacral agenesis. The dietary control of diabetes is discussed in Chapter 10.

Phenylketonuria

A history of phenylketonuria in the mother requires a return to a tyrosine-restricted diet during pregnancy to prevent related complication in the fetus.

Human Immunodeficiency Virus

Human immunodeficiency virus (HIV) and other viruses are transmissible in breast milk. Breast-feeding is contraindicated in HIV-positive women.

CLINICAL HIGHLIGHTS

Dietary recommendations for pregnancy and lactation vary to some extent with the prepregnant weight, age, and nutritional status of individual women. Assuming near-optimal prepregnancy weight and nutritional status and biologic maturity at conception, most women following a prudent diet during pregnancy would be able to meet their macronutrient recommendations. In such a diet, 25% to 30% of calories come from fat, 60% from carbohydrate, and 15% from protein. Energy consumption should be increased approximately 300 kcal per day during pregnancy and 500 kcal per day during lactation.

The use of multivitamin/multimineral supplements beginning several months before conception and throughout pregnancy and lactation is indicated. Low- or non-fat dairy products should be eaten regularly as a source of calcium, and red meat should be eaten as a source of heme iron, provided fat and protein intake is in compliance with guidelines. Vegetarian women may require iron supplementation in addition to a prenatal vitamin; such supplementation generally is not required in omnivorous women.

Vegans may require calcium supplementation, as is true of other women without regular intake of dairy products. Vitamin B_6 and gingerroot have been used with success in the management of pregnancy-related nausea and appear to be safe. A graded program of exercise and caloric restriction post partum is required to restore prepregnancy weight. Most women in the United States retain up to 5.5 lb after each pregnancy, a factor contributing to the prevalence of obesity among women. Management of diet and the degree of weight gain during pregnancy are thought to be preferable to an exclusive focus on postpartum weight loss. When maternal weight gain is insufficient during pregnancy, the risk of low birth weight is increased; therefore, diet should be managed to ensure that energy intake is neither excessive nor deficient.

REFERENCES

1. McGanity W, Dawson E, Fogelman A. Embryonic development, pregnancy, and lactation. In: Shils ME.
2. Woodall AA, Ames B. Nutritional prevention of DNA damage to sperm and consequent risk reduction in birth defects and cancer in offspring. In: Bendich A, Deckelbaum RJ, eds. *Preventive nutrition: the comprehensive guide for health professionals.* Totowa, NJ: Humana Press, 1997.
3. McVeagh P, Miller J. Human milk oligosaccharides: only the breast. *J Paediatr Child Health* 1997;33: 281–286.
4. Emmett P, Rogers I. Properties of human milk and their relationship with maternal nutrition. *Early Hum Dev* 1997;49:s7–s28.
5. Bates C, Prentice A. Breast milk as a source of vitamins, essential minerals and trace elements. *Pharmacol Ther* 1994;62:193–220.
6. Picciano M. Human milk: nutritional aspects of a dynamic food. *Biol Neonate* 1998;74:84–93.

7. Jensen R, Ferris A, Lammi-Keefe C. Lipids in human milk and infant formulas. *Annu Rev Nutr* 1992;12:417–441.

8. Park M, Namgung R, Kim D, et al. Bone mineral content is not reduced despite low vitamin D status in breast milk-fed infants versus cow's milk based formula-fed infants. *J Pediatr* 1998;132:641–645.

9. Laskey M, Prentice A, Hanratty L, et al. Bone changes after 3 mo of lactation: influence of calcium intake, breast-milk output, and vitamin D-receptor genotype. *Am J Clin Nutr* 1998;67:685–692.

10. Mackey A, Picciano M, Mitchell D, et al. Self-selected diets of lactating women often fail to meet dietary recommendations. *J Am Diet Assoc* 1998;98:297–302.

11. Francois C, Connor S, Wander R, et al. Acute effects of dietary fatty acids on the fatty acids of human milk. *Am J Clin Nutr* 1998;67:301–308.

12. Huisman M, Beusekom CV, Lanting C, et al. Triglycerides, fatty acids, sterols, mono- and disaccharides and sugar alcohols in human milk and current types of infant formula milk. *Eur J Clin Nutr* 1996;50:255–226.

13. Uauy R, Andraca ID. Human milk and breast feeding for optimal mental development. *J Nutr* 1995;125:2278s–2280s.

14. Dewey K. Effects of maternal caloric restriction and exercise during lactation. *J Nutr* 1998;128:386s–389s.

15. Lovelady C, Garner K, Moreno K, et al. The effect of weight loss in overweight, lactating women on the growth of their infants. *N Engl J Med* 2000;342:449–453.

16. Butte N. Dieting and exercise in overweight, lactating women. *N Engl J Med* 2000;342:502–503.

17. Winkvist A, Rasmussen K. Impact of lactation on maternal body weight and body composition. *J Mammary Gland Biol Neoplasia* 1999;4:309–318.

18. Vandenplas Y. Myths and facts about breastfeeding: does it prevent later atopic disease? *Acta Paediatr* 1997;86:1283–1287.

19. Garofalo R, Goldman A. Cytokines, chemokines, and colony-stimulating factors in human milk: the 1997 update. *Biol Neonate* 1998;74:134–142.

20. Hamosh M. Protective function of proteins and lipids in human milk. *Biol Neonate* 1998;74:163–176.

21. Kling P, Sullivan T, Roberts R, et al. Human milk as a potential enteral source of erythropoietin. *Pediatr Res* 1998;43:216–221.

22. Sarwar G, Botting H, Davis T, et al. Free amino acids in milks of human subjects, other primates and non-primates. *Br J Nutr* 1998;79:129–131.

23. Mennella J. Mother's milk: a medium for early flavor experiences. *J Hum Lact* 1995;11:39–45.

24. Mennella J, Beauchamp G. Early flavor experiences: research update. *Nutr Rev* 1998;56:205–211.

25. Mennella J, Beauchamp G. The effects of repeated exposure to garlic-flavored milk on the nursling's behavior. *Pediatr Res* 1993;34:805–808.

26. Mennella J. Infants' suckling responses to the flavor of alcohol in mothers' milk. *Alcohol Clin Exp Res* 1997;21:581–585.

27. Mennella J, Beauchamp G. The transfer of alcohol to human milk. Effects on flavor and the infant's behavior. *N Engl J Med* 1991;325:981–985.

28. Mennella J, Gerrish C. Effects of exposure to alcohol in mother's milk on infant sleep. *Pediatrics* 1998;101:E2.

29. Schieve L, Cogswell M, Scanlon K. An empiric evaluation of the Institute of Medicine's pregnancy weight gain guidelines by race. *Obstet Gynecol* 1998;91:878–884.

30. Hamaoui E, Hamaoui M. Nutritional assessment and support during pregnancy. *Gastroenterol Clin North Am* 1998;27:89–121.

31. Czeizel A. Folic acid-containing multivitamins and primary prevention of birth defects. In: Bendich A, Deckelbaum RJ, eds. *Preventive nutrition: the comprehensive guide for health professionals.* Totowa, NJ: Humana Press, 1997.

32. Locksmith G, Duff P. Preventing neural tube defects: the importance of periconceptual folic acid supplements. *Obstet Gynecol* 1998;91:1027–1034.

33. Flynn A. Minerals and trace elements in milk. *Adv Food Nutr Res* 1992;36:209–252.

34. Scholl T, Hediger M. Maternal nutrition and preterm delivery. In: Bendich A, Deckelbaum RJ, eds. *Preventive nutrition: the comprehensive guide for health professionals.* Totowa, NJ: Humana Press, 1997.

35. Murray M. *Encyclopedia of nutritional supplements.* Rocklin, CA: Prima Publishing, 1996.

36. Alaejos MS, Romero CD. Selenium in human lactation. *Nutr Rev* 1995;53:159–166.

37. Ortega R, Andres P, Martinez R, et al. Zinc levels in maternal milk: the influences of nutritional status with respect to zinc during the third trimester of pregnancy. *Eur J Clin Nutr* 1997;51:253–258.

38. Petridou E, Koussouri M, Toupadaki N, et al. Diet during pregnancy and the risk of cerebral palsy. *Br J Nutr* 1998;79:407–412.

39. Eaton S, Konner M. Paleolithic nutrition revisited: a twelve-year retrospective on its nature and implications. *Eur J Clin Nutr* 1997;51:207–216.

40. Fischer-Rasmussen W, Kjaer S, Dahl C, et al. Ginger treatment of hyperemesis gravidarum. *Eur J Obstet Gynecol Reprod Biol* 1990;38:19.

BIBLIOGRAPHY

See "Sources for All Chapters."

Dietz WH, Stern L, eds. *American Academy of Pediatrics guide to your child's nutrition.* New York: Villard Books (Random House, Inc.), 1999

Tamborlane WV, ed. *The Yale guide to children's nutrition.* New Haven, CT: Yale University Press, 1997.

Kleinman RE, ed. *Committee on Nutrition, American Academy of Pediatrics. Pediatric nutrition handbook,* 4th ed. Elk Grove Village, IL: American Academy of Pediatrics, 1998.

Duffy VB, Bartoshuk LM, Striegel-Moore R, et al. Taste changes across pregnancy. *Ann N Y Acad Sci* 1998; 855:805–809.

Institute of Medicine. *Nutrition during pregnancy.* Washington, DC: National Academy Press, 1990.

Institute of Medicine. *Nutrition during lactation.* Washington, DC: National Academy Press, 1991.

Koletzko B, Aggett PJ, Bindels JG, et al. Growth, development and differentiation: a functional food science approach. *Br J Nutr* 1998;80[Suppl 1]:s5–s45.

26

Diet and the Menstrual Cycle

INTRODUCTION

Variations in food intake and preference occur during the normal menstrual cycle. Even more extreme variations are characteristic of the premenstrual syndrome (PMS), particularly the subtype in which food cravings are a predominant feature. Hormonal variation during the menstrual cycle induces changes in taste perception, nutrient metabolism, and the thermic effect of food. The intake pattern of macronutrients and micronutrients influences symptoms associated with the menstrual cycle in both normal and pathologic states. Dietary management of PMS often is possible.

OVERVIEW

The normal menstrual cycle is approximately 28 days in length and consists of three phases: menstruation, the follicular phase, and the luteal phase. During menstruation, levels of the pituitary gonadotrophins, luteinizing hormone and follicle-stimulating hormone, as well as the ovarian hormones estradiol and progesterone, are at baseline levels. When the endometrium has sloughed completely, the follicular phase begins as estradiol levels begin to rise. Estradiol levels peak just before the midpoint of the cycle (day 14), inducing a surge in levels of the gonadotrophins. This surge, in turn, induces a transient fall in estradiol levels. Progesterone levels rise slowly throughout the follicular phase. Ovulation, induced by the midcycle surge in gonadotrophins, occurs on or about day 14, and represents the division between

the follicular and luteal phases. In the luteal phase, gonadotrophin levels return quickly to baseline, as estradiol levels begin to rise again while progesterone levels continue to rise, now at a somewhat accelerated rate. Estradiol peaks for a second time, and progesterone for the first time, at or near the midpoint of the luteal phase. If implantation occurs, progesterone levels are maintained and continue to rise. In the absence of implantation, levels of both estradiol and progesterone fall toward baseline, inducing menstruation approximately 14 days after ovulation. The phases of the menstrual cycle are summarized in Table 26.1.

The recurrent hormonal fluctuations associated with the menstrual cycle interact with diet in important ways. Appetite, hunger, satiety, cravings, and aversions all vary with the cycle. These variations are subtle in many women but quite profound in others. In the most extreme manifestation, PMS is associated with typified food preferences thought to represent an attempt at self-treatment.

The converse situation also is true, that is, dietary pattern potentially influences the menstrual cycle. Estrogen is metabolized in adipose tissue, and levels are affected by both excessive and deficient adiposity.

Variation in eating pattern and appetite is a well-recognized occurrence even in normal menstrual cycles. There is evidence that with variation in steroid hormone levels, there is corresponding, albeit modest, variation in taste thresholds (1,2). The extent to which seemingly subtle alterations in taste perception govern the variations in food preference and intake throughout the menstrual cycle

TABLE 26.1. *Phases of the prototypical menstrual cycle*

Phase	Approximate timing	Gonadotrophins (LH and FSH)	Estradiol	Progesterone
Menstruation	Days 1–3	Baseline level	Baseline level	Baseline level
Follicular phase	Days 3–14	Baseline level	Gradual rise/peak	Gradual rise
Ovulation	Day 14	Surge	Abrupt fall	Gradual rise
Luteal phase	Days 14–28	Baseline level	Gradual rise/second peak followed by a decline to baseline	Faster rise/peak followed by a decline to baseline

FSH, follicle-stimulating hormone; LH, luteinizing hormone.

currently is uncertain. Also uncertain at present is whether gustatory thresholds change more profoundly in women with PMS. To date, there is no clear association between dietary pattern and the risk of dysmenorrhea (3).

Premenstrual syndrome, a constellation of monthly symptoms, occurs in the luteal phase of the cycle. Severe symptoms occur in up to 10% of all susceptible women; up to 40% experience less severe symptoms (4). Premenstrual symptoms consistent with the syndrome occur in up to 60% of women (5). Recent survey data suggest that the majority of these women are receiving suboptimal care from primary care physicians (6).

There are four distinct symptom complexes implied by the rubric of PMS: anxiety is prominent in one, depression in another, food cravings in another, and hyperhydration (bloating) in the fourth. Each variant of PMS has been associated with distinct physiologic disturbances; therefore, treatment strategies vary with syndrome. When anxiety is predominant, estrogen tends to be high and progesterone low; there is evidence supporting the use of supplemental pyridoxine. Food cravings have been shown to respond to magnesium supplementation. Hyperhydration may be associated with elevated aldosterone levels; avoidance of caffeine and nicotine, restriction of sodium, and supplementation with pyridoxine and vitamin E have been advocated. Physical activity has consistently been reported to confer modest benefit.

Treatment strategies remain controversial, however, as most available evidence is preliminary. In a study of the hyperhydration variant of PMS, Olson and colleagues (7) found the syndrome to be associated with urinary sodium loss rather than retention; sodium restriction was not found to be beneficial. A trial of progesterone supplementation failed to show any benefit with regard to cyclical craving of chocolate and/or sweets (8).

The evidence supporting a therapeutic role for pyridoxine has been criticized for its methodologic limitations. Nonetheless, in a systematic review, Wyatt and colleagues (9) found evidence supporting use of up to 100 mg per day of B_6 in the treatment of PMS, particularly with depressive symptoms.

The understanding of the pathophysiology of the several subtypes of PMS is still quite limited. The possibility that the variants are mechanistically distinct suggests that intervention trials that failed to target a particular PMS variant were treating a heterogeneous group and, therefore, subject to type II error. Studies of PMS are increasingly focusing on subject groups homogeneous with regard to symptom complex.

Serotonin levels are thought to be related to symptoms of PMS (see Chapter 32), a hypothesis that would account for the carbohydrate craving experienced by some women. Consistent with this theory is evidence that selective serotonin reuptake inhibitors (SSRIs) relieve symptoms in many women and apparently more effectively than other commonly used classes of medications and nutriceuticals (10). The benefit of SSRIs apparently is greatest when dysphoric or depressive symptoms are predominant (11).

Evidence appears to be particularly strong for a role of calcium metabolism in PMS. In 1995, Thys-Jacobs and Alvir (12) demonstrated that although total and ionized calcium levels varied predictably throughout the menstrual cycle in subjects with PMS and in matched controls, only the subjects with PMS experienced a midcycle surge in levels of intact parathyroid hormone. The authors interpreted these data to indicate that a transient, secondary hyperparathyroid state was implicated in the pathogenesis of PMS. Following up on this finding, Thys-Jacobs and colleagues (13) conducted a randomized trial of calcium supplementation involving more than 450 women. Compared with placebo, supplementation with 1,200 mg per day of elemental calcium resulted in a significant reduction in all symptoms of PMS.

Related evidence suggests that impaired calcium homeostasis may be an important element in the pathophysiology of polycystic ovarian syndrome (14).

Although in the aggregate less compelling than the evidence for calcium, there is evidence of a therapeutic effect of magnesium as well (15). Facchinetti and colleagues (16) studied a high-magnesium yeast product (Sillix Donna) in a double-blind, placebo-controlled, randomized trial and found a statistically and clinically significant reduction in PMS symptoms over the 6-month study period. Walker et al. (17) found a daily dose of 200 mg of magnesium oxide reduced symptoms of hyperhydration by the second month of administration in a randomized, double-blind, crossover trial of 38 women; no significant effect was seen on other symptom categories. Cocoa, and therefore chocolate, is a relatively rich source of magnesium, suggesting one possible reason why chocolate craving is apparently common both in PMS and the normal menstrual cycle. There is suggestive evidence of a role for manganese supplementation as well (18).

There has been interest in the use of essential fatty acids in the treatment of PMS, and evening primrose oil, which is rich in γ-linolenic acid, has been advocated. In a randomized, crossover trial, Collins and colleagues (19) found no benefit of essential fatty acid supplementation in 27 women with PMS.

Leptin levels have been shown to vary throughout the menstrual cycle, suggesting a role in the changes in appetite and occurrence of cravings. In an observational study, however, Paolisso et al. (20) found that although both leptin and food intake varied throughout the menstrual cycle in 16 healthy women, the two were discordant in time.

Vegetarianism has been reported to be associated with an increased propensity for amenorrhea, oligomenorrhea, and anovulation. However, studies to date have been limited by sampling bias (21). Although there are various mechanisms by which a vegetarian diet could lead to menstrual irregularities, the most plausible is loss of body fat. Strict vegetarian diets are associated with both amenorrhea and weight loss beyond recommended levels (22).

Competitive athletics in adolescent girls is associated with amenorrhea due to the energy demands of training and, in some, associated eating disorders thought to be induced by the pressure to remain thin. However, the occurrence of menstrual irregularities in female athletes without disordered eating is well established; the term "exercise-related menstrual irregularities" has been applied (23). The exact mechanisms responsible for exercise-related menstrual irregularities remain under investigation.

The reduction of body fat associated with intense training apparently disrupts the menstrual cycle via effects on estrogen metabolism and possibly via effects on cortisol and leptin (24). The nutritional requirements associated with competitive athletics are discussed in Chapter 30; the prevention of osteoporosis is discussed in Chapter 13. Amenorrhea in adolescent girls is a clear indication of a risk for potentially irreversible osteopenia. Although management should focus on the restoration of adequate nutrition and energy balance, oral contraceptives are indicated when the patient is resistant to such interventions, or when primary or secondary amenorrhea persist despite these actions.

Isoflavones in soy and other foods are known to exert selective estrogen effects, generating clinical and popular interest in such foods as a natural means to replace ovarian hormones or modify disease risk. Data from supplementation trials are beginning to accumulate. In a randomized crossover study of 14 premenopausal women, Duncan and colleagues (25) found that even high-level isoflavone supplementation induced no significant changes in menstrual cycle length, endometrial histology, or plasma estrogen levels. Using similar methods in 12 healthy premenopausal women, Xu et al. (26) found that soy protein supplementation decreased urinary excretion of endogenous estrogens, while increasing excretion of soy phytoestrogens. A significant increase in the ratio of 2-hydroxyestrone to 16α-hydroxyestrone was observed, suggesting a mechanism by which phytoestrogens might reduce cancer risk (26).

CLINICAL HIGHLIGHTS

The normal menstrual cycle produces changes in metabolism and taste that result in variations in food intake pattern. This tendency becomes extreme in the craving variant of PMS. Such cravings may respond to supplemental magnesium in particular, although data are preliminary. All variants of PMS may respond to calcium supplementation, which should be attempted in most patients, given its safety and other potential benefits. Supplementation with calcium and magnesium, and a multivitamin with minerals, appears appropriate given available evidence. Available evidence suggests that a daily dose of calcium in the range of 1,000 to 1,500 mg is appropriate for a therapeutic trial.

If this strategy is ineffective, a trial of pyridoxine of approximately 100 mg per day appears to be justified; whether such intervention should be combined or applied separately has not yet been addressed and must rely on clinical judgment. Combination therapy is not precluded by any potential toxicity. A diet rich in complex carbohydrates may be beneficial in ameliorating depressive symptoms of PMS through a serotonergic mechanism. When depressive symptoms are pronounced or refractory to dietary interventions, SSRIs should be used as indicated. Physical activity, avoidance of nicotine, and restricted intake of caffeine may offer benefit in PMS and are indicated on other grounds. By judiciously selecting and combining available therapies, clinicians may hope to alleviate symptoms in the great majority of patients with PMS.

REFERENCES

1. Kuga M, Ikeda M, Suzuki K. Gustatory changes associated with the menstrual cycle. *Physiol Behav* 1999;66:317–322.
2. Alberti-Fidanza A, Fruttini D, Servili M. Gustatory and food habit changes during the menstrual cycle. *Int J Vitam Nutr Res* 1998;68:149–153.
3. Di Cintio E, Parazzini F, Tozzi L, et al. Dietary habits, reproductive and menstrual factors and risk of dysmenorrhoea. *Eur J Epidemiol* 1997;13:925–930.
4. Ugarriza DN, Klingner S, O'Brien S. Premenstrual syndrome: diagnosis and intervention. *Nurs Pract* 1998;23:40, 45, 49–52.
5. Singh BB, Berman BM, Simpson RL, et al. Incidence of premenstrual syndrome and remedy usage: a national probability sample study. *Altern Ther Health Med* 1998;4:75–79.
6. Kraemer GR, Kraemer RR. Premenstrual syndrome: diagnosis and treatment experiences. *J Womens Health* 1998;7:893.
7. Olson BR, Forman MR, Lanza E, et al. Relation between sodium balance and menstrual cycle symptoms in normal women. *Ann Intern Med* 1996;125:564–567.
8. Michener W, Rozin P, Freeman E, et al. The role of low progesterone and tension as triggers of perimenstrual chocolate and sweets craving: some negative experimental evidence. *Physiol Behav* 1999;67:417–420.
9. Wyatt KM, Dimmock PW, Jones PW, et al. Efficacy of vitamin B_6 in the treatment of premenstrual syndrome: a systematic review. *BMJ* 1999;318:1375–1381.
10. Diegoli MS, da Fonseca AM, Diegoli CA, et al. A double-blind trial of four medications to treat severe premenstrual syndrome. *Int J Gynaecol Obstet* 1998;62:63–67.
11. Yonkers KA, Halbreich U, Freeman E, et al. Symptomatic improvement of premenstrual dysphoric

disorder with sertraline treatment. A randomized controlled trial. Sertraline premenstrual dysphoric collaborative study group. *JAMA* 1997;278:983–988.

12. Thys-Jacobs S, Alvir MJ. Calcium-regulating hormones across the menstrual cycle: evidence of a secondary hyperparathyroidism in women with PMS. *J Clin Endocrinol Metab* 1995;80:2227–2232.

13. Thys-Jacobs S, Starkey P, Bernstein D, et al. Calcium carbonate and the premenstrual syndrome: effects on premenstrual and menstrual symptoms. Premenstrual Syndrome Study Group. *Am J Obstet Gynecol* 1998;179:444–452.

14. Thys-Jacobs S, Donovan D, Papadopoulos A, et al. Vitamin D and calcium dysregulation in the polycystic ovarian syndrome. *Steroids* 1999;64:430–435.

15. Facchinetti F, Borella P, Sances G, et al. Oral magnesium successfully relieves premenstrual mood changes. *Obstet Gynecol* 1991;78:177–181.

16. Facchinetti F, Nappi RE, Sances MG, et al. Effects of a yeast-based dietary supplementation on premenstrual syndrome. A double-blind placebo-controlled study. *Gynecol Obstet Invest* 1997;43:120–124.

17. Walker AF, De Souza MC, Vickers MF, et al. Magnesium supplementation alleviates premenstrual symptoms of fluid retention. *J Womens Health* 1998;7:1157–1165.

18. Penland JG, Johnson PE. Dietary calcium and manganese effects on menstrual cycle symptoms. *Am J Obstet Gynecol* 1993;168:1417–1423.

19. Collins A, Cerin A, Coleman G, et al. Essential fatty acids in the treatment of premenstrual syndrome. *Obstet Gynecol* 1993;81:93–98.

20. Paolisso G, Rizzo MR, Mazziotti G, et al. Lack of association between changes in plasma leptin concentration and in food intake during the menstrual cycle. *Eur J Clin Invest* 1999;29:490–495.

21. Barr SI. Vegetarianism and menstrual cycle disturbances: is there an association? *Am J Clin Nutr* 1999;70[3 Suppl]:549s–554s.

22. Koebnick C, Strassner C, Hoffmann I, et al. Consequences of a long-term raw food diet on body weight and menstruation: results of a questionnaire survey. *Ann Nutr Metab* 1999;43:69–79.

23. De Cree C. Sex steroid metabolism and menstrual irregularities in the exercising female. A review. *Sports Med* 1998;25:369–406.

24. Warren MP, Stiehl AL. Exercise and female adolescents: effects on the reproductive and skeletal systems. *J Am Med Womens Assoc* 1999;54:115–130.

25. Duncan AM, Merz BE, Xu X, et al. Soy isoflavones exert modest hormonal effects in premenopausal women. *J Clin Endocrinol Metab* 1999;84:192.

26. Xu X, Duncan AM, Merz BE, et al. Effects of soy isoflavones on estrogen and phytoestrogen metabolism in premenopausal women. *Cancer Epidemiol Biomarkers Prev* 1998;7:1101.

BIBLIOGRAPHY

See "Sources for All Chapters."

Barnhart KT, Freeman EW, Soundheimer SJ. A clinician's guide to the premenstrual syndrome. *Med Clin North Am* 1995;79:1457–1472.

Dye L, Blundell JE. Menstrual cycle and appetite control: implications for weight regulation. *Hum Reprod* 1997;12:1142–1151.

Freeman EW, Halbreich U. Premenstrual syndromes. *Psychopharmacol Bull* 1998;34:291.

27

Diet and Early Development: Pediatric Nutrition

INTRODUCTION

Physical and cognitive development is rapid during infancy and early childhood, which imposes extreme metabolic demands. The provision of adequate nutrition from birth is fundamental to the maintenance of normal growth and development. Infants are subject to certain specific micronutrient deficiencies, and they have requirements different from those of adults for macronutrients, particularly protein.

The health benefits of breast-feeding (see Chapter 25) during the first 6 months of life are increasingly clear. Although the principal goal of nutrition management in early childhood is the preservation of optimal growth and development, children in the United States and other developed countries are increasingly susceptible to the adverse effects of dietary excess, particularly obesity (see Chapter 5). As a result, there is intense interest regarding the age at which dietary restrictions might first be safely imposed.

In general, restriction of macronutrients (dietary fat being of particular concern) is discouraged before age 2, with increasing evidence that restrictions comparable to those recommended for adults may be safe and appropriate after age 2. The establishment of health-promoting diet and activity patterns in childhood may be of particular importance, as preferences established early in life tend to persist (see Chapters 36 and 41).

OVERVIEW

Diet

The importance of adequate nutrition to normal growth and development during the neonatal period and early childhood is well established and largely self-evident. Basal metabolic rate is higher in infants and children than in adults; the nutritional needs to support growth are superimposed on the higher basal metabolism, resulting in considerably higher energy and nutrient requirements per unit body weight.

The average term infant triples in weight and doubles in length during the first year of life. Consequently, energy requirements in early childhood are very high. Newborns require three to four times more energy per unit body weight than do adults: 90 to 120 kcal/kg/day compared to 30 to 40 kcal/kg/day for adults. Inefficiency of intestinal absorption contributes to this difference.

As a result of a child's rapid growth, protein requirements are higher in infancy than in adulthood. Total protein requirement is greater than the additive needs for essential amino acids by a factor of two to three. Protein intake of 2.0 to 2.2 g/kg/day is recommended, compared with 0.8 to 1.0 g/kg/day for adults who engage in moderate levels of physical activity.

Infants require protein of high biologic value to ensure adequate consumption of essential amino acids (leucine, isoleucine, valine, threonine, methionine, phenylalanine, tryptophan, lysine, and histidine). Cysteine and tyrosine also are recognized as essential dietary proteins in infancy, although not beyond the first 6 months of life. The reason is unclear in the case of tyrosine, whereas for cysteine there is a well-characterized delay in the maturity of the enzymatic pathway that converts methionine to cysteine. The minimal intake necessary to provide the indicated amounts of all essential amino acids would provide half or less of total protein requirements, indicating the importance of both quantity and quality of dietary protein.

The protein composition of human milk is ideal for infants. Breast milk provides on average 1 g of protein per 100 mL. Therefore, to achieve the recommended intake of 2.0 to 2.2 g/kg/day, infants need to consume approximately 200 mL of breast milk per kilogram per day. This level exceeds the intake of many infants, yet protein deficiency generally does not occur in breast-fed infants. Apparently, any limitations in the quantity of breast milk protein consumed are compensated by the digestibility and quality of protein in breast milk (see Chapter 25). Currently available infant formulas contain all amino acids essential for infants and, therefore, provide protein of comparable quality to that of breast milk.

Need for carbohydrate and fat in infancy is restricted to those levels necessary to prevent ketosis and fatty acid deficiency, respectively. Total intake of carbohydrate and fat generally are adequate whenever total energy intake is appropriate.

Recommended dietary allowances (RDAs) have been established for essential nutrients for both the first and second 6-month intervals of life (Table 27.1). Iron deficiency is the most common nutrient deficiency in early childhood. Iron absorption from breast milk apparently is particularly efficient, as iron deficiency rarely occurs in breast-fed infants despite the lower levels of iron in breast milk than in formula (1). Increased use of iron-fortified infant formula

among babies who were not breast-fed has substantially reduced the incidence of iron deficiency in this age group. Iron requirements may be related to vitamin E and polyunsaturated fat content of the diet. Supplementation is recommended in infants who are not breast-fed until age 2. Vitamin deficiencies are rare in adequately nourished infants. Vitamin K is provided by injection at or near the time of birth to prevent neonatal hemorrhage; subsequently, deficiency is uncommon.

An intake of 75 to 100 mL fluid per kilogram per day is considered adequate for the first years of life, but 150 mL is preferred as a defense against dehydration. A well-nourished infant generally easily meets the recommended intake with either breast milk or formula. The fluid consumption of infants allows for the intake of the recommended 150 mL/kg/day of water.

The nutrient recommendations for infants 6 to 12 months of age are based largely on extrapolation from the first 6-month period; less is known about the nutrient needs of infants 6 to 12 months old. There currently is debate regarding the optimal level of energy intake, with some recommending a reduction from 95 to 85 kcal/kg/day (1). Adequate growth apparently is maintained at the lower energy-intake level.

By 6 months of age, gastrointestinal physiology is substantially mature, and infants metabolize most nutrients is comparably to adults. Nutrient needs can be met with breast milk or formula, but most authorities advocate the gradual introduction of solid foods beginning at or around 6 months. As infant foods begin to replace breast milk or formula, the nutrient density of the diet is apt to decline, and the introduction of a multivitamin supplement is indicated (1). Completion of weaning to solid food by 1 year of age is common practice and is appropriate.

Breast milk is widely considered the optimal means of nourishing newborns, barring contraindications such as communicable disease in the mother. The properties of breast milk are discussed in greater detail in

TABLE 27.1. *Recommended nutrient intake in infancy/childhood*

Nutrient	0–6 mo	6–12 mo	1–3 yr	4–6 yr	7–10 yr
Protein (g)	13	14	16	24	28
Vitamin A (μg RE)	375	375	400	500	700
Vitamin D (μg)	7.5	10	10	10	10
Vitamin E (mg TE)	3	4	6	7	7
Vitamin K (μg)	5	10	15	20	30
Vitamin C (mg)	30	35	40	45	45
Thiamine (mg)	0.3	0.4	0.7	0.9	1
Riboflavin (mg)	0.4	0.5	0.8	1.1	1.2
Niacin (mg NE)	5	6	9	12	13
Vitamin B_6 (mg)	0.3	0.6	1.0	1.1	1.4
Folate (μg)	25	35	50	75	100
Vitamin B_{12} (μg)	0.3	0.5	0.7	1.0	1.4
Calcium (mg)	400	600	800	800	800
Phosphorus (mg)	300	500	800	800	800
Magnesium (mg)	40	60	80	120	170
Iron (mg)	6	10	10	10	10
Zinc (mg)	5	5	10	10	10
Iodine (μg)	40	50	70	90	120
Selenium (μg)	10	15	20	20	30
Biotin (μg)	10	15	20	25	30
Pantothenic acid (mg)	2	3	3	3–4	4–5
Copper (mg)	0.4–0.6	0.6–0.7	0.7–1.0	1.0–1.5	1.0–2.0
Manganese (mg)	0.3–0.6	0.6–1.0	1.0–1.5	1.5–2.0	2.0–3.0
Fluoride (mg)	0.1–0.5	0.2–1.0	0.5–1.5	1.0–2.5	1.5–2.5
Chromium (μg)	10–40	20–60	20–80	30–120	50–200
Molybdenum (μg)	15–30	20–40	25–50	30–75	50–150

NE, niacin equivalent equal 1 mg of dietary niacin or 60 mg of dietary tryptophan; RE, retinol equivalent; TE, α-tocopherol equivalent.

Values are derived from National Research Council. *Recommended dietary allowances,* 10th ed. Washington, DC: National Academy Press, 1989. For ongoing revisions of dietary reference intakes by the National Research Council, see http://www.nas.edu/nrc/.

Chapter 25. Breast milk has lower calcium and phosphorus than bovine milk. Although breast-fed infants have a less mineralized skeleton at several months of age, there is no evidence that this is harmful. Bone density during the first several months of life is lower in breast-fed than formula-fed infants, because of the lower calcium and phosphorus of breast milk. Differences in bone density do not persist beyond infancy. Breast-feeding also is associated with transient hyperbilirubinemia during the first few days of life; if extreme, phototherapy is indicated to prevent kernicterus.

The protein content of breast milk seems lower than ideal, yet, as noted, breast-fed infants rarely display evidence of protein deficiency. The particular advantages of breast-feeding relate to the development of immune function and resistance to infection, development of the intestinal tract, and psychological bonding between mother and infant (see Chapter 25). There is increasing evidence that breast-feeding reduces the risk of childhood infections, and that prolonged breast-feeding may protect against later obesity (2).

The principal hazard of breast-feeding is the issue of supply; infants must be followed closely during the first few days to weeks of life to ensure normal growth. The adequacy of breast-feeding can be assessed by preprandial and postprandial weighings; every milliliter of milk consumed should add 1 g of weight.

There are concerns about converting from breast milk to bovine milk (rather than formula) as the principal source of nutrition after 6 months. The practice results in protein and sodium intake well above recommendations, and iron and linoleic acid intake well below. Deficiency of essential fatty acids is the most significant concern regarding the use of bovine milk (whole or reduced fat) as the staple after 6 months.

Formulas generally are based on either unmodified or modified bovine milk protein. Bovine milk can be modified so that the whey-to-casein ratio approximates that of human milk. There is no clear evidence that either is superior. For infants intolerant of bovine milk protein, the protein can be hydrolyzed, or soy protein can be substituted.

Soy-based formulas are appropriate for infants with lactose intolerance (see Chapter 17).

Formulas based on bovine milk protein typically provide 1.5 g of protein per 100 mL, or 50% more protein than breast milk. The nutrient composition of commercial formulas is otherwise very comparable to that of breast milk (Table 27.2). Provided a sanitary water supply is available, the safety of formula generally is not of concern. Properly nourished, the healthy infant should double in weight by 4 to 5 months of age, and triple in weight by 12 months. Demand feeding is the preferred method of ensuring adequate energy intake.

TABLE 27.2. *Composition of commonly available commercial formulas compared to that of breast milk*

Nutrient (quantity per liter)	Human milk	Similac (Ross)	Enfamil (Mead Johnson)	Prosobee[a] (Mead Johnson)	Isomil[a] (Ross)
Energy (kcal)	680	676	680	660	660
Protein (g)	10.5	14.5	14.2	19.7	16.1
Fat (g)	39	36.5	35.8	34.8	35.8
Percent polyunsaturated	14.2	37	29	18.8	23.5
Percent monounsaturated	41.6	17	16	37.6	38.3
Percent saturated	44.2	46	55	42.5	32.7
Carbohydrate (g)	72	72.3	73.7	65.6	67.6
Calcium (mg)	280	492	528	690	690
Phosphorus (mg)	140	380	358	540	490
Magnesium (mg)	35	41	54	70	50
Iron (mg)	0.3	12.2	12.2	11.8	11.8
Zinc (mg)	1.2	5.1	6.8	7.9	4.9
Manganese (μg)	6	34	101	NA	160
Copper (μg)	252	610	507	490	490
Iodine (μg)	110	95	68	NA	NA
Sodium (mg)	179.4	184	184	240	290
Potassium (mg)	526.5	706	729	790	710
Vitamin A (μg)	675	676	630	590	590
Vitamin D (μg)	0.5	10	10.8	NA	NA
Vitamin E (IU)	4	20	13.6	9.7	13.2
Vitamin K (μg)	2.1	54	54	NA	NA
Thiamine (μg)	210	680	541	530	390
Riboflavin (μg)	350	1,010	947	590	590
Pyridoxine (μg)	205	410	406	NA	NA
Vitamin B$_{12}$ (μg)	0.5	1.7	2.0	2.0	3
Niacin (mg)	1.5	7.1	6.8	6.6	8.9
Folate (μg)	50	100	108	110	100
Pantothenic acid (mg)	1.8	3	3.4	NA	4.9
Vitamin C (mg)	40	60	81.2	79	59
Biotin (μg)	4	30	20.3	NA	NA

[a] Soy-based formulas.
NA, not available in the sources used.
Values are derived from American Academy of Pediatrics. *Pediatric nutrition handbook,* 4th ed. Elk Grove Village, IL: American Academy of Pediatrics.1998; and USDA Nutrient Database for Standard Reference, Release 13, November 1999: http://www.nal.usda.gov/.

Inclusion of cow's milk in the diets of infants 6 to 12 months old appears to be fairly common practice in the United States. The result is elevated intake of protein and sodium relative to the RDAs. Protein and sodium consumption is higher still in infants fed fat-reduced milk. There is interest in the role of preventing hypertension in adulthood by restricting sodium intake in childhood, but the data are only preliminary (see Chapter 7). The substitution of skim for whole milk in this age group does not confer any known benefit, nor does it appear to reduce total energy intake as a result of compensation for the missing calories (1). The substitution of bovine milk for formula tends to reduce the iron level in the diet, and skim milk will reduce the intake of linoleic acid below recommended levels.

Children over the age of 1 year will tend to eat an appropriate variety of foods/nutrients when provided access to them. Balance may not be achieved on any given day; however, provided the child continues to be provided reasonable food choices, balance will be achieved over several days' time. Parents should be reassured that a balanced diet need not be measured on a per-meal or even per-day basis. A reasonable approach is to avoid any major distinction between snacks and meals, so that healthy food can be eaten when the child is hungry, and meal size can be adjusted to account for snacking.

The prudence of advocating the same diet for adults and children has been challenged. Evidence is lacking that dietary restrictions in childhood prevent chronic disease in adults (3). Obtaining such evidence, however, is a daunting challenge. Indirect, epidemiologic, and inferential evidence may be the best guidance available. The safety of the American Heart Association step 1 diet for children over the age of 2 has received fairly widespread support (4).

The epidemiology of nutrition-related health problems in children changed dramatically in the latter half of the 20th century. Childhood obesity is considerably more common in the United States than is growth retardation (5). Most children still consume fat in excess of recommendations and fail to consume the recommended quantities of fruits and vegetables. National surveys have revealed excessive intake of both total and saturated fat in children over the age of 1 year (6). Dietary fat intake was excessive in children as young as 6 months in the Bogalusa Heart Study, which also demonstrated important racial differences in dietary patterns in young children, with African-American children consuming more total energy and fat than their white counterparts (7).

Therefore, from a population perspective, there appears to be little potential harm and considerable potential gain in promoting the dietary pattern recommended for adults to school-age children as well (5). Dietary intervention has been shown to lower the high cholesterol levels common among children in Finland, with levels rising again on resumption of the habitual diet (8). Controversy over the optimal dietary recommendations for young children has persisted for more than a decade (9).

In Canada, a working group was convened from the membership of the Canadian Paediatric Society and Health Canada to address the appropriateness of adult nutritional guidelines for children. The group concluded that the provision of adequate energy and nutrients to ensure growth and development should be the highest priority, and that, during childhood, foods should not be eliminated on the basis of fat content (10).

The group advocates a transition during childhood to a diet with 30% or less of calories from fat, and 10% or less of calories from saturated fat (10). Dietary guidelines need not be specifically advocated as a priority until linear growth has stopped. The Canadian guidelines encourage a common eating pattern for families, with the implication that the fat content in the diets of children might decline, and encourage the promotion of regular physical activity and fruit and vegetable consumption during childhood (11).

Proponents of the restriction of dietary fat beginning at age 2 cite evidence that atherosclerosis begins in childhood, and that a diet with not more than 30% of calories from fat beginning at age 2 is compatible with optimal growth (12). Others in the United States argue for the Canadian approach, with a gradual transition to lower fat intake and attention to the type and distribution of dietary fat (13).

Further support for advocating dietary fat restriction in particular for young children comes from epidemiologic data in Italy. A recent rise in the saturated fat consumption has been noted in a population with a traditionally health-promoting "Mediterranean" diet (14). A study of 100 Finnish school children demonstrated that the intake of several important nutrients tended to be lower among the children with the highest fat intake (15). Further, this study suggested that the diets of young children are quite diverse, so that offering dietary recommendations was unlikely to "disrupt" a traditional dietary pattern chosen by families for their young children.

Efforts to resolve the debate regarding the safety of fat restriction in early childhood have resulted in controlled intervention studies. Niinikoski et al. (16) conducted a randomized, prospective study (STRIP: The Special Turku Coronary Risk Factor Intervention Project for Babies) in which more than five hundred 7-month-olds were assigned either to a dietary counseling intervention aimed at reducing fat intake and promoting compliance with adult dietary guidelines or to a control group.

At 3 years, cholesterol was lower in the intervention subjects (significantly in males, not significantly in females) than the controls, with no discernible differences in height, weight, or rate of growth (17). Dietary counseling in the study was aimed at keeping fat intake between 30% and 35% of calories, achieving an intake ratio of polyunsaturated to monounsaturated to saturated fatty acid of 1:1:1, and reducing salt intake while maintaining energy consumption. The intervention produced significant reductions in total and saturated fat intake by 13

months, and this effect was sustained thereafter (17). Of note is that growth was preserved despite a decline in energy intake associated with the intervention. Although the debate in the United States and Canada has focused on the safety of restricting dietary fat after age 2, this study suggests that such an intervention may be safe even at a much earlier age (16).

Another intervention trial (CATCH: The Child and Adolescent Trial for Cardiovascular Health) examined the effects of a multidisciplinary program emphasizing change in school nutrition on cardiac risk factors in children beginning in third grade (18). The study lowered fat intake significantly, while lowering serum cholesterol minimally. Growth and development were unaffected.

A comparable age group was studied in the Dietary Intervention Study in Children (DISC), which randomly assigned 8- to 10-year-old children with low-density lipoprotein cholesterol above the 80th percentile to usual care or more intensive counseling (19). The intervention significantly lowered total and saturated fat intake and low-density lipoprotein cholesterol levels, with no adverse effects on growth and development.

A pathology study of adolescents and young adults who died of trauma demonstrated that elevated serum lipids, as well as smoking, influence the development of early signs of atherosclerosis in adolescents. Elevated serum lipids probably contribute to early lesions of atherosclerosis in children 10 to 14 years old and may begin to do so in children between the ages of 3 and 9 years (20,21).

Thus, there is increasing evidence that efforts to modify the diets of children to reduce long-term cardiovascular risk are likely to be safe. Whether such diets reduce long-term risk is less clear. Obviously, evidence of long-term outcome effects is difficult to obtain. To be considered in the debate is the importance of providing a single, consistent, dietary pattern for a family, as well as the issue of dietary patterns tracking over time. Data from the Bogalusa Heart Study demonstrate that there is tracking, between the ages of 6 months and 4 years, of both dietary pattern and cardiovascular risk factors (22).

In light of these considerations, it appears that the recommendation in the United States to advocate a similar diet for everyone over the age of 2 years is reasonable and safe, and it may offer long-term benefits. Although there is some evidence that a comparable diet may be safe even before age 2, consensus opinion in the United States and prudence argue against the imposition of macronutrient restrictions in this age group. Conclusive evidence of benefit from early dietary modification efforts will accrue very slowly.

Nutrients and Nutriceuticals

n-3 Fatty Acids

Long-chain polyunsaturated fatty acids are particularly concentrated in the brain and retina. Eicosapentaenoic acid and docosahexaenoic acid (DHA) are relatively abundant in human breast milk and prominently incorporated into the developing brain (23). Docosahexaenoic acid in particular is considered essential to healthy brain development (24). Impaired cognitive development in premature babies may be related in part to insufficient availability of DHA during a critical period of brain development (25).

Breast-feeding is associated with enhancement of IQ and visual acuity in infants (26). The apparent health benefits of breast-feeding relative to formula feeding may be related in part to the DHA content of breast milk. Increasingly, long-chain polyunsaturated fatty acids, including DHA, are being added to commercial formulas (27). Although the essential fatty acid α-linolenic acid is a precursor to DHA as well as to eicosapentaenoic acid, conversion to DHA in particular appears to be limited and variable. The putative benefits of DHA apparently require that it be administered directly in the diet (28). Although health benefits of DHA supplementation are likely on the basis of confluent lines of evidence, the benefits are not yet conclusive (29).

TOPICS OF SPECIAL INTEREST

Low-birth-weight Infants

Approximately 7% of all infants born in the United States weigh less than 2,500 g. The energy reserves of a term infant of normal size are enough to withstand nearly 1 month of starvation, whereas those of a 1,000-g infant would last only 4 to 5 days. Adequate nutrition is likely to be critical to normal cognitive development in premature and low-birth-weight (LBW) infants in particular. The caloric and protein density of formula generally allows for more rapid catch-up growth, but evidence to date suggests that breast milk may reduce the risk of infections and confer a range of other benefits as well, including superior visual acuity and cognition.

Energy needs of LBW infants are estimated to be 120 kcal/kg/day. Protein intake and weight gain are directly related in LBW infants; a protein intake of about 3 g/kg/day is recommended. For a variety of reasons, insensible water loss of LBW infants tends to be approximately twice that of term infants; fluid intake of approximately 140 mL/kg/day is recommended. Higher fluid intake can increase the risk of patent ductus arteriosus. A team of specialists invariably is involved in the nutritional management of LBW infants, and the details of such management are beyond the scope of this text.

CLINICAL HIGHLIGHTS

The provision of optimal nutrition during infancy and early childhood is of vital importance to growth and development and likely is related to a wide array of health outcomes in later life. The establishment of good nutriture for an infant begins while *in utero,* during which time maternal dietary practices may influence fetal metabolism (see Chapter 25).

The most reliable way to ensure optimal nutrition for a newborn is breast-feeding. Therefore, clinicians should routinely encourage breast-feeding for a period of 6 months unless the practice is contraindicated by communicable disease. This advice is based on the confluence of multiple lines of evidence.

The maintenance of salutary maternal nutrition during lactation is of importance to the health of both mother and baby (see Chapter 25). Although commercial infant formulas provide generally balanced nutrition, there is concern that they are deficient in long-chain polyunsaturated fatty acids, particularly DHA. As evidence of the importance of DHA and other essential fatty acids continues to accrue, the composition of commercial formulas will likely be revised. In the interim, there is preliminary evidence that cognition and vision are enhanced by breast-feeding as compared to formula feeding.

Weaning to solid food generally should begin at approximately 6 months; earlier weaning may increase the risk of food allergies (see Chapter 17). Weaning from breast milk or formula generally is complete by around 12 months, although such practices are culturally determined; medically, weaning at 12 months is appropriate.

Children generally will self-select foods that meet micronutrient requirements when provided with an array of healthy food choices; this practice is to be encouraged. Children also reliably meet their energy needs, although energy intake may vary considerably by meal and even day. Parents should be reassured in this regard and discouraged from placing too great an emphasis on "plate cleaning"; whether or not such a practice contributes to later obesity is unknown, but an association is plausible.

Controversy persists regarding the optimal timing for approximating adult dietary guidelines in children. There is evidence that adult dietary recommendations are safe for children as young as 7 months of age, although few in the United States would endorse such a practice.

Evidence is more definitive that the imposition of such guidelines beginning at age 2 is safe and reasonable. Taking this approach provides the added benefit of unifying family dietary practices earlier. There is evidence that dietary preferences established in childhood tend to persist (see Chapter 36), highlighting the importance of establishing a prudent dietary pattern early. Therefore, the diet that should be advocated to adults and older children to promote health (see Chapter 40) may be provided promptly, or approximated gradually, in children beginning at age 2. Micronutrient supplementation with a multivitamin/mineral tailored for children is a reasonable practice. Regular consumption of fish should be encouraged. The consistent intake of DHA may offer considerable health benefits, which is supported by preliminary, but accumulating, evidence.

REFERENCES

1. Heird W. Nutritional requirements during infancy. In: Ziegler EE, Filer LJ Jr., eds. *Present knowledge in nutrition*, 7th ed. Washington, DC: ILSI Press, 1996.
2. von Kries R, Koletzko B, Sauerwald T, et al. Breast feeding and obesity: cross sectional study. *Br Med J* 1999;319:147–150.
3. Lifshitz F. Children on adult diets: is it harmful? Is it healthful? *J Am Coll Nutr* 1992;11:84s.
4. Dobrin-Seckler B, Deckelbaum R. Safety of the American Heart Association step 1 diet in childhood. *Ann N Y Acad Sci* 1991;623:263.
5. Kennedy E, Powell R. Changing eating patterns of American children: a view from 1996. *J Am Coll Nutr* 1997;16:524.
6. Kimm S, Gergen P, Malloy M, et al. Dietary patterns of US children: implications for disease prevention. *Prevent Med* 1990;19:432.
7. Nicklas T, Farris R, Major C, et al. Dietary intakes. *Pediatrics* 1987;80[Suppl]:797.
8. Vartiainen E, Puska P, Pietinen P, et al. Effects of dietary fat modifications on serum lipids and blood pressure in children. *Acta Paediatr Scand* 1986; 75:396.
9. Taras HL, Nader P, Sallis JF, et al. Early childhood diet: recommendations of pediatric health care. *J Am Diet Assoc* 1988;88:1417.
10. Joint Working Group of the Canadian Paediatric Society and Health Canada. Nutrition recommendations update: dietary fats and children. *Nutr Rev* 1995;53:367.
11. Zlotkin S. A review of the Canadian "Nutrition Recommendations Update: Dietary Fat and Children." *J Nutr* 1996;126:1022s.

12. Kleinman R, Finberg L, Klish W, et al. Dietary guidelines for children: US recommendations. *J Nutr* 1996;126:1028s.

13. Lifshitz F, Tarim O. Considerations about dietary fat restrictions for children. *J Nutr* 1996;126:1031s.

14. Greco L, Musmarra R, Franzese C, et al. Early childhood feeding practices in southern Italy: is the Mediterranean diet becoming obsolete? Study of 450 children aged 6–32 months in Campania, Italy. *Acta Paediatr* 1998;87:250.

15. Rasanen L, Ylonen K. Food consumption and nutrient intake of one- to two-year-old Finnish children. *Acta Paediatr* 1992;81:7.

16. Niinikoski H, Viikari J, Ronnemaa T, et al. Prospective randomized trial of low-saturated-fat, low-cholesterol diet during the first 3 years of life. The STRIP Baby Project. *Circulation* 1996;94:1386.

17. Niinikoski H, Lapinleimu H, Viikari J, et al. Growth until 3 years of age in a prospective, randomized trial with reduced saturated fat and cholesterol. *Pediatrics* 1997;99:687.

18. Luepker R, et al. Outcomes of a field trial to improve children's dietary patterns and physical activity. The Child and Adolescent Trial for Cardiovascular Health (CATCH). *JAMA* 1996;275:768.

19. Writing Group for the DISC collaborative research group. Efficacy and safety of lowering dietary intake of fat and cholesterol in children with elevated low-density lipoprotein cholesterol. The Dietary Intervention Study in Children (DISC). *JAMA* 1995; 273:1429.

20. McGill H, McMahan C, Malcolm G, et al. Effects of serum lipoproteins and smoking on atherosclerosis in young men and women. The PDAY Research Group. Pathological determinants of atherosclerosis in youth. *Arterioscler Thromb Vasc Biol* 1997;17:95.

21. McGill H. Nutrition in early life and cardiovascular disease. *Curr Opin Lipidol* 1998;9:23.

22. Nicklas T, Farris R, Smoak C, et al. Dietary factors relate to cardiovascular risk factors in early life. Bogalusa Heart Study. *Arteriosclerosis* 1988;8:193.

23. Koletzko B, Rodriguez-Palmero M. Polyunsaturated fatty acids in human milk and their role in early infant development. *J Mammary Gland Biol Neoplasia* 1999;4:269.

24. Horrocks L, Yeo Y. Health benefits of docosahexaenoic acid. *Pharmacol Res* 1999;40:211.

25. Gordon N. Nutrition and cognitive function. *Brain Dev* 1997;19:165.

26. Golding J, Rogers I, Emmett P. Association between breast feeding, child development and behaviour. *Early Hum Dev* 1997;49[Suppl]:s175.

27. Smith K. Recent developments in infant formulae: 1—the addition of LCPs. *Prof Care Mother Child* 1998;8:151,154.

28. Gerster H. Can adults adequately convert alpha-linolenic acid (18:3n-3) to eicosapentaenoic acid (20:5n-3) and docosahexaenoic acid (22:6n-3)? *Int J Vitamin Nutr Res* 1998;68:159.

29. Morley R. Nutrition and cognitive development. *Nutrition* 1998;14:752–754.

BIBLIOGRAPHY

See "Sources for All Chapters."

American Academy of Pediatrics. *Pediatric nutrition handbook,* 4th ed. Elk Grove Village, IL: American Academy of Pediatrics, 1998.

Dietz WH, Stern L, eds. *Guide to your child's nutrition. American Academy of Pediatrics.* New York: Random House, 1999.

Koletzko B, Aggett PJ, Bindels JG, et al. Growth, development and differentiation: a functional food science approach. *Br J Nutr* 1998;80[Suppl 1]:s5–s45.

Lanting CI, Boersma ER. Lipids in infant nutrition and their impact on later development. *Curr Opin Lipidol* 1996;7:43.

Tamborlane WV, ed. *The Yale guide to children's nutrition.* New Haven, CT: Yale University Press, 1997.

28

Diet and Adolescence

INTRODUCTION

The nutritional requirements of adolescence differ from those of childhood by virtue of the adolescent's larger body size and advent of sexual maturation. They differ as well from those of adulthood, because of the metabolic demands of rapid growth. As a result, the recommended dietary allowances (RDAs), and now dietary reference intakes (DRIs), for adolescence differ from those of other periods of the lifecycle (Table 28.1). Nutrients of particular importance to all adolescents appear to be magnesium, zinc, and calcium. With the advent of menses, adolescent girls become particularly subject to iron deficiency.

Specific aspects of diet, health, and adolescence relate to physical activity patterns and issues of body image. Relatively sedentary adolescents are at risk of obesity because nutrient energy intake exceeds need. Adolescent obesity anticipates adult obesity. Similarly, the combination of inactivity and a diet excessive in processed and fast food high in fat, sugar, salt, and calories predisposes to elevations of cholesterol, insulin, and possibly blood pressure.

Many adolescents participate in competitive sports and, therefore, are at potential risk of inadequate nutrient intake. Inadequate nutrients and energy are particularly problematic in those participating in sports requiring low body weight, such as wrestling, crew, gymnastics, and ballet.

Body image is of particular importance to adolescents and may result in extreme efforts to control or modify diet. The adoption of vegetarianism by an adolescent may mask a weight-loss effort and, if so, may result in a nutritionally unbalanced diet. Eating disorders, considered psychiatric rather than truly nutritional disorders, are typically manifest in adolescence.

OVERVIEW

Factors influencing changes in dietary pattern at adolescence are both physiologic and social. Physiologically, energy and nutrient requirements are driven up by increasing body size and the advent of sexual maturation, including menarche in girls. Socially, adolescence affords opportunity for food selection independent of parental guidance, often for the first time. Such choices often are made on the basis of prevailing patterns in peer groups. Adolescents are particularly resistant to health promotion messages, likely a consequence of the need to exercise autonomy. Typical dietary patterns in adolescents are influenced by targeted advertising and industry promotions and, therefore, emphasize commercial products, such as sodas and fast foods, rather than unprocessed foods.

As a consequence, dietary patterns established in adolescence may initiate susceptibility to obesity, hyperlipidemia, hypertension, and other chronic disease. The common preoccupation with body image during adolescence, particularly among girls, along with the psychosocial pressures of this period are related to the development of eating disorders. Both anorexia and bulimia nervosa are typically first revealed in adolescence; these are discussed further in Chapter 23.

TABLE 28.1. *Recommended dietary allowances (average daily intakes) for adolescents*

Nutrient	Ages 11–14 yr		Ages 15–18 yr		Ages 19–24 yr	
	Female	Male	Female	Male	Female	Male
Energy[a]						
—kcal	2,200	2,500	2,200	3,000	2,200	2,900
—kcal/cm	14.0	15.9	13.5	17.0	13.4	16.4
Protein (g)	46	45	44	59	46	58
Vitamin A[f] (μg RE)	1,000	800	1,000	800	1,000	800
Vitamin D (μg)	10	10	10	10	10	10
Vitamin E (mg TE)	8	10	8	10	8	10
Vitamin K (μg)	45	45	55	65	60	70
Vitamin C[b,f] (mg)	50	50	60	60	60	60
Thiamine (mg)	1.1	1.3	1.1	1.5	1.1	1.5
Riboflavin (mg)	1.3	1.5	1.3	1.8	1.3	1.7
Niacin (mg NE)	15	17	15	20	15	19
Vitamin B$_6$ (mg)	1.4	1.7	1.5	2.0	1.6	2.0
Folate[c] (μg)	150	150	180	200	180	200
Vitamin B$_{12}$ (μg)	2.0	2.0	2.0	2.0	2.0	2.0
Calcium[d,f] (mg)	1,200	1,200	1,200	1,200	1,200	1,200
Phosphorus (mg)	1,200	1,200	1,200	1,200	1,200	1,200
Magnesium (mg)	280	270	300	400	280	350
Iron[e,f] (mg)	15	12	15	12	15	10
Zinc[f] (mg)	12	15	12	15	12	15
Iodine (μg)	150	150	150	150	150	150
Selenium (μg)	45	40	50	50	55	70

[a] Energy intake is expressed as the average daily need assuming average height, and the average need per centimeter of height.

[b] The recommended intake of vitamin C has been increased for adults from 60 to 200 mg per day.

[c] Daily intake of about 400 μg is recommended before conception to prevent neural tube defects. This intake is advisable in adolescent girls planning or at risk of becoming pregnant.

[d] Calcium supplementation may be particularly important in adolescent girls unless the diet is very calcium-dense. An intake of 1,500 mg per day may be better than the RDA of 1,200 mg. During pregnancy and lactation, the calcium requirements of adolescent girls are even higher.

[e] Iron intake of 18 mg per day in both sexes now is generally recommended. Supplementation in adolescent girls may be indicated. Monitoring of the complete blood count after menarche is indicated, but has low sensitivity for early iron deficiency. If an individual adolescent is believed to be at risk of deficiency, serum ferritin should be assayed.

[f] Nutrients for which adolescent intake is most likely to fall short of recommendations.

NE, niacin equivalents equals 1 mg of dietary niacin or 60 mg of dietary tryptophan; RE, retinol equivalent; TE, α-tocopherol equivalent.

Adapted from National Research Council. *Recommended dietary allowances,* 10th ed. Washington, DC: National Academy Press, 1989 and from dietary reference intake updates available from the National Research Council at http://www.nas.edu/nrc/.

Topics of importance in the dietary management of health during adolescence include obesity, hypertension, diabetes, osteoporosis, vegetarian diets, athletic activity, and eating disorders (each addressed in its own chapter), as well as the nutritional demands of rapid growth. Although adolescents' energy requirements are high because of their rapid growth, the recommended dietary pattern is the same as that for adults. Recommendations call for calories predominantly from complex carbohydrates, but adolescents in developed countries tend to have diets particularly high in fat and sugar. The short-term risks of such a dietary pattern are modest, but the persistence of this pattern beyond adolescence is not uncommon and clearly is associated with the prevailing chronic diseases of adulthood.

In the United States, the maximal rate of growth in height for girls occurs between the ages of 10 and 13, whereas for boys it is between the ages of 12 and 15. The adolescent growth spurt contributes approximately

15% to 20% to adult height and 45% to 50% to adult weight. The growth during adolescence reduces the proportion of total body mass contributed by adipose tissue in boys but increases it in girls. Body fat in girls rises during adolescence from 10% to between 20% and 24%. A divergence in adiposity at adolescence contributes to the diverging nutritional requirements of males and females at this stage of life. By the end of adolescence, lean body mass in males on average is double that of females.

In girls, peak calorie intake typically occurs in the year of menarche. In boys, calorie intake continues to rise throughout the growth spurt, generally peaking near 3,400 kcal at about age 16. The divergence in lean body mass results in a marked divergence in macronutrient needs. The average daily caloric requirement per unit height rises during adolescence for boys, while actually falling for girls because of the increasing proportion and lower metabolic demand of body fat.

The adequacy of energy intake in adolescents can be assessed by determination of body mass index and comparison to age-appropriate reference ranges (1). Inadequate energy intake in adolescents, if mild, tends to delay the growth spurt rather than prevent attainment of normal height. While recommended dietary allowances were developed and dietary reference intakes are being developed on the basis of chronologic age, the developmental stage is a more reliable index of actual needs. The Tanner scale of sexual maturity is widely used and can guide nutritional recommendations to adolescents.

Protein intake in adolescents in the United States is more likely to exceed than to fall short of recommendations. However, if protein deficiency is suspected because of dietary restrictions, prealbumin and retinol-binding protein are useful laboratory assays that provide high sensitivity for subclinical protein malnutrition.

Inadequate calcium intake during adolescence contributes to the risk of osteoporosis and fractures in later life (see Chapter 13). With the onset of menarche, girls become susceptible to iron deficiency; serum ferritin is the most reliable measure of iron stores. Zinc deficiency is apparently common in US adolescents, and inclusion in the diet of zinc-rich foods (see Nutrient Reference Data Tables in Section III) or zinc supplementation (in a multivitamin/mineral) is appropriate.

In general, the dietary fiber intake of the US population is well below recommendations. Concern has been expressed that high intake of fiber could interfere with the absorption of nutrients needed to maintain normal growth during childhood and adolescence. Williams and colleagues (2) have recommended that a level of intake equal to age plus 5 to 10 g per day will be beneficial to children, without increasing the risk of micronutrient deficiencies.

Cardiac risk factors established in adolescence or earlier are known to track into adulthood. Assessment of tobacco use and of serum lipids, body mass index, blood pressure, physical activity level, and habitual diet are indicated in adolescence to reverse or prevent developing risk for cardiovascular disease in adulthood (3). Excess energy and fat intake is common in children and adolescents in the United States, contributing to obesity as well as adult risk of cardiac events (4,5). Dietary health promotion in the school setting may be particularly important (6,7).

Simons-Morton and Obarzanek (8) reviewed the literature on diet and blood pressure in children and adolescents. They concluded that the data, although limited in both quantity and quality, support an association with dietary sodium. Translating recommendations into practice may be particularly difficult with adolescent patients (see Chapter 41). Dietary counseling in adolescence is more likely to be influential if it emphasizes appearance rather than long-term health effects to which adolescents generally feel relatively invulnerable.

In general, physical activity is beneficial to health and complementary to the health-promoting effects of prudent diet. Competitive athletics in adolescent girls, however, can inhibit or reverse the appropriate rise in adiposity necessary for estrogen metabolism and normal menses (9). Amenorrhea in particular is associated with reduced peak bone mass, stress fractures, and increased risk of osteoporosis years later. In the treatment of adolescent amenorrhea, reductions in training or increases in energy intake or both and oral contraceptives may be indicated to restore menses and maintain normal bone mineralization (9).

Although the subject is of considerable interest to adolescents and their parents, there is no convincing evidence of a link between diet and acne.

CLINICAL HIGHLIGHTS

In the United States, the average adolescent is at greater risk of nutritional excess and obesity than of macronutrient deficiencies. But even in the context of overnutrition, deficiencies of select micronutrients appear to be quite common. Deficiencies of iron, calcium, zinc, vitamin A, and vitamin C are particularly common, although other nutrients probably are not consumed at truly optimal levels. Although a balanced diet provides the needed micronutrients, social pressures at adolescence tend to favor a particular pattern of dietary imbalance, with excessive intake of processed and fast foods, and consequently sugar, salt, and fat. A multivitamin/mineral supplement is an appropriate recommendation, although clearly not compensatory for an imprudent dietary pattern.

Energy requirements of athletes may not be met. This is particularly problematic for girls, who as a result may fail to develop the necessary body fat mass to maintain menses. The resultant disruption of bone mineralization may be irreversible. Calcium supplementation, control of energy expenditure, and supplemental energy intake are all indicated to maintain menses and protect the bones of female athletes. In more extreme cases, oral contraceptives should be used as well.

Eating disorders often emerge at adoles-

cence, and a high level of suspicion facilitates early detection. Management is specialized, relying in particular on expert and often multidisciplinary psychiatric care.

Risk factors for cardiovascular disease often develop during adolescence and, if so, track into adulthood. Therefore, efforts to identify and modify risk factors for cardiovascular and other chronic disease in adolescents are clearly indicated.

Modification of adolescent dietary patterns to promote health will be most effective if environmental as well as behavioral factors are addressed. The same overall dietary pattern recommended for health promotion in adults (see Chapter 40) is appropriate for adolescents, but translating such recommendations into practice represents a particular challenge with this age group.

REFERENCES

1. American Academy of Pediatrics. *Pediatric nutrition handbook,* 4th ed. Elk Grove Village, IL: American Academy of Pediatrics, 1998.
2. Williams CL, Bollella M, Wynder EL. A new recommendation for dietary fiber in childhood. *Pediatrics* 1995;96:985–988.
3. Gidding SS. Preventive pediatric cardiology. Tobacco, cholesterol, obesity, and physical activity. *Pediatr Clin North Am* 1999;46:253–262.
4. Berenson GS, Srinivasan SR, Nicklas TA. Atherosclerosis: a nutritional disease of childhood. *Am J Cardiol* 1998;82:22T–29T.
5. Bronner YL. Nutritional status outcomes for children: ethnic, cultural, and environmental contexts. *J Am Diet Assoc* 1996;96:891–903.
6. Lytle LA. Lessons from the Child and Adolescent Trial for Cardiovascular Health (CATCH): interventions with children. *Curr Opin Lipidol* 1998;9:29–33.
7. Guidelines for school health programs to promote lifelong healthy eating. Centers for Disease Control and Prevention. *MMWR Morb Mortal Wkly Rep* 1996;45:1–41.
8. Simons-Morton DG, Obarzanek E. Diet and blood pressure in children and adolescents. *Pediatr Nephrol* 1997;11:244–249.
9. Warren MP, Stiehl AL. Exercise and female adolescents: effects on the reproductive and skeletal systems. *J Am Womens Assoc* 1999;54:115.

BIBLIOGRAPHY

See "Sources for All Chapters."
Adams LB. An overview of adolescent eating behavior

barriers to implementing dietary guidelines. *Ann N Y Acad Sci* 1997;817:36–48.

Dietz WH, Stern L, eds. *American Academy of Pediatrics guide to your child's nutrition.* New York: Villard Books (Random House, Inc.), 1999.

Jacobson MS, Rees JM, Golden NH, et al., eds. Adolescent nutritional disorders. Prevention and treatment. In: *Annals of the New York Academy of Sciences, Volume 817.* New York: The New York Academy of Sciences, 1997.

Neumark-Sztainer D, Story M, Perry C, et al. Factors influencing food choices of adolescents: findings from focus-group discussion with adolescents. *J Am Diet Assoc* 1999;99:929–937.

Story M, Neumark-Sztainer D. Promoting healthy eating and physical activity in adolescents. *Adolesc Med* 1999;10:109.

Tamborlane WV, ed. *The Yale guide to children's nutrition.* New Haven, CT: Yale University Press, 1997.

29

Diet and Senescence

INTRODUCTION

Nutritional factors play important roles in the process of aging. Requirements for energy and specific nutrients change as a result of altered metabolism, diminished energy expenditure, and changes in behavioral patterns. The optimal adjustments in micronutrient intake for individuals older than 65, or the so-called "older old," greater than age 80, are uncertain, but progress is being made in this area of study and new recommendations are being generated.

Even more fundamental than the modified energy needs of older age is the role nutrition appears to play in the physiology of aging. Oxidation is emerging as an important aspect of cellular aging; therefore, dietary prooxidants and antioxidants may influence the nature and pace of the aging process itself. Animal studies demonstrated convincing extension of the lifespan with reduced energy intake, provided micronutrient adequacy is maintained.

Nutritional recommendations may be made with some confidence both to older patients trying to maintain health and to younger patients seeking ways to forestall the effects of aging. The importance of optimal nutrition for the elderly population continues to increase with the size of this population and the prolongation of life expectancy.

OVERVIEW

Diet

Life expectancy is steadily increasing and may soon reach 85 to 90 years (1). Current projections suggest that by the year 2030, as much as 20% of the US population will be 65 or older (2).

Assigning particular physiologic characteristics to the process of aging is a complex and controversial process. Cellular degradation and a putative limit to the replicative capacity of DNA appear to be key components. Whatever the natural pace of aging might be, it is clearly influenced, in humans and other species, by environmental stressors. Among such stressors are not only infectious disease and trauma, but also nutrient excess and deficiency.

Daily energy consumption is driven largely by resting metabolic rate (RMR), which accounts for 60% to 75% of the total (3). An additional 10% is accounted for by postprandial thermogenesis, the thermic effect of food. The energy consumed as fuel for physical activity can vary by nearly 30-fold, from a low of approximately 100 kcal per day (3).

Aging is associated with reductions in RMR, postprandial thermogenesis, and physical activity, with declines in activity disproportionately responsible for reduced energy expenditure (3). People older than 65 initially are subject to weight gain and obesity because they tend to maintain the energy intake of their younger years and reduce their expenditure. The older old are increasingly subject to weight loss and the sequelae of malnutrition, as a result of reduced intake. The decline in RMR associated with aging is the result of reduced fat-free body mass, as well as the effects of reduced physical activity. Studies suggest that the association between age and declining RMR begins at around age 40 in men (3).

The capacity to measure the energy requirements of different age groups has been enhanced by application of the doubly labeled water method, an accurate means of measuring total daily energy expenditure. Use of the method has clarified the importance of variability in physical activity in the variability of energy requirements among the elderly, with physical activity influencing RMR (3). Use of the doubly labeled water method suggests that energy requirements of the elderly may, in general, have been underestimated (4). Such methods also suggest that an age-related increase in body fat may be largely attributable to reduced physical activity (4,5). The potential hazards of both undernutrition and overnutrition in the elderly have been noted (6). Energy requirements generally decline with age, predominantly because of a loss of lean body mass and associated change in metabolic rate, as well as reductions in energy expenditure in physical activity (7). There is evidence that basal metabolic rate declines with age to some degree; some reduction in RMR not attributable to declines in physical activity or fat-free mass is apparent (8).

A regimen of regular physical activity can, to varying degrees, preserve lean body mass in the elderly and will naturally result in higher energy requirements, while conferring a host of health benefits as is true in younger age groups. A study of 11 healthy women with a mean age of 73 revealed that, with maintenance of physical activity, energy expenditure was not reduced as a product of age (9). The authors emphasize that the effects of aging on energy requirements and body composition are quite variable and modified substantially by general health and physical activity (9).

Although in general energy requirements decline with age, in part or whole because of diminished physical activity and consequent loss of lean body mass, there is evidence that energy intake goes down disproportionately. Consequently, many elderly, particularly those living alone and homebound, are undernourished (10). Factors influencing reduced energy intake in elderly individuals include changes in olfaction or taste, poor dentition, dysphagia, constipation, and anorexia (see Chapter 36).

Aging is associated with a substantial increase in proportional body fat, along with a loss of lean body mass (11) up to age 65 or so, after which body fat content declines as well. Negative energy balance and particularly negative nitrogen balance are common problems in the elderly. As energy intake falls, protein requirements to avoid negative nitrogen balance rise (11).

Undernutrition in the elderly appears to be secondary not only to underestimates of energy requirements in this age group but also to a relative inability of elderly individuals to maintain a constant energy balance. In a study comparing the adaptive responses of younger and older men to periods of overfeeding and underfeeding, Roberts (11) reported that compensation occurred only in the younger men.

Protein requirements tend to rise in the elderly, especially those with limited mobility. Both inactivity and reduced muscle mass tend to result in negative nitrogen balance, requiring increased protein consumption to compensate (7). Protein requirements remain relatively stable in elderly people whose functional status and activity are preserved. Increased protein is needed particularly when demands rise in the context of injury or illness, both of which are common in the elderly. There is no evidence that protein intake above 0.8 g/kg accelerates a decline in renal function in elderly people who show no evidence of renal insufficiency (7). For elderly people in whom renal insufficiency is established, protein restriction may be indicated (see Chapter 11).

Because many protein-rich foods have a high nutrient content in general, their consumption by elderly should be encouraged (7). Protein intake in the elderly in the United States is generally near the recommended 0.8 to 1 g/kg/day. When energy intake is inadequate, however, negative nitrogen balance occurs even with putatively adequate protein intake. Carbohydrate and fat intake guidelines for the elderly do not differ from those for younger adults.

Whereas protein deficiency appears not to be a problem in most elderly people who live independently, protein malnutrition is common among those living in institutions (12). The maintenance of nitrogen balance is strongly influenced by total energy intake.

Even when a person's weight stays consistent, energy requirements decline with advancing age, whereas protein requirements remain fairly constant or increase (12). Therefore, the maintenance of adequate protein nutriture requires that the percent of calories from protein rises over time. For example, 56 g per day of protein would be required to provide 0.8 g/kg/day to a 70-kg individual. At an energy intake of 2,500 kcal, protein would constitute 9% of calories. At a reduced energy intake of 1,800 kcal, protein would constitute over 12% of calories (12).

Whereas the maintenance of adequate nutritional intake in the elderly is a priority, calorie restriction over time is associated with longevity in most species studied (13). A variety of mechanisms have been proposed. In virtually all species studied to date, caloric restriction appears to lower body temperature, reduce basal metabolic rate, and reduce signs of oxidative injury to cells, organelles, and DNA (14).

The effects of restricted energy intake result not only in optimizing survival (i.e., raising mean survival to nearer the predicted maximum) but in extending the natural lifespan as well. Data derived from studies of primates are not yet available, but are being generated in on-going studies (14). A recent report suggests that obesity poses less risk of premature mortality to older subjects than to younger (15). However, only those individuals who have already avoided early mortality live to experience obesity late in life, and obesity at earlier ages clearly is associated with increased risk of premature mortality (see Chapter 5).

There is, to date, no confirmatory evidence in humans that energy restriction extends survival, nor evidence that caloric restriction initiated in old age is beneficial. If beneficial in humans, energy restriction must be accompanied by nutrient supplementation to prevent deficiencies.

Arguments for restricting dietary fat intake and for modifying the contributions of various fats to the diet have been made throughout this text (see Chapters 5, 6, and 40). As the maintenance of adequate energy and micronutrient intake in the elderly often is of paramount importance, efforts to restrict fat intake in elderly patients whose fat intake was not previously restricted are likely to be justified only when in response to some specific health risk or need. In elderly subjects already adhering to a fat-restricted diet, there is likely to be little reason to increase fat intake, provided weight maintenance is satisfactory (7). In either case, supplementation of fat-soluble vitamins is likely to be prudent.

The reduction in physical activity associated with age and resultant decline in energy consumption lead to reduced intake of micronutrients unless the nutrient density of the diet is intentionally altered. The decline in micronutrient intake places the elderly at risk of subtle deficiencies, with potentially important implications for health (12).

In the population over 65 years old, 80% have one or more chronic medical conditions requiring use of prescription drugs. Both the disease state and the pharmacotherapy may influence metabolism (12). The wide variation in the state of health and the rate of aging, producing extreme heterogeneity among the elderly with regard to energy and nutrient requirements, limiting the utility of broad, age-specific recommendations (12).

In the same individual, skeletal muscle is approximately 40% less at age 70 than during early adulthood (12), resulting in declines in RMR of 1% to 2% per decade beginning at age 25. Reductions in caloric expenditure made for the sake of avoiding obesity require commensurate reductions in energy consumption, but at the risk of reducing consumption of essential micronutrients.

Between age 25 and 75, a person would have to reduce energy consumption by 25% to maintain energy balance and avoid excessive body fat. But the maintenance of a comparably nutrient-dense diet over time would then result in the 25% reduction in the intake of micronutrients.

For some nutrients, intake generally is sufficiently abundant so that such a reduction would preserve adequacy. For others, such a reduction might lower intake below the desired threshold. Intake levels of copper, zinc, chromium, calcium, and vitamin D during adulthood typically do not allow for a 25% reduction, thus placing the elderly at risk of deficiency (see later).

The recommended daily intake levels of vitamins and minerals are under revision by the Food and Nutrition Board of the National Research Council, and efforts continue to generate specific guidelines for the elderly. The latest recommendations can be found on the Web at http://www.nas.edu/nrc/.

There is evidence that deficiencies of vitamins C, B_6, and B_{12} are fairly prevalent among elderly in the United States. On this basis, supplementation, at least with the doses provided by a multivitamin, seems prudent (7).

In general, deficiency of fat-soluble vitamins is infrequent because of large tissue stores. One exception in the elderly appears to be vitamin D, the levels of which decline with age because of decreased consumption, decreased sun exposure, and decreased efficiency of the body's ability to convert provitamin D to the active form (7).

To date, there is little evidence that mineral requirements change with age, other than in response to metabolic disturbances associated with disease or treatment (e.g., diuretic use). Iron requirements tend to decline somewhat with age; the potential benefits of calcium consumption in excess of 800 mg per day remains a subject of controversy (7). The recommended dietary allowance

(RDA) for vitamin A may be too high for the elderly, as absorption appears to increase with age (12).

In a 1997 review of the nutritional needs of the elderly, Blumberg (16) recommended eggs as a dietary source of the macronutrients and micronutrients often deficient in older adults. Nutrient density is of particular importance in the diets of the elderly, given reduced energy intake and largely preserved or increased micronutrient and protein requirements (16,17).

In 1998, Saltzman and Russell (18) reviewed age-dependent change in gastrointestinal physiology. The principal changes cited include achlorhydria secondary to atrophic gastritis, almost invariably due to *Helicobacter pylori* infection, and lactose intolerance. The former can impair absorption of iron, folate, calcium, vitamin K, and vitamin B_{12}, whereas the latter may contribute to poor calcium nutriture (18). With these exceptions, gastrointestinal function is well preserved with aging and generally is not the limiting factor in the maintenance of optimal nutritional status.

Serum glucose levels tend to rise with age, and suggestions have been made for age-specific thresholds for defining fasting hyperglycemia (7). Age-related glucose intolerance may be compensated by relative restriction of simple sugar intake.

Complex carbohydrates should be prioritized as a source of fiber, both soluble and insoluble, and of micronutrients. Dietary fiber intake in the United States is approximately 12 g per day among adults, whereas the recommended amount is 25 to 30 g per day. Reductions of energy consumption by elderly patients are likely to result in low fiber intake as well. The elderly are particularly susceptible to constipation and are apt to benefit from increased consumption of dietary fiber.

The more rapid intestinal transit time that comes with increased fiber consumption, however, may reduce mineral absorption, increasing the risk of deficiencies in the elderly. Therefore, increased nutrient density or supplementation is indicated when fiber intake is augmented (12). Fruits, vegetables, and cereal grains may offer protection against constipation, diverticulosis, and nutrient deficiencies. Dentition should be assessed in making such recommendations; ability to eat fruit and vegetables may be impaired in elderly with poor dentition (7).

Aging is associated with a decline in immune function, as well as greater susceptibility to an array of micronutrient deficiencies. In a study of institutionalized elderly with evidence of micronutrient deficiencies, multivitamin supplementation (B complex, vitamins C and E, and β-carotene) for a period of 10 weeks significantly enhanced immune function as gauged by cutaneous hypersensitivity reactions to injected antigens (19).

Mazari and Lesourd (20) studied the effects of age and nutritional status on cell-mediated immunity. Although T-cell function was reduced in elderly people compared with young adults, the differences were much greater among the elderly with one or more indications of nutritional impairment. The authors conclude that some of what has traditionally been considered an age-dependent decline in immune function is, in fact, nutrition dependent.

Elderly patients are particularly subject to dehydration and its sequelae, because of reduced body water, diminished renal concentrating ability, diminished thirst, insensitivity to antidiuretic hormone, and susceptibility to orthostatic hypotension due to reduced autonomic tone. Thirst is not a very reliable index of hydration status among elderly.

Recommendations to maintain optimal fluid status are for fluid intake of 30 mL per kilogram of actual weight, 1 mL per kilocalorie consumed, or 1,500 mL per day, whichever is higher, is generally appropriate under conditions of typical daily activity (7,12).

Kerstetter et al. (12) offer a practical approach that does not require patients to measure their fluid intake so precisely. Maximal concentration of urine at age 90 is estimated at 800 mosmol/L, down from 1,200 mosmol/L at younger age. Therefore, in the elderly, fluid intake should be maintained at a level that allows for the excretion of approximately 1,200 mosmol of solute waste per day. This amount would require at least 1.5 L of urine produced per day for the very elderly. At this concentration, the urine appears light yellow. Therefore, a level of fluid intake that results in urine that is consistently light yellow implies adequate hydration status (12).

In an article on the potential benefits of complementary medicine to an aging population, Bland (21) characterizes the functional declines of aging in discrete categories, such as impaired mitochondrial function related to oxidative stresses, glycation of functional proteins, chronic inflammation, and impaired methylation.

Many of the physiologic changes of aging are nutrient responsive. Mitochondrial function may be influenced by a range of nutrients, including ubiquinone, n-acetylcysteine, lipoic acid, creatine, vitamin E, and n-acetyl-carnitine (21). Glycation may be reduced by improved glucose tolerance, potentially influenced by intake of chromium, magnesium, and other nutrients (21) (see Chapter 10). Inflammation may be reduced by augmenting intake of n-3 fatty acids and by other interventions. Methylation is supported by adequate intake of B vitamins and can be tracked by the level of plasma homocysteine (21). Although the evidence for various nutritional interventions in efforts to curtail adverse effects of aging varies, many "complementary" or "alternative" practices are consistent with the weight of available evidence in the scientific literature.

Nutrients and Nutriceuticals

Vitamin D

Actual or suspected lactose intolerance, as well as prevailing social patterns, tend to limit milk consumption by the elderly. Fortified dairy products and seafood—intake of which in the elderly tends to be low—are the principal dietary sources of vitamin D.

The skin's ability to manufacture vitamin D with exposure to sunlight becomes less efficient with age, and the elderly tend to reduce their amount of sun exposure. Therefore, vitamin D deficiency appears to be fairly widespread among the older population. Deficiency of vitamin D leads to impaired calcium absorption, compounding the generally inadequate calcium intake in this age group. Supplementation with 400 IU of vitamin D alone or as part of a multivitamin is a prudent precaution against deficiency and accelerated osteopenia.

Vitamin C

The RDA for vitamin C is undergoing upward revision from 60 to 200 mg per day. There is no specific evidence that deficiency occurs more commonly among the elderly, or that supplementation is beneficial. However, for the same reasons that intake up to 500 mg per day (see Chapter 40 and Nutrient Reference Data Table, Section III) may be beneficial to other age groups, intake in this range may offer benefits to the elderly as well.

Vitamin B₆

The RDA for vitamin B_6 is 2 mg per day in men and 1.6 mg per day in women. Recent evidence suggests this level is too low. Intake of vitamin B_6 among the elderly often fails to meet the RDA. Low intake of vitamin B_6 may contribute to elevations of serum homocysteine and accelerated atherosclerosis. A vitamin B_6 supplement of 2 mg per day is indicated for the elderly; most multivitamins provide this dose.

Vitamin B₁₂

Atrophic gastritis is more prevalent in the elderly and, therefore, so is B_{12} deficiency. In individuals with atrophic gastritis, B_{12} must be supplemented parenterally because intrinsic factor is lacking. Less severe B_{12} deficiency due to poor diet also may occur and may contribute to cognitive impairment, anemia, or elevated homocysteine levels in older people. B_{12} supplementation in a multivitamin is reasonable and appropriate for elderly individuals.

Folate

Folate deficiency does not appear to be a particular problem associated with aging. However, low folate intake will occur when the diet is poor and may contribute to elevations in homocysteine. Folate supplementation in the form of a multivitamin is appropriate.

Calcium

Calcium intake throughout life tends to be lower than recommended, especially for women (see Chapter 13). The elderly are particularly susceptible to osteoporosis and related fracture. Adequate calcium intake may forestall osteoporotic fracture, but it cannot restore bone density already lost. Calcium intake also is associated with reduced risk of colon cancer (see Chapter 12) and reduction in blood pressure (see Chapter 7). Reduced-fat dairy products are preferable as dietary sources of calcium, but supplementation with up to 1,000 mg per day may offer benefits. Calcium absorption declines with age, particularly after age 60 or so (12). This decline in function is compounded by vitamin D deficiency. Marginal intake of both vitamin D and calcium contributes to age-related bone loss and the risk of fracture.

Copper

The density of copper in the average American diet is approximately 0.6 mg per 1,000 kcal (12). To meet the RDA of 1.5 to 3.0 mg per day, 2,500 kcal are required. As the elderly often need and consume fewer calories than this amount, copper deficiency is probable. Copper is needed for hematopoiesis, and deficiency can result in both anemia and neutropenia.

Chromium

The typical American diet provides approximately 15 μg per 1,000 kcal of chromium, whereas an intake of 50 to 200 μg per day is recommended. At the prevailing level of chromium density, more than 2,500 kcal per day would be required to meet recommended intake, placing the elderly at particular risk for deficiency. Deficiency of chromium impairs glucose and insulin metabolism, produces elevations of serum triglycerides, and is associated with peripheral neuropathy (12).

Zinc

Zinc intake is below the recommended level for adults in the United States, and the gap is greater for the elderly. Zinc appears to affect immunity. As immune dysfunction is characteristic of aging and may result in life-threatening infections, efforts to maintain optimal immune function are important.

Consumption of less than 10 mg per day by elderly individuals may impair immunity, wound healing, and the acuity of taste and smell (12). The average diet provides approximately 5 mg of zinc per 1,000 kcal; therefore, 3,000 kcal would be required to provide the recommended 12 to 15 mg per day.

Zinc is abundant in poultry, fish, and meat, and diets rich in these sources may provide a greater density of zinc. However, increased meat consumption generally is precluded by efforts to limit fat intake and promote fruit and vegetable consumption. Zinc supplementation of 15 mg per day is a reasonable precaution; this level is provided by most multivitamin and mineral supplements.

Iron

Iron requirements decline with age for women, because of the cessation of monthly blood loss following menopause. Even though iron absorption declines with age, iron stores tend to increase (12).

Magnesium

Magnesium intake in developed countries often is marginal in all age groups. Intake in the range of 4 mg/kg/day is common, whereas 6 mg/kg/day is considered more appropriate (22). Deficiency is particularly likely among the elderly, due to reduced intake, depletion associated with chronic disease states such as type II diabetes mellitus, and impaired gastrointestinal absorption. Clinical consequences may include sleep disturbance, cognitive impairment, and myalgias (22). Although the results of trials demonstrating sustained benefit of magnesium supplementation are lacking to date, the use of diet or supplements to achieve an intake level greater than 5 mg/kg/day appears justified (22).

CLINICAL HIGHLIGHTS

Aging is associated with a loss of lean body mass and an increase in body fat, up until the sixth decade. Thereafter, both lean mass and fat mass diminish. Energy requirements tend to decline with age, in part because of reduced physical activity and in part because of the loss of metabolically active tissue. Nutrient and energy intake, however, tend to decline disproportionately to energy needs, so that many elderly are undernourished.

Energy deficiency in the elderly results in negative nitrogen balance with accelerated muscle loss. Deficiencies of micronutrients, particularly of B vitamins, vitamin D, and certain minerals, such as zinc, are very common. Use of prescription medications may compound age-related changes in olfaction, taste, and gastrointestinal motility, contributing to poor dietary intake.

Emphasis in primary care should be on the maintenance of weight and especially preservation of lean body mass. Elderly people should be encouraged to become or remain physically active as their functional status permits. Periodic assessment of dietary intake, informally or via referral to a dietitian, may be helpful in ensuring maintenance of adequate nutriture. A multivitamin/mineral supplement is a low-cost and safe means of protecting elderly patients against several common micronutrient deficiencies, although specific evidence of benefit from such a practice is lacking.

An effort to increase the nutrient density of the diet is a valid, although more difficult, alternative, and the two practices are complementary rather than mutually exclusive. Common sequelae of aging, such as cognitive and immunologic deficits, may be due in part to nutrient deficiencies and, therefore, are potentially preventable or reversible. There is convincing evidence to support supplementing the diets of elderly patients with zinc, chromium, magnesium, calcium, and possibly copper, along with vitamins. There is some suggestive evidence that nutrients not traditionally included on the RDA lists, such as ubiquinone (coenzyme Q_{10}) and lipoic acid, may offer benefits for elderly patients.

As patients age, the short-term functional benefits of adequate nutriture may need to be compared with any long-term consequences of specific dietary practices. For example, whereas the cholesterol content of eggs may be an important consideration in younger adults at long-term risk for coronary disease, the nutrient density of eggs may provide benefits in excess of any risks for elderly patients. A diet rich in a variety of fruits and vegetables offers the same array of benefits to the elderly as to younger age groups.

REFERENCES

1. Olshansky SJ, Carnes BA, Cassel CK. In search of Methuselah: estimating the upper limits to human longevity. *Science* 1990;250:634.
2. Roush W. Live long and prosper? *Science* 1996;273:42.
3. Poehlman ET. Energy expenditure and requirements in aging humans. *J Nutr* 1992;122:2057.
4. Roberts SB, Dallal GE. Effects of age on energy balance. *Am J Clin Nutr* 1998;68[Suppl]:975s.
5. Roberts SB, Young VR, Fuss P, et al. What are the energy needs of elderly adults? *Int J Obes* 1992;16:969.
6. Hosoya N. Nutrient requirements of the elderly: an overview. *Nutr Rev* 1992;50:447.
7. Chernoff R. Effects of age on nutrient requirements. *Clin Geriatr Med* 1995;11:641.
8. Pannemans DLE, Westerterp KR. Energy expenditure, physical activity and basal metabolic rate of elderly subjects. *Br J Nutr* 1995;73:571.
9. Reilly JJ, Lord A, Bunker VW, et al. Energy balance in healthy elderly women. *Br J Nutr* 1993;69:21.
10. Ausman LM, Russell RM. Nutrition in the elderly. In: Shils.
11. Roberts SB. Effects of aging on energy requirements and the control of food intake in men. *J Gerontol* 1995;50A:101.
12. Kerstetter JE, Holthausen BA, Fitz PA. Nutrition and nutritional requirements for the older adult. *Dysphagia* 1993;8:51.
13. Masoro EJ. Caloric restriction. *Aging Clin Exp Res* 1998;10:173.
14. Weindruch R, Sohal RS. Caloric intake and aging. *N Engl J Med* 1997;337:986.
15. Bender R, Jockel KH, Trautner C, et al. Effect of age on excess mortality in obesity. *JAMA* 1999;281:1498.
16. Blumberg J. Nutritional needs of seniors. *J Am Coll Nutr* 1997;16:517.
17. Rigler S. A clinical approach to proper nutrition in the elderly. *Kans Med* 1998;98:20.
18. Saltzman JR, Russell RM. The aging gut. Nutritional issues. *Gastroenterol Clin North Am* 1998;27:309.
19. Buzina-Suboticanec K, Buzina R, Stavljenic A, et al. Aging, nutritional status and immune response. *Int J Vitam Nutr Res* 1998;68:133.
20. Mazari L, Lesourd BM. Nutritional influences on immune response in healthy aged persons. *Mech Ageing Dev* 1998;104:25.
21. Bland JS. The use of complementary medicine for healthy aging. *Altern Ther Health Med* 1998;4:42.
22. Durlach J, Bac P, Durlach V, et al. Magnesium status and aging: an update. *Magnes Res* 1997;11:25.

BIBLIOGRAPHY

See "Sources for All Chapters."

Morley JE, Glick Z, Rubenstein LZ, eds. *Geriatric nutrition. A comprehensive review*, 2nd ed. New York: Raven Press, 1995.

Rolls BJ. Do chemosensory changes influence food intake in the elderly? *Physiol Behav* 1999;66:193.

Yeh SS, Schuster MW. Geriatric cachexia: the role of cytokines. *Am J Clin Nutr* 1999;70:183.

Hetherington MM. Taste and appetite regulation in the elderly. *Proc Nutr Soc* 1998;57:625.

30

Diet and Athletic Performance

INTRODUCTION

The role of diet in optimizing athletic performance has long been a topic of considerable interest, a natural extrapolation of efforts to optimize dietary health. Diet provides the fuel that is burned to sustain physical activity, and it seems reasonable that alterations in the fuel will influence the efficiency of that combustion. Although the recommended daily allowance of protein is not adjusted on the basis of physical activity, sports enthusiasts and competitive athletes generally perceive a need for increased protein intake. Recent evidence supports this position, but is preliminary.

A variety of micronutrients play defined roles in energy metabolism and have received attention as potential enhancers of athletic performance, among them are carnitine, creatine, boron, coenzyme Q_{10}, and other nutriceutical agents such as dehydroepiandrosterone (DHEA). Evidence of enhanced athletic performance in response to supplementation exists for some of these substances, but is generally both inconsistent and of marginal quality to date. That the overall adequacy of diet can influence physical performance in an athlete, as well as in general, is beyond dispute.

OVERVIEW

Diet

In general, the US population engages in too little physical activity and consumes too many calories. Therefore, although sufficient calorie intake is a fundamental requirement to maintain physical activity, it is not a concern for the majority of patients. Individuals engaging in extremely intense physical activity for extended periods, particularly competitive endurance athletes, may actually need to make an effort to meet energy requirements. For the most part, little evidence exists that the dietary pattern for physically active individuals should be altered from that generally recommended for health promotion. However, fat is the most calorically dense macronutrient, and fat restriction may be untenable in athletes with high energy expenditure. The average calorie requirements of a sedentary, 70-kg male adult are estimated at approximately 2,400 kcal. Studies in human athletes have demonstrated 24-hour expenditures of more than 10,000 calories, and a maximal sustainable expenditure of up to 12,000 kcal is estimated on the basis of animal research (1). The energy demands of various representative physical activities are shown in Table 30.1.

In the United States, carbohydrate is the predominant energy source and is readily oxidized to support physical activity. Studies generally suggest that monosaccharides and polysaccharides are comparable energy sources, although glucose is metabolized somewhat more efficiently than are other sugars. Preliminary studies suggest that carbohydrate sources with a low glycemic index, such as lentils, may support endurance better than foods with a high glycemic index, such as potatoes (see Chapter 10). The low

TABLE 30.1. *Energy expenditure of some representative physical activities*[a]

Activity	METs[b] (multiples of RMR)	kcal/min
Resting (sitting or lying down)	1.0	1.2–1.7
Sweeping	1.5	1.8–2.6
Driving (car)	2.0	2.4–3.4
Walking slowly (2 mph)	2.0–3.5	2.8–4
Cycling slowly (6 mph)	2.0–3.5	2.8–4
Horseback riding (walk)	2.5	3–4.2
Volleyball	3.0	3.5
Mopping	3.5	4.2–6.0
Golf	4.0–5.0	4.2–5.8
Swimming slowly	4.0–5.0	4.2–5.8
Walking moderately fast (3 mph)	4.0–5.0	4.2–5.8
Baseball	4.5	5.4–7.6
Cycling moderately fast (12 mph)	4.5–9.0	6–8.3
Dancing	4.5–9.0	6–8.3
Skiing	4.5–9.0	6–8.3
Skating	4.5–9.0	6–8.3
Walking fast (4.5 mph)	4.5–9.0	6–8.3
Swimming moderately fast	4.5–9.0	6–8.3
Tennis (singles)	6.0	7.7
Chopping wood	6.5	7.8–11
Shoveling	7.0	8.4–12
Digging	7.5	9–12.8
Cross-country skiing	7.5–12	8.5–12.5
Jogging	7.5–12	8.5–12.5
Football	9.0	9.1
Basketball	9.0	9.8
Running	15	12.7–16.7
Running at 4-min mile pace	30	36–51
Swimming (crawl) fast	30	36–51

[a] All values are estimates and based on a prototypical 70-kg male. Energy expenditure generally is lower in women and higher in larger individuals. MET and kilocalorie values derived from different sources may not correspond exactly.

[b] A MET is the rate of energy expenditure at rest, attributable to the resting (or basal) metabolic rate (RMR). Whereas resting energy expenditure varies with body size and habitus, a MET generally is accepted to equal approximately 3.5 mL/kg/min of oxygen consumption. The energy expenditure at 1 MET generally varies over the range from 1.2 to 1.7 kcal/min. The intensity of exercise can be measured relative to the RMR in METs.

Derived from Ensminger AH, Ensminger M, Konlande J, et al. *The concise encyclopedia of foods and nutrition.* Boca Raton, FL: CRC Press, 1995. Wilmore JH, Costill DL. *Physiology of sport and exercise. Human kinetics.* Champaign, IL: 1994; American College of Sports Medicine. *Resource manual for guidelines for exercise testing and prescription,* 2nd ed. Philadelphia: Williams & Wilkins, 1993; Burke L, Deakin V, eds. *Clinical sports nutrition.* Sydney, Australia: McGraw-Hill Book Company, 1994; McArdle WD, Katch FI, Katch VL. *Sports exercise nutrition.* Baltimore: Lippincott Williams & Wilkins, 1999.

glycemic index may favor reconstitution of muscle glycogen following exercise.

Carbohydrate loading apparently is of no benefit for exercise of short or moderate duration. When high-intensity exercise lasts for more than 90 minutes, muscle glycogen depletion tends to occur. A modest benefit

of carbohydrate loading under such circumstances is probable (2), although not certain (3). Sustained elevations in muscle glycogen following several days of carbohydrate loading have been reported (4).

There is some suggestion that a short period of high fat intake may enhance fat oxidation, spare carbohydrate, and delay fatigue (5), but the evidence is inconclusive. Concern has been raised about fat loading, both on the basis of limited evidence and because the practice is at odds with dietary practices for health promotion (6). There is some evidence that the effects of carbohydrate loading differ by gender, with less evidence of benefit in women (7). Thus, controversy persists regarding optimal alterations of diet for the enhancement of sustained, high-intensity exercise. The preponderance of evidence generally supports the prevailing practice of carbohydrate loading for endurance sports such as marathon running.

Endurance training enhances fatty acid utilization in muscle; if fat intake is sustained at a high level, the efficiency of fat oxidation improves with time (1). There is some evidence that high fat intake may delay time to exhaustion with moderate-intensity exercise. Fat loading tends to spare muscle glycogen stores during exercise (8).

High fat intake is the most efficient means for meeting very high energy requirements associated with extreme exertion, such as endurance training or mountain-climbing expeditions. The health hazards to the general public of high dietary fat intake should be borne in mind, and recommendations for individual athletes to increase dietary fat intake should be made judiciously. Studies characterizing the ideal profile of fatty acids in a high-fat diet designed for athletic performance are lacking to date.

Evidence in other areas suggests the virtue of prioritizing intake of monounsaturated fatty acids and a mixture of n-3 and n-6 polyunsaturates in a ratio of 1:1 to 1:4. Saturated and trans fatty acid intake should be kept proportionately low (see Chapters 2, 6, and 40). The evidence for a role of high-fat diets in influencing athletic performance other than by meeting high energy requirements is equivocal (8).

Dietary protein is of particular interest to bodybuilders and other athletes involved in strength training and is the most commonly used ergogenic aid (9). An intake of 3 g protein for every 4 g of carbohydrate is touted to promote health and enhance athletic performance in the book *Enter the Zone* by Barry Sears (10). Despite its popularity, the Zone diet is not supported by evidence accessible in the peer-reviewed literature. An evaluation by Cheuvront (11) suggests the Zone diet is more likely to compromise than enhance athletic performance.

The role of increasing dietary protein in augmenting contribute to muscle mass and strength remains controversial. Some studies have demonstrated benefit with protein intake three or more times the recommended dietary allowance of 0.75 g/kg/day. Consensus is emerging that moderate increases in protein intake may be indicated for athletes. Intake in the range from 1.2 to 1.4 g/kg/day is recommended for endurance athletes, and from 1.7 to 1.8 g/kg/day for athletes engaged in strength training (12). This level of intake may be optimal in terms of the athletic effort, but the long-term effects of such a diet on specific health outcomes and chronic disease risk have not been adequately studied. Therefore, an athlete should prepare to modify dietary intake to meet prevailing recommendations whenever he or she tapers the level of physical activity. The use of amino acid beverages and supplementation with specific classes of amino acids are popular practices that currently lack convincing scientific support (9).

Although notable as a modern phenomenon, the proclivity to seek performance enhancement by altering diet is ancient. In antiquity, such practices were rooted in what is easily seen today as superstition, such as the belief that eating the heart of an enemy would impart courage (9).

Although modern practices are more likely to derive from science than superstition, interest in performance-enhancing dietary regimens consistently runs ahead of available evidence. So-called ergogenic aids often are promoted on the basis of animal or *in vitro* data, before human interventions can be conducted (8). Although the quality of evidence to support certain ergogenic supplements has improved, the financial imperative and loose regulation driving the promotion of such products warrant cautious skepticism (13).

Nutrients and Nutriceuticals

Creatine

Creatine phosphate in muscle donates phosphate to adenosine diphosphate to reconstitute adenosine triphosphate. The intent of creatine supplementation is to increase energy storage in muscle as a means to enhance performance. There is some evidence of benefit in high-intensity, short-term exercise, but currently little evidence of benefit in endurance activities (8). A double-blind, randomized trial in college football players demonstrated significant benefits of creatine supplementation in muscle mass and sprint performance. Over the 28 days of supplementation with creatine 15.75 g per day, no adverse effects were reported (14). The preponderance of evidence suggests some benefit in high-intensity, repetitive activities and in muscle building (15). Creatine appears to be safe in doses commonly used (see Nutrient Reference Data Table, Section III).

Carnitine

Carnitine participates in the transport of long-chain fatty acids into mitochondria and is thought to spare muscle glycogen by facilitating fat oxidation (8). Carnitine supplementation also may increase levels of coenzyme A, enhancing the efficiency of the Krebs cycle. The evidence to date suggesting that carnitine may enhance athletic performance is inconclusive (8) (see Nutrient Reference Data Table, Section III).

Bicarbonate

Bicarbonate loading is used as an ergogenic aid in the belief that it will buffer lactic acid accumulated in muscle and prevent or delay muscle fatigue and dysfunction. The evidence suggests that bicarbonate does enhance performance, provided the activity is brief (i.e., several minutes) and intense, but not too brief (e.g., 30 seconds), and that the dose of bicarbonate is adequate (300 mg/kg sodium bicarbonate) (8,16,17). In particular, bicarbonate loading may enhance recovery time between repeated bouts of short, high-intensity activity, such as sprinting, by neutralizing muscle lactate (8). There is some suggestion that the benefit attributed to bicarbonate may instead be due to the effects of a sodium load on intravascular volume (8).

Dehydroepiandrosterone (DHEA)

Dehydroepiandrosterone is a steroid hormone with potential for both estrogenic and androgenic effects (18). There is interest in the role of DHEA in enhancing athletic performance, but to date no reliable data on which to base a conclusion are available. There is a general consensus that data from human intervention trials with DHEA are inadequate to support its use as a supplement for an ergogenic effect or other putative benefits (19,20).

Caffeine

Caffeine, taken alone, is considered a drug rather than a nutrient and is banned by the International Olympic Committee. Caffeine functions as a stimulant, possibly increasing adrenergic tone. It may enhance fat oxidation and sparing of muscle glycogen. Evidence suggesting that endurance is increased by caffeine supplementation is convincing (8). Most studies to date have enrolled only men, so effects on athletic performance in women are speculative.

Chromium Picolinate

Chromium functions as a cofactor in the metabolism of glucose and protein, principally by enhancing insulin action. Chromium picolinate is reputed to enhance energy metabolism in muscle and thereby improve strength and stamina. There is some evidence to suggest that exercise may increase urinary losses of chromium, and strenuous activity is associated with the excretion of minerals in sweat. No convincing evidence exists to date, however, of enhanced athletic performance attributable to chromium supplementation. There is evidence from randomized and crossover trials of the failure of chromium supplementation to enhance the effects of resistance training on muscle size and strength (21–23). Thus, the popular notion that chromium picolinate is an ergogenic aid must be considered unsubstantiated.

Coenzyme Q_{10}

Coenzyme Q_{10} functions in mitochondrial electron transfer and therefore is fundamental to energy metabolism in all cells. There is new interest in the potential role of coenzyme Q_{10} supplementation in the enhancement of athletic performance. Although the evidence is relatively strong for a therapeutic role of coenzyme Q_{10} in certain pathologic states (see Chapter 6 and Section III), evidence is lacking of an ergogenic effect. There is some uncertainty whether supplementation significantly influences levels of the nutrient in muscle (24).

CLINICAL HIGHLIGHTS

Although interest in the potential for dietary manipulations to enhance athletic performance is widespread and long-standing, evidence of such effects is sparse. A dietary pattern associated with health promotion (see Chapter 40) is, for the most part, associated with optimal functional status as well.

Small deviations from a health-promoting diet, however, may be conducive to enhancements in strength or endurance. Although the recommended protein intake for healthy adults is approximately 0.8 g/kg/day, a level twice that much may support muscle development with resistance training and clearly is safe over the short term. A protein intake above 2 g/kg/day may support strength as opposed to endurance training, and there is limited evidence that an intake as high as 2.5 g/kg/day may facilitate bodybuilding. The long-term health effects of protein intake at this level are uncertain; a return to more moderate intake once the period of intense training is over is indicated.

Although the protein consumed should be of high biologic value (see Chapter 3), there is no evidence to support the use of protein formulas or modified, commercial protein products. Studies of putatively ergogenic nutrients have largely been negative, although there is some evidence of improved endurance with creatine supplementation. The evidence that bicarbonate loading enhances tolerance of short bouts of high-intensity exercise is fairly convincing. Caffeine enhances endurance; of note, the International Olympic Committee considers it a drug rather than a nutrient. High carbohydrate ingestion for several days before an endurance event seems likely to delay fatigue by sustaining muscle glycogen stores, with the evidence of benefit more convincing in men than in women.

REFERENCES

1. Buskirk E. Exercise. In: Ziegler E, Filer FJ, eds. *Present knowledge in nutrition,* 7th ed. Washington, DC: ILSI Press, 1996.
2. Hawley J, Schabort E, Noakes T, et al. Carbohydrate-loading and exercise performance. An update. *Sports Med* 1997;24:73–81.
3. Zant RV, Lemon P. Preexercise sugar feeding does not alter prolonged exercise muscle glycogen or protein catabolism. *Can J Appl Physiol* 1997;22:268.
4. Goforth HJ, Arnall D, Bennett B, et al. Persistence of supercompensated muscle glycogen in trained subjects after carbohydrate loading. *J Appl Physiol* 1997;82:342–347.
5. Lambert E, Hawley J, Goedecke J, et al. Nutritional strategies for promoting fat utilization and delaying the onset of fatigue during prolonged exercise. *J Sports Sci* 1997;15:315–324.
6. Sherman W, Leenders N. Fat loading: the next magic bullet? *Int J Sport Nutr* 1995;5[Suppl]:s1–s12.
7. Tarnopolsky M, Atkinson S, Phillips S, et al. Carbohydrate loading and metabolism during exercise in men and women. *J Appl Physiol* 1995;78:1360–1368.
8. Clarkson P. Nutrition for improved sports performance. Current issues on ergogenic aids. *Sports Med* 1996;21:393–401.
9. Applegate E, Grivetti L. Search for the competitive

edge: a history of dietary fads and supplements. *J Nutr* 1997;127:869s–873s.

10. Sears B, Lawren B. *Enter the zone*. New York: Regan Books, 1995.

11. Cheuvront S. The zone diet and athletic performance. *Sports Med* 1999;27:213–228.

12. Lemon W. Is increased dietary protein necessary or beneficial for individuals with a physically active lifestyle? *Nutr Rev* 1996;54:s169–s175.

13. Beltz S, Doering P. Efficacy of nutritional supplements used by athletes. *Clin Pharm* 1993;12: 900–908.

14. Kreider R, Ferreira M, Wilson M, et al. Effects of creatine supplementation on body composition, strength, and sprint performance. *Med Sci Sports Exerc* 1998;30:73–82.

15. Volek J, Kraemer W. Creatine supplementation: its effect on human muscular performance and body composition. *J Strength Condition Res* 1996;10: 200–210.

16. McNaughton L, Backx K, Palmer G, et al. Effects of chronic bicarbonate ingestion on the performance of high-intensity work. *Eur J Appl Physiol* 1999;80:333–336.

17. McNaughton L, Dalton B, Palmer G. Sodium bicarbonate can be used as an ergogenic aid in high-intensity, competitive cycle ergometry of 1 h duration. *Eur J Appl Physiol* 1999;80:64–69.

18. Ebeling P, Koivisto V. Physiological importance of dehydroepiandrosterone. *Lancet* 1994;343:1479–1481.

19. Katz S, Morales A. Dehydroepiandrosterone (DHEA) and DHEA-sulfate (DS) as therapeutic options in menopause. *Semin Reprod Endocrinol* 1998;16:161–170.

20. Khorram O. DHEA: a hormone with multiple effects. *Curr Opin Obstet Gynecol* 1996;8:351–354.

21. Campbell W, Joseph L, Davey S, et al. Effects of resistance training and chromium picolinate on body composition and skeletal muscle in older men. *J Appl Physiol* 1999;86:29–39.

22. Hallmark M, Reynolds T, DeSouza C, et al. Effects of chromium and resistive training on muscle strength and body composition. *Med Sci Sports Exerc* 1996;28:139–144.

23. Walker L, Bemben M, Bemben D, et al. Chromium picolinate effects on body composition and muscular performance in wrestlers. *Med Sci Sports Exerc* 1998;30:1730–1737.

24. Svensson M, Malm C, Tonkonogi M, et al. Effect of Q_{10} supplementation on tissue Q_{10} levels and adenine nucleotide catabolism during high-intensity exercise. *Int J Sport Nutr* 1999;9:166–180.

BIBLIOGRAPHY

See "Sources for All Chapters."

Burke L, Deakin V, eds. *Clinical sports nutrition.* Sydney, Australia: McGraw-Hill Book Company, 1994.

McArdle WD, Katch FI, Katch VL. *Sports exercise nutrition.* Baltimore: Lippincott Williams & Wilkins, 1999.

31

Endocrine Effects of Diet: Phytoestrogens

INTRODUCTION

Natural constituents of foods with hormonal effects are widespread. Phytoestrogens are a diverse group of naturally occurring food chemicals with varying degrees of estrogen agonism and antagonism. There is particular interest in use of phytoestrogens, in food or as concentrated supplements, to modify both the symptoms and sequelae associated with menopause. Isoflavones in soy have been studied most extensively to date.

OVERVIEW

The principal classes of phytoestrogens include isoflavones, lignans, and coumestans. Both soybeans and flaxseeds are particularly rich sources of phytoestrogens. Phytoestrogens are widespread in plants; their distribution has been reviewed (1). The presence of phytoestrogens in whole-grain products may be responsible for some of the health benefits associated with their regular consumption (2).

The various effects of phytoestrogens, a mix of estrogen agonism and antagonism, mimic those of synthetic selective estrogen receptor modulators (SERMs), raising the possibility that natural products could be used as substitutes for synthetic SERMs (3,4). Isoflavones in soy and other foods are known to exert selective estrogen effects,

generating both clinical and popular interest in such foods as a natural means to replace ovarian hormones or modify disease risk. Data from supplementation trials are beginning to accumulate. In a randomized cross-over study of 14 premenopausal women, Duncan and colleagues (5) found that even high-level isoflavone supplementation induced no significant changes in menstrual cycle length, endometrial histology, or plasma estrogen levels. Albertazzi and colleagues (6) studied the effects of supplementing diet with 60 g of soy powder daily for 3 months. They measured urine and blood phytoestrogen levels and the frequency of hot flushes in a randomized, placebo-controlled trial of 104 postmenopausal women (6). Soy supplementation significantly raised levels of genistein and other phytoestrogens, but these levels did not correlate with the frequency of hot flushes or vaginal maturation indexes.

Many herbs are used to treat aspects of women's health related to hormonal function; the mechanism by which such herbs exert their effects often is through agonism or antagonism of estrogen receptors (7). Chinese herbal preparations traditionally used for management of menopause-related symptoms have been found to contain phytoestrogens. In some instances, the potency is commensurate with that of conventional hormone replacement therapy (HRT) (8).

Trials of phytoestrogens for the amelioration of menopausal symptoms have yielded mixed results to date (9). The evidence available suggests that up to two thirds of women will experience some relief from hot flushes by using phytoestrogenic supplements, although relatively few can be expected to gain relief from vaginal dryness (10).

The mixed agonist/antagonist properties of many estrogenic herbs have led to uncertainty about their potential influence on the risk of breast cancer. Using breast cancer cell lines, Dixon-Shanies and Shaikh (11) found the phytoestrogens genistein, daidzein, biochanin A, and coumesterol from hops; black cohosh; and vitex inhibited cell growth. The results suggest that such compounds might contribute to the prevention of breast cancer in humans. The effects of phytoestrogen-containing herbal preparations on breast cancer risk are inadequately studied to date (7).

In a randomized crossover trial of 12 healthy premenopausal women, Xu et al. (12) found that soy protein supplementation decreased urinary excretion of endogenous estrogens, while increasing excretion of soy phytoestrogens. A significant increase in the ratio of 2-hydroxyestrone to 16α-hydroxyestrone was observed, suggesting a mechanism by which phytoestrogens might reduce cancer risk (12).

Phytoestrogens, including genistein, have been shown to inhibit tumor cell proliferation and angiogenesis, possibly contributing an important mechanism by which fruits and vegetables in the diet mitigate cancer risk (13). A role for genistein has been proposed in the prevention of prostate cancer (14,15) and breast cancer (15), although evidence of this effect is based on animal research and epidemiologic associations and therefore is quite preliminary. Clinical trials of genistein and other phytoestrogens in prostate cancer prevention have been proposed (16).

There is preliminary evidence of cardiovascular benefits of soy phytoestrogens, apparently with comparable effects in men and women (17). Specific mechanisms include lowering of low-density lipoprotein, raising of high-density lipoprotein and apoprotein A-1, inhibition of low-density lipoprotein oxidation, and salutary effects on vascular reactivity (17,18). In a randomized crossover trial of 51 perimenopausal women, Washburn and colleagues (19) demonstrated reductions in total cholesterol, blood pressure, and vasomotor symptoms in response to daily intake of 34 mg of soy phytoestrogens. Effects on cardiovascular risk indexes suggest a probable reduction of cardiac risk, but this hypothesis is as yet unproved.

Phytoestrogens have been identified in hops, and consequently beer (20) and wine (21). Some of the putative health benefits of moderate alcohol consumption may be attributable to phytoestrogen effects.

Data are limited on the role of naturally occurring isoflavones, principally from soy, on the rate of postmenopausal bone resorption. Available data suggest a probable benefit of including soy in the diet (22). A synthetic isoflavone analogue, ipriflavone, has been shown to preserve bone density (22). There currently is insufficient evidence to characterize the effect of phytoestrogen supplements on the preservation of bone density (10,23,24).

Phytoestrogens have been shown to influence sexual differentiation in animal models (9). Even though some soy-based infant formulas are very rich in phytoestrogens, no adverse effects in humans have been reported (9). Human breast milk contains negligible concentrations of isoflavones (25). There is speculation that early exposure to soy phytoestrogens may reduce the risk of certain chronic diseases later in life (25).

In vitro studies of cultured adrenal cortical cells suggest that phytoestrogen consumption reduces cortisol production, while increasing the production of androgens (26). Similar effects are seen with a lactovegetarian diet (27).

One of the limiting factors in efforts to gauge the potential benefits of phytoestrogens has been their exclusion from standard measures of diet composition (28), but measurement instruments that will permit tracking of phytoestrogen intake have now been developed. A rapid proliferation of pertinent literature is likely in the near future.

CLINICAL HIGHLIGHTS

Phytoestrogens act as selective estrogen receptor agonists and antagonists, in much the same way as SERMs. The possibility that foods containing phytoestrogens, or concentrated supplements, could be used to ameliorate symptoms and sequelae of menopause is supported by available evidence, much of which is preliminary. A diet rich in a variety of plant foods, particularly soybeans, flaxseeds, and whole grains, is advisable on other grounds and will provide a rich supply of the best-studied phytoestrogens. Such a diet, via the effects of both phytoestrogens and other beneficial constituents, appears likely to reduce the risk of breast cancer, prostate cancer, cardiovascular disease, and possibly other cancers and osteoporosis. There currently is insufficient evidence to recommend phytoestrogens as an alternative to HRT with estrogen, estrogen/progesterone in combination, or a SERM. However, on-going and future studies may provide such evidence. For those patients committed to use of phytoestrogens as an alternative to HRT, dosing is a matter of conjecture. Clinical benefits have been seen with daily doses of soy protein of 60 g and with 30 to 40 mg of soy isoflavones.

REFERENCES

1. Mazur W. Phytoestrogen content in foods. *Baillieres Clin Endocrinol Metab* 1998;12:729–742.
2. Slavin J, Martini M, Jacobs DJ, et al. Plausible mechanisms for the protectiveness of whole grains. *Am J Clin Nutr* 1999;70:459s–463s.
3. Brzezinski A, Debi A. Phytoestrogens: the "natural" selective estrogen receptor modulators? *Eur J Obstet Gynecol Reprod Biol* 1999;85:47–51.
4. Fitzpatrick L. Selective estrogen receptor modula-

tors and phytoestrogens: new therapies for the post-menopausal women. *Mayo Clin Proc* 1999;74: 601–607.
5. Duncan A, Merz B, Xu X, et al. Soy isoflavones exert modest hormonal effects in premenopausal women. *J Clin Endocrinol Metab* 1999;84:192–197.
6. Albertazzi P, Pansini F, Bottazzi M, et al. Dietary soy supplementation and phytoestrogen levels. *Obstet Gynecol* 1999;94:229–231.
7. Wade C, Kronenberg F, Kelly A, et al. Hormone-modulating herbs: implications for women's health. *J Am Med Womens Assoc* 1999;54:181–183.
8. Shiizaki K, Goto K, Ishige A, et al. Bioassay of phytoestrogen in herbal medicine used for post-menopausal disorder using transformed MCF-7 cells. *Phytother Res* 1999;13:498–503.
9. Whitten P, Naftolin F. Reproductive actions of phytoestrogens. *Baillieres Clin Endocrinol Metab* 1998;12:667–690.
10. Eden J. Phytoestrogens and the menopause. *Baillieres Clin Endocrinol Metab* 1998;12:581–587.
11. Dixon-Shanies D, Shaikh N. Growth inhibition of human breast cancer cells by herbs and phytoestrogens. *Oncol Rep* 1999;6:1383–1387.
12. Xu X, Duncan A, Merz B, et al. Effects of soy isoflavones on estrogen and phytoestrogen metabolism in premenopausal women. *Cancer Epidemiol Biomarkers Prev* 1998;7:1101–1108.
13. Fotsis T, Pepper M, Montesano R, et al. Phytoestrogens and inhibition of angiogenesis. *Baillieres Clin Endocrinol Metab* 1998;12:649–666.
14. Griffiths K, Denis L, Turkes A, et al. Phytoestrogens and diseases of the prostate gland. *Baillieres Clin Endocrinol Metab* 1998;12:625–647.
15. Stephens F. The rising incidence of breast cancer in women and prostate cancer in men. Dietary influences: a possible preventive role for nature's sex hormone modifiers—the phytoestrogens. *Oncol Rep* 1999;6:865–870.
16. Moyad M. Soy, disease prevention, and prostate cancer. *Semin Urol Oncol* 1999;17:97–102.
17. Clarkson T, Anthony M. Phytoestrogens and coronary heart disease. *Baillieres Clin Endocrinol Metab* 1998;12:589–604.
18. Cassidy A, Griffin B. Phyto-estrogens: a potential role in the prevention of CHD? *Proc Nutr Soc* 1999; 58:193–199.
19. Washburn S, Burke G, Morgan T, et al. Effect of soy protein supplementation on serum lipoproteins, blood pressure, and menopausal symptoms in perimenopausal women. *Menopause* 1999;6:7–13.
20. Milligan S, Kalita J, Heyerick A, et al. Identification of a potent phytoestrogen in hops (Humulus lupulus L.) and beer. *J Clin Endocrinol Metab* 1999;84:2249–2252.
21. Calabrese G. Nonalcoholic compounds of wine: the phytoestrogen resveratrol and moderate red wine consumption during menopause. *Drugs Exp Clin Res* 1999;25:111–114.
22. Scheiber M, Rebar R. Isoflavones and postmenopausal bone health: a viable alternative to estrogen therapy? *Menopause* 1999;6:233–241.
23. Anderson J, Garner S. Phytoestrogens and bone. *Baillieres Clin Endocrinol Metab* 1998;12:543–557.

24. Garner D, Olmstead M, Bohr Y, et al. The eating attitudes test: psychometric features and clinical correlates. *Psychol Med* 1982;12:871–878.
25. Setchell K, Zimmer-Nechemias L, Cai J, et al. Isoflavone content of infant formulas and the metabolic fate of these phytoestrogens in early life. *Am J Clin Nutr* 1998;68:1453s–1461s.
26. Meisano S, Katz S, Lee J, et al. Phytoestrogens alter adrenocortical function: genistein and diadzein suppress glucocorticoid and stimulate androgen production by cultured adrenal cortical cells. *J Clin Endocrinol Metab* 1999;84:2443–2448.
27. Remer T, Pietrzik K, Manz F. Short-term impact of a lactovegetarian diet on adrenocortical activity and adrenal androgens. *J Clin Endocrinol Metab* 1998;83:2132–2137.
28. Pillow P, Duphorne C, Chang S, et al. Development of a database for assessing dietary phytoestrogen intake. *Nutr Cancer* 1999;33:3–19.

BIBLIOGRAPHY

See "Sources for All Chapters."

Keller C, Fullerton J, Mobley C. Supplemental and complementary alternatives to hormone replacement therapy. *J Am Acad Nurse Pract* 1999;11:187.

Setchell KD, Cassidy A. Dietary isoflavones: biological effects and relevance to human health. *J Nutr* 1999;129:758s.

Humfrey CD. Phytoestrogens and human health effects: weighting up the current evidence. *Nat Toxins* 1998;6:51.

Setchell KD. Phytoestrogens: the biochemistry, physiology, and implications for human health of soy isoflavones. *Am J Clin Nutr* 1998;68[6 Suppl]:1333s.

Davis SR, Dalais FS, Simpson ER, et al. Phytoestrogens in health and disease. *Recent Prog Horm Res* 1999;54:185.

32

Diet, Sleep–Wake Cycles, and Mood

INTRODUCTION

A potential role for both macronutrients and micronutrients in the regulation of the sleep–wake cycle and mood is of clinical and popular interest. The interaction between diet and mood has the potential to ameliorate or compound affective disorders, eating disorders, and weight gain/obesity. Dietary patterns may influence the quality of nighttime sleep, the propensity for daytime somnolence, vigilance, and concentration.

The role of dietary protein and carbohydrate in the metabolism of serotonin is of particular importance. Pharmacologic manipulation of brain serotonin levels using selective serotonin reuptake inhibitors (SSRIs) has the potential to influence food cravings and dietary patterns as well as affect. Although the literature on nutrition, sleep, and mood is extensive, most studies involve small numbers of subjects. The importance of diet to sleep and mood is increasingly clear, whereas evidence to support specific therapeutic interventions remains largely preliminary to date.

OVERVIEW

In a variety of ways, dietary pattern and nutrients can influence somnolence, alertness, and the adequacy of sleep. The specific neural mechanisms controlling patterns of sleep and wakefulness are under active investigation (1–3). Alterations in levels of neurotransmitters, particularly serotonin, are clearly involved and influenced by diet.

The amino acid tryptophan is converted into serotonin, which plays an important role in regulating sleep and mood. Tryptophan is thought to be the soporific substance in the time-honored glass of warm milk. It is also relatively abundant in meat and fish. Tryptophan supplements were available until they were banned by the Food and Drug Administration following an outbreak of the eosinophilia-myalgia syndrome induced by contaminated batches of L-tryptophan from Japan. Experimentally induced tryptophan depletion has been shown to disrupt the pattern of the sleep electroencephalogram (4).

The ingestion of carbohydrate triggers an insulin release that facilitates the deposition of circulating amino acids into skeletal muscle. However, the effect is selective, causing the levels of branched-chain amino acids in circulation to fall by as much as 40%, while negligibly affecting levels of tryptophan. The level of tryptophan in the brain is determined in part by its competition with other amino acids; the lower the level of other neutral amino acids presented to the blood–brain barrier, the greater the brain uptake of tryptophan. The greater the uptake of tryptophan, the more serotonin is produced. Elevations in serotonin enhance mood and promote sleepiness.

Deficiencies of B complex vitamins are associated with neuropsychiatric disturbances, including delirium and psychosis. Nominal deficiencies may be involved in mood disturbance; evidence of B vitamin deficiencies in the US population has been increasing.

Nutrient-poor diets high in refined carbohydrate and processed sugar are particularly likely to induce such B vitamin deficiency states. The avoidance of such patterns, and compensation with a daily multivitamin, may confer benefit to mood in susceptible individuals.

Seasonal affective disorder (SAD) tends to result in a craving for carbohydrate. The condition is associated with elevated levels of tyrosine and impaired serotonin metabolism. Melatonin was initially implicated, but more recent data refute this concept (5,6). Light (particularly sunlight) exposure is helpful, as is intake of complex carbohydrates to elevate levels of serotonin. In a randomized, double-blind, placebo-controlled crossover trial of 44 healthy adults, Lansdowne et al. (7) reported a significant improvement in the symptoms of SAD when subjects were supplemented with vitamin D_3.

The tendency of patients to use carbohydrate and fat to influence serotonin production is associated with weight gain and obesity (8). Therefore, use of SSRIs may be helpful in the management of obesity in select patients, particularly those with symptoms of depression and carbohydrate craving (8). Melatonin therapy for SAD, insomnia, or jet lag is supported by principally anecdotal evidence (9). A recent randomized trial of melatonin for jet lag showed no benefit (10).

In a study of nine women with a history of food cravings, Gendall and colleagues (11) found that subjects who ate high-protein meals experienced a greater tendency to binge on carbohydrate than after consuming a high-carbohydrate or mixed meal. The authors suggest that sensory-specific satiety or a serotonergic mechanism might be involved.

The night-eating syndrome consists of insomnia, hyperphagia at night, and anorexia in the morning. The condition has been shown to be associated with a blunted nocturnal rise in melatonin and leptin levels and elevated levels of plasma cortisol (12). Features of somnambulism and disordered eating may be concurrent (13), and treatment for both may be indicated.

Chocolate is associated with a stronger pleasure response than most other foods. Chocolate craving in some women, particularly associated with menstrual cycle variations (see Chapter 26), is strong enough to have been labeled "addiction." Although chocolate ingestion in self-labeled "chocolate addicts" is pleasurable, the guilt associated with ingestion obviates any genuine mood enhancement (14). Recent evidence supports use of the term "chocolate addiction," revealing close parallels with other well-characterized addictive states (15).

The effects of macronutrient distribution on both mood and somnolence remain under investigation. In a study of intragastric infusions in nine healthy adult subjects, Wells and colleagues (16) demonstrated the induction of sleepiness by infusion of lipid as compared with either sucrose or saline. In a crossover trial of 16 adults, somnolence was induced by both a high-fat and a high-carbohydrate test meal (17). In a study of ten adults, Orr and colleagues (18) found that sleep latency was reduced by a solid meal, regardless of composition, compared with an isocaloric liquid meal or water. However, some evidence suggests that high-fat meals induce more somnolence, possibly related to the release of cholecystokinin (19).

There may be considerable interindividual variability in susceptibility to postprandial somnolence (20). When a midday meal was compared to a fast in 21 healthy men, time to onset of sleep was comparable, but sleep duration was longer in the fed state (21). A high-carbohydrate meal has been shown to counter the stimulatory effects of a bout of exercise (22). Although obstructive sleep apnea occurs in normal-weight individuals, it is more common in the obese. The sleep fragmentation and other sequelae of the syndrome may be ascribed in large measure to excess energy intake (23).

In a comparison of 24 stress-prone to 24 control subjects, Markus and colleagues (24) demonstrated that a high-carbohydrate meal, leading to increased brain serotonin levels, mitigated the effects of induced stress in the predisposed subjects. In a randomized crossover trial comparing carbohydrate-craving obese subjects to matched controls, however, Toornvliet et al. (25) found no evidence of mood enhancement with high-carbohydrate meals.

Currently, popular diet books emphasize the restriction of dietary carbohydrate, and especially sugar, in efforts to improve weight control and overall health. However, Surwit and colleagues (26) demonstrated that with comparable caloric restriction, high- and low-sucrose diets for 6 weeks resulted in comparable degrees of weight loss in obese women, with no discernible differences in emotional affect between groups.

Depression, hunger, and negative mood decreased in both groups, and vigilance and positive mood increased, suggesting that these benefits may result from weight loss per se.

In a study of night-shift workers, Paz and Berry (27) found only modest differences in mood and performance when meal composition was varied. Mood and performance were optimized by meals containing a macronutrient distribution (55% carbohydrate, 18% protein, and 27% fat) closely matching prevailing nutritional guidelines, as compared with meals higher in either protein or carbohydrate (27). There is suggestive evidence that high-fat meals may induce a particular decline in postprandial alertness and concentration (28) as compared with isocaloric meals higher in carbohydrate.

Several studies suggest a potential role for dietary fat and serum lipids in mood regulation. Kaplan and colleagues (29) reported evidence that cholesterol reduction in monkeys leads to serotonin depletion in the brain, precipitating aggressive behavior. The authors suggest this as a possible explanation for the association between cholesterol lowering in humans and the increased risk of traumatic death (29). Wells and colleagues (30) found that converting subjects from a 41% fat-energy to a 25% fat-energy diet for

a period of 1 month was associated with adverse changes in mood, including more anger/hostility. These effects were independent of any change in plasma cholesterol (30).

Pain perception has been shown to be attenuated in the fed as compared with the fasting state, with dietary fat apparently particularly effective at mitigating pain (31). The fasted, or energy-restricted state, however, has not produced consistently deleterious effects. A study in soldiers has shown that 30 days of relative calorie deficiency had no adverse effects on mood or performance as compared with a control condition (32). Similarly, in a study of healthy female volunteers, Green and colleagues (33) showed that a fast for up to 24 hours has minimal effects on concentration and cognitive function (33).

Alcohol and caffeine ingestion can interfere with sleep, particularly in the elderly (34). Low alcohol consumption may enhance sleep, but higher intake disrupts sleep patterns. Alcohol in breast milk alters the sleep–wake pattern and generally reduces the total duration of sleep in infants (35).

Valerian is an herb traditionally used to make tea for treating insomnia. Apparently effective as a mild tranquilizer, the sleep-inducing chemical in valerian is as yet unidentified. The tea has a bitter and rather unpleasant taste. Valerian root extract is available; 150 to 300 mg approximately 30 minutes before bedtime is recommended. (Some alternative medicine sources recommend 500 mg of magnesium taken 30 minutes before bedtime.) Some traditional somnolents may exert only a placebo effect. In a double-blind, placebo-controlled study of lemongrass, a common ingredient in sleep-promoting herbal tea, no sedative-hypnotic effects were demonstrated (36).

The herb St. John's wort, or hypericum, is advocated for use in depression. The mechanism is believed to be serotonergic, but it is not yet known with certainty. Although there is some evidence to support its use in dysthymic states, hypericum has not been compared with conventional pharmaceuticals in the treatment of depression. Deltito and Beyer (37) have made recommendations for evidence-based use of hypericum.

CLINICAL HIGHLIGHTS

Diet and nutrients influence mood, somnolence, and wakefulness in a variety of ways, many of which are poorly understood at present. The role of food intake on levels of serotonin in the brain has emerged as a mechanism of particular importance. What is known of this pathway suggests that a diet rich in complex carbohydrates, consistent with prevailing recommendations, is appropriate to maintain appropriate serotonin levels. Perturbations in serotonin metabolism may account for both affective and eating disorders, and in such situations pharmacotherapy with SSRIs may be indicated.

Contrary to the view advanced by many popular diet books, high levels of dietary protein have not been shown to enhance energy levels or sense of well-being. Meals high in fat are associated with particularly pronounced postprandial somnolence. Animal research suggests that extreme dietary fat restriction, however, resulting in reduced plasma lipoprotein levels, may favor aggressiveness. Such findings would support the macronutrient distribution advocated throughout the text, with approximately 55% to 60% of calories from predominantly complex carbohydrate, 20% to 25% from fat, and 15% to 20% from protein (see Chapter 39).

Sleep adequate in quantity and quality is supported by the avoidance of excess caffeine or alcohol in the diet. Sleep apnea often is consequent to obesity; therefore, avoidance of excess energy consumption and overweight is important in efforts to ensure normal sleep patterns. A large midday meal induces postprandial somnolence independent of meal composition, whereas smaller snacks throughout the day actually tend to promote alertness. Thus, the food intake pattern conducive to daytime alertness is that supported by other lines of evidence (see

Chapters 5, 10, and 41 indicating the value of distributing calories in small meals).

Finally, mood may be influenced by intense cravings for food, sharing characteristics of addiction; chocolate appears to be the most important example. Chocolate craving varies with the phase of the menstrual cycle, as discussed in Chapter 26. In general, control of such cravings is facilitated by consistent, moderate consumption of the craved food in a fed rather than fasted state.

REFERENCES

1. Kayama Y, Koyama Y. Brainstem neural mechanisms of sleep and wakefulness. *Eur Urol* 1998; 33s3:12–15.
2. Xi M, Morales F, Chase M. Evidence that wakefulness and REM sleep are controlled by a GABAergic pontine mechanism. *J Neurophysiol* 1999; 82:2015–2019.
3. Gottesmann C. The neurophysiology of sleep and waking: intracerebral connections, functioning and ascending influences of the medulla oblongata. *Prog Neurobiol* 1999;59:1–54.
4. Voderholzer U, Hornyak M, Thiel B, et al. Impact of experimentally induced serotonin deficiency by tryptophan depletion on sleep EEG in healthy subjects. *Neuropsychopharmacology* 1998;18:112–124.
5. Partonen T, Lonnqvist J. Seasonal affective disorder. *Lancet* 1998;352:1369–1374.
6. Partonen T, Vakkuri O, Lonnqvist J. Suppression of melatonin secretion by bright light in seasonal affective disorder. *Biol Psychatr* 1997;42:509–513.
7. Lansdowne A, Provost S. Vitamin D₃ enhances mood in healthy subjects during winter. *Psychopharmacology* 1998;135:319–323.
8. Wurtman R, Wurtman J. Brain serotonin, carbohydrate-craving, obesity and depression. *Obes Res* 1995;[Suppl 4]:477s–480s.
9. Avery D, Lenz M, Landis C. Guidelines for prescribing melatonin. *Ann Med* 1998;30:122–130.
10. Spitzer R, Terman M, Williams J, et al. Jet lag: clinical features, validation of a new syndrome-specific scale, and lack of response to melatonin in a randomized, double-blind trial. *Am J Psychaitr* 1999;156:1392–1396.
11. Gendall K, Joyce P, Abbott R. The effects of meal composition on subsequent cravings and binge eating. *Addict Behav* 1999;24:305–315.
12. Birketvedt G, Florholmen J, Sundsfjord J, et al. Behavioral and neuroendocrine characteristics of the night-eating syndrome. *JAMA* 1999;282: 657–663.
13. Winkelman J. Clinical and polysomnographic features of sleep-related eating disorder. *J Clin Psychiatry* 1998;59:14–19.
14. Macdiarmid J, Hetherington M. Mood modulation by food: an exploration of affect and cravings in

"chocolate addicts." *Br J Clin Psychol* 1995;34: 129–138.

15. Tuomisto T, Heterington M, Morris M, et al. Psychological and physiological characteristics of sweet food "addiction." *Int J Eat Disord* 1999;25:169–175.

16. Wells A, Read N, Macdonald I. Effects of carbohydrate and lipid on resting energy expenditure, heart rate, sleepiness, and mood. *Physiol Behav* 1998; 63:621–628.

17. Wells A, Read N, Idzikowski C, et al. Effects of meals on objective and subjective measures of daytime sleepiness. *J Appl Physiol* 1998;84:507–515.

18. Orr W, Shadid G, Harnish M, et al. Meal composition and its effect on postprandial sleepiness. *Physiol Behav* 1997;62:709–712.

19. Wells A, Read N, Uvnas-Moberg K, et al. Influences of fat and carbohydrate on postprandial sleepiness, mood, and hormones. *Physiol Behav* 1997; 61:679–686.

20. Monk T, Buysse D, Reynolds CR, et al. Circadian determinants of the postlunch dip in performance. *Chronobiol Int* 1996;14:123–133.

21. Zammit G, Kolevzon A, Fauci M, et al. Postprandial sleep in healthy men. *Sleep* 1995;18:229–231.

22. Verger P, Lagarde D, Betejat D, et al. Influence of the composition of a meal taken after physical exercise on mood, vigilance, performance. *Physiol Behav* 1998;64:317–322.

23. Day R, Gerhardstein R, Lumley A, et al. The behavioral morbidity of obstructive sleep apnea. *Prog Cardiovasc Dis* 1999;41:341–354.

24. Markus CR, Panhuysen G, Tuiten A, et al. Does carbohydrate-rich, protein-poor food prevent a deterioration of mood and cognitive performance of stress-prone subjects when subjected to a stressful task? *Appetite* 1998;31:49.

25. Toornvliet A, Pijl H, Tuinenberg J, et al. Psychological and metabolic responses of carbohydrate craving obese patients to carbohydrate, fat, and protein-rich meals. *Int J Obes Relat Metab Disord* 1997; 21:860–864.

26. Surwit R, Feinglos M, McCaskill C, et al. Metabolic and behavioral effects of a high-sucrose diet during weight loss. *Am J Clin Nutr* 1997;65:908–915.

27. Paz A, Berry E. Effect of meal composition on alertness and performance of hospital night-shift workers. Do mood and performance have different determinants? *Ann Nutr Metab* 1997;41:291–298.

28. Wells A, Read N, Craig A. Influences of dietary and intraduodenal lipid on alertness, mood, and sustained concentration. *Br J Nutr* 1995;74:115–123.

29. Kaplan J, Muldoon M, Manuck S, et al. Assessing the observed relationship between low cholesterol and violence-related mortality. Implications for suicide risk. *Ann N Y Acad Sci* 1997;836:57–80.

30. Wells A, Read N, Laugharne J, et al. Alterations in mood after changing to a low-fat diet. *Br J Nutr* 1998;79:23–30.

31. Zmarzty S, Wells A, Read N. The influence of food on pain perception in healthy human volunteers. *Physiol Behav* 1997;62:185–191.

32. Shukitt-Hale B, Askew E, Lieberman H. Effects of 30 days of undernutrition on reaction time, moods, and symptoms. *Physiol Behav* 1997;62:783–789.

33. Green M, Elliman N, Rogers P. Lack of effect of short-term fasting on cognitive function. *J Psychiatr Res* 1995;29:245–253.

34. Neubauer D. Sleep problems in the elderly. *Am Fam Physician* 1999;59:2551–2558, 2559–2560.

35. Mennella J, Gerrish C. Effects of exposure to alcohol in mother's milk on infant sleep. *Pediatrics* 1998;101:E2.

36. Leite J, Seabra MdL, Maluf E, et al. Pharmacology of lemongrass (Cymbopogon citratus Stapf). III. Assessment of eventual toxic, hypnotic and anciolytic effects on humans. *J Ethnopharmacol* 1986;17: 75–83.

37. Deltito J, Beyer D. The scientific, quasi-scientific and popular literature on the use of St. John's wort in the treatment of depression. *J Affect Disord* 1998;51:345–351.

BIBLIOGRAPHY

See "Sources for All Chapters."

Garcia-Garcia F, Drucker-Colin R. Endogenous and exogenous factors on sleep-wake cycle regulation. *Prog Neurobiol* 1999;58:297–314.

Keenan SA. Normal human sleep. *Respir Care Clin North Am* 1999;5:319–331.

Kurzer MS. Women, food, and mood. *Nutr Rev* 1997;55:268–276.

Breakey J. The role of diet and behavior in childhood. *J Paediatr Child Health* 1997;33:190–194.

Kanarek R. Psychological effects of snacks and altered meal frequency. *Br J Nutr* 1997;77[Suppl 1]:s105–s118, s118–s120.

Kirkwood CK. Management of insomnia. *J Am Pharm Assoc* 1999;39:688–696.

Christensen L. The effect of carbohydrates on affect. *Nutrition* 1997;13:503–514.

Toornvliet AC, Pijl H, Tuinenburg JC, et al. Psychological and metabolic responses of carbohydrate craving obese patients to carbohydrate, fat and protein-rich meals. *Int J Obes Metab Disord* 1997;21:860–864.

Bellisle F, Blundell JE, Dye L, et al. Functional food science and behavior and psychological functions. *Br J Nutr* 1998;80[Suppl 1]:s173–s193.

33

Diet and Cognitive Function

INTRODUCTION

The importance of nutritional status in the development of the brain and normal cognitive function is indisputable; developmental issues are discussed in Chapters 25 and 27. Although there is considerable interest in the role of diet in the age-related decline in mental capacity, the evidence linking specific dietary patterns and practices to the prevention or promotion of such decline is at best suggestive. More definitive evidence of such associations is likely to accrue quite slowly.

The study of diet and cognition is hampered by difficulty in the establishment of temporal relationships (i.e., change in mental status may influence diet rather than the other way around) and the difficulty in obtaining accurate dietary intake data from individuals with cognitive deficits. Despite these limitations, available data support general recommendations for maintenance of lean body mass (i.e., the prevention of ongoing weight loss), intake of adequate but not excessive calories, and abundant intake of antioxidant vitamins, B vitamins, and minerals.

There is evidence supporting increased consumption of fruits and vegetables, as well as n-3 fatty acids from fish. Intake of total fat, saturated fat, and cholesterol should be moderate. Although the strength of these associations in the literature on cognitive function is modest, such recommendations may be made on the basis of evidence in other areas of health promotion and maintenance.

OVERVIEW

Diet

Antiaging properties of antioxidant nutrients have stimulated interest in the role these nutrients might play in the enhancement and preservation of cognitive ability. Further, oxidative injury is recognized in neurodegenerative conditions. Animal studies suggest that dietary supplementation with fruit or vegetable extracts rich in antioxidants, or with isolated vitamin E, may retard age-related declines in cognitive function and basic neurophysiology (1). Evidence of benefit of dietary antioxidants in preservation of neurocognitive function in humans is inconsistent and limited to date (2).

Observational studies, both prospective and retrospective, have relied on serum measures, supplements, and dietary intake to gauge antioxidant exposure (2). Suggestions of benefit from such studies have emerged for vitamins E and C. One randomized trial demonstrated a delay in institutionalization due to dementia with the administration of either selegiline or high-dose vitamin E (3). A small cohort study in Australia suggested that high intake of vitamin C might preserve cognitive function (4).

Difficulties in assessing the relationship between antioxidants and cognitive impairment include the possibility that cognitive impairment alters dietary intake, as well as the inherent difficulty in obtaining accurate dietary intake data from cognitively impaired individuals. A cross-sectional study of more than 5,000 elderly found a specific positive association between β-carotene intake and cognitive function, with an odds ratio of nearly 2 (5). The β-carotene intake was estimated using a food-frequency questionnaire and, therefore, represented whole foods rather than the nutrient in isolation. The study could not determine the temporal sequence responsible for the association.

In one of the few prospective studies of cognitive function, no significant evidence was found linking either moderate alcohol consumption or cigarette smoking to cognitive decline in either men or women (6). A potential beneficial effect of moderate alcohol intake on cognitive function among individuals with cardiovascular disease risk factors, such as diabetes mellitus, has been reported (7); the same study suggested harmful effects of smoking on cognition in those with diabetes or cardiovascular disease. The mechanism for such effects is conjectured to be inhibition or promotion of atherosclerosis in the cerebrovasculature (see Chapter 9). Data from other sources suggest a link between risk factors for vascular disease and cognitive impairment (8).

The association between overall dietary pattern and cognitive function was assessed in five cohorts of men from the Seven Countries study. Dietary pattern was summarized by applying the healthy diet index (HDI), established by the World Health Organization. Although there was a suggestion of association between "healthier" diets and better cognition among the more than 1,000 subjects, statistical significance was not achieved (9).

Data on dietary intake and cognitive function from nearly 400 elderly men in the Zutphen Elderly Study suggest that high intake of linoleic acid (polyunsaturated, n-6) may accelerate cognitive decline, whereas fish consumption, and consequent n-3 polyunsaturated fat intake, may be protective (10).

The study found no evidence of an effect by a variety of antioxidant nutrients. Evaluation of diet and cognitive function in 278 subjects from the Italian Longitudinal Study on Aging demonstrated a significant protective effect of total monounsaturated fatty acid intake, with an odds ratio of 0.24 for the highest quartile of intake (11). A study of dietary intake and cognitive function in 260 elderly in Spain found positive associations between cognitive impairment and intake of total fat, saturated fat, and cholesterol, and protective effects of carbohydrate, fiber, total vitamins, and minerals (12).

Associations have been reported between caloric restriction in the context of intentional weight loss and deficits in cognitive function. A controlled intervention trial comparing a group of 14 obese women on a severely calorie-restricted diet to 11 controls revealed significant decline in simple reaction time among the intervention subjects, but showed no evidence of deficits in attention or immediate recall (13). In a study of 70 women engaged in varying efforts to restrict calorie intake, deficits in recall and task planning were associated with preoccupation with dieting and body habitus, rather than calorie restriction per se (14). A cohort study of Seventh Day Adventists in California revealed a significant positive association between total calorie intake and cognitive decline over the subsequent 15 years (15). Thus, the results of studies attributing cognitive deficits associated with dieting to the calorie-restricted diet should be interpreted cautiously.

There is fairly consistent evidence that iron deficiency anemia, the most common anemia in the United States, is associated with cognitive impairment. In a study of 14 obese women, Kretsch and colleagues (16) demonstrated that severe caloric restriction for 15 weeks resulted in signs of iron deficiency despite supplementation. The measures of serum iron and transferrin saturation, as well as of hemoglobin, had strong negative associations with concentration ability (16).

A case-control study of Alzheimer's disease demonstrated higher energy intake among cases than controls but revealed the higher calorie intake was necessary to maintain weight, suggesting those with the disease have higher energy requirements (17). Another case-control study suggests that Alzheimer's disease is associated with hyperhomocystinemia, but not particularly with deficient intake of B vitamins (18). The direction of any causal relationship cannot be determined from this study; elevated homocysteine may contribute to Alzheimer's disease, or the other way around. The potential benefits of B vitamin (B_{12}, folate, and B_6) supplementation on cognition, or on Alzheimer's disease specifically, have not been adequately studied to date to allow for reliable recommendations.

The effects of dietary carbohydrate on tryptophan levels have been linked to both stress tolerance and short-term cognition (19). Responding to stress is associated with activity in the serotonergic systems in the brain. Low levels of serotonin are implicated in disorders of mood (see Chapter 32) and are associated with certain aspects of cognition as well. Dietary tryptophan serves as a precursor to serotonin; thus, serum tryptophan can influence the quantity of serotonin in the brain. Insulin facilitates the entry of large neutral amino acids, with the exception of tryptophan, into skeletal muscle.

In response to carbohydrate ingestion and an insulin spike, the ratio of tryptophan to other large amino acids rises, theoretically raising the relative availability of tryptophan for use by the brain; ingestion of protein will tend to have the opposite effect (19). In a controlled comparison of high-carbohydrate and high-protein meals in stress-prone and non–stress-prone subjects, Markus and colleagues (19) demonstrated that carbohydrate loading raised the proportion of tryptophan in serum and preserved cognitive function during stress in the stress-prone subjects.

Diet and childhood development is discussed in Chapter 27. There appear to be implications for adult cognition and cognitive deficits of childhood nutriture. Advantages of breast-feeding in the cognitive development of both preterm and term infants have been reported with good consistency (20). The developmental effects of breast milk seem to pertain in particular to its composition of essential fatty acids, both n-3 and n-6 (20). Breast milk is discussed in greater detail in Chapter 25.

Nutrients and Nutriceuticals

Ginkgo Biloba

Ginkgo biloba is extracted from the leaves of the ginkgo tree, which can live as long as 4,000 years (21). Leaf extract, used as a tonic in China for more than 1,000 years, contains antioxidant flavonoids and terpenoids. One of the constituents of standard preparations, ginkgolide B, exerts an inhibitory effect on platelets (22) by antagonizing platelet-activating factor (23). This moiety is responsible for the principal toxicity of the extract, an increased bleeding propensity, particularly in patients taking aspirin (23).

The benefits of ginkgo biloba in dementia have been demonstrated in a number of small controlled randomized trials (24). Effects on brain function are supported by evidence from electroencephalography of a stimulatory effect of the extract (24).

One of the more rigorous studies to date enrolled more than 300 subjects with vascular or Alzheimer's dementia and randomly assigned them to receive active supplement or placebo (25). In this trial, subjects receiving the active agent had better cognitive performance as measured by a performance instrument and as evaluated by caregivers. However, an instrument relying on the clinician's impression demonstrated no difference. In addition, subjects were eliminated from the analysis subsequent to randomization, and the results analyzed excluded those of many participants who dropped out early (25). On the basis of available data, the conclusion that ginkgo biloba is effective in dementia cannot be reached with certainty, but the extract does appear promising and worthy of judicious use and further investigation. The magnitude of any benefit appears to be small (22).

There is considerable variability in constituent density in the leaves, and standardized preparation is important for consistent dosing (21). The typical dose for dementia is 40 to 80 mg of the standardized extract (Egb761 or LI1370) taken two to three times daily.

CLINICAL HIGHLIGHTS

Overall evidence linking dietary practices to cognitive function or decline is limited in quality and quantity; however, consistencies that form the basis for counseling have been reported in the literature. Patients should be encouraged to establish stable dietary patterns that facilitate maintenance of near ideal body weight; both obesity and persistent efforts at weight loss appear to be disadvantageous. The health benefits of weight loss in overweight patients, however, more than justify any modest impairment of cognitive function such efforts may impose (see Chapter 5).

Generous intake of vegetables and fruits appears to be beneficial, perhaps because of multiple effects. Supplements of vitamin E or C (or both), if indicated for other purposes, may contribute to preservation of cognitive function. Smoking should be avoided, but moderate alcohol consumption may confer modest benefit. Systematic modification of risk factors for cardiovascular disease (see Chapter 6) and cerebrovascular disease (see Chapter 9) appears to be important in the maintenance of cognitive ability.

Beneficial effects of ginkgo biloba appear to be real but, if so, are likely modest. The extract should be used cautiously in patients taking aspirin or anticoagulants, to avoid increased risk of bleeding.

REFERENCES

1. Joseph J, Shukitt-Hale B, Denisova N, et al. Long-term dietary strawberry, spinach, or vitamin E supplementation retards the onset of age-related neuronal signal-transduction and cognitive behavioral deficits. *J Neursci* 1998;18:8047–8055.
2. Launer L, Kalmijn S. Anti-oxidants and cognitive function: a review of clinical and epidemiologic studies. *J Neural Transm Suppl* 1998;53:1–8.
3. Sano M, Ernesto C, Thomas R, et al. A controlled trial of selegiline, alpha-tocopherol, or both as treatment for Alzheimer's disease. *N Engl J Med* 1997;336:1216–1222.
4. Paleologos M, Cumming R, Lazarus R. Cohort study of vitamin C intake and cognitive impairment. *Am J Epidemiol* 1998;148:45–50.
5. Jama J, Launer L, Witteman J, et al. Dietary antioxidants and cognitive function in a population-based sample of older persons. The Rotterdam Study. *Am J Epidemiol* 1996;144:275–280.
6. Edelstein S, Kritz-Silverstein D, Barrett-Connor E. Prospective association of smoking and alcohol use with cognitive function in an elderly cohort. *J Womens Health* 1998;7:1271–1281.
7. Launer L, Feskens E, Kalmijn S, et al. Smoking, drinking, and thinking. The Zutphen Elderly Study. *Am J Epidemiol* 1996;143:219–227.
8. Kilander L, Nyman H, Boberg M, et al. Cognitive function, vascular risk factors and education. A cross-sectional study based on a cohort of 70-year-old men. *J Intern Med* 1997;242:313–321.
9. Huijbregts P, Feskens E, Rasanen L, et al. Dietary patterns and cognitive function in elderly men in Finland, Italy and The Netherlands. *Eur J Clin Nutr* 1998;52:826–831.
10. Kalmijn S, Feskens E, Launer L, et al. Polyunsaturated fatty acids, antioxidants, and cognitive function in very old men. *Am J Epidemiol* 1997;145:33–41.
11. Capurso A, Solfrizzi V, Panza F, et al. Dietary patterns and cognitive functions in elderly subjects. *Aging Clin Exp Res* 1997;9:45–47.
12. Ortega R, Requejo A, Andres P, et al. Dietary intake and cognitive function in a group of elderly people. *Am J Clin Nutr* 1997;66:803–809.
13. Kretsch M, Green M, Fong A, et al. Cognitive effects of a long-term weight reducing diet. *Int J Obes* 1997;21:14–21.
14. Green M, Rogers P. Impairments in working memory associated with spontaneous dieting behaviour. *Psychol Med* 1998;28:1063–1070.
15. Fraser G, Singh P, Bennett H. Variables associated with cognitive function in elderly California Seventh-day Adventists. *Am J Epidemiol* 1996;143:1181–1190.
16. Kretsch M, Fong A, Green M, et al. Cognitive function, iron status, and hemoglobin concentration in obese dieting women. *Eur J Clin Nutr* 1998;52:512–518.
17. Spindler A, Renvall M, Nichols J, et al. Nutritional status of patients with Alzheimer's disease: a 1-year study. *J Am Diet Assoc* 1996;96:1013–1018.
18. McCaddon A, Davies G, Hudson P, et al. Total serum homocysteine in senile dementia of alzheimer type. *Int J Psychiatr* 1998;13:235–239.
19. Markus C, Panhuysen G, Tuiten A, et al. Does carbohydrate-rich, protein-poor food prevent a deterioration of mood and cognitive performance of

stress-prone subjects when subjected to a stressful task? *Appetite* 1998;31:49–65.

20. Gordon N. Nutrition and cognitive function. *Brain Dev* 1997;19:165–170.

21. Pang Z, Pan F, He S. Ginkgo biloba L.: history, current status, and future prospects. *J Altern Complement Med* 1996;2:359–363.

22. Ginkgo biloba for dementia. *Med Lett* 1998; 40:63–64.

23. Ginkgo biloba. *Altern Med Rev* 1998;3:54–57.

24. Maurer K, Ihl R, Dierks T, et al. Clinical efficacy of Ginkgo biloba special extract Egb 761 in dementia of the Alzheimer type. *J Psychiatr Res* 1997; 31:645–655.

25. LeBars P, Katz M, Berman N, et al. A placebo-controlled, double-blind, randomized trial of an extract of Ginkgo biloba for dementia. *JAMA* 1997;278:1327–1332.

See "Sources for All Chapters."

34

Diet and Vision

INTRODUCTION

The two leading causes of visual impairment in older adults are age-related macular degeneration and cataracts. Approximately 7% of individuals over age 75 have impaired vision due to macular degeneration, and 40% in this age group have cataracts that impair vision (1,2). As the population ages, the public health impact of these conditions is rising.

Photocoagulation is effective for treatment of advanced macular degeneration in only a minority of patients. Because it is safe and generally effective, cataract extraction has become the most common surgery performed in people over age 60 in the United States and thus represents an enormous public health burden. Cataract is both more prevalent and more disabling in developing than in developed countries; worldwide, cataract accounts for 50% of all blindness (3). There is, therefore, well-founded interest in preventive strategies for both diseases.

Both conditions have been linked to cumulative oxidative injury. In the lens, reactive oxygen species damage crystallin proteins. In the macula, peroxidation of polyunsaturated fatty acids in photoreceptor cells may lead to degeneration. Dietary factors have the potential to accelerate or retard the development of impaired visual acuity and blindness with aging. Studies of antioxidants in diet and supplement form suggest a possible benefit.

Ocular complications of diabetes mellitus resulting in impaired vision may be forestalled by dietary practices that improve glycemic control. This topic is addressed in Chapter 10.

OVERVIEW

The lens is composed of proteins that are retained throughout life, migrating toward the lens center or nucleus. Damage to the proteins from exposure to light and oxygen accumulates over time. Vitamin C is concentrated in the lens (2), and levels in the lens and eye compartments apparently are responsive to dietary intake (1). Levels generally decline with aging, and low levels have been associated with cataract formation (2).

Overall, the evidence linking specific nutrients to cataract prevention is preliminary. The evidence is suggestive for vitamins C and E, as well as the carotenoids. The evidence of a protective effect is more convincing for a diet rich in fruits and vegetable than for specific nutrients (2). Smoking has been implicated in cataract formation.

Thus, dietary and lifestyle recommendations that may be made with confidence for other reasons, such as smoking cessation and increased fruit and vegetable consumption, offer the promise of reduced cataract risk as well (2). Although not definitive, the evidence suggests that vitamin C supplementation in the range of 500 mg per day may offer additional benefit. The results of on-going and future intervention trials will be required before more definitive recommendations can be made with security.

The retina, in general, and the macula, in particular, may be susceptible to oxidative injury because of their concentration of unsaturated fatty acids. The antioxidant effects of vitamins C and E, the carotenoids, as well as zinc, copper, and selenium may play a role in protecting the macula from injury caused by singlet oxygen, which is generated by light absorption (1). Zinc and copper are cofactors to superoxide dismutase; selenium is needed for the action of glutathione peroxidase.

Evidence derived from animal models, case-control, observational-cohort, and occasional randomized trials clearly supports a role for nutritional factors in the course of macular degeneration. The evidence is most convincing that, among the antioxidants, lutein and zeaxanthin are protective (1). Lutein and zeaxanthin are carotenoids found abundantly in dark green vegetables; they have no provitamin A activity, but they have been associated with protection against macular degeneration; they are preferentially taken up by the macula (1).

Carotenoids are a diverse family of pigments, some with and some without provitamin A activity (see Nutrient Reference Data Table, Section III). Both β-carotene and α-carotene are moderate antioxidants with provitamin A activity. Although essential for eye function as a component of rhodopsin, which is the visual pigment of rod cells in the retina, vitamin A does not appear to play a role in the development or prevention of macular degeneration.

Preliminary evidence supports a protective role of zinc supplementation. Deficiencies in habitual intake of several nutrients were reported in an evaluation of a representative population of elderly subjects (ages 65 to 85) in Maryland; zinc deficiency was particularly common (4). Risk factors, dietary and other, for coronary artery disease are correlated with the risk of macular degeneration as well. Postmenopausal estrogen replacement appears to be protective, as does intake of n-3 fatty acid (1). There is interest in the possible role of dietary supplementation with long-chain polyunsaturated fatty acids, especially of the n-3 class, in the development and protection of the macula (5,6). The evidence in support of dietary n-3 fatty acids is inconclusive (6).

Although the nutrient-specific data to date are preliminary, general dietary recommendations for the prevention of macular degeneration may be made with some confidence. A diet rich in green, leafy vegetables will provide abundant lutein and zeaxanthin, and should be encouraged. Other fruits and vegetables may provide additional benefits and should be consumed to promote health in any event. A large, population-based study of the visually impaired in Finland revealed a convincing association between eye disease, particularly macular degeneration, and cancer (7). The authors conclude that age-related eye disease and various cancers share risk factors, particularly smoking and diet.

The benefit of vitamin E or C and of several minerals remains uncertain, but multivitamin/mineral supplementation, advocated on other grounds, may confer protection against macular degeneration. Cardiovascular disease risk factor modification, including smoking cessation and postmenopausal hormone replacement therapy, may be protective of the macula as well.

Christen (8) reviewed the literature on prevention of macular degeneration and cataract. Cross-sectional, case-control, and prospective observational studies produced variable results but are generally compatible with a modest benefit of high antioxidant intake in the form of supplements or food on age-related eye disease. More conclusive evidence, and specification of nutrient and dose, awaits completion of on-going randomized trials (8). Brown and colleagues (9) reviewed the same literature and offered specific "reasonable" doses for daily supplementation that may offer benefit to eye health with little risk of toxicity. Suggested supplements include 1 mg of vitamin A, 500 to 1,000 mg of vitamin C, 300 mg of vitamin E, and 20 mg of zinc; other recommendations mirror the recommended dietary allowances (9).

CLINICAL HIGHLIGHTS

Definitive evidence of nutrient-specific protection of the lens or macula is as yet unavailable, although evidence from various sources strongly suggests that generous antioxidant intake from diet is protective. A diet rich in green, leafy vegetables should be recommended as primary prevention of age-related eye disease. Smoking cessation is clearly indicated for this and other clinical goals. Supplementation with a multivitamin/mineral tablet may be beneficial, especially in those over age 50 or with less-than-judicious diets.

As discussed elsewhere (see Chapter 15 and Section III), zinc deficiency may be widespread in the United States; use of a daily mineral supplement is supported by the potential role of zinc in protection of both the macula and the lens. Patients with a particular interest in prevention of eye disease should consider supplementation with vitamin C 500 mg and vitamin E 400 to 800 IU, although evidence of benefit is at best suggestive.

Inclusion in the diet of n-3 fatty acids from fish or plant sources is advisable on general principles and may prove to be of benefit to vision (see Chapter 40). Intake of this class of fat may be particularly important to the eyes, as it appears to be for cognitive development, during infancy (see Chapters 25 and 27). The dietary pattern tentatively associated with protection of vision, rich in fruits and vegetables, is advisable on general principles and may be recommended with conviction.

REFERENCES

1. Hung S, Seddon J. The relationship between nutritional factors and age-related macular degeneration. In: Bendich A, Deckelbaum R, eds. *Preventive nutrition.* Totowa, NJ: Humana Press, 1997.
2. Taylor A, Jacques P. Antioxidant status and risk for cataract. In: Bendich A, Deckelbaum R, eds. *Preventive nutrition.* Totowa, NJ: Humana Press, 1997.
3. Javitt J, Wang F, West S. Blindness due to cataract: epidemiology and prevention. *Annu Rev Public Health* 1996;17:159.
4. Cid-Ruzafa J, Calulfield L, Barron Y, et al. Nutrient intakes and adequacy among an older population on the eastern shore of Maryland: the Salisbury Eye Evaluation. *J Am Diet Assoc* 1999;99:564.
5. Birch E, Hoffman D, Uauy R, et al. Visual acuity and the essentiality of docosahexaenoic acid and arachidonic acid in the diet of term infants. *Pediatr Res* 1998;44:201.
6. Gibson R, Makrides M. Polyunsaturated fatty acids and infant visual development: a critical appraisal of randomized clinical trials. *Lipids* 1999;34:179.
7. Pukkala E, Verkasalo P, Ojamo M, et al. Visual impairment and cancer: a population-based cohort study in Finland. *Cancer Causes Control* 1999;10:13.
8. Christen W. Antioxidant vitamins and age-related eye disease. *Proc Assoc Am Physicians* 1999;111:16.
9. Brown N, Bron A, Harding J, et al. Nutrition supplements and the eye. *Eye* 1998;12:127.

See "Sources for All Chapters."

35

Diet and Dentition

INTRODUCTION

The associations among diet, the oral cavity, and health are diverse and bidirectional. A variety of nutrient deficiencies are reflected in the oral cavity, with inflammation of the buccal and glossal mucous membranes. Nutrition influences immunocompetence (see Chapter 15), which in turn influences the degree to which bacteria in the oral cavity contribute to tooth decay and caries. Poor dentition, particularly in the elderly, may play a role in malnutrition, with restriction in the variety and quantity of food attributable to mechanical limitations. Nutrition, through site-specific and systemic effects, plays a role in the development and maintenance of dental health.

OVERVIEW

Diet

Teeth are composed of an outer layer of enamel and an inner layer of dentin surrounding the pulp. Erosion of the outer mineralized layers leads to the formation of cavities, or caries. Dental caries, an infectious disease of the oral cavity and teeth, remains a considerable public health problem despite declines over recent decades attributable primarily to fluoridation of the water supply and of dentifrices; it is the most common, chronic infectious disease of humans. At least 50% of children still develop dental caries and the prevalence of the disease rises with age, so that very few adults are caries-free.

The pathogenesis of dental caries involves demineralization of the tooth surface, a period of equilibration, and remineralization. The process appears to span nearly 18 months; therefore, the opportunity exists to arrest and reverse caries before a clinically overt cavity is formed.

The four factors influencing the development of caries, other than genetically induced susceptibility, are mouth bacteria, fermentable dietary carbohydrate, deficient exposure to fluoride and other dietary minerals, and the volume and composition of saliva. Plaque is composed of oral bacterial flora, polysaccharides, and salivary proteins. The predominant bacterial species is *Streptococcus mutans*. Plaque bathes and—without consistent oral hygienic practice—adheres to teeth.

Ingested carbohydrate is metabolized (fermented) to organic acids, including lactic, butyric, acetic, formic, and propionic. A decline in plaque pH ensues, with dissolution of tooth surface enamel at a pH between 5.3 and 5.7. Any acid can lead to tooth demineralization and the formation of caries. Eating disorders that include purging (self-induced vomiting) have serious consequences for dental health because of the frequent exposure of teeth to gastric acid (1). This issue is addressed in Chapter 23.

A variety of epidemiologic studies, including the natural experiments imposed by periods of shortage (e.g., World War II) reveal that dietary sugars are implicated in the etiology of dental caries. Plaque formation is accelerated when sucrose is present.

Streptococcus mutans elaborates polysaccharides in the presence of sucrose that facilitate adhesion of bacteria to dental surfaces. Other commonly ingested sugars behave like sucrose and precipitate a comparable fall in the pH of plaque.

Because of their several properties, dried fruits, cereals, cookies, crackers, chips, and breads all contribute to the formation of caries. Although they contain concentrated sugars, fresh fruits tend to be of low cariogenic potential because of their high water content and the presence of citric acid, which is a sialagogue. Foods containing citrate stimulate saliva production and may be beneficial if only moderate citrate is ingested.

Saliva plays an important role in the prevention of caries; xerostomic patients develop caries at particularly high rates. Saliva mobilizes food particles, directly buffers acid in plaque, depresses bacterial counts, and promotes remineralization by transporting calcium, phosphorus, and fluoride. The acid content of fruit may inhibit bacterial fermentation, but when high, as it is in lemons and oranges, may directly erode enamel.

Meats, hard cheeses, nuts, and most vegetables appear to be uninvolved in the formation of caries. Certain hard cheeses prevent dietary sugar from lowering plaque pH by as yet uncertain means. The implication is that certain foods may specifically protect tooth enamel from the effects of sugars in other foods.

The adherence of starchy foods to the teeth contributes to cariogenesis; the role of starches in caries has been convincingly established (2). Refined and processed grains contain modified starch susceptible to the action of salivary amylase. The release of maltose results, and its fermentation lowers plaque pH and contributes to demineralization. Processed foods high in starch tend to adhere to teeth for protracted periods and thus may contribute disproportionately to cavity formation. Of note, dietary starch present in vegetables is noncariogenic.

The frequency of meals or snacks containing starch or sugar correlates directly with the formation of caries. Foods that adhere to teeth eaten between meals increase the risk in particular. Food sequence is influential as well. When sugar-containing foods are consumed at the end of a meal or snack, they produce the most protracted fall in plaque pH; other foods eaten after sources of starch or sugar can immediately attenuate their effects.

Although sugar in solution adheres less to teeth surfaces than does sugar from solids, sweetened drinks are associated with increased risk of caries. The risk appears to be comparable for juices and sodas. The potential benefits of artificial sweeteners are under investigation (see Chapter 38). Even though they lack sugar, diet sodas that are acidic may be as damaging to teeth as nondiet varieties; the acid content contributes directly to demineralization (3). Sugar alcohols, such as mannitol and sorbitol, are fermented more slowly than monosaccharides and disaccharides, and they are less cariogenic, although bacterial acclimation appears to occur if habitual intake is high.

Xylitol is not cariogenic. Saccharin has been found to inhibit tooth decay in animal studies. Animal studies of aspartame indicate that it plays no role in the development of caries. Chewing gum sweetened with noncariogenic substances such as xylitol has a protective effect by stimulating the production and flow of saliva that neutralizes bacterial acids, dislodging trapped food particles, and reducing plaque.

Although moderation of dietary sugar intake may be beneficial to dental health and is advisable on other grounds, greater benefit to dentition may be achieved by consistently brushing with a fluoride toothpaste at least twice per day (4). Naturally, these practices need not be mutually exclusive, and their benefits are likely to be additive.

During tooth development, protein calorie malnutrition can retard tooth eruption and reduce tooth size. Vitamin A deficiency during development results in malformed teeth. Deficiencies of vitamin D, calcium, or phosphorus impair tooth mineralization. The availability of fluoride in sufficient but not excessive quantity strengthens tooth enamel; excess mottles the teeth. Iodine deficiency delays tooth eruption and alters growth patterns. Protein/calorie malnutrition and vitamin A, vitamin D, calcium, fluoride, and iodine deficiencies are all implicated in the development of caries. Vitamin C deficiency has been implicated in impaired tooth development and possibly in the development of caries.

Infants and toddlers between the ages of 1 and 2 are at risk of baby-bottle tooth decay (5), which results when they are allowed to fall asleep drinking milk or formula from a bottle. The pooling of sugar-containing fluid around the teeth produces a characteristic, and sometimes severe, pattern of tooth decay. The condition is avoided by limiting nighttime and naptime fluid intake to water after the teeth have erupted. Human breast milk is apparently not cariogenic (6). The diet to which infants are weaned is considered to influence dentition over both the short and long term. An emphasis in the literature has been placed on the avoidance of sugar-containing beverages between meals and at bedtime (7).

Older adults with receding gingiva are at risk for caries over exposed surfaces of tooth roots. These surfaces lack enamel and are susceptible to caries at an accelerated rate. Implicated foods include sweetened beverages and starches. Care of the gingiva is fundamental to the prevention of this condition.

Gingivitis, inflammation of the gums, and periodontitis, a more serious infectious process involving the attachment apparatus of the tooth, are thought to be influenced by nutritional status, but specific associations have not be demonstrated. Because both processes are infectious and inflammatory, the relationship between diet and immune function (see Chapter 15) is apt to be pertinent. Thus, nutritional adequacy with regard to immune function likely plays a role in the health of the gingiva and periodontal tissues, indirectly if not directly.

Tooth decay and loss impacts nutritional status (8,9). Approximately 40% of adults over the age of 65 in the United States are edentulous. Many medications reduce saliva production, and for this reason as many as 50% of the elderly have iatrogenically induced reductions in saliva production. Reduction of saliva can accelerate tooth decay, as well as interfere with the functioning of dentures if already placed. The stimulation of saliva through the use of chewing gums containing xylitol may be compensatory.

Maintenance of oral health is essential to maintaining good nutritional patterns and thereby reducing risk for a variety of chronic diseases in elderly adults (10). Masticatory ability in individuals with partial or complete dentures generally is reduced to approximately 20% of normal.

Data from an observational study of more than 1,200 male veterans indicate that poor dentition is associated with reduced intake of many vitamins, minerals, protein, and fiber. The diets of those with compromised and intact dentition differed both qualitatively and quantitatively (11). The study revealed that subjects with compromised dentition avoid eating nutrient-dense foods considered difficult to chew, including fruits, vegetables, nuts, and meats (11). Fortunately, for a variety of reasons, the prevalence of tooth loss in the elderly is decreasing over time (11). Dental health correlates to some extent with education level and the consistency of dental care. Krall and colleagues (11) suggest that some variation in diet previously attributed to education level may be confounded by dentition status.

Nutrients and Nutriceuticals

Fluoride

A reduction in the rate of dental caries attributable to water and dentifrice fluoridation is irrefutable. Fluoride is incorporated into the hydroxyapatite of teeth, rendering tooth mineral less susceptible to demineralization. Fluoride also inhibits the replication and enzymes of *S. mutans*. A substantial decrease in the risk of caries for both children and adults is associated with fluoride at a dose of one part per million in the drinking water. This dose, studied extensively, is not associated with any known adverse health effects. The incorporation of fluoride into bone may confer benefit as well (see Chapter 13).

When water is not fluoridated, fluoride supplementation for children is indicated; the dose recommended is 0.05 mg/kg/day. Fluoride supplementation is recommended for infants breast-fed beyond 6 months, beginning at that age, as the fluoride content of breast milk is low. Prenatal supplementation is of uncertain benefit. Fluorosis results when fluoride intake is excessive. Because young children will swallow a portion of toothpaste used, small amounts should be dispensed to prevent excess fluoride ingestion.

CLINICAL HIGHLIGHTS

Diet influences dentition, and dentition and the health of the oral cavity influence diet. The dietary factors most important in the pathogenesis of dental caries are the sugar and starch content of the diet, the conclusion of meals and eating snacks with foods high in processed starch or sugar, and the frequency of snacks containing such foods.

The incidence of dental caries can be reduced by limiting sugar intake, avoiding sugary or starchy snacks, using chewing gum sweetened with xylitol or other nonfermentable sweeteners, and frequent brushing to remove trapped food particles. Dietary adequacy in general is important to optimize immune function and the health of the buccal and lingual mucosae. A multivitamin supplement may be of benefit, particularly in individuals past the age of 50.

Fluoride intake over years greatly influences susceptibility to caries. The fluoride content of patients' drinking water should be addressed in primary care; physicians should advise supplementation when the water fluoride is low. Virtually all municipal or public water supplies are fluoridated; private wells generally, of course, are not. Children should be weaned to diets that are moderate in sugar content and, in particular, should not be allowed to take a sweetened beverage in a bottle to bed. Careful attention to the dentition of aging adults is essential to the preservation of native teeth, which in turn influences the adequacy, in terms of quality and quantity, of the overall diet.

REFERENCES

1. Milosevic A, Brodie D, Slade P. Dental erosion, oral hygiene, and nutrition in eating disorders. *Int J Eat Disord* 1997;21:195.
2. Kashket S, Zhang J, Houte JV. Accumulation of fermentable sugars and metabolic acids in food particles that become entrapped on the dentition. *J Dent Res* 1996;75:1885.
3. Thomas B. *Nutrition in primary care. A handbook for health professionals.* Oxford, England: Blackwell Science, 1996.
4. Gibson S, Williams S. Dental caries in pre-school children: association with social class, toothbrushing habit and consumption of sugars and sugar-containing foods. Further analysis of data from the National Diet and Nutrition Survey of children aged 1.5–4.5 years. *Caries Res* 1999;33:101.
5. Sonis A, Castle J, Duggan C. Infant nutrition: implications for somatic growth, adult onset disease, and oral health. *Curr Opin Pediatr* 1997;9:289.
6. Erickson P, Mazhari E. Investigation of the role of human breast milk in caries development. *Pediatr Dent* 1999;21:86.
7. Holt R, Moynihan P. The weaning diet and dental health. *Br Dent J* 1996;181:254.
8. Ettinger R. Changing dietary patterns with changing dentition: how do people cope? *Spec Care Dent* 1998;18:33.
9. Papas A, Palmer C, Rounds M, et al. The effects of denture status on nutrition. *Spec Care Dent* 1998;18:17.
10. Saunders M. Nutrition and oral health in the elderly. *Dent Clin North Am* 1997;41:681.
11. Krall E, Hayes C, Garcia R. How dentition status and masticatory function affect nutrient intake. *J Am Dent Assoc* 1998;129:1261.

BIBLIOGRAPHY

See "Sources for All Chapters."
DePaola DP, Faine MP, Vogel RI. Nutrition in relation to dental medicine. In: Shils ME.
Rugg-Dunn AJ, Nunn JH. *Nutrition, diet, and oral health.* Oxford, England: Oxford University Press, 1999.

36

Hunger, Appetite, Taste, and Satiety

INTRODUCTION

Control over the process of energy and nutrient intake is vital to the survival of an individual and a species. Minimally, food intake is influenced by hunger, the sensations induced by a deficit in readily metabolizable energy sources. But it also is influenced by appetite, a desire for food influenced by cravings for specific tastes and/or nutrients, and the palatability, familiarity, and availability of specific foods. Also important is satiety, the sensation that whatever impulses have led to food consumption have been satisfied.

In humans, food intake is the product of physiologic, psychological, and sociologic factors that defy simple classification. The conditions of endemic and epidemic obesity increasingly common in industrialized countries, while ascribable to an imbalance in the regulation of energy intake, are less readily ascribed to a particular component of the complex governing systems. There is evidence that redundant processes in humans govern energy intake, a state that may have conferred survival benefit throughout human prehistory, when the adequacy of dietary energy often was in question.

The properties of specific foods and the physiologic responses evoked by their consumption appear to have implications for the regulation of energy intake, although simple explanations are elusive and perhaps ill advised. Sufficient insights and evidence have accumulated to permit clinical recommendations that may be expected to contribute to salutary energy balance.

OVERVIEW

Physiologic defenses against undernutrition are far more robust than those against overnutrition (1). Even so, were physiology alone responsible for nutrient energy consumption, food intake would begin with hunger and end with satiety. The characteristic physical sensations of hunger and fullness, however, are one part of a complex interplay of physiologic and nonphysiologic factors governing the quantity, frequency, and variety of food intake (2–4). Food consumption may be in excess of that required to meet energy needs when the food is particularly palatable or the social context is conducive to overindulgence. Food intake may fail to meet the demands of hunger, even when ingestible energy is abundantly available, if the food is unfamiliar or unpalatable.

Food intake is regulated by the response of the brain to the extensive variety of pertinent signals. The specific brain regions relevant to energy regulation appear to reside in the hypothalamus. The ventromedial hypothalamus appears to be important in the generation of satiety, whereas hunger is in part regulated by the lateral hypothalamus. Other sites in the brain appear to be involved as well. Redundancy in central regulation of energy intake may confer a survival advantage, but obviously complicates efforts to isolate genetic or metabolic defects responsible for perturbations of energy balance, such as those leading to obesity or severe anorexia.

Body energy requirements are clearly one factor driving hunger and appetite. The availability of nutrient energy is reflected in diet-induced thermogenesis, the generation of heat for a period of approximately 6 hours following ingestion due to the metabolic work of digestion and activation of the sympathetic nervous system. A rise in body temperature due to diet-induced, or postprandial, thermogenesis signals the adequacy of nutrient energy supplies, whereas a decline in temperature between meals is an indication of declining energy supplies, and a stimulus to hunger.

An interaction among core body temperature, heat generation by brown adipose tissue, and serum glucose levels has been theorized to influence hunger and consequent energy intake. When core temperature falls, heat generation by brown fat increases, with resultant extraction of glucose from serum. Relative hypoglycemia is likely a stimulus for ingestion. With ingestion, core temperature rises, reducing the metabolic activity of brown fat, providing a stimulus for meal termination. Postprandial thermogenesis may influence the initiation and termination of meals, as well as their size and frequency. The evidence for the role of this mechanism in the control of food intake is preliminary.

Satiety is influenced by signals from stretch receptors in the stomach and by the delivery of nutrient energy to the duodenum. The effects of ingestion on satiety are mediated by the vagus nerve and by gut hormones. Ten gut hormones have been shown to influence satiety, and the best studied to date is cholecystokinin, which shortens the duration of feeding. The entry of gastric chyme into the duodenum is a stimulus for the release of cholecystokinin. Cholecystokinin slows gastric emptying, increasing the signals to gastric stretch receptors and contributing to a sense of satiety. Cholecystokinin also may provide direct signaling of satiety to the brain. Macronutrient absorption in the small bowel stimulates the vagus nerve, which also signals satiety to the brain.

The signals of satiety delivered before or during nutrient absorption are reinforced by postabsorptive signals. Nutrient entry into the portal vein results in signals of satiety from the liver to the brain via the vagus nerve. The mechanisms of signal exchange between liver and central nervous system are uncertain. Circulating levels of glucose, insulin, and amino acids may all contribute to satiety.

The flavor of foods is perceived as the combination of taste, smell, and chemical stimuli, each activating different systems. Taste is mediated by taste buds, clustered in fungiform papillae over the anterior tongue and foliate papillae on the posterior tongue. The gustatory system is innervated by branches of the seventh and tenth cranial nerves.

Whether the range of tastes discerned is reducible to four taste categories (e.g., sweet, sour, salty, bitter) remains controversial, although this view prevails. Olfaction is mediated by neurons in the nasal cavities that are components of the first cranial nerve and lead directly to the olfactory bulb in the brain. The chemical properties and physiologic responses that permit the discernment of diverse smells remain speculative.

Finally, there is a somatosensory component to taste, responsible for the perception of chemical irritants such as capsaicin. This system is subtended primarily by the trigeminal nerve. There may be some overlap between the perception of chemical irritants and the perception of temperature in the oral cavity (e.g., spicy is perceived as "hot"; menthol is perceived as "cold"). Whereas the function of the chemosensory tissues influences food intake, nutritional status also influences the activity of these tissues, which are metabolically active and have a high rate of cellular turnover.

Cravings represent an extreme expression of appetite, although not necessarily hunger, often occurring in a particular social or physiologic context, such as during pregnancy, at a party, or at a particular stage of the menstrual cycle. The predominant example of food craving is for chocolate (5). Many theories have been advanced to account for various food cravings under various circumstances, but none is conclusive. Cognitive processing of chemosensory properties of food results in interpretations that determine the hedonic properties, or the capacity of food to induce pleasure.

The role of genetic factors in regulating energy balance, and consequently body weight, is a subject of intense interest. The ob gene, originally identified in mice in 1994, has been cloned from humans. The gene encodes for leptin, a protein produced by adipocytes that acts as a satiety signal (6). Whereas obese mice homozygous for ob gene mutations are deficient in leptin (7), in obese humans, leptin levels correlate positively with percent body fat (8).

Appetite and energy regulation also are influenced by neuropeptide Y, a product of the hypothalamus that stimulates appetite by elevating levels of insulin and glucocorticoids (7). In turn, insulin and cortisol stimulate release of leptin, completing an inhibitory feedback pathway between adipose tissue and the hypothalamus. Insensitivity to leptin appears to be the defect resulting from ob gene mutation in humans and is a potential contributor to disordered energy regulation and obesity (7) (see Chapter 5).

Many of the factors influencing dietary intake patterns appear to be heritable, in whole or in part (9). There is genetic variation in taste perception, generally measured as sensitivity to 6-n-propylthiouracil (10). Recent evidence fails to support the hypothesis that such variation translates into predictable pleasure responses to dietary sugar (10).

Physical activity can induce an energy deficit comparable to fasting. However, the effects of physical activity on appetite appear to be distinct. Limited evidence suggests that fasting increases hunger, whereas exercise may not (11,12).

Aging is associated with apparently minor reductions in taste and smell sensitivity in healthy individuals, but memory deficits, comorbidity, and medication use are issues that compound nutriture in older people. The elderly may be subject to nutritional deficiencies due to declines in taste, olfaction, or the regulation of appetite, complicated by

social factors that may limit dietary diversity (13).

Dietary preferences are strongly influenced by cultural factors (14). The physiology of appetite regulation interacts with an array of social and behavioral influences on dietary selection in producing a particular dietary pattern (2). There is reason to believe that early food exposures may play an important role in establishing lifelong preferences, possibly during specific developmental periods (15), although much remains uncertain to date.

Diet

Appetite begins with anticipation of food intake. The cephalic phase of appetite includes increased sensation of hunger, as well as metabolic responses preparatory to the act of ingestion. Satiety is mediated by sensory, social, ingestive, and postabsorptive stimuli. Sensory factors that influence a person's appetite and food intake include a food's taste (sweet, sour, salty, and bitter), smell, texture, appearance, and familiarity.

Foods tend to be more desirable when they are consumed in limited amount, with the pleasure derived from a particular food generally decreasing as the quantity of that food eaten rises. As the variety available within a single meal increases, energy intake (compared to single-food meals) greatly increases as well (16). This effect is apparently due to sensory-specific satiety, the capacity of satiety centers in the hypothalamus to register satiety differentially by category of taste. The variety of foods constantly available in developed countries may be a factor contributing to augmented appetite, energy excess, and obesity.

Levels of serotonin, norepinephrine, and endogenous opiates are thought to influence appetite. Serotonin levels are raised by the ingestion of tryptophan. Transport of tryptophan across the blood–brain barrier is dependent on the concentration of tryptophan relative to that of other large neutral amino acids. A protein meal rich in other large neutral amino acids actually decreases brain uptake of tryptophan.

Carbohydrate ingestion stimulates insulin release. Whereas insulin enhances tissue uptake of amino acids, the effect on tryptophan is limited because of albumin binding of tryptophan. Therefore, carbohydrate meals tend to increase the circulating concentration, and thereby the brain uptake, of tryptophan.

Evidence has been summarized that appetite and its resolution are to some extent taste or food specific (17). This condition has been termed "sensory-specific satiety" (16). Various studies suggest that appetite persists longer, and more total calories are consumed, when food is available in variety. Conversely, satiety is reached sooner and with less total energy consumption when a single food is available. This response is very rapid, so that differential intake is noted during a single meal, as well as over time.

The satiety thresholds for different tastes are thought to be distinct, with that for sweet highest, explaining the desirability of dessert at the end of a meal. A teleologic view of this condition suggests it motivated the effort required of our ancestors to maintain dietary diversity and defend themselves against micronutrient deficiencies (16). In a nutritional environment with variety available in constant abundance, sensory-specific satiety is thought to contribute to excessive nutrient consumption and obesity (16).

This situation is compounded by food industry manipulations, such as the addition of sugar to foods perceived as salty (e.g., ketchup), and the addition of salt to foods perceived as sweet (e.g., breakfast cereals, desserts); satiety may be delayed by within-food taste variety. Viewed via an understanding of the factors governing appetite, obesity is more readily ascribed to a toxic nutritional environment than to impaired restraint on the part of an individual (18).

The principal determinant of hunger is energy need, independent of energy source. The consistency of appetite and hunger in regulating energy intake in individuals has been shown. Louis-Sylvestre and colleagues (19) studied a group of 17 adolescent males and demonstrated that, over the course of hours to days, precise compensation occurred for the administration of calorie-modified foods so that energy intake remained constant. This consistency may explain why fat- or calorie-reduced products appear to have limited potential for weight control. There is some evidence, however, that the source of nutrient energy—carbohydrate, protein, or fat—influences perceptions of hunger and satiety. The existence of nutrient-specific hunger remains uncertain but seems likely. There is evidence that hunger is stimulated by nutritional variety and suppressed by nutritional monotony.

Considerable evidence from animal studies indicates the tendency to maintain a constant protein intake despite variations in the protein density of the diets offered. Some evidence exists of protein regulation in humans, but it is less conclusive. There is no evidence in either animals or humans that carbohydrate consumption is regulated per se, as might be expected, given that there is no true dietary requirement for carbohydrate other than the trivial amount required to prevent ketosis.

The available evidence in sum suggests that regulation of macronutrients, particularly fat and protein, may be a component of appetite, but that regulation is of lesser priority than the maintenance of adequate energy intake. Animal studies have demonstrated adaptive dietary intake patterns in response to induced micronutrient deficiencies. Without a condition of gross deficiency, it is unknown whether regulation of micronutrient intake plays a role in influencing appetite and intake patterns.

Dietary Carbohydrate

Evidence from both animal and human studies that declines in serum glucose trigger hunger and food intake is inconclusive. Regulation of food intake in response to the serum glucose level is known as the "glucostatic" theory. Although there has been some evidence to support variations in hunger corresponding to variations in serum glucose (20), animal studies have shown hunger to persist despite hyperglycemia and to abate despite hypoglycemia. Most evidence suggests that if serum glucose influences appetite, the effect is indirect.

Some evidence suggests that sudden declines in serum glucose predict food intake. Other studies suggest that glucose utilization in the brain, or in the liver, may be the determining factor. Insulin action in the central nervous system suppresses food intake. Insulin is believed to inhibit the synthesis of neuropeptide Y, which is a potent stimulus to hunger, in the arcuate nucleus. Reductions in serum glucose and consequently insulin are associated with increases in neuropeptide Y release.

Carbohydrate is less readily stored than fat, less calorically dense, and generally more satiating; nonetheless, ingestion of carbohydrate may contribute substantially to obesity. Sugar in particular may stimulate appetite and be subject to a higher satiety threshold than other nutrients (21). Individuals with depression, and particularly those with seasonal affective disorder, may develop a carbohydrate craving. This tendency has been postulated to be a response to low levels of brain serotonin. Low serotonin may be causally related to both depression and excessive hunger.

Carbohydrate ingestion increases brain uptake of tryptophan, a serotonin precursor. Some variability in the satiating effects of carbohydrates has been demonstrated; fructose suppresses food intake more than other sugars do. In general, slowly absorbed carbohydrates that result in small, sustained elevations of glucose and insulin are more satiating than rapidly absorbed carbohydrates. This fact suggests that carbohydrate sources rich in fiber, and especially soluble fiber, are more satiating in general than low-fiber sources.

Dietary Protein

The role of circulating amino acids on satiety is uncertain. The aminostatic theory posits that protein status dominates in control of appetite. There is interest in tryptophan as a precursor to serotonin synthesis, and in tyrosine and histidine as precursors to catecholamines and histamine, respectively, as these compounds suppress appetite. To date, no direct evidence of specific amino acid effects on satiety has been established.

When a diverse source of nutrients is available, protein intake generally constitutes approximately 15% of total calories, suggesting that a protein-specific appetite may be operative. The need for amino acid ingestion would be the putative teleologic basis for a protein appetite. When administered at energy doses comparable to those of either carbohydrate or fat, protein is more satiating. Various high-protein diets have been advocated for rapid weight loss, but evidence of sustained benefit is lacking (see Chapter 5). As noted, selective ingestion of protein may contribute to a preferential appetite for carbohydrate.

Dietary Fat

The lipostatic theory links stores of body fat to regulation of food intake. The release of leptin by adipocytes may be the mediating messenger (22). Leptin binds to receptors on cells in the hypothalamus responsible for the production and release of neuropeptide Y; reduced secretion of neuropeptide Y suppresses appetite (22). Reduced levels of neuropeptide Y stimulate release of norepinephrine, which in turn influences insulin levels and action. The actions of leptin are complex and incompletely understood; some effects may be mediated by interleukin 1 or prostaglandins, or both (23).

Leptin levels vary directly both with fat mass and satiety. The relationship between leptin and satiety apparently is maintained, although perhaps weakened, even in obese individuals (24).

A preference for dietary fat among obese individuals has been suggested (25), but the role of taste differences or altered hedonic responses to food in the etiology of obesity remains controversial. Fat is the most energy-dense macronutrient, providing 9 kcal/g. The storage of ingested fat in adipose tissue requires less energy than that of other macronutrients.

Ingested fat induces satiety, but there is evidence it does so less effectively than carbohydrate. The energy density of fat, the facility with which it is stored, and its limited satiating effects may all partly explain the epidemiologic link between diets high in fat and obesity. A preference for dietary fat can be induced by morphine and suppressed with opiate antagonists, indicating that fat ingestion is reinforced through endogenous opiate production (25).

Physiologic habituation to high fat intake, in the form of enhanced oxidation, has been demonstrated in animals, suggesting that dietary fat may be more rewarding when habitual intake is high (26). In addition to physiologic adaptation, the familiarity of a high-fat diet has been shown to produce preference (27). Postingestive effects of dietary fat also have been shown to influence preference (28). In humans, both sugar and dairy fat have been shown to induce dose-dependent pleasure ratings, with the fat not revealing an upper threshold (29). The association of sugar and fat in the diet may contribute to excess energy intake, with sugar serving as a vehicle for the calorie density of fat (30).

Macronutrients and Satiety

There is known to be considerable variability in the satiating capacity of different foods. Holt and colleagues (31) reported results of a feeding experiment in 41 adult subjects, where satiety was indicated both by subjective scales and subsequent *ad libitum* food intake. Satiety was positively associated with the weight of food and its water, fiber, and protein content, and negatively correlated with palatability and fat content (31).

Holt and colleagues (32) reported data from a study of the effects of different breakfasts on subsequent food intake in 14 adult subjects. The study showed higher subsequent energy intake after a high-fat than a high-fiber, high-carbohydrate breakfast, suggesting the greater satiating capacity of carbohydrate and fiber. Protein is thought to be the most satiating of the macronutrient classes, and fat the least (33,34). In a comparison of isoenergetic meals of differing composition, Poppitt and colleagues (35) found protein to be significantly more satiating than other macronutrients and to reduce subsequent *ad libitum* intake of a meal of fixed composition.

Some evidence suggests, however, that craving for carbohydrate may be induced by meals exclusively high in protein, at least in certain individuals (36). On balance, the available evidence supports a diet adequate in protein and high in complex, fiber-rich carbohydrate as a way of maximizing satiety and optimizing appetite control. High intake of dietary fat is least conducive to control of appetite and regulation of weight (37,38). In studies of beverages, volume appears to be an independent mediator of satiety (39).

Nutrients and Nutriceuticals

Vitamin A

Vitamin A deficiency is associated with impairment of taste and smell that may lead to or exacerbate malnutrition. The condition is reversible with vitamin A supplementation (40).

B Vitamins

Atrophy of taste buds occurs with various B vitamin deficiencies, as does glossitis. The condition is quickly reversed with B vitamin supplementation.

Copper

Copper deficiency is associated with reduced sensitivity to the taste of salt and a relative salt craving. Copper repletion reverses the condition.

Zinc

Zinc deficiency may impair taste, but definitive evidence in humans is lacking.

Salt

Preferences for salt have been proved malleable in response to habitual exposure. Exposure to high- or low-salt diets over a period of 6 to 8 weeks has been shown to alter preferences.

CLINICAL HIGHLIGHTS

The capacity of clinicians to influence health outcomes in their patients by means of dietary manipulation is ultimately dependent on the patients' capacity to change dietary patterns. This capacity, in turn, is dependent on the factors that govern dietary patterns and dietary preferences in the first place. Appetite, hunger, and satiety are mediated by a complex array of biopsychosocial factors.

Although neither patient nor clinician is able to directly control much of the physiology of appetite, compensations may be built into dietary practices to defend against specific vulnerabilities. When the principal threat to health is excess dietary intake, diet may be manipulated to optimize its satiating properties and minimize the stimulation of appetite. Among the many pertinent strategies (see Chapters 5 and 41) are increasing intake of fiber and complex carbohydrate, avoiding excessive variety within a given day or meal, optimizing protein intake, and restricting dietary fat intake. The effects of volume on satiety support the common practice of drinking water before a meal to help curb appetite. Conversely, when appetite is poor and dietary intake is inadequate, restricting fiber, increasing variety, and increasing fat intake may provide some compensation (see Chapter 24).

Efforts should be made to encourage par-

ents to establish judicious eating habits early in their children, as dietary habits may be increasingly resistant to change over time. Creativity in the use of ingredients can be used to reduce the fat, sugar, salt, and calorie content of foods while preserving familiar aspects of the diet important in the provision of pleasure (see Section III).

Patients who have been provided with information about the physiology of appetite may be able to make better use of nutrition labels to guard against manipulative food industry practices. A shared understanding between patient and clinician of the complex and largely involuntary nature of appetite and satiety is supportive of counseling that is practical, productive, and humane (see Chapter 41).

REFERENCES

1. Blundell J, King N. Overconsumption as a cause of weight gain: behavioural-physiological interactions in the control of food intake (appetite). *Ciba Found Symp* 1996;201:138–154.
2. Nestle M, Wing R, Birch L, et al. Behavioral and social influences on food choice. *Nutr Rev* 1998; 56:s50–s74.
3. Glanz K, Basil M, Maibach E, et al. Why Americans eat what they do: taste, nutrition, cost, convenience, and weight control concerns as influences on food consumption. *J Am Diet Assoc* 1998;98:1118–1126.
4. Drewnowski A. Taste preferences and food intake. *Annu Rev Nutr* 1997;17:237–253.
5. Gibson E, Desmond E. Chocolate craving and hunger state: implications for the acquisition and expression of appetite and food choice. *Appetite* 1999;32:219–240.
6. Coleman R, Herrmann T. Nutritional regulation of leptin in humans. *Diabetologia* 1999;42:639–646.
7. Rohner-Jeanrenaud F, Jeanrenaud B. Obesity, leptin, and the brain. *N Engl J Med* 1996;334:324–332.
8. Considine R, Sinha M, Heiman M, et al. Serum immunoreactive-leptin concentrations in normal-weight and obese humans. *N Engl J Med* 1996; 334:292–295.
9. Castro JD. Behavioral genetics of food intake regulation in free-living humans. *Nutrition* 1999;15: 550–554.
10. Drewnowski A, Hernderson S, Shore A, et al. Nontasters, tasters, and supertasters of 6-n-propylthiouracil (PROP) and hedonic response to sweet. *Physiol Behav* 1997;62:649–655.
11. Hubert P, King N, Blundell J. Uncoupling the effects of energy expenditure and energy intake: appetite response to short-term energy deficit induced by meal omission and physical activity. *Appetite* 1998;31:9–19.

12. King N. What processes are involved in the appetite response to moderate increases in exercise-induced energy expenditure? *Proc Nutr Soc* 1999;58: 107–113.

13. Rolls B. Do chemosensory changes influence food intake in the elderly? *Physiol Behav* 1999; 66:193–197.

14. Axelson M. The impact of culture on food-related behavior. *Annu Rev Nutr* 1986;6:345–363.

15. Mennella J, Beauchamp G. Early flavor experiences: research update. *Nutr Rev* 1998;56:205–211.

16. Rolls B. Sensory-specific satiety. *Nutr Rev* 1986; 44:93–101.

17. Rolls B. Experimental analyses of the effects in a meal on human feeding. *Am J Clin Nutr* 1985;42: 932–939.

18. Rogers P. Eating habits and appetite control: a psychobiological perspective. *Proc Nutr Soc* 1999; 58:59–67.

19. Louis-Sylvestre J, Tournier A, Verger P, et al. Learned caloric adjustment of human intake. *Appetite* 1989;1:95–103.

20. Melanson K, Westerterp-Plantenga M, Saris W, et al. Blood glucose patterns and appetite in time-blinded humans: carbohydrate vs. fat. *Am J Physiol* 1999;277:R337–R345.

21. Drewnowski A. Energy intake and sensory properties of food. *Am J Clin Nutr* 1995;62:1081s–1085s.

22. Lonnquist F, Nordfors L, Schalling M. Leptin and its potential role in human obesity. *J Intern Med* 1999;245:643–652.

23. Luheshi G, Gardner J, Rushforth D, et al. Leptin action on food intake and body temperature are mediated by IL-1. *Proc Natl Acad Sci U S A* 1999;96:7047–7052.

24. Heini A, Lara-Castro C, Kirk K, et al. Association of leptin and hunger-satiety ratings in obese women. *Int J Obes Relat Metab Disord* 1998;22:1084–1087.

25. Drewnowski A. Why do we like fat? *J Am Diet Assoc* 1997;97[Suppl]:s58–s62.

26. Reed D, Tordoff M. Enhanced acceptance and metabolism of fats by rats fed a high-fat diet. *Am J Physiol* 1991;261:R1084–R1088.

27. Warwick Z, Schiffman S, Anderson J. Relationship of dietary fat content to food preferences in young rats. *Physiol Behav* 1990;48:581–586.

28. Lucas F, Sclafani A. Flavor preferences conditioned by intragastric fat infusions in rats. *Physiol Behav* 1989;46:403–412.

29. Drewnowski A, Greenwood M. Cream and sugar: human preferences for high-fat foods. *Physiol Behav* 1983;30:629–633.

30. Emmett P, Heaton K. Is extrinsic sugar a vehicle for dietary fat? *Lancet* 1995;345:1537–1540.

31. Holt S, Miller J, Petocz P, et al. A satiety index of common foods. *Eur J Clin Nutr* 1995;49:675–690.

32. Holt S, Delargy H, Lawton C, et al. The effects of high-carbohydrate vs. high-fat breakfasts on feelings of fullness and alertness, and subsequent food intake. *Int J Food Sci Nutr* 1999;50:13–28.

33. Stubbs R. Peripheral signals affecting food intake. *Nutrition* 1999;15:614–625.

34. Westerterp-Plantenga M, Rolland V, Wilson S, et al. Satiety related to 24 h diet-induced thermogenesis during high protein/carbohydrate vs. high fat diets measured in a respiration chamber. *Eur J Clin Nutr* 1999;53:495–502.

35. Poppitt S, McCormack D, Buffenstein R. Short-term effects of macronutrient preloads on appetite and energy intake in lean women. *Physiol Behav* 1998;64:279–285.

36. Gendall K, Joyce P, Abbott R. The effects of meal composition on subsequent cravings and binge eating. *Addict Behav* 1999;24:305–315.

37. Rolls B, Bell E. Intake of fat and carbohydrate: role of energy density. *Eur J Clin Nutr* 1999;53:s166–s173.

38. Drewnowski A. Energy density, palatability, and satiety: implications for weight control. *Nutr Rev* 1998;56:347–353.

39. Rolls B, Castellanos V, Halford J, et al. Volume of food consumed affects satiety in men. *Am J Clin Nutr* 1998;67:1170–1177.

40. Mattes RD, Kare MR. Nutrition and the chemical senses. In: Shils ME, Olson JA, Shike M, eds. *Modern nutrition in health and disease*, 8th ed. Philadelphia: Lea & Febiger, 1994.

BIBLIOGRAPHY

See "Sources for All Chapters."

Blundell JE, Stubbs RJ. High and low carbohydrate and fat intakes: limits imposed by appetite and palatability and their implications for energy balance. *Eur J Clin Nutr* 1999;53[Suppl 1]:s148–s165.

Drewnowski A. Intense sweeteners and energy density of foods: implications for weight control. *Eur J Clin Nutr* 1999;53:757–763.

Duffy VB, Bartoshuk LM, Striegel-Moore R, et al. Taste changes across pregnancy. *Ann N Y Acad Sci* 1998;855:805–809.

Flatt JP. What do we most need to learn about food intake regulation? *Obes Res* 1998;6:307–310.

Hetherington MM. Taste and appetite regulation in the elderly. *Proc Nutr Soc* 1998;57:625–631.

Kostas G. Low-fat and delicious: can we break the taste barrier? *J Am Diet Assoc* 1997;97[7 Suppl]:s88–s92.

MacBeth H, ed. *Food preferences and taste*. Providence, RI: Berghahn Books, 1997.

Reed DR, Bachmanov AA, Beauchamp GK, et al. Heritable variation in food preferences and their contribution to obesity. *Behav Genet* 1997;27:373–387.

Rogers PJ. Eating habits and appetite control: a psychobiological perspective. *Proc Nutr Soc* 1999;58:59–67.

Rolls BJ, Bell EA. Intake of fat and carbohydrate: role of energy density. *Eur J Clin Nutr* 1999;53[Suppl 1]:s166–s173.

Rolls ET. Taste and olfactory processing in the brain and its relation to the control of eating. *Crit Rev Neurobiol* 1997;11:263–287.

Seeley RJ, Schwartz MW. Neuroendocrine regulation of food intake. *Acta Paediatr Suppl* 1999;88:58–61.

37

Vegetarianism, Veganism, and Macrobiotic Diets

INTRODUCTION

Dietary recommendations for health promotion and disease prevention consistently emphasize the importance of a diet relatively rich in fruits, vegetables, and whole grains. Thus, a vegetarian diet offers apparent health benefits, but the partial or complete exclusion of animal products from the diet does not ensure optimal or even balanced nutrition. Strict vegetarians are at potential risk of micronutrient or even protein deficiencies. A vegetarian diet based on processed rather than natural foods may combine the excesses of the western diet with the risk of such deficiencies.

Because vegetarianism is increasingly popular in western countries as a result of personal ethics or health concerns, the clinician should be prepared to distinguish prudent from imprudent vegetarian diets and offer advice as required to promote dietary balance. The potential health benefits of a nutritionally adequate vegetarian diet appear to be considerable.

OVERVIEW

Vegetarianism is a generic term encompassing a small variety of distinct dietary patterns. The term itself generally implies at least a relative avoidance of meat in the diet. Veganism is strict avoidance of all animal products, including eggs and dairy foods. Lactovegetarianism permits consumption of dairy products, but not eggs. Lactoovovegetarianism permits consumption of dairy products and eggs. Pescovegetarianism, a seldom-used term, refers to diets that permit fish but not other animal products. In common usage, "vegetarianism" may refer to any of these patterns or to the exclusion of only red meat. More restrictive patterns, such as macrobiotic diets, typically are bound by a religious or cultural belief system that stipulates the dietary exclusions.

Plant foods tend to be relatively high in fiber and consequently low in calories per unit volume. When caloric excess is more of a threat than caloric deficiency, this tends to be one of the benefits of vegetarianism, reducing the risk of obesity. Vegetarians are, on average, leaner than their omnivorous counterparts. Energy may be deficient, however, when metabolic demand is high, due to growth or activity. Thus, inclusion in the diets of vegetarian children of some calorically dense foods, such as nuts, peanut butter, avocados (one of only two "high-fat" fruits, the other being the olive), and vegetable oils may be particularly important.

Protein is widely distributed in the food supply, and total protein deficiency is unlikely to be induced by a balanced vegetarian diet. A greater risk, when dairy products and eggs are excluded from the diet along with meat, is deficiency of one or more essential amino acids, which can be avoided by balanced selection of protein sources. Beans, peas, and lentils have an excellent amino acid profile, including lysine; grains are complementary, serving as a good source of methionine (see Chapters 3 and 4). The amino acid profile of soybeans is nearly as complete as that of egg albumin, making this a particularly valuable food for vegans.

Inclusion of cereals, as well as beans, peas, or lentils; nuts or seeds; and vegetables in the daily diet is likely to ensure adequate amino acid intake. Efficient use of essential amino acids requires that all essential amino acids be present simultaneously (see Chapter 3); therefore, balanced intake must be consistent.

The fat content of vegetarian diets tends to be lower than that of corresponding omnivorous diets, but not invariably so. When dairy is included in the diet, the substitution of cheese for meat can result in high intake of saturated fat. When fat intake is kept at moderate levels, the exclusion of fish from the diet may elevate the ratio of n-6 to n-3 fatty acids. The inclusion of flaxseeds and linseeds and their oils will add α-linolenic acid to the diet and help prevent imbalance of essential fatty acids.

Several micronutrient deficiencies may result from vegetarian practices. Plant foods are less concentrated sources of iron and zinc than is meat, and the quantity present generally is less readily absorbed. Intake can be adequate when a balanced and diverse diet is maintained and absorption enhanced by concomitant intake of vitamin C. A study among Australian men comparing nearly 50 vegetarians to 25 omnivores found higher iron intake among the vegetarians, but significantly higher ferritin levels in the omnivores, suggesting the importance of dietary source and absorption (1).

Diets excluding all animal products will be subject to calcium deficiency. Although calcium is present in many vegetables, oxalate binding limits absorption and bioavailability. In vegans, calcium supplementation generally should be encouraged. Vitamin B_{12}, found only in animal foods, is apt to be deficient in vegan diets as well; supplementation is prudent. The inclusion of dairy products or eggs in the diet will help maintain adequate B_{12} stores. Vitamin D is absent from plant foods, but needs can be met by synthesis in the skin with sufficient sun exposure. Nonetheless, supplementation is prudent for vegans, particularly in temperate climates. The possibility of iodine deficiency has been raised (2), but it is an unlikely hazard if iodized salt is included in the diet.

When a vegetarian diet is based largely on processed foods, which apparently is a particular tendency among adolescents (see Chapter 28), the fiber content may be low, and the content of simple sugar may be high. Such a diet offers the potential hazards of animal food exclusions from the diet without the attendant benefits of well-practiced vegetarianism and generally should be discouraged.

Vegetarianism is increasingly popular among adolescents for reasons related to health and body image, as well as philosophy and ecology (3). There is some suggestion from survey research that vegetarianism in adolescents may be a means of masking an effort at dietary restraint (4) or even a tendency toward an eating disorder (5) (see Chapter 23).

Veganism places young children in particular at risk of nutrient deficiencies (see Chapter 27). Soy-based infant formulas can meet the nutrient needs of infants who are not breast-fed or who are weaned. As vegan infants advance to solid foods, the principles outlined earlier provide some guidance. Particular effort should be made to ensure adequate intake of dietary fat. Cholesterol, which is found only in animal products, will be absent from the diet. The general practice of referring vegan families to a dietitian for tailored advice is appropriate.

States of high metabolic demand may expose adults to the same hazards of overly restrictive diets as children. Pregnancy, lactation, chronic disease, trauma, acute infection, and high levels of physical activity require heightened attention to ensure adequate intake of energy, protein, and micronutrients. The possibility of both clinical and subclinical disturbances in the menstrual cycle attributed to vegetarianism have been reported, but evidence is inconclusive (6). If such disturbances exist, low body fat content is one putative explanation, with resultant reduction in estradiol levels.

A vegetarian diet has been used in the context of a randomized pilot study in subjects with noninsulin-dependent diabetes mellitus (7). Compared with a conventional low-fat diet, the vegan diet used in the study produced significant reductions in weight, fasting glucose levels, and the need for medication over a 12-week period.

Although generally associated with reduced risk of cardiovascular disease, vegetarianism often is associated with other lifestyle practices, such as the avoidance of smoking, and physical activity that complicate attribution. In a study that matched for other aspects of lifestyle between vegetarians and omnivores, Mezzano and colleagues (8) reported elevated homocysteine and enhanced platelet aggregability in the vegetarians. A study of similar design conducted in an African population demonstrated reduced levels of fibrinolytic activity and elevated fibrinogen in omnivores compared with vegetarians (9).

A small, short-term intervention demonstrated that the addition of plant sources of n-3 fatty acids to the diet of vegetarians can alter platelet phospholipids, although effects on markers of thrombotic risk were not observed (10). Veganism has been reported to produce a more favorable lipid profile than lactoovovegetarianism among African-American Seventh Day Adventists (11). The clinical significance of the reported alterations of serum markers of cardiovascular risk is uncertain.

Inconsistency in the reported effects of vegetarianism on serum parameters of cardiovascular risk emphasizes the need for well-controlled studies of clinically impor-

tant outcomes. In the interim, observational data suggest a benefit of vegetarianism on both cardiovascular and all-cause mortality (12,13). A study of elderly women in China, for example, found that vegetarianism was associated with a reduced rate of ischemic heart disease, although vegetarians were less likely than matched omnivores to smoke (14). The vegetarians in this study were subject to anemia due to deficiencies of vitamin B_{12} or iron, or both.

The macrobiotic diet, which was developed by a Japanese spiritualist, is actually a series of ten increasingly restricted diets. Adherents begin with a diverse and balanced diet, then progress in stages to a diet that excludes all but cereal grains, ostensibly in pursuit of spiritual purity. Vitamin B_{12} deficiency has been shown to persist following a macrobiotic diet, even after conversion to more mainstream dietary patterns (15). An association with reduced bone mass also has been reported (16). The upper levels of the diet have resulted in overt cases of nutritional deficiency and even death, and, from a health care perspective, are to be adamantly discouraged.

CLINICAL HIGHLIGHTS

Observational data suggest that vegetarianism is associated with reduced risk of various chronic diseases and all-cause mortality. Such findings are potentially confounded by other health-promoting behaviors often associated with vegetarianism. Studies of serum markers of cardiovascular risk are conflicting and inconclusive, although most suggest a benefit of plant-based diets.

Whether vegetarianism is nutritionally optimal or simply superior to prevailing dietary patterns in the West is uncertain. Strict veganism poses some risk of micronutrient deficiencies, particularly of zinc, iron, calcium, and vitamins B_{12} and D. A diverse and balanced vegan diet that meets all nutrient needs, however, is readily achievable. Adolescents appear to be at particular risk of unbalanced vegetarian practices and should receive dietary counseling; routine referral to a dietitian is appropriate.

All vegetarian patients should be interviewed briefly to ascertain whether the diet is based on a balanced distribution of plant-based foods or on a preponderance of processed foods. In the latter instance, the patient is subject to the excesses of the western diet and to nutrient deficiencies as well and should be counseled accordingly. For both reasons, if the patient is not well informed about the protein and nutrient content of plant foods, referring the patient to print and web-based sources of information (see Section III) and to a dietitian for detailed counseling is warranted. The optimal distribution of nutrient intake for health promotion (see Chapter 40) is achievable with a vegetarian diet. Although a plant-based diet is rich in many micronutrients, certain deficiencies are particularly probable. A daily multivitamin/mineral supplement is advisable, as is additional calcium supplementation (see Table, Section III) if dairy is excluded from the diet.

REFERENCES

1. Wilson AK, Ball MJ. Nutrient intake and iron status of Australian male vegetarians. *Eur J Clin Nutr* 1999;53:189.
2. Remer T, Neubert A, Manz F. Increased iodine deficiency with vegetarian nutrition. *Br J Nutr* 1999;81:45–49.
3. Johnston PK, Haddad E, Sabate J. The vegetarian adolescent. *Adolesc Med* 1992;3:417–438.
4. Martins Y, Pliner P, O'Connor R. Restrained eating among vegetarians: does a vegetarian eating style mask concerns about weight? *Appetite* 1999; 32:145–154.
5. Neumark-Sztainer D, Story M, Resnick MD, et al. Adolescent vegetarians. A behavioral profile of a school-based population in Minnesota. *Arch Pediatr Adolesc Med* 1997;151:833–838.
6. Barr SI. Vegetarianism and menstrual cycle disturbances: is there an association? *Am J Clin Nutr* 1999;70:549s–554s.
7. Nicholson AS, Sklar M, Barnard ND, et al. Toward improved management of NIDDM: A randomized, controlled, pilot intervention using a lowfat, vegetarian diet. *Prev Med* 1999;29:87–91.
8. Mezzano D, Munoz X, Martinez C, et al. Vegetarians and cardiovascular risk factors: hemostasis, inflammatory markers and plasma homocysteine. *Thromb Haemost* 1999;81:913–917.
9. Famodu AA, Osilesi O, Makinde YO, et al. The influence of a vegetarian diet on haemostatic factors for cardiovascular disease in Africans. *Thromb Res* 1999;95:31–36.
10. Li D, Sinclair A, Wilson A, et al. Effect of dietary alpha-linolenic acid on thrombotic risk factors in vegetarian men. *Am J Clin Nutr* 1999;69:872–882.
11. Toohey ML, Harris MA, DeWitt W, et al. Cardiovascular disease risk factors are lower in African-American vegans compared to lacto-ovo-vegetarians. *J Am Coll Nutr* 1998;17:425–434.
12. Key TJ, Thorogood M, Appleby PN, et al. Dietary habits and mortality in 11,000 vegetarians and health conscious people: results of a 17 year follow up. *BMJ* 1996;313:775–779.
13. Frentzel-Beyme R, Chang-Claude J. Vegetarian diets and colon cancer: the German experience. *Am J Clin Nutr* 1994;59:1143s–1152s.
14. Woo J, Kwok T, Ho SC, et al. Nutritional status of elderly Chinese vegetarians. *Age Ageing* 1998;27: 455–461.
15. van Dusseldorp M, Schneede J, Refsum H, et al. Risk of persistent cobalamin deficiency in adolescents fed a macrobiotic diet in early life. *Am J Clin Nutr* 1999;69:664–671.
16. Parsons TJ, van Dusseldorp M, van der Vliet M, et al. Reduced bone mass in Dutch adolescents fed a macrobiotic diet in early life. *J Bone Miner Res* 1997;12:1486–1494.

BIBLIOGRAPHY

See "Sources for All Chapters."
Dwyer JT. Health aspects of vegetarian diets. *Am J Clin Nutr* 1988;48:712–738.
Hackett A, Nathan I, Burgess L. Is a vegetarian diet adequate for children? *Nutr Health* 1998;12:189–195.
Sanders TA. Vegetarian diets and children. *Pediatr Clin North Am* 1995;42:955–965.

38

Macronutrient Food Substitutes

INTRODUCTION

Macronutrient substitutes generally are used to replace either sugar or fat in the diet. The intent of such substitutions is to reduce caloric intake, dental caries, and chronic disease risk, and to improve glucose and insulin metabolism and serum lipid levels. Carbohydrate substitutes may be used to replace starch as well as sugar. Fat is replaced with other macronutrients (protein or carbohydrate) modified to mimic the sensory characteristics of fat; synthetic substitutes that replace fat on a gram-for-gram basis but provide fewer or even no calories; or reduced-calorie fat molecules. Sugar substitutes are divided into nonnutritive intense sweeteners and nutritive bulk sweeteners.

OVERVIEW

Sweeteners/Sugar Substitutes

Sugar substitution generally is intended either to reduce calorie intake or to avoid cariogenic exposures to sucrose. A causal role for dietary sugar in attention-deficit disorder of children does not appear to be substantiated (1); thus, sugar substitution is not of therapeutic value in that disorder.

Nonnutritive Sweeteners

Nonnutritive intense sweeteners work particularly well in beverages, as the loss of sugar bulk does not compromise the product.

Intense sweeteners commonly used in the United States include saccharin, aspartame, and acesulfame-K; sucralose also is approved for use (2). A variety of plant-derived intense sweeteners are used in other countries and are under study (2).

Saccharin is a synthetic compound with sweetness intensity up to 500 times that of sugar. It becomes bitter with heating, and for that reason it can only be used in foods served cool. Animal studies with doses far beyond those expected in humans have raised concern about carcinogenicity, but there are no human epidemiologic data to support an association. The extrapolation of animal data regarding the carcinogenicity of saccharin to humans may not be justified based both on dose and mechanism (3). Saccharin is excreted unmetabolized in urine and egested in stool. The FDA has removed saccharin from its list of carcinogens.

Aspartame is composed of two amino acids. Metabolism of aspartame yields phenylalanine and aspartic acid. Unlike saccharin, aspartame provides some nutrient energy, although very little. Like saccharin, it does not tolerate heat and is limited to foods served cool. Aspartame is approximately 160 times as sweet as sugar. Because it contains phenylalanine, it is contraindicated in phenylketonuria.

The metabolism of phenylalanine to norepinephrine and epinephrine has raised concern that aspartame ingestion could alter neurotransmitter levels and result in neurotoxicity; no data support this theoretical concern.

Acesulfame-K is a synthetic compound nearly 200 times as sweet as sugar. It often is used in combination with other synthetic sweeteners in processed foods. Unlike saccharin and aspartame, acesulfame-K is stable when heated. Commercially prepared sugar substitutes often are combinations of natural sugar and an intense sweetener.

Bulking Agents

In solid foods, sugar provides both sweetness and bulk/texture; therefore, substitution calls for both intense sweeteners and bulking agents. Polyols, or sugar alcohols, are hydrogenated simple sugar analogues. They tend to be used in candies and gum. Sugar alcohols are less bioavailable in the upper gastrointestinal tract than are the parent sugars. As a result, such sugars reach, and are fermented in, the large bowel. Sugar fermentation in the colon produces heat, gaseous waste such as methane, and short-chain fatty acids, thus releasing less usable energy than sugar absorption in the small bowel. Commonly used sugar alcohols include sorbitol, with an estimated energy content of 2.6 kcal/g; xylitol, with 2.4 kcal/g; and isomalt, with 2.0 kcal/g.

Sugar alcohols are less cariogenic than glucose or sucrose. Use of sorbitol and xylitol in chewing gum prevents the generation of cariogenic acid (4). Xylitol has antibacterial effects, reducing colony counts of *Streptococcus mutans* (4). Evidence that xylitol is noncariogenic is clear, but evidence of an actual preventive or therapeutic effect is only preliminary (5).

Sorbitol is directly oxidized to fructose and does not appreciably raise serum glucose or insulin levels. At high doses, sorbitol has a laxative effect due to its slow absorption. Erythritol is a bulking agent sugar with no caloric value. Other bulking agent sugar substitutes include the sugar alcohols lactitol and maltitol, reduced starch hydrolysates, fructooligosaccharides, and polydextrose.

A variety of natural fibers are used as bulking agents. Galctomannans derived from guar gum and locust bean gum often are used in reduced-fat or reduced calorie foods to restore texture and consistency. Cellulose, derived from the cell walls of plants, is used as a noncaloric bulking agent. Some forms of starch are resistant to digestive enzymes and are of potential use as bulking agents. Resistant starch may offer health benefits comparable to those of dietary fiber. Guar, pectin, and inulin are commonly used carbohydrate bulking agents. Resistant starch in the large bowel increases bacterial mass, reduces transit time, and increases levels of butyrate, which is known to have antiproliferative properties. Therefore, resistant starches may reduce colon cancer risk by several mechanisms.

Fat Substitutes

Availability, familiarity, and selectivity mediate food choice, as do anticipation and expectation based on taste, color, texture, and odor (6). The use of macronutrient substitutes is directed at preserving the familiarity of traditional foods, a factor known to be a powerful determinant of dietary preference (7). The rate of introduction of fat-reduced foods by the food industry accelerated markedly during the 1990s, and thousands of products now are available (7). By reducing the energy density of foods, macronutrient substitutes generally raise the nutrient density of the diet (the ratio of micronutrients per unit energy).

The principal rationale for fat substitution is to reduce an individual's fat intake and the energy density of food to help prevent obesity and the development of chronic diseases. Energy excess in the diet has differential effects on the metabolic processing of macronutrients. Oxidation of both carbohydrate and protein is augmented when energy is ingested in excess of need (8). In contrast, fat intake in excess of energy needs does not lead to enhanced oxidation, but rather to enhanced storage.

Obesity on a population basis is consistently associated with high-fat dietary patterns. Increasing adiposity does promote fat oxidation, so that a new equilibrium state is established (8). Relatively high intake of dietary fat is associated with enhanced efficiency in fat metabolism so that fat is more readily stored in adipose tissue.

Although the use of fat substitutes to reduce dietary fat is based in part on the goal of reducing chronic disease, to date there is no direct evidence that fat substitution is associated with reduced disease risk. The available evidence suggests that fat substitutes are generally effective at reducing fat intake, but not necessarily at reducing calorie intake, as compensation may occur. The use of intense sweeteners may result in caloric compensation as well (9).

There is some evidence that satiety may depend more on food mass than calories, resulting in reduced energy consumption when food is made relatively dilute in calories.

Population survey data indicate that nearly 90% of consumers eat fat-reduced products, and nearly 80% do so within any 2-week period (9). Modified foods apparently are used more often than exercise as a weight-loss strategy (9). Increased dietary fat consumption, as well as increased intake of animal protein, is consistently associated with the greater dietary variety that accompanies rising gross national product and per capita income. There currently is no evidence to indicate that a society can revert back to a simpler, less varied, less energy-dense diet once the "western" pattern has been assumed (9). Therefore, food modification as one aspect of efforts to modify the nutritional environment is seemingly justified (9).

The three categories of fat replacers are fat mimetics, fat substitutes, and low-calorie fats.

Fat in foods confers many properties beyond energy density, including effects on flavor and palatability, and creaminess and mouth feel. Ingredient substitutions in fat-reduced foods often are directed at restoring these characteristics to foods.

Fat mimetics are nonfat constituents of foods that replace fats, mimic the properties

fats confer, and add fewer calories than the fats they replace. Examples include starches, cellulose, pectin, proteins, dextrins, polydextrose, and other products. Fat mimetics often are useful in desserts and spreads, but generally of less use in foods that require frying or other high-temperature preparation. Fat mimetics range from 0 to 4 kcal/g.

Reduced-calorie fats are triglycerides modified to deliver less than the 9 kcal/g of most naturally occurring fats. Medium-chain triglycerides provide 7 to 8 kcal/g. Other commercially produced low-calorie fats are poorly absorbed because they are composed of fatty acids of varying chain lengths attached to glycerol. The calorie content of such products as Caprenin (Procter & Gamble) and Salatrim (Nabisco) is approximately 5 kcal/g. Soluble fibers used as fat substitutes confer health benefits independent of fat replacement, such as cholesterol reduction and reduced postprandial insulin release (10). For some individuals, processed fat-reduced foods could become a significant source of soluble fiber.

Limited evidence from dietary intervention trials of short duration and studies of consumer behavior reviewed by Mela (11) suggests that compensation for energy reduction resulting from macronutrient substitutions is consistent. Fat substitutes do not result in compensatory fat intake, however, and the reduced energy density of the diet apparently is associated with modest weight loss (11). Dietary fat reduction is helpful in long-term maintenance of weight loss, and fat substitutes may be useful in this context (12). Evidence that macronutrient substitutes adversely affect micronutrient intake is generally limited, with some evidence of beneficial effects (13). Consumption of fat-reduced products is much less commonly reported by African-Americans than by non-Hispanic whites (13).

The substitution of skim milk for whole milk and of lean meats for beef reduces intake of fat and saturated fat, but not to recommended levels (14). Therefore, additional dietary modifications are required to achieve recommended dietary patterns. Consistent substitution of fat-reduced or nonfat foods for their standard-fat counterparts would achieve fat intake goals, according to computer modeling (14). Evidence is fairly convincing that fat substitutes sustainably lower fat intake, but their effect on energy intake is as yet uncertain (15). Children may be particularly adept at compensating for the calorie reductions associated with macronutrient substitutes, although the compensation may not be complete (16). As is true of adults, energy compensation in children is not specific to the macronutrient class being manipulated.

The most studied fat substitute to date is the sucrose polyester olestra developed by Procter & Gamble. Variations in the length of the fatty acids esterified can alter the melting point and other physical properties of the product. Because it is essentially indigestible, olestra passes through the gastrointestinal tract carrying fat-soluble micronutrients with it. Approved by the Food and Drug Administration for use in snack foods, olestra is controversial because of the potential for gastrointestinal upset and the leaching of fat-soluble nutrients. A variety of products derived from alterations of fat molecules is under development.

In a randomized, double-blind, placebo-controlled crossover trial of 51 adults, Hill and colleagues (17) demonstrated that olestra resulted in significant reductions in fat and energy intake over a 14-day period. Subjects compensated for 15% of the fat and 20% of the energy reduction. In a placebo-controlled study of more than 3,000 volunteers, snack foods containing olestra eaten *ad libitum* did not produce any more gastrointestinal symptoms than those containing standard fat (18).

Miller et al. (19) found that fat and energy intake were reduced by consumption of olestra-containing chips rather than standard chips whether or not informative nutrition labels were provided. Cotton and colleagues (20) demonstrated that the degree of compensation is increased when the dietary fat reduction is more extreme. When fat intake was reduced by means of olestra from 32% to 20% of calories, subjects compensated for 74% of the energy deficit on the following day (20).

Olestra decreases absorption of vitamins A, D, E, and K, but this effect is at least partially compensated by the fortification of olestra-containing foods with fat-soluble vitamins (21). Most evidence suggests that olestra-containing snack foods, when consumed under ordinary circumstances, do not produce any more gastrointestinal symptoms than standard products (21). Concern has been expressed, however, regarding the intensity of Procter & Gamble's campaign to win support for the product (22).

Food substitutes based on unique chemical properties must generally be approved by the Food and Drug Administration through a process known as a food additive petition (FAP). Relatively minor modifications of natural foods may be approved through a less arduous process in which the product is labeled as GRAS ("generally recognized as safe") (see www.FDA.gov for more information).

CLINICAL HIGHLIGHTS

There is convincing evidence that judicious use of macronutrient substitutes can provide distinct health benefits. Sugar substitutes are of principal value in reducing the risk of dental caries, although the use of sugar substitutes to reduce energy intake also is of potential value. Fat substitution is beneficial in reducing both the fat content of the diet and total energy intake. Evidence that macronutrient substitutions contribute to sustainable weight loss is suggestive.

Recommendations to patients should emphasize a dietary pattern based largely on whole grains, vegetables, and fruits. In such a context, the use of macronutrient substitutes in processed foods may help to further reduce fat and energy intake; to increase the nutrient density of the diet; to increase dietary fiber; and to attenuate various risk factors for chronic disease. Therefore, such substitutions should be encouraged as an adjuvant, but certainly not an alternative, to efforts at achieving a salutary dietary pattern.

REFERENCES

1. Baxter P. Attention-deficit hyperactivity disorder in children. *Curr Opin Pediatr* 1995;7:381–386.
2. Kinghorn A, Kaneda N, Baeck N, et al. Noncariogenic intense natural sweeteners. *Med Res Rev* 1998;18:347–360.
3. Cohen S. Human relevance of animal carcinogenicity studies. *Regul Toxicol Pharmacol* 1995;21:75–80.
4. Edgar W. Sugar substitutes, chewing gum and dental caries—a review. *Br Dent J* 1998;184:29–32.
5. Scheie A, Fejerskov O. Xylitol in caries prevention: what is the evidence for clinical efficacy? *Oral Dis* 1998;4:268–278.
6. Grivetti L. Social determinants of food intake. In: Anderson G, Rolls B, Steffen D, eds. *Nutritional implications of macronutrient substitutes. Annals of the New York Academy of Sciences.* New York: The New York Academy of Sciences, 1997.
7. Anderson G. Nutritional and health aspects of macronutrient substitution. In: Anderson G, Rolls B, Steffen D, eds. *Nutritional implications of macronutrient substitutes. Annals of the New York Academy of Sciences.* New York: The New York Academy of Sciences, 1997.
8. Tartaranni P, Ravussin E. Effect of fat intake on energy balance. In: Anderson G, Rolls B, Steffen D, eds. *Nutritional implications of macronutrient substitutes. Annals of the New York Academy of Sciences.* New York: The New York Academy of Sciences, 1997.
9. Anderson G, Rolls B, Steffen D, eds. *Nutritional implications of macronutrient substitutes. Annals of the New York Academy of Sciences.* New York: The New York Academy of Sciences, 1997.
10. Behall K. Dietary fiber: nutritional lessons for macronutrient substitutes. In: Anderson G, Rolls B, Steffen D, eds. *Nutritional implications of macronutrient substitutes. Annals of the New York Academy of Sciences.* New York: The New York Academy of Sciences, 1997.
11. Mela D. Impact of macronutrient-substituted foods on food choice and dietary intake. In: Anderson G, Rolls B, Steffen D, eds. *Nutritional implications of macronutrient substitutes. Annals of the New York Academy of Sciences.* New York: The New York Academy of Sciences, 1997.
12. Peters J. Nutritional aspects of macronutrient-substitute intake. In: Anderson G, Rolls B, Steffen D, eds. *Nutritional implications of macronutrient substitutes. Annals of the New York Academy of Sciences.* New York: The New York Academy of Sciences, 1997.
13. Heimbach J, van der Riet B, Egan S. Impact of the use of reduced-fat foods on nutrient adequacy. In: Anderson G, Rolls B, Steffen D, eds. *Nutritional implications of macronutrient substitutes. Annals of the New York Academy of Sciences.* New York: The New York Academy of Sciences, 1997.
14. Morgan R, Sigman-Grant M, Taylor D, et al. Impact of macronutrient substitutes on the composition of the diet and U.S. food supply. In: Anderson G, Rolls B, Steffen D, eds. *Nutritional implications of macronutrient substitutes. Annals of the New York Academy of Sciences.* New York: The New York Academy of Sciences, 1997.
15. Lawton C, Blundell J. The role of reduced fat diets and fat substitutes in the regulation of energy and fat intake and body weight. *Curr Opin Lipidol* 1998;9:41–45.
16. Birch L, Fisher J. Food intake regulation in children. Fat and sugar substitutes and intake. In: Anderson G, Rolls B, Steffen D, eds. *Nutritional implications of macronutrient substitutes. Annals of the New York Academy of Sciences.* New York: The New York Academy of Sciences, 1997.
17. Hill J, Seagle H, Johnson S, et al. Effects of 14 d of covert substitution of olestra for conventional fat on spontaneous food intake. *Am J Clin Nutr* 1998;67:1178–1185.
18. Sandler R, Zorich N, Filloon T, et al. Gastrointestinal symptoms in 3181 volunteers ingesting snack foods containing olestra or triglycerides. A 6-week randomized, placebo-controlled trial. *Ann Intern Med* 1999;130:253–261.
19. Miller DL, Castellanos VH, Shide DJ, et al. Effect of fat-free potato chips with and without nutrition labels on fat and energy intakes. *Am J Clin Nutr* 1998;68:282.
20. Cotton J, Weststrate J, Blundell J. Replacement of dietary fat with sucrose polyester: effects on energy intake and appetite control in nonobese males. *Am J Clin Nutr* 1996;63:891–896.
21. Thomson A, Hunt R, Zorich N. Review article: olestra and gastrointestinal safety. *Aliment Pharmacol Ther* 1998;12:1185–1200.
22. Nestle M. The selling of Olestra. *Public Health* 1998;113:508–520.

BIBLIOGRAPHY

See "Sources for All Chapters."

Blundell JE, Green SM. Effect of sucrose and sweeteners on appetite and energy intake. *Int J Obes Relat Metab Disord* 1996;20[Suppl 2]:s12.

Drewnowski A. Intense sweeteners and energy density of foods: implications for weight control. *Eur J Clin Nutr* 1999;53:757.

Kinghorn AD, Kaneda N, Baek NI, et al. Noncariogenic intense natural sweeteners. *Med Res Rev* 1998;18:347.

SECTION II

Principles of Dietary Counseling

39

Evolutionary Biology, Culture and Determinants of Human Behavior

If the presence of certain airborne toxins led researchers to conclude that human health would be promoted were we all to breathe under water, we as clinicians would surely hesitate before offering that advice to our patients. The salient fact that we cannot breathe under water would, and should, concern us more than the putative benefits of doing so. Even if a science developed that made it possible to distinguish—by virtue of depth, temperature, and content—optimal from less optimal water, the futility of such inquiry would impress us more than any such insights.

The fact is, we cannot breathe in water (while other species can), simply because we have not been designed to do so by the forces of evolution. Encouraging our patients to breathe in ways they cannot is not unlike encouraging them to eat in ways they cannot.

Among the environmental forces shaping the adaptation of species, diet, no less than air, has played a premier role (1–3). Only food, water, and air have been at work on our physiology from both without and within. Although the role of diet in evolution was clear to Darwin and seems self-evident now, much of dietary counseling and nutrition policy ignore its implications.

The conventional practice of nutrition counseling relies principally on an understanding of what patients should be advised to eat. That information becomes essential once we know why people eat as they do and understand what impediments must be overcome to change dietary behavior. But it is of decidedly less value with these questions unanswered. Limited success in the promotion of health and the amelioration of disease through the provision of dietary counseling (4–7) is cause not to renounce responsibilities in this area, but rather to reconsider how they can be fulfilled.

The adaptations of our own species are less apparent to us than those of others and consequently are readily overlooked. Consider for a moment a polar bear in its natural habitat. Better still, consider 1,000 polar bears, and transplant them all to Morocco. Let their perspicuous demise play itself briefly in your mind, as you consider its cause and obvious remedy. Now consider 1,000 people, or better still several hundred million, in their natural habitat. No particular scene springs readily to mind, for our apparent mastery of the environment has obscured our relationship with it. But although our ingenuity has largely allowed us to overcome the constraints of climate, we have fared less well in our excursions beyond the bounds of the native human diet (3). Much of the chronic disease burden and the majority of deaths in the industrialized world are directly or indirectly linked to a lifestyle and a diet at odds with human physiology (8–10).

For most species, the limits of tolerance are blatantly displayed in anatomic variation: the length of a coat, the presence of gills, the shape of a beak. If we generally overlook the limits of human environmental tolerance, it is because our frailties are concealed from view. We, less visibly but otherwise no less than any species, are well suited for a particular environment and ill suited for others. To compensate for incompatibilities between human health and the prevailing environment, those incompatibilities must be understood. To modify human dietary behavior, we must know why we eat as we do (11).

Prehuman history, and consequently the origins of human dietary behavior, can be traced back reliably at least 4 million years (2). By examining fossilized teeth and fossilized human feces (coprolites) and by studying scanning electron microscopy of dental wear patterns, paleoanthropologists have gained considerable insight into prehuman nutrition.

The earliest identifiable human progenitors were arboreal, and they were predominantly if not exclusively herbivorous (2,3). Over hundreds of thousands of years, prehuman primates increased in size and descended from the trees. As the cranial vault grew and intellect increased, our ancestors came together in cooperative groups, began to use first bone and then stone implements, and were able to scavenge successfully. Australopithecines began to use bone implements and were able to add meat to the diet through scavenging nearly 4 million years ago. Prehuman advances have been characterized by the nature of tools devised and used. Most of the 4-million-year-long human evolutionary period, characterized by the use of rough stone implements, is known as the Paleolithic; the Neolithic period was ushered in by the manufacture of polished stone implements, little more than 10,000 years ago (12).

Advanced australopithecines ultimately were supplanted by *Homo erectus,* the first member of the genus *Homo,* which dates back approximately 2 million years; the genus included the species habilis, erectus, and sapiens. *Homo habilis* scavenged more successfully than its predecessors, but had limited success in hunting. The greater cranial capacity of *H. erectus* permitted the planning and organizing necessary to ambush large game. Our ancestors became successful hunters in the time of *H. erectus* and continued to refine their skills thereafter. Hunting became particularly important during the ascendancy of the species sapiens, in particular *Homo sapiens neanderthalensis.* The earliest members of *H. sapiens* date back some 300,000 years: *H. sapiens neanderthalensis* approximately 100,000 years, Cro-Magnon humans as much as 50,000 years ago, and modern *H. sapiens sapiens* approximately 30,000 years (13,14).

Although our ancestors became increasingly successful at hunting over time, studies of both the fossil record and modern-day hunter-gatherers suggest that early hominids obtained no more than 30% to 40% of total calories from hunting, with the remainder obtained through gathering. Nonetheless, even a partial dependency on the hunt meant that as soon as prehumans began to eat more than vegetable matter, food supply was always in question. A large kill might supply an abundance of food for a brief period, but invariably it was followed by periods of famine. The cyclical redundancy of feast and famine was among the salient characteristics of the nutritional environment to which our ancestors adapted, characterizing more than 99% of the hominid era on earth (15).

A pattern of eating in excess of caloric need and storing fat to endure periods of relative deprivation is observed in modern hunter-gatherers and is thought likely to have characterized the Paleolithic period as well (16). Because of the harsh survival demands of their world, including malnutrition, our ancestors lived a truncated life by modern standards; 19 of 20 Neanderthals (middle Paleolithic) were dead by the time they were 40; ten of them by the age of 20 (2).

An increasing reliance on meat in the diet did not expose our ancestors to the type of dietary fat implicated in the chronic disease burden of developed countries. Although at times prehistoric hunters consumed a great deal of meat (17), they consumed very different meat than we do today. Modern beef cattle are 25% to 30% fat by weight, whereas the average fat content of free-living African herbivores, thought to be representative of their ancestors, is 3.9% (3). Further, the flesh of wild game contains more than five times more polyunsaturated fat per gram than is found in modern meat, and it contains n-3 (omega-3) fatty acids, which are almost completely absent from domestic beef (3).

Paleolithic humans consumed far more fiber than we do, more calcium, a sixth of the current US intake of sodium, and abundant vitamins from the variety of plant foods consumed. They generally ate much less fat than we do, although the amount varied with time and place (17), and they may have even exceeded our intake of cholesterol from consumption of meat, eggs, organs, and bone marrow (2,3). Western society, over the course of recent decades, has progressively consumed more fat, less starch, more sugar, and less grains and fiber (18), further distancing us from the diet of our ancestry. Public response to the proliferation of nutritional recommendations has not reversed this trend (19).

Also noteworthy is the dramatic decline in caloric expenditure since the Paleolithic. Our ancestors are estimated to have consumed more calories than we do, but to have burned more than twice as many in the performance of work (3). Skeletal remains indicate that despite high caloric consumption, our ancestors were consistently lean. A discrepancy between caloric intake and expenditure, and the consequent advent of obesity, is a modern phenomenon with origins in the industrial revolution (3). The impact of energy-saving devices on caloric expenditure has accelerated over the course of recent decades. Data in Great Britain reveal a 65% decline in work-related caloric expenditure since the 1950s (20).

The point of origin of human civilization is subject to debate, but the weight of evidence continues to favor Mesopotamia (2,21). Agriculture developed approximately 12,000 years ago in the delta of the Tigris and Euphrates rivers in what is now Iraq. Sumerians formalized agriculture based on irrigation, permitting the establishment of a reliable food supply for the first time in history.

A predictable food supply gave rise to unprecedented population density. Repeated cycles of irrigation caused salt to precipitate in the soil, destroying its fertility. For the first time, the nutritional needs of a human population exceeded the potential yield from hunting and gathering. The large, concentrated population that agriculture had sustained was compelled to spread out in search of adequate sustenance, giving rise to a human diaspora that ultimately colonized the planet and initiated trade, exploration, and conquest.

The notable nutritional consequence of human dispersion was dietary variation due largely to variations in climate and soil. Each new excursion resulted in the failure of certain established crops and the successful cultivation of new staples. Whereas barley was the principal grain in Mesopotamia, wheat flourished in Egypt, and bread was invented there (2,22).

Naturally, as humanity spread west, it also spread east. The reliance on millet and rice in the diets of eastern Asia reflects the early success of these crops there (23). Each interaction of human population and food supply left an indelible imprint on culture. The need to regulate the distribution of water in irrigation ditches along the banks of the Nile gave rise to centralized regulation that evolved into the pharaonic system of government. Legends developed around the public works of early Chinese leaders committed to producing more arable land to support a growing population.

In ancient Greece, a distinct culture by 1200 BC, olive trees were widely planted to replace trees felled to build houses and ships primarily because olive trees grew well over superficial limestone characteristic of Greece. A demand for oil in cooking resulted in reliance on the olive as a source because it happened to be readily available. The now recognized health benefits of monounsaturated fatty acids (MUFAs) were introduced into the Mediterranean diet by happenstance. By the fourth century BC, a privileged class in Greece was enjoying a relatively rich diet; this group may have unknowingly benefited from the influence of monounsaturated fatty acids (24).

In ancient Rome, the need to feed a swelling population fostered conquest and further territorial expansion. Greater class distinctions encouraged a taste for the exotic among the wealthy. For the first time, dietary excess became a public health problem, albeit for a select group. The origins of "processing" are traced to Rome and may reflect a preference for heavily seasoned food as a result of nearly universal lead poisoning and a resultant blunting of taste (25).

Medieval Europe with its feudal system was profoundly influenced by food supply. Bread was a mainstay of the diet, and the word "lord" derives from the old English word "hlaford," meaning "keeper of the bread." Throughout the medieval period, shortages of food were frequent in late winter, and various pests decimated crops at regular intervals. The dense concentration of European populations, the lack of animal proteins in the diets of serfs, and widespread crop shortages were reflected in human stature. Human beings, both in the new world and old, were on average 6 inches shorter than their hunting ancestors (26). Average height reached the level of the earliest humans again only after the industrial revolution. In the Americas, corn thrived and became a staple. The tomato initially was discovered as a "weed" in the corn fields of ancient central America (27).

The human diaspora has served largely to obscure the link between humanity and dietary adaptations about which generalizations can be made. The marked variations in diets around the globe in the modern era have concealed our common origins and our generally common dietary preferences. An obvious example is the Far East. The current ascendancy of the western or American dietary pattern as the global preference reveals our shared taste for sugar, salt, and fat and is a predictable consequence of our common origins (2,28).

The process of natural selection during the Paleolithic era remains an essential consideration in human dietary behavior, as the human genome is essentially unchanged for thousands and perhaps tens of thousands of years (2,3,29,30). The current nutritional environment is one to which humanity has not had adequate time to adapt genetically (30a). We are still characterized by the endowment of evolution, however irrelevant that legacy may now seem. The recent work of anthropologists reveals, for example, that men generally perform better than women in judging distance and throwing accurately, and that this ability is genetically sex-linked in a way that suggests it must have conferred an advantage that worked primarily through the male. Similarly, studies suggest that women see better in dim light and have sharper hearing. Such attributes would have served them well when they were searching for edible plants or tracking small game (2).

The prevailing diet of our distant ancestors remains the principal determinant of our nutritional physiology. The diet and the nutritional environment to which our ancestors adapted still dictate our preferences, tendencies, and aversions. That humanity adapted genetically to nutritional, environmental pressures, may explain, in part, the prevalence of chronic disease in modern society.

In 1962, Neel (15) postulated that genes associated with type II diabetes mellitus were too prevalent in the gene pool to comply with conventional paradigms of genetic disease. Invoking the sickle cell gene as an analogy, Neel (15) proposed that the "gene" for diabetes provided a survival advantage in the prevailing nutritional environment of human prehistory. The metabolically efficient individual, able to process and store energy optimally in times of plenty, almost certainly was best suited to endure periods of deprivation. The genotype, which under conditions of dietary excess manifests as obesity and type II diabetes, may have been the salvation of our nutritionally insecure ancestors (15).

This concept has since been embraced more broadly. As stated by Eaton and Konner (31) in an article on Paleolithic nutrition reported in the *New England Journal of Medicine* in 1985, "diets available to preagricultural human beings [determine]...the nutrition for which human beings are in essence genetically programmed." The authors contend that the divergence of humanity from the dietary pattern to which it adapted has significant implications for health (31).

The imprint of evolution remains readily apparent in the idiosyncrasies of modern human dietary behavior and nutritional physiology. Perhaps the single most important example is the nearly universal tendency to gain weight easily and to lose it with considerably more difficulty. Vulnerability to weight gain may be mediated in part through elevated sensory preferences for calorie-dense food (see Chapter 36). Such a preference, which, like Neel's purported gene for diabetes, promotes obesity under conditions of sustained nutritional abundance, may have conveyed a survival advantage during millennia of subsistence and recurrent privation (15,32).

Recent studies have begun to elucidate a genetic basis for obesity (see Chapter 5). But genes responsible for a condition now affecting more than one half of the adult population in the United States, and lower but rising proportions in all developed countries, cannot simply be labeled "defective." The same metabolic thriftiness responsible for epidemic obesity was likely essential to the survival of our ancestors in a world of dietary deprivation. This common susceptibility to weight gain has been dramatically revealed in the experience of the Pima Indians of the American southwest. Adapted to a desert diet unusually low in fat and sugar and unusually high in soluble fiber derived from mesquite, the Pimas had, until the 1940s, a health profile typical of that of other indigent groups. After World War II, the government expanded support for native Americans and provided the Pimas with, among other trappings of modern society, the typical American diet. Government support also resulted in a decrease in the caloric expenditure required for self-preservation.

In the ensuing 5 decades, the Pimas have gone on to develop the highest rates of obesity and type II diabetes of any population known (33). Although extensive study of this group has advanced our understanding of metabolic rate, the genetics of obesity, and the pathophysiology of the insulin resistance syndrome, perhaps the most interesting finding is the most intuitive. When the Pimas resume consumption of their native diet, their health problems tend to dissipate (33).

The tendency to overeat calories may derive in part from the adaptive "feasting" of our ancestors when food was available. The overconsumption of calories may be not so much a problem of self-discipline as a problem of unprecedented access to calories. The problem of dietary excess is compounded by the variety of foods constantly available to modern consumers.

Sensory-specific satiety is the tendency to become satiated by consumption of a particular food and to consume more total calories when food is available in greater variety (see Chapter 36). Satiety is thought to derive from the interplay of characteristics inherent in food and the concurrent nutritional state of the body. The expression of satiety influences nutrient intake and energy balance.

The potential teleologic advantage of sensory-specific satiety, as posited by Rolls (34), is as incentive for the requisite dietary diversity to satisfy micronutrient requirements. Under current nutritional conditions of constant variety within and between meals, however, the tendency favors caloric overindulgence (34). Satiety thresholds are higher for sweets than for other foods, a fact that may account for the consumption of dessert at the end of the meal in most cultures: when satiety is attained, sugar remains desirable (35). Craving for sweetness may have had adaptive value as long as fruits and wild honey were the only available sweet foods, for they are a quick, convenient source of calories. In addition, naturally sweet foods are less apt to be toxic than are foods with a bland or bitter taste (2).

The incorporation of new foods into our ancestral diet was contingent on negotiation of the "omnivore's paradox": although food sampling was essential to prevent nutrient deficiencies, any previously untried food represented potential danger. In reaction to these pressures, a natural curiosity developed toward new foods, whereas the degree of preference was associated with familiarity (36). Sweet food may have more readily negotiated the paradox than food associated with other flavors, because of the consistency with which such food proved to be safe (2). The innate preference for sweet taste demonstrated by human infants (37) highlights an involuntary aspect of dietary selection.

The boundaries of individual control over dietary selection in an environment of constantly abundant food have not been established. Classic experiments by Clara Davis (38,39) revealed the ability of human infants to meet metabolic needs by self-selection of diet, but only when a variety of "simple, fresh, unsophisticated foods" was made readily available. Davis and reviewers of her work concur that were children exposed to less nutritious choices, the quality of their diets would suffer (38–40). Laboratory rats that were exposed to a "supermarket diet" in addition to standard chow become obese (40–42). Unrestricted access to high-calorie, marginally nutritious foods may promote the development of obesity in children (40). Injudicious dietary patterns established early in life may contribute to the later development of heart disease, hypertension, and cancer (40,43).

Our fondness for dietary fat may derive from its prehistoric importance as a dense source of needed calories. As noted earlier, the fat available to our ancestors appears free of the ill effects of the fat we consume today. Preference for high-fat food apparently is mediated by metabolic, sensory, and sociocultural factors (see Chapter 36). There is evidence that ingestion of sugar and fat may stimulate pleasure by activation of the endogenous opioid peptide system. Consequently, there may be analogies between the intake of dietary fat and addiction (44).

Fats endow foods with a range of sensory characteristics and play a significant role in determining overall palatability. Improved socioeconomic status is associated with increased consumption of animal fats. Attempts to reduce the fat consumption of individuals or groups have been only partly successful, perhaps because of a failure to recognize that the regulation of fat consumption may have a physiologic as well as a psychological basis (44).

Studies in rats have demonstrated preferences for flavors coupled to the intragastric infusion of fat. Preference for fat was uncoupled from prior flavor preference, and the effect was enhanced by calorie deprivation (42). Generally, rats select high-fat (30% to 80%) diets when given a choice between low-fat and high-fat chow (45). The preference for high levels of dietary fat can be attributed to both the orosensory and nutritive properties of fat. Rats may have an innate attraction to the flavor of fat, but also learn to prefer fat-associated flavors based on the postingestive effects of fat. Human studies support a similar affinity for dietary fat (see Chapter 36). Fat is less readily perceived in solid foods and, therefore, more readily accepted even by subjects educated to be fat averse (46). In a study of 30 human subjects conducted over 10 days' time, Mela and Sacchetti (47) found a correlation between fat preference and adiposity.

Innate and physiologically mediated food preferences are reinforced by environmental exposures. The convenient availability of a particular food has always been a significant determinant of its selection, and familiarity is an important element in food preference (11,48). The innate predilection for sweet is modulated by experience. In an experimental setting, infants fed sweetened water exhibited a greater preference for sucrose solutions than others not previously exposed (37).

There is substantial animal evidence that familiarity is a principal determinant of dietary preferences (49). Geyer and Kare (49) studied young rats and mice and noted that the animals exhibit selective preference for the solid diet of the female from whom they received milk. The authors suggest that dietary selection by the nurturing female may be reflected in the taste of her milk.

Reed and Tordoff (50) fed nutritionally complete, isocaloric diets of differing fat composition to two groups of rats and reported that animals acclimated to the high-fat diet demonstrated greater acceptance of, and preference for, this preparation. In a similar study of weanling rats, Warwick and colleagues (51) demonstrated that 4 weeks of exposure to a high-fat diet engendered preference for high-fat preparations. In addition, rats that subsequently were crossed over to the control diet sustained the preferences for high fat generated during the earlier period. The authors suggest that sensory preferences acquired during early development may be more resistant to change than preferences acquired later (51).

In addition to the available research, there is the universally available empirical evidence that diverse human cultures have evolved preferences for a wide range of diets. That the palatability of such diets often is culturally limited and defined suggests that familiarity is significant. Human diets incorporate a spectrum of innately unpalatable tastes. Mechanisms responsible for the development of preference for an innately unpalatable substance remain largely unknown (37). One apparent mediator of preference for a particular taste is its association with a context of appropriate, or familiar, food. Preference for this context, itself, appears to be culturally mediated (37).

The differences between dietary patterns in the United States and Japan, for example, have been ascribed to disparate tastes and preferences (44). As the standard of living among Japanese has risen, however, the pop-ularity of meat and imported fast foods has increased in proportion to their accessibility (44). Nutritional differences between the Japanese and American diets, and among diets globally, are waning (52,53). Universal dietary preferences evidently predominate over cultural patterns as nutrient-dilute, energy-dense foods become available (52,53).

Food and culture have always interacted, but whether functionally or dysfunctionally has been a matter of circumstance (35,54). Anthropologists believe that the acquisition of food may have shaped early religious beliefs, with late Neolithic period hunters/herders expressing their dependence on a variety of animals in the creation myth, and early agricultural societies expressing their preoccupation with the seasonal demise and restoration of their food supply in resurrection myths (2). A preoccupation with the acquisition of food has clearly resounded through the ages. Success as a hunter was the principal means of gauging status in early tribal societies. In medieval Europe, control of land and the food it could produce gave rise to noble status. To this day, we link status to the acquisition of food, as evidenced by such phrases as "earning the dough," "winning the bread," and "bringing home the bacon" (35,55).

Thus, genetic evolution and cultural history have cultivated human dietary preferences that are well suited for a world in which food is difficult to acquire. The endemic and epidemic health problems of modern societies are in large measure traceable to our lack of defenses against dietary excess. Constant nutritional abundance, unknown to both human physiology and human culture for 4 million years, has become a modern vulnerability.

The physiologic tendencies endowed by evolution, such as innate preferences for sugar and fat and sensory-specific satiety, are compounded by overt and covert activities of the food industry. Overtly, the food industry spends billions of dollars in advertisements promoting the taste and convenience of fast and processed foods. The basis for preferring fat-dense, sweet, and salty food has already been addressed; other mediators of preference are familiarity and convenience (see Chapter 36). A destructive cycle is created as foods are produced that stimulate our shared preferences for sugar, salt, and fat, and then familiarity with such foods is promoted through advertising. The role of healthful foods in the prevailing diet in the United States is increasingly threatened by their marginalization in the popular food culture.

In addition to advertising through the media, the food industry consistently presents information on food package labels to their maximal advantage and often to the detriment of the consumer, our patients. Bold lettering, for example, often implies that the absence of a certain ingredient, such as cholesterol, offers health benefits. Such labeling, however, often appears on products that are naturally free of cholesterol (i.e., all plant-based products) but rich in saturated or trans fat. Trans fat, thus far, need not be listed separately on nutrition labels (although that fact soon may change; the Food and Drug Administration and Congress are being vigorously lobbied on this issue as of February 2000).

Packages boasting an absence of the highly saturated tropical oils often contain products in which these oils have been replaced by partially hydrogenated fat. Fat-modified dairy products indicate how much fat they contain by weight (e.g., 2% milk) rather than how much fat was removed from the original product (e.g., 50% in the case of 2% milk). Whatever nutrient has most recently captured the public imagination as a means to promote health is named in bold letters on every package of processed foods. In fact, it generally makes a far more modest contribution to the actual composition of the food (the "contains oat bran" period is a good example). A public preoccupation with the health-promoting properties of nature has resulted in widespread labeling of foods as "natural." Cheese, bacon, whole milk, cream, and butter may be "natural," but the

benefits in promoting them as such accrue only to their producers, not to our patients.

The food industry exploits prevailing vulnerabilities of consumers in a more subtle or covert manner as well. The addition of sugar to such foods as tomato ketchup or processed meats, which would not generally fit into the cultural category of sweet foods, may exert subliminal pressure on the consumer to over-indulge because of sensory-specific satiety and resultant undermining of self-restraint (35). The addition of salt to such foods as breakfast cereals, often in amounts comparable to those in salty snack foods, may exert a similar pressure, even though the taste of salt in such products is largely masked. Whereas an innate preference for sweet and a high associated satiety threshold are thought to have guided our ancestors toward such sources of readily available calories as fruits and wild honey, these traits have been rendered maladaptive by environmental change. With the proliferation of factory-sweetened foods and processed sugar, the guiding hand of evolution is misdirected toward temptation and overindulgence (35). In modern western society, therefore, cultural patterns exacerbate physiologic tendencies, further undermining the capacity of our patients to select a health-promoting diet (35,55).

There are clearly aspects of diet-related behavior that are predominantly nonvolitional. Voluntary restriction of fat and sugar intake appears to be at odds with 4 million years of genetic adaptation and psychobehavioral conditioning. The same may be true for salt restriction. Kumanyika (56) reported that the intensity and cost of interventions necessary to achieve compliance with a sodium guideline of 3,000 mg per day are prohibitive given the prevailing US diet. Encouraging individual responsibility for diet without distinguishing volitional from nonvolitional factors is likely to be detrimental in two ways.

First, frustration and duress will ensue as individuals fail in their efforts to master nonvolitional factors. The psychological consequences of obesity, the societal pressure against it, and the prevailing preoccupation with often unsuccessful dieting have been described by Brownell (57) and others (58) (see Chapter 5). Second, efforts to develop effective strategies for modifying diet, based on both individual counseling and alteration of the food supply, will receive insufficient emphasis so long as a "blame the victim" tendency prevails (see Chapter 41).

Primary care providers must understand the diverse impediments to dietary modification and view that understanding as the basis for more artful counseling, rather than as cause for pessimism. The public health stakes are simply too high for us to abandon our efforts at promoting nutritional health (8). Nutrition is of critical importance in the pathogenesis of the most prevalent chronic diseases in the United States, as well as obesity. National nutrition objectives in the United States for the year 2010 are predicated on the conviction that changes in diet and lifestyle can reduce or prevent prevalent causes of morbidity and mortality.

The main conclusion of the 1988 Surgeon General's Report on Nutrition and Health is that overconsumption, particularly of foods high in fats, is a major health concern for Americans (9). Healthy People 2000 and 2010 advances the objective of reducing dietary fat intake to 30% or less of total calories for all individuals over age 2. Although the trend from the second and third National Health and Nutrition Examination Surveys (NHANES II and III) (see Chapter 5) suggests some progress toward this goal, there is a long way to go, and there is some evidence that we have overestimated the progress made thus far (59,60).

Dietary guidelines have been generated, and disseminated, with the presumption that individuals have both the will and capacity to modify dietary selection, independent of environmental constraints. There is ample cause to question this conviction (61). There is an obvious conflict in a culture that exposes children to "junk food" and then encourages them to eat well (62). Fundamentally, our patients are threatened by a toxic nutritional environment (47,62–65). The constant temptations of dietary variety, of sugar, salt, and fat, are compounded by the conveniences of modern society and the resultant progressive decline in activity levels.

An understanding of the determinants of human dietary preference and selection is a prerequisite to dietary modification. Just as limited success in smoking cessation counseling has fostered greater efforts in this area, the limited successes of dietary counseling imply a need for greater efforts. Only an approach to dietary health that accommodates the physiologic characteristics and cultural predispositions with which humanity has been endowed has meaningful hope of success. As is the case for smoking, changing dietary behaviors likely will require multiple interventions and certainly will require an understanding of the obstacles to such change.

Whereas admonishments to quit smoking are sufficient motivation for some patients, others require alternative interventions, such as nicotine replacement. Advising nicotine-addicted patients to quit smoking was less successful before nicotine addiction was recognized. Similarly, means to reduce dietary fat intake have been devised on the basis of an understanding of dietary preferences; substitution of low-fat ingredients in the preparation of otherwise familiar food is one such method (66).

Participants in the Women's Health Trial, surveyed 1 year after the termination of the trial to assess maintenance of learned, low-fat dietary patterns, persisted in ingredient substitution and recipe modification, whereas efforts at avoiding fat and replacing high-fat food were less well maintained (66a). Low-fat substitutions in food preparation may reduce fat intake while preserving the basic structure of the diet and its culturally important "meaning" (67). Further, establishing familiarity with a fat-reduced diet may be difficult, but, once achieved, may substantially enhance acceptance and even preference. Participants in this study acclimated to a low-fat diet reported actual physical discomfort and aversion associated with high-fat meals (66).

Given the physiologic impulses with which millennia of evolution have endowed humanity, a prevailing preference for calorically dense food, for refined sugar, processed carbohydrate, and fat, is what would be expected. To the extent that the nutritional environment accommodates these impulses, they are generally indulged. Education and enhancement of individual motivation are most likely to achieve behavioral change when accompanied by environmental modification (48,68).

Although primary care providers can do little to modify the food supply, more effective dietary counseling will contribute to interim progress. There is evidence that the public receives most of its nutrition information from media sources (69–71), but that most people trust nutrition information from a personal physician or health care provider more than from any other source (70). There also is evidence, albeit limited, that dietary counseling by primary care providers meaningfully influences dietary behavior (7).

An approach to human nutrition based in part on evolutionary biology has certain limitations: (i) we have at best imperfect knowledge of what/how our ancestors ate; (ii) our ancestors lived a relatively short lifespan; and (iii) we have limited knowledge of the nutrition-related health problems to which our ancestors may have been subject. The diet favored by natural selection for a 40-year lifespan is not necessarily optimal for a lifespan nearly twice as long. Yet our knowledge of our ancestors' diets is useful in explaining our dietary tendencies and preferences, even if it fails to identify the optimal diet for health promotion.

Zoo animals, by way of analogy, may live longer in captivity than their wild counterparts. But the wild condition is what explains the physiology of the captive animal. The native state, whether it is optimal in every way, is highly informative of appropriate environmental conditions, diet included. Consideration of evolutionary biology is valuable in emphasizing the relevance of our adaptation to a particular nutritional environment and our struggles in attempting to adapt to a very different one.

The adaptations of our ancestors, and the interplay of physiology, psychology, and culture, may thus explain our nutritional failings and inform our attempts to characterize the optimal diet for our patients. Whereas the health-promoting properties of the n-3 fatty acids have only recently begun to generate interest, the markedly higher intake of this fat by our ancestors may explain its compatibility with our metabolism.

An understanding of why we eat as we do, and what impedes and promotes dietary change, is an essential element in promoting nutritional health. Such an understanding, shared with patients, alleviates feelings of personal failure in attempts to improve diet. Advising our patients what to eat, without addressing the diverse impediments to dietary modification, our shared vulnerabilities, cravings, and aversions, may be comparable to encouraging polar bears in North Africa simply to stop retaining heat. By addressing the obstacles to nutritional health and working with our patients to circumvent them, we may hope to see our efforts at dietary counseling translate into appreciable improvements in the public health.

REFERENCES

1. Darwin C. *Origin of species.* New York: Avenel Books, 1979.
2. Tannahill R. *Food in history.* London, England: Penguin Books, 1988.
3. Eaton S, Konner M. Paleolithic nutrition revisited: a twelve-year retrospective on its nature and implications. *Eur J Clin Nutr* 1997;51:207–216.
4. Glanz K. Review of nutritional attitudes and counseling practices of primary care physicians. *Am J Clin Nutr* 1997;65:2016s–2019s.
5. Kushner R. Barriers to providing nutrition counseling by physicians: a survey of primary care practitioners. *Prev Med* 1995;24:546–552.
6. Lazarus K. Nutrition practices of family physicians after education by a physician nutrition specialist. *Am J Clin Nutr* 1997;65:2007s–2009s.
7. Nawaz H, Adams M, Katz DL. Weight loss counseling by health care providers. *Am J Public Health* 1999;89:764–767.

8. McGinnis J, Foege W. Actual causes of death in the United States. *JAMA* 1993;270:2207–2212.

9. US Department of Health and Human Services. *The Surgeon General's report on nutrition and health.* Washington, DC: US Government Printing Office, 1988.

10. US Department of Health and Human Services. *Healthy people 2000.* Washington, DC: US Government Printing Office, 1991.

11. Glanz K, Basil M, Maibach E, et al. Why Americans eat what they do: taste, nutrition, cost, convenience, and weight control concerns as influences on food consumption. *J Am Diet Assoc* 1998;98:1118–1126.

12. Eaton S, Konner M, Shostak M. Stone agers in the fast lane: chronic degenerative diseases in evolutionary perspective. *Am J Med* 1988;84:739–749.

13. Hippel AV. Human evolutionary biology: human anatomy and physiology from an evolutionary perspective. Anchorage, AL: Stone Age Press,1998.

14. Howell F. *Early man.* New York: Time Life Books, 1971.

15. Neel J. Diabetes mellitus: a "thrifty" genotype rendered detrimental by "progress"? *Am J Hum Genet* 1962;14:353–362.

16. Eaton S, Konner M, Garn S. From the Miocene to olestra: A historical perspective on fat consumption. *J Am Diet Assoc* 1997;97:s54–s57.

17. Garn S. From the Miocene to olestra: A historical perspective on fat consumption. *J Am Diet Assoc* 1997;97:s54–s57.

18. Gortner W. Nutrition in the United States, 1900 to 1974. *Cancer Res* 1975;35:3246–3253.

19. Nestle M. Promoting health and preventing disease: national nutrition objectives for 1990 and 2000. *Nutr Today* 1988:26–30.

20. Ministry of Agriculture, Fisheries and Foods. *Household food consumption and expenditure, with a study of trends over the period 1940–1990.* London: HMSO, 1990.

21. Kramer S. *Cradle of civilization.* New York: Time-Life Books, 1967.

22. Casson L. *Ancient Egypt.* New York: Time-Life Books, 1965.

23. Schafer E. *Ancient China.* New York: Time Life Books, 1967.

24. Bowra C. *Classical Greece.* New York: Time-Life Books, 1965.

25. Hadas M. *Imperial Rome.* New York: Time-Life Books, 1965.

26. Simons G. *Barbarian Europe.* New York: Time-Life Books, 1968.

27. Leonard J. *Ancient America.* New York: Time-Life Books, 1967.

28. Nestle M, Wing R, Birch L, et al. Behavioral and social influences on food choice. *Nutr Rev* 1998;56:s50–s74.

29. Eaton S, Eaton S III, Konner M, et al. An evolutionary perspective enhances understanding of human nutritional requirements. *J Nutr* 1996;126:1732–1740.

30. Neel J. *Physician to the gene pool.* New York: John Wiley, 1994:302, 315.

30a. Cavalli-Sforza LL. Human evolution and nutrition. In: Walcher DN, Kretchmer N, eds. *Food, nutrition and evolution. Food as an environmental factor in the genesis of human variability.* Masson Publishing USA, Inc., 1981;1–7.

31. Eaton S, Konner M. Paleolithic nutrition. A consideration of its nature and current implications. *N Engl J Med* 1985;312:283.

32. Pettitt D, Lisse J, Knowler W, et al. Mortality as a function of obesity and diabetes mellitus. *Am J Epidemiol* 1982;115:359–366.

33. Fox C, Esparza J, Nicolson M, et al. Is a low leptin concentration, a low resting metabolic rate, or both the expression of the "thrifty genotype"? Results from Mexican Pima Indians. *Am J Clin Nutr* 1998;68:1053–1057.

34. Rolls B. Sensory-specific satiety. *Nutr Rev* 1986;44:93–101.

35. Fischler C. Food preferences, nutritional wisdom, and sociocultural evolution. In: Walcher D, Kretchmer N, eds. *Food, nutrition and evolution. Food as an environmental factor in the genesis of human variability.* Masson Publishing USA, 1981:59–67.

36. Rozin P. The selection of foods by rats, humans and other animals. In: Rosenblatt J, Hinde R, Shaw E, et al., eds. *Advances in the study of behavior.* New York: Academic Press, 1981.

37. Beauchamp G. Ontogenesis of taste preferences. In: Walcher D, Kretchmer N, eds. *Food, nutrition and evolution. Food as an environmental factor in the genesis of human variability.* Masson Publishing USA, 1981:49–57.

38. Davis C. Clara Davis revisited. *Nutr Rev* 1987;45.

39. Davis C. Self-selection of diet by newly weaned infants. *Am J Dis Child* 1992;36:651–79.

40. Story M, Brown J. Do young children instinctively know what to eat? *N Engl J Med* 1987;316:103–106.

41. Drewnowski A, Kirth C, Rahaim J. Taste preferences in human obesity: environmental and familial factors. *Am J Clin Nutr* 1991;54:635–641.

42. Lucas F, Sclafani A. Flavor preferences conditioned by intragastric fat infusions in rats. *Physiol Behav* 1989;46:403–412.

43. Johnston F. Health implications of childhood obesity. *Ann Intern Med* 1985;103:1068–1072.

44. Drewnowski A. Nutritional perspectives on biobehavioral models of dietary change. In: Henderson MM, Bowen DJ, DeRoos KK, et al., eds. *Promoting dietary change in communities: applying existing models of dietary change to population-based interventions.* Seattle, WA: Cancer Prevention Research Program, Fred Hutchinson Cancer Research Center, 1992:96–109.

45. Sclafani A. Psychobiology of fat appetite. In: Henderson MM, Bowen DJ, DeRoos KK, et al., eds. *Promoting dietary change in communities: applying existing models of dietary change to population-based interventions.* Seattle, WA: Cancer Prevention Research Program, Fred Hutchinson Cancer Research Center, 1992:82–95.

46. Drewnowski A, Shrager E, Lipsky C, et al. Sugar and fat: sensory and hedonic evaluation of liquid and solid foods. *Physiol Behav* 1989;45:177–183.

47. Mela D, Sacchetti D. Sensory preferences for fats: relationships with diet and body composition. *Am J Clin Nutr* 1991;53:908–915.

48. Glanz K. Food supply modifications to promote population-based dietary change. In: Henderson

MM, Bowen DJ, DeRoos KK, et al., eds. *Promoting dietary change in communities: applying existing models of dietary change to population-based interventions.* Seattle, WA: Cancer Prevention Research Program, Fred Hutchinson Cancer Research Center, 1992:195–204.

49. Geyer L, Kare M. Taste and food selection in the weaning on nonprimate mammals. In: Walcher D, Kretchmer N, eds. *Food, nutrition and evolution. Food as an environmental factor in the genesis of human variability.* Masson Publishing, 1981:68–82.

50. Reed D, Tordoff M. Enhanced acceptance and metabolism of fats by rats fed a high-fat diet. *Am J Physiol* 1991;261:R1084–R1088.

51. Warwick Z, Schiffman S, Anderson J. Relationship of dietary fat content to food preferences in young rats. *Physiol Behav* 1990;48:581–586.

52. Lands W, Hamazaki T, Yamazaki K, et al. Changing dietary patterns. *Am J Clin Nutr* 1990;51:991–993.

53. Drewnowski A, Popkin B. The nutrition transition: new trends in the global diet. *Nutr Rev* 1997; 55:31–43.

54. Beidler L, et al. *Sweeteners: issues and uncertainties.* Washington, DC: Academy Forum, National Academy of Sciences, 1979.

55. Axelson M. The impact of culture on food-related behavior. *Annu Rev Nutr* 1986;6:345–363.

56. Kumanyika S. Behavioral aspects of intervention strategies to reduce dietary sodium. *Hypertension* 1991;17:i90–i95.

57. Brownell K. The psychology and physiology of obesity: implications for screening and treatment. *J Am Diet Assoc* 1984;84:406–414.

58. Wadden TA, Stunkard AJ. Social and psychological consequences of obesity. *Ann Intern Med* 1985; 103:1062–1067.

59. Katz DL, Brunner RL, St Jeor ST, et al. Dietary fat consumption in a cohort of American adults, 1985–1991: covariates, secular trends, and compliance with guidelines. *Am J Health Promotion* 1998;12:382–390.

60. Kennedy E, Bowman S, Powell R. Dietary-fat intake in the US population. *J Am Coll Nutr* 1999; 18:207–212.

61. Institute of Medicine. Improving America's diet and health: from recommendation to action. Washington, DC: National Academy Press, 1991.

62. Galanter R. To the victim belong the flaws. *Am J Public Health* 1977;67:1025–1026.

63. Milio N. Health, nutrition and public policy. *Nurs Outlook* 1991;39:6–9.

64. Becker M. The tyranny of health promotion. *Public Health Rev* 1986;14:15–25.

65. Cohen C, Cohen E. Health education: panacea, pernicious or pointless? *N Engl J Med* 1978;299: 718–720.

66. Kristal A. Public health implications of biobehavioral models. In: Henderson MM, Bowen DJ, DeRoos KK, et al., eds. *Promoting dietary change in communities: applying existing models of dietary change to population-based interventions.* Seattle, WA: Cancer Prevention Research Program, Fred Hutchinson Cancer Research Center, 1992:126–135.

66a. Kristal AR. Public health implications of biobehavioral models. In: Henderson MM, Bowen DJ, DeRoos KK, et al. *Promoting dietary change in communities: Applying existing models of dietary change to population-based interventions.* Proceedings of a Conference. Seattle, WA: Cancer Prevention Research Program. Fred Hutchinson Cancer Center, 1992;126–135.

67. Kinne S. Policy interventions on nutrition. In: Henderson MM, Bowen DJ, DeRoos KK, et al., eds. *Promoting dietary change in communities: applying existing models of dietary change to population-based interventions.* Seattle, WA: Cancer Prevention Research Center, 1992:205–213.

68. Glanz K. Environmental interventions to promote healthy eating: a review of models, programs and evidence. *Health Educ Q* 1988;15:395–415.

69. Achterberg C. Qualitative research: what do we know about teaching good nutritional habits? *J Nutr* 1994;124:1808s–1812s.

70. Hiddink G, Hautvast J, van Woerkum CM, et al. Consumers' expectations about nutrition guidance: the importance of the primary care physicians. *Am J Clin Nutr* 1997;65:1974s–1979s.

71. Abusabha R, Peacock J, Achterberg C. How to make nutrition education more meaningful through facilitated group discussions. *J Am Diet Assoc* 1999;99:72–76.

BIBLIOGRAPHY

See "Sources for All Chapters."

Milton K. Nutritional characteristics of wild primate foods: do the diets of our closest living relatives have lessons for us? *Nutrition* 1999;15:488–498.

40

Dietary Recommendations for Health Promotion and Disease Prevention

The achievement of health promotion through diet has two prerequisites: i) a reliable and consistent base of evidence on which to make dietary recommendations, and ii) reliable means of translating the evidence in support of a particular dietary pattern into behavior. There are, at present, certain controversies and uncertainties concerning the former; challenges to the latter are considerably more formidable. Nonetheless, the potential benefits of successful dietary health promotion justify a vigorous approach in clinical practice.

Heart disease, the leading killer of adults in the United States, is amenable to dramatic risk reduction through diet, by a variety of mechanisms (see Chapter 6). The estimate of Doll and Peto that more than a third of all cancers are potentially preventable through dietary manipulations is widely accepted (1), if not wholly substantiated (see Chapter 12). Obesity in the United States, increasingly a hybrid endemic and epidemic threat to both adults and children, is directly linked to diet and activity patterns (see Chapter 5). Stroke, hypertension, diabetes, pregnancy outcomes, degenerative arthritis, and innumerable other diseases, as well as general perceptions of well-being, are responsive to dietary influences.

There currently is considerably more consensus than controversy with regard to a health-promoting diet. Controversy persists, and arises, in areas of on-going study, such

as the health effects of specific nutrients, or the optimal diet for the prevention or reversal of specific diseases. Therefore, such controversies tend to be nutrient or disease specific. An extensive review of the diverse influences of diet on health serves to mitigate such controversies by providing contiguous lines of evidence that ultimately function as a Venn diagram, encircling an area of overlapping recommendations.

Behavior change often is facilitated in the context of established disease; individuals with disease perceive risk more acutely and therefore are more motivated to change behavior. Dietary recommendations in the setting of clinical disease are similar to those for health promotion, but they may be more extreme both in response to the greater acuity and in response to the patient's greater willingness to adhere to recommendations. The clustering of risk factors for various chronic diseases, and of the diseases themselves, requires that dietary manipulations for secondary and tertiary prevention not be overly disease specific. Therefore, although specific dietary intervention may be targeted to a single disease, the dietary pattern remains consistent with recommendations for general health promotion.

This chapter will characterize the dietary recommendations that may be offered with confidence in the delivery of clinical care to virtually all patients, as well as those who may be added in the setting of established disease or risk factors for disease. Recommendations are divided into those that are established as the consensus view of the nutrition community, and those supported by confluent lines of evidence, but as yet not achieving consensus endorsement. This latter category represents, in essence, unrecognized consensus disclosed only on exhaustive review of a diverse literature.

DIETARY RECOMMENDATIONS FOR HEALTH PROMOTION

Consensus Recommendations

Consensus regarding the optimal diet for the maintenance and promotion of health is reflected in guidelines generated by expert bodies including the US Surgeon General, the American Heart Association, the American Cancer Society, and the National Cancer Institute (NCI). These guidelines differ only in subtleties, and all reflect the convergence of evidence for the prevention of diverse diseases. The prescription of various diets for the prevention of particular diseases has largely been supplanted by the "one diet" that is thought to prevent multiple diseases by enhancing health.

The recommended diet is schematically represented by the food pyramid. The foundation of the recommended diet is cereal grains. Fruits and vegetables should be consumed in variety and abundance, with NCI's "5 a day" representing a minimal

Food Guide Pyramid
A Guide to Daily Food Choices

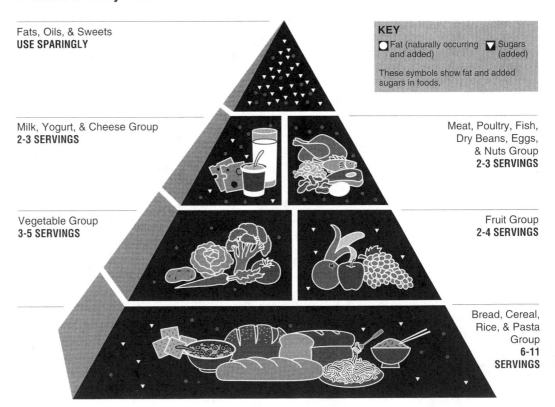

Fats, Oils, & Sweets
USE SPARINGLY

KEY
⭘ Fat (naturally occurring and added)   ▼ Sugars (added)

These symbols show fat and added sugars in foods.

Milk, Yogurt, & Cheese Group
2-3 SERVINGS

Meat, Poultry, Fish, Dry Beans, Eggs, & Nuts Group
2-3 SERVINGS

Vegetable Group
3-5 SERVINGS

Fruit Group
2-4 SERVINGS

Bread, Cereal, Rice, & Pasta Group
6-11 SERVINGS

recommendation. The consumption of fat-restricted and preferably fat-free dairy products is advisable to increase calcium intake; intake of full-fat dairy products should be restricted. Meats generally should be eaten as peripherals to vegetable-based meals. Lean meats should be chosen preferentially, and fish consumption should receive particular emphasis. Fatty, dark-meat fish, such as salmon, is particularly rich in ω-3 fatty acids and should be prioritized. Poultry should be eaten without skin, and white meat should be consumed preferentially. The consumption of red meat generally should be limited, and lean cuts should be selected. Beans and legumes should be eaten regularly as an alternative protein source to meat. Seeds and nuts should be eaten in variety, but in modest quantities because of their caloric density. Highly refined foods, sweets, and oils should be used sparingly.

With regard to macronutrient distribution, guidelines call for 30% of total calories from fat, 55% to 60% from carbohydrate, and 10% to 15% from protein. More specific recommendations with regard to fat generally suggest an intake of monounsaturates at approximately 10% to 15% of total calories, polyunsaturates at approximately 10% of total calories, and saturated fat below 10% of total calories and preferably lower still. Specific recommendations for the intake of trans fat are lacking, but the evidence suggests that trans and saturated fat should be combined and collectively restricted to less than 10% of total caloric intake. Total calorie consumption should be that required to maintain a healthful body weight. People should consume at least 30 g of dietary fiber daily, a figure reached by complying with recommendations for abundant intake of grains, beans, fruits, and vegetables. Sodium intake should be restricted to not more than 3 g per day, a figure supported by recommendations to eat processed foods sparingly. Alcohol consumption should be modest, not exceeding 15 g of ethanol per day for women or 30 g per day for men.

Recommendations Supported by Confluent Evidence

Dietary Fat

Perhaps the area of greatest controversy in nutrition at present is the relative benefits of a diet severely restricted in total fat (i.e., less than 10% of total calories) as compared with a diet with liberal fat intake, but relatively rich in polyunsaturated and monounsaturated fatty acids (see Chapters 2 and 6). Recent results reported by Ornish et al. (1a) provide additional support for the extremely low-fat diet, at least for the prevention of cardiovascular events. Results from the Lyons Heart Study offer similar support for the Mediterranean diet (2).

The current estimates of Paleolithic intake suggest that we are adapted to a fat intake of approximately 25% of total calories (3), which is below the typical level in the United States today and below the liberal fat intake of Mediterranean countries, but well above the intake advocated by Ornish and others. Further, our ancestral intake of trans fat was negligible, and intake of saturated fatty acids is thought to have made up less than 5% of total calories.

Nearly half of the fat in our "natural" diets derived from polyunsaturated fat, with an n-3 to n-6 ratio between 1:1 and 1:4. The other half derived from monounsaturated fat. There is preliminary evidence of a benefit of supplementing n-3 fatty acid intake in areas ranging from cognitive development (see Chapter 33) to the control of rheumatoid arthritis (see Chapter 18). Although definitive evidence of n-3 fatty acid deficiency or of the benefits of supplementation may be lacking for any single disease, the weight of evidence overwhelmingly suggests a prevailing relative deficiency in the modern Western diet.

On this basis, a recommendation may be made to consume approximately 25% of total calories as fat, in a nearly even distribution between polyunsaturates and monounsaturates. The combination of trans fat and saturated fat should be kept below 5% of total calories, an effect that can be achieved in part by following the consensus recommendations specified above.

Unless fish consumption is very consistent, however, n-3 fatty acid intake is apt to be lower than optimal given the near-complete elimination of n-3 fatty acids from the flesh of domestic food animals. Consumption of soybeans and seeds, particularly flaxseeds, as a means of raising n-3 fatty acid intake is recommended. The use of flaxseed oil, totaling about 1 tablespoon per day for adults, is an easy way to increase n-3 consumption. The fat and calories added to the diet in the form of ω-3 polyunsaturated fat should be compensated by reduced intake of fat from other sources.

Dietary Protein

Although the evidence that high intake of dietary protein is harmful in the context of impaired renal function and that protein consumption may accelerate the age-related decline in glomerular filtration rate is convincing, the harmful effects of protein independent of other lifestyle and dietary hazards are uncertain. If the overall dietary pattern is judicious, a relatively higher protein intake may be tolerated without sequelae. Even in studies of competitive athletes, however, there is little evidence of benefit from very high protein intake.

The available evidence in the aggregate supports protein consumption in the range from 0.6 to 1 g per kilogram body weight in adults. Intakes up to approximately 2 g per kilogram may offer some advantages to vigorously active individuals, although this is uncertain (see Chapter 30). Higher intakes appear to be ill advised (see Chapters 3, 11, and 30). High-protein diets advocated for control of insulin resistance and weight loss are not supported by evidence of long-term health benefits and, in general, should be discouraged in favor of the pattern described (see Chapters 5 and 10).

Dietary Fiber

A diet consistent with consensus recommendations will result in considerably greater fiber intake than is typical in the United States. Although recommendations include a fiber intake of approximately 30 g per day, the weight of evidence also supports a specific effort to increase consumption of soluble fiber. Soluble fiber is found abundantly in beans and legumes, and in a variety of fruits, vegetables, and in particular grains. Consumption of soluble fiber tends to lower serum lipids and reduce the postprandial rise in both glucose and insulin. A specific recommendation to consume a variety of beans, lentils, apples, and oat-based products is supported by the available evidence.

Micronutrient Supplements

Nominal micronutrient deficiencies persist despite the abundance of the US diet. Elevated homocysteine levels are reduced with supplements of vitamin B_6 and folate. Folate supplementation before conception reduces the incidence among neonates of neural tube defects. Supplements of zinc appear to enhance immune function, and chromium supplements improve insulin metabolism.

Teleologically, we may be adapted to a higher intake of micronutrients given the higher energy needs of our physically active ancestors and the calorie-dilute, nutrient-dense foods available to them. In addition, there is a large body of confluent evidence suggesting, although as yet not clearly establishing, a benefit of antioxidant supplementation, and in particular, a combination of fat- and water-soluble antioxidants.

Given the lack of discernible toxicity and the potential benefits, the consumption of a multivitamin/multimineral supplement by all adults is a reasonable recommendation. Patients should be discouraged from using such a supplement as justification to comply less completely with dietary recommendations. The benefits of micronutrient supplementation are not nearly as well established as the benefits of a dietary pattern approximating recommendations. Inclusion of antioxidants in the supplement may offer specific benefits. Specific supplementation with high doses of single nutrients lacks supporting evidence for primary prevention, but may be appropriate for more targeted disease prevention efforts.

Distribution of Meals

There is limited evidence that the consumption of frequent, small meals precipitates less insulin release than does the consumption of comparable calories in larger meals spaced further apart. In addition, for the majority of adults who would benefit from at least modest weight loss, frequent snacking may blunt appetite and help prevent bingeing. As discussed in Chapter 41, the psychological benefits of frequent eating may be considerable for patients working at weight loss or weight maintenance.

Energy Restriction

The evidence that total energy restriction may reduce all-cause morbidity and mortality is provocative, although not definitive for humans. Long-term compliance with low-energy diets is unlikely in all but the most highly motivated individuals; therefore, this recommendation is of limited practical value for health promotion. In the context of established disease, the benefits of energy restriction may be sufficient to outweigh the inconvenience.

RECOMMENDATIONS FOR DISEASE PREVENTION

Cardiovascular Disease

Patients with established coronary artery disease are encouraged to comply with dietary recommendations offered by the American Heart Association (4,5) (see Chapter 6). However, the American Heart Association step 1 guidelines, and even the more restrictive step 2 guidelines, modify the prevailing US diet less than is optimal for the prevention of coronary events. Events have been prevented both by an extremely fat-restricted diet (1a) and by a Mediterranean dietary pattern (6).

The rate of recurrent myocardial infarction has been reduced with vitamin E supplementation (CHAOS) (6a). Vitamins E and C have been shown to improve endothelial function (7). A substantial body of evidence suggests that coenzyme Q_{10} supplementation may be beneficial to patients with ischemic heart disease, and especially those with congestive heart failure. The beneficial effects of antioxidant-rich plant products, and of modest alcohol intake, are convincingly established.

In light of all currently available evidence, patients at high risk for, or with known, coronary artery disease should be encouraged to adopt a basic dietary pattern matching that advocated for health promotion. Total fat intake should be reduced from the current US mean of 34% to approximately 25% of calories. A particular emphasis should be placed on the reduction of saturated and trans fat intake, as well as the intake of cholesterol. Frequent fish consumption, inclusion of flaxseeds in baked goods, and use of flaxseed oil on salad should be encouraged. Cooking should be done with olive and/or canola oil.

A multivitamin/multimineral supplement is recommended, as is an additional 500 mg of vitamin C and 400 to 800 IU of vitamin E per day. Coenzyme Q_{10}, at a dose of approximately 1 mg per pound of body weight (2 mg per kg), should be recommended in patients with congestive heart failure and may offer benefits to patients with coronary artery disease with preserved left ventricular function.

Consumption of one alcoholic beverage per day is recommended; men may benefit from up to two drinks. Although the benefits of alcohol pertain to all ethanol, polyphenols in the skins of grapes have antioxidant properties; therefore, red wine may offer additional benefits. Patients with hyperlipidemia should make a particular effort to increase intake of soluble fiber. They may do so by eating oatmeal, and particularly oat bran, consistently with breakfast; by eating oat-based breads and baked goods; and by eating beans, lentils, and apples. There may be benefits in distributing calories over many small meals rather than several larger ones. Limited evidence suggests that frequent, small meals precipitate the release of less insulin than do larger meals spaced further apart. The distribution of meals also may affect weight maintenance.

Cerebrovascular Disease

Cardiovascular disease and cerebrovascular disease share risk factors. Despite one study suggesting that high fat intake may reduce the risk of stroke (8), the weight of evidence favors comparable recommendations for the prevention of all sequelae of atherosclerotic disease (see Chapters 6, 9, and 18). There is insufficient basis to justify modifying the recommendations for prevention of cardiovascular disease in patients at risk for, or with a history of, cerebrovascular disease. The only caveat here pertains to patients with a history of intracranial bleeding, in whom fish oil and possibly vitamin E should be avoided, depending on the etiology of the bleed, to avoid platelet inhibition.

The best established means of preventing first or recurrent stroke is blood pressure control. The dietary recommendations for the control of blood pressure are provided in Chapter 7. In general, a generous intake of calcium, magnesium, and potassium and a restricted intake of sodium are recommended. A diet adhering to the pattern described for health promotion will facilitate control of blood pressure (9).

Diabetes Mellitus

In direct comparison, a Mediterranean diet has been shown to ameliorate serum glucose levels more effectively than a high-carbohydrate diet (see Chapter 10); therefore, the diet described for health promotion is indicated as well for the control of diabetes. A particular effort should be made to supplement intake of soluble fiber by frequent inclusion in the diet of beans, lentils, grains, and apples. The consumption of soluble fiber in meals may serve to blunt the glycemic effect of other foods.

The metabolic advantages of frequent, small meals have been suggested, and this pattern may offer additional advantages with regard to weight control (see Chapter 41). Therefore, frequent consumption of small meals or snacks, including foods rich in soluble fiber, may be a particularly beneficial approach. This is only true provided "snacking" redistributes, rather than increases, total daily calorie intake, and that the foods chosen are appropriate (e.g., fresh fruit, dried fruit, fresh vegetables, whole-grain products, nonfat dairy). The benefits of supplementation with chromium 200 μg per day are under investigation. At a minimum, the chromium provided in a multivitamin/multimineral supplement may offer some benefit (see Chapter 10).

Cancer

The maintenance of ideal body weight, low total energy consumption, and intake of a variety of fruits and vegetables appear to offer protection against a wide range of, perhaps even most, cancers. These recommendations are consistent with those for health promotion and the prevention of other leading diseases. One departure is alcohol, which may reduce the risk of cardiovascular disease, but appears to promote cancers of the breast, head, neck, and other sites. Women at high risk of breast cancer, or individuals with a cancer history, are advised to abstain from alcohol. In such individuals also at risk for, or suffering from, heart disease, alternative means should be sought to provide the benefits of alcohol. Specifically, exercise and avoidance of refined carbohydrate may raise high-density lipoprotein, whereas aspirin, vitamin E, and n-3 fatty acids may inhibit platelet aggregation.

The benefits of energy restriction appear to pertain particularly to cancer prevention. Patients at high risk for, or with a history of, cancer should be encouraged to restrict calories to bring weight down to near ideal. In such situations, the use of micronutrient supplements is particularly important. In advanced cancer, nutritional goals should be shifted to weight maintenance, and energy restriction should be abandoned.

Inflammatory Diseases

Although food intolerance may play a role for some individuals in the etiology of chronic inflammatory and autoimmune diseases, there is no evidence of such an association for the majority of patients. The most promising nutritional approach to chronic inflammation is supplemented intake of n-3 fatty acids (see Chapter 18). Therefore, the dietary recommendations for health promotion need not be altered for patients at risk for, or with, chronic inflammatory conditions. Use of nutriceutical proteoglycans, such as glucosamine sulfate, for control of pain and inflammation is supported by satisfactory evidence and should be considered along with use of pharmaceutical products.

Infectious Disease

The principal effect of nutrition on the course of infectious disease is mediated through effects on immune system function. The one exception is in chronic infectious disease, such as acquired immunodeficiency syndrome, where cachexia may become an independent threat to health. A variety of micronutrients serve as cofactors in metabolic activities germane to immune function. Certain minerals important to the immune system, including zinc and magnesium, tend to be at nominal levels in the typical American diet.

A micronutrient supplement including minerals is indicated for the prevention of infectious disease and in all individuals with chronic infectious disease. The increased metabolic demands of infection, particularly when fever is present, require increased energy intake to maintain body mass. There is no evidence to suggest that the overall dietary pattern recommended for health promotion should be altered for purposes of preventing or managing infectious disease.

Renal Insufficiency

The most widely supported dietary manipulation for the management of renal insufficiency is restriction of protein to 0.6 g/kg. This intake level is consistent with recommendations for health promotion and, therefore, may be advocated to all patients. The leading causes of renal failure in the United States are diabetes mellitus and hypertension, both of which are amenable to dietary management as described earlier and elsewhere (see Chapters 7 and 10).

Liver Disease

The principal dietary manipulations in patients with chronic liver disease are protein restriction and avoidance of alcohol. Moderate protein restriction is advisable for health promotion, whereas the optimal dose of dietary ethanol varies with individual circumstances. Thus, patients with liver disease should, for the most part, adhere to a diet consistent with recommendations for health promotion, while abstaining from alcohol. Supplementation with B vitamins generally is indicated and is provided if a multivitamin is taken daily. Preliminary evidence for nutriceuticals such as silymarin is discussed elsewhere (see Chapter 21).

SUMMARY

The myriad effects of nutrition on health outcomes are documented in a vast literature of widely divergent quality. In certain vital areas, consensus has yet to develop. Sufficient evidence has been gathered, however, to permit the generation of dietary recommendations for health promotion and disease prevention with considerable confidence.

The single most important principle in dietary health promotion is the same dietary pattern is appropriate for the prevention of most diseases. Patients with cardiovascular disease often have diabetes, also may have cerebrovascular disease, often have hypertension, may have renal insufficiency, may have had or have cancer, and are constantly vulnerable to infectious disease. If each disease required a different diet, consistent recommendations could not be made to an individual, let alone a population. The emergence of a "one diet" approach to nutritional health is a logical outgrowth of confluent lines of evidence and the clinical imperative for consistent and practicable advice. The benefits of a health-promoting diet should be combined with regular physical activity for maximal benefit; a sedentary lifestyle may undermine many of the potential health benefits of an otherwise salutary dietary pattern.

All patients, with or without chronic disease or risk factors, should be encouraged to comply with the health-promoting diet detailed earlier in this chapter. Patients with one or more predominant risk factors or diseases may benefit from modest disease- or factor-specific dietary adjustments. Although the advice may not change much with the development of disease, the conviction and frequency with which counseling is provided, and the willingness of the patient to change, should both increase.

REFERENCES

1. Doll R, Peto R. The causes of cancer: quantitative estimates of avoidable risks of cancer in the United States today. *J Natl Cancer Inst* 1981;66:119–308.
1a. Ornish D, Scherwitz L, Billings J, et al. Intensive lifestyle changes for reversal of coronary heart disease. *JAMA* 1998;280:2001–2007.
2. Lorgeril MD. Mediterranean diet in the prevention of coronary heart disease. *Nutrition* 1998;14:55–57.
3. Eaton S, Konner M. Paleolithic nutrition revisited: a twelve-year retrospective on its nature and implications. *Eur J Clin Nutr* 1997;51:207–216.
4. Geil P, Anderson J, Gustafson N. Women and men with hypercholesterolemia respond similarly to an American Heart Association step 1 diet. *J Am Diet Assoc* 1995;95:436–441.
5. Schaefer E, Lichtenstein A, Lamon-Fava S, et al. Efficacy of a National Cholesterol Education Program Step 2 diet in normolipidemic and hypercholesterolemic middle-aged and elderly men and women. *Arterioscler Thromb Vasc Biol* 1995;15:1079–1085.
6. Lorgeril Md, Salen P, Martin J, et al. Mediterranean diet, traditional risk factors, and the rate of cardiovascular complications after myocardial infarction: final report of the Lyon Diet Heart Study. *Circulation* 1999;99:779–785.
6a. Stephens NG, Parsons A, Schofield PM, et al. Randomised controlled trial of vitamin E in patients with coronary disease: Cambridge Heart Antioxidant Study (CHAOS). *Lancet* 1996;347:781–786.
7. Plotnick GD, Corretti M, Vogel RA. Effect of antioxidant vitamins on the transient impairment of endothelium-dependent brachial artery vasoactivity following a single high-fat meal. *JAMA* 1997;278:1682–1686.
8. Gillman M, Cupples L, Millen B, et al. Inverse association of dietary fat with development of ischemic stroke in men. *JAMA* 1997;278:2145–2150.
9. Moore T, Vollmer W, Appel L, et al. Effect of dietary patterns on ambulatory blood pressure: results from the Dietary Approaches to Stop Hypertension (DASH) Trial. DASH Collaborative Research Group. *Hypertension* 1999;34:472–477.

BIBLIOGRAPHY

See "Sources for All Chapters."
Willett WC, Sacks F, Trichopoulou A, et al. Mediterranean diet pyramid: a cultural model for healthy eating. *Am J Clin Nutr* 1995;61[6 Suppl]:1402s–1406s.

41

Dietary Counseling in Clinical Practice

INTRODUCTION

Dietary and lifestyle patterns are predicated on many other considerations than health (1). Given that human dietary metabolism and preferences are derivatives, largely, of the very different environment of prehistory (see Chapter 39), and that the modern nutritional environment has developed to satisfy preferences, health problems resulting from dietary excess are not surprising.

Given the multiple influences on dietary selection, and the fact that health is generally not the dominant concern, professional guidance is clearly required to encourage and guide individual efforts to approximate a health-promoting dietary pattern. Such efforts must play out at the complex interface of medicine and lifestyle, physiology and sociology, anthropology and evolutionary biology, and psychology and metabolism. Of fundamental importance to such efforts is the understanding that any effort to change individual behavior requires talking individuals out of the behavioral pattern they have selected, or into another they have not. Thus, effective dietary counseling leans heavily on the power of persuasion.

Attempting to talk our patients into behavioral patterns they have rejected (or not considered) may seem a potentially thankless task. However, the aggregate toll of diet-related health problems is enormous. Dietary practices divergent from recommendations are considered the second leading cause of preventable death in the United States, behind tobacco use (2). Because, however, everyone eats while only a minority of the population uses tobacco, in the aggregate the health effects of nutrition are likely to be far greater. Even when not discernibly contributing to the development or prevention of a particular disease, nutrition plays a role in lifelong health, influencing appearance, functional status, self-esteem, socialization, energy level, athletic performance, susceptibility to infection, and possibly independent of morbidity, longevity. Therefore, the potential for dietary practices to modify health is tremendous and universally applicable. Consequently, routine counseling to promote healthy eating is encouraged by the US Preventive Services Task Force (3).

There are, however, numerous impediments to the delivery of effective dietary counseling. Expertise in clinical nutrition traditionally has been the purview of dietitians, to whom only a minority of patients are ever referred. For the physician to provide pertinent counseling has been precluded above all by the lack of nutrition education in most medical schools (4–6), but also by time pressure, competing demands, and lack of conviction, inspired by lack of evidence, that the effort would be productive (7–10).

There is, however, simply too much at stake for the clinician not to engage in at least limited efforts at dietary counseling; the impediments to such counseling are surmountable. As to the lack of nutrition training, it is the explicit intent of this text to provide the base of information needed for counseling. There is evidence that physician training in nutrition enhances counseling (9). As for time constraints, this chapter provides guidelines for counseling of varying scope and intensity. Limited, but nonetheless valuable, dietary guidance can be offered in only several minutes. When more extensive counseling is required, the time commitment can be spread over a number of office visits, and much of the work can be delegated to a dietary consultant. Finally, as for the issue of effectiveness, there is evidence that physician nutrition counseling does influence patient behavior (10–13). Such evidence is limited in part because the scope of research and clinical effort in this area has been limited. But lack of evidence of effect is not the same as evidence of lack of effect. Lack of evidence for dietary counseling in primary care has resulted in a lack of perceived efficacy on the part of clinicians. The resultant tendency to assign low priority to such counseling in the context of brief, dense clinical encounters has resulted in relative neglect of dietary counseling by physicians. With less counseling, there is less effective counseling and, therefore, less evidence of effect. The degenerating cycle thus produced is incompatible with the importance of diet to health. There is, as well, some evidence that such counseling as does occur often is misdirected (14).

The single most common clinical condition seen in primary care practices is obesity (15). Diet is fundamental to the management and prevention of cardiovascular diseases, diabetes, cancer, and hypertension. Thus, any controversies regarding dietary counseling in primary care should be devoted to how, not whether or why. There is reason to believe, on the basis of both judgment and empirical evidence, that greater commitment to nutrition counseling in clinical practice would lead to greater effectiveness and greater effect.

A limited assessment of dietary pattern should be routinely incorporated into every history and physical examination. A brief overview of a health-promoting diet should be provided on such occasions as well (see Chapter 40). Dietary counseling should always be linked to advice about physical activity, as the health benefits of each support those of the other; there is evidence that physician counseling effectively promotes physical activity (16). Difficulties involved in making dietary and other lifestyle changes should be discussed briefly. When more involved dietary counseling is indicated as part of weight loss or disease management efforts, the counseling generally should be shared with a dietitian. In such circumstances, the physician's role is to reinforce the detailed counseling provided by the dietitian; situate diet in the overall clinical plan; and encourage the patient's efforts by applying realistic behavior modification principles that distinguish between responsibility and blame, the reasons why, and the methods how.

Fundamental to all efforts at health promotion in clinical care is an understanding of the factors governing behavior and its modification. An overview of behavior modification principles and models is provided as a foundation on which all dietary counseling efforts should rest. A novel approach to behavior modification, synthesized from established models specifically to offer the efficiency and focus required in the context of clinical practice, is introduced (16a). This model is used to identify the patient's need for additional motivation to change, assistance in overcoming the resistance to change, or both. Means of meeting the patient's needs in both categories are discussed. Finally, a discrete list of steps in dietary counseling is provided to facilitate application in the widest possible range of clinical practice settings.

BEHAVIOR MODIFICATION THEORY AND APPLICATION

Relevant Principles

The science of effective dietary modification is in its infancy. Although the standards of evidence-based practice challenge us to advance the science, patients in need of advice today can ill afford to wait for the results of incremental progress in that regard. Therefore, as has traditionally been the case with clinical practice, a mature art may shore up an immature science until the latter has developed.

The science of dietary counseling borrows heavily from the generic science of behavior modification. Best studied of the behaviors physicians strive to change, in part because of its relative simplicity, is tobacco use, particularly cigarette smoking (17–19). Predominant behavioral models in attempts to promote health through behavior modification are the stages of change model of Prochaska and DiClemente (20); the social-cognitive model, including the concepts of self-efficacy, self-esteem, and locus of control (21); and the health beliefs model (22–25). All have relevance to dietary change. There is expanding literature to suggest that by matching dietary counseling efforts to the patient's "stage of change," significant improvements in the efficacy of counseling are likely (26–28).

The stages of change, or transtheoretical model, stipulates that behavior change proceeds through a predictable series of stages, including precontemplation, contemplation, preparation, action, and maintenance; and that, to varying degrees, needs to facilitate behavior change are similar among subjects in a particular stage (29). Included during the maintenance stage is the occasional lapse to the prior behavioral pattern, while termination, in which there is no temptation to return to the modified behavior, represents success. A potentially complex variety of factors influence the progression of individuals from one stage to the next (30), including their level of knowledge, motivation, and health beliefs; factors influencing progress may vary by stage (31,32).

Social cognitive theory is pertinent to the transition from one stage to the next. Self-efficacy refers to the capacity an individual believes himself or herself to have to initiate a desired change (33). Movement from one stage of change to the next is precluded if the patient, despite a will to initiate change,

is not convinced of his or her ability to do so. Self-efficacy can be an impediment to change either because the patient has never known/believed he or she had the capacity to make a particular change, or because prior attempts to make and maintain a particular change have failed. Implications of these two situations differ, as discussed later. In the former, the patient may merely require information; in the latter, the patient requires support in overcoming the perception of past failure and targeted strategies for overcoming the previously encountered impediments to change. Self-esteem is apt to suffer as a result of failed attempts at behavior change, leading to diminished self-efficacy (21).

Related to the concept of self-efficacy is the locus of control (21). Locus of control is either internal or external. An external locus of control implies that an individual believes the capacity to change circumstances resides without rather than within. This orientation typically occurs when one has not been able to influence the environment, but rather has been reactive to it. A prototypical example is children living under violent circumstances, who become fatalistic about their own survival, believing they can do little to influence it (34). For reasons that are largely self-evident, an external locus of control is associated with low self-esteem and low self-efficacy (21), although self-efficacy may be the more reliable predictor of change in diet-related behavior.

Although not obviously like living in violence, the pervasive struggle with diet is similar in some important ways. Most people living in violence have heard about right and wrong, but experience teaches them the opposite of the rhetoric. This also is true of diet, where most of our patients have heard what constitutes a healthful diet, but find adhering to it difficult if not impossible. The tendency to engage in behavior one knows or believes to be wrong cultivates feelings of guilt, self-doubt, and, ultimately, apathy. Recurrent failure in efforts to achieve the demands of authority, conscience, or perceived norms destroys self-esteem. This is true whether the behavior is physical violence or dietary indulgence. In a chaotic environment, one loses a sense of control, and control becomes external. Many of our patients have an empirical belief that dietary change simply is not possible. This external locus of control is vulnerable to exploitation. Knowing that a resolution of the conflict with diet can only come from without, many eagerly await the next wonder diet or miracle drug. The pervasive struggle with food and dietary control, and the common sense of failure and frustration among our patients in efforts to improve diet, support the success of manipulative practices by the food industry, publishing industry, and weight loss industries.

A third behavior modification model with relevance to dietary counseling is the health beliefs model (22,35). This model stipulates that behavior change will occur when, and only when: (i) an individual believes the consequences of not changing behavior are significant, i.e., the condition to be avoided is perceived as serious; (ii) an individual believes that he or she is personally at risk of adverse outcomes unless behavior is changed; (iii) an individual believes that the particular behavior change of interest is effective in preventing or improving the adverse outcome(s) in question; and (iv) the individual perceives the change as feasible. The constituent parts of this final criterion vary with the situation, but may include accessibility, availability, cost, convenience, safety, familiarity, and understanding. Feasibility, or the perception of it, is of course influenced by self-efficacy and locus of control, indicating the interdependence of behavior change models (36).

Synthesis of elements from various behavior modification models to characterize, and influence, the processes of change more effectively is of increasing interest (37). To that end, the governance of behavior maintenance and behavior change can be distilled down into two opposing forces: (i) desire for change, or motivation, and (ii) resistance to change, or difficulty. Believing in the importance of the condition to be avoided, in per-

sonal risk, and in the utility of the change are all components, or prerequisites, of motivation (38,39). A change believed to modify meaningfully a substantial, personal risk is desirable. Such a change, however, will only occur if the resultant motivation exceeds the aggregate resistance (whatever the nature or source of that resistance).

In this regard, the established behavior change models are informative. To effect a change, one must be capable of change. Individuals with an external locus of control cannot change their behavior until or unless they learn that they have the capacity to do so. The stages of change model represents sequential assessments of the balance between resistance and motivation. When the difficulty is perceived to exceed the rewards of change, one is unwilling to change and fails to advance to the action stage. With new information or experience, motivation for change may rise as the perceived difficulty remains constant. As the gap between the two narrows, one perceives the potential for change and becomes contemplative. Change is attempted whenever motivation, at least temporarily, exceeds the recognized resistance. The behavior change is maintained until or unless difficulty overtakes motivation, at which time relapse occurs. A more realistic, or at least more practiced, assessment of both difficulty and motivation are the result of unsuccessful attempts at change. These attempts either serve as the necessary preparation for sustainable change or lead to frustration.

The complexities of diet make behavior change particularly difficult. The well-known slogan of drug control efforts in the United States, "Just say no," is clearly impertinent when it comes to diet. Diet cannot be avoided, but it must be managed. The need to struggle with the desired behavior change on a continuous basis is more than most people can manage successfully. Consequently, the rate of compliance with dietary recommendations is apparently very low (40,41).

In primary care practice, most (but certainly not all) patients will be fairly motivated to select a health-promoting diet. This is true either because the patients are already sick and therefore motivated by the perception of personal risk, or they are seeking primary care despite being well, in which case they are seeking preventive and health-promotion services. The most common nutrition-related problem seen in primary care is obesity, and it is the one most likely to have led to prior efforts to change diet. Obese adults seeking primary care are unlikely to need motivation for dietary change. Failure to change diet in most patients is the result not of inadequate motivation, but of excessive difficulty. The only ways to produce change under such circumstances are to reduce the difficulty or increase motivation further.

Often, motivation can be raised, and specific methods of motivational interviewing have been developed (38,39). As noted by Botelho and Skinner, "advice giving," a relatively ineffective means of raising motivation, has tended to predominate in clinical practice (38). Minimally, motivation for dietary change requires knowledge of the link between diet and health. This is achieved by informing patients of the hazards of an injudicious diet and the benefits of a more healthful diet as a routine part of primary care delivery. Although patients often are informed in this area, they also frequently are misinformed, and important knowledge gaps prevail (42–44). There are particular opportunities for motivating patients with prior illness; disease-specific counseling often is more effective than health promotion (22).

An especially important aspect of raising motivation to change is reestablishing self-esteem and self-efficacy when they have been lost, and, as a related effort, cultivating an internal locus of control. Paradoxically, one of the ways to reestablish a patient's self-efficacy is to inform him or her how much of dietary behavior is beyond individual control (see Chapter 39). This approach requires that the practitioner, and patient, distinguish between responsibility and blame. Patients with repeated, unsuccessful efforts at changing diet (usually to lose weight) must be taught that

factors beyond their control contrive to prevent such change. Specifically, these factors include, at a minimum: an innate preference for sweet food; activation of endogenous opioid receptors by both dietary sugar and fat; a tendency to binge eat, which is characteristic of most omnivorous species and hunter-gatherer tribes; sensory-specific satiety; a frugal metabolism designed for protracted famine and occasional feast; unrealistic societal ideals for both male and female physique; reliance on food as a means to gratify, nurture, reward, punish, and soothe; reliance on food as the cornerstone of virtually all social occasions; active sabotage by others unsuccessful at dietary modification; deceptive labeling by food manufacturers; confusing and conflicting reports on diet and health in the popular press and media; the sociologic link between food and status, captured in the vernacular as "making dough," being the "bread winner," and "bringing home the bacon"; perceptions of food as security; instinctive fear of hunger; the inconvenience of eating differently from the majority; the proliferation of convenience technologies and the resultant decline in physical activity levels; reluctance to try unfamiliar food; lack of culturally sanctioned restraint with regard to food; and disintegration of the social context constraining and defining appropriate dietary behavior. Each of these factors is either the direct product of physiologic adaptations to the forces of natural selection or the result of sociologic, psychological, religious, and cultural evolution.

There are two reasons why a brief discussion of these exonerating factors is essential. First, by alleviating patients of their feelings of failure and futility, lost motivation for dietary change can be rediscovered. However, to prevent failure from recurring yet again, the balance between motivation and difficulty must be fundamentally altered. To do this, difficulty in changing diet must be reduced. This can only be achieved if the impediments to sustainable dietary change are recognized by both practitioner and patient, and if strategies tailored to overcome them are designed and implemented.

Patient-specific dietary counseling should only begin after the initial steps outlined earlier have been addressed. In this way, one avoids the risk of simply telling patients, again, to do something they cannot. Such is the nature of the largely unsuccessful dietary counseling traditionally offered in primary care. However, advice about what to and what not to eat is precisely what most of our patients least need. This information may require some clarification, but is readily available. For patients to change their diets, they need us to explain: (i) why it is so difficult to change diet; (ii) why they are not at fault for the difficulty; and (iii) what strategies can serve to reduce the difficulty and make sustainable change possible.

Application of Behavior Modification Theory in Clinical Practice

Although the established models of behavior change are invaluable to the developing science of effective dietary modification, a novel construct tailored to the clinical practice setting may be useful to the busy clinician. Fundamentally, behavior change may be reduced to the tension between desire for change, or motivation, and resistance to change, or the difficulty involved in altering behavior. In this model, the outcome of attempts to change diet (or other behaviors) is determined by the relative force applied by motivation and difficulty, as shown in the following formulae:

1. Capacity to change diet or sustain change = aggregate motivation − aggregate difficulty, where the difference must be positive
2. Inability to initiate or sustain dietary change = aggregate difficulty − aggregate motivation, where the difference must be positive
3. Tendency to relapse after change varies directly with difficulty and indirectly with motivation; relapse will occur when difficulty meets or exceeds motivation.

Believing in the importance of the condition to be avoided, in personal risk, and in the efficacy of the change are all components of motivation. A change believed to modify meaningfully a substantial, personal risk is desirable. Such a change, however, will only occur if the resultant motivation exceeds resistance. In this regard, the other models are informative. To effect a change, one must be capable of change. Individuals with an external locus of control cannot change their behavior until or unless they learn that they have the capacity to do so (45).

For convenience, this simple construct is referred to as the *pressure system model* (PSM) (16a), which derives its name from meteorology, where differences in barometric pressure determine the direction in which wind blows. Air is pushed from a high-pressure system toward a low-pressure system; changes in relative pressure can reverse or stifle the movement of air. In the PSM, the same is true of behavior change.

The initial contribution of the PSM is its capacity to separate two fundamental goals of behavioral counseling, raising motivation and overcoming resistance. Either effort may serve to produce the desired behavior change: movement will proceed from high to low, however the difference in relative "pressure" is achieved. This concept is displayed schematically in Fig. 1.

The conventional approach to behavioral counseling in primary care is to raise motivation (38). Patients are apprised of the health risks associated with the maintenance of smoking, alcohol consumption, illicit drug use, or sedentary lifestyle, and of the benefits of changing such behaviors. As shown in Fig. 1, when motivation can be raised above resistance, behavior change will occur.

Generally unaddressed in counseling efforts, however, are the fixed impediments to behavior change. A schedule that does not readily accommodate exercise may overcome motivation for physical activity. A fellow household member's smoking may overcome an individual's motivation to quit. The convenience and familiarity of fast food, and uncertainty about how to change patterns

**Situations in Which Change
Will Not Occur:**

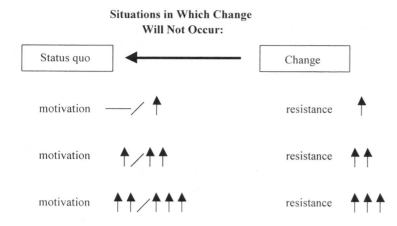

FIG. 1. Schematic representation of the pressure system model. The relative force of motivation and resistance, represented by arrows, determines whether desired behavior change occurs or whether the *status quo* is maintained. A horizontal line indicates neutrality, a single arrow modest force, two arrows moderate force, and three arrows strong force.

of shopping and cooking, may overcome an individual's desire to improve their diet (1). As shown in Fig. 1, even if motivation is fairly high, change cannot occur if resistance to change is higher still. While counseling may serve to raise motivation, the level may fail to exceed resistance.

The insidious danger in this traditional approach to counseling is the tendency to actually or at least apparently "blame the victim" of behavioral risk factors (46–50). While an unmotivated patient may be encouraged by a clinician's efforts to motivate, an already motivated patient is apt to experience frustration when change does not occur. That frustration generally is shared by the practitioner, adversely affecting the relationship (51). The PSM serves as a reminder that motivation is not infinitely malleable, and that when resistance is great enough, motivation alone cannot produce behavior change. This encourages both patient and provider to engage in the productive process of identifying impediments to change that may be surmountable, instead of the unproductive process of self-recrimination.

The second contribution of the PSM is its capacity to define the appropriate focus of counseling efforts based on discrete and easily recognized clinical scenarios. This progression from theoretical construct to clinical algorithm renders the model practical under the constraints of primary care practice.

The stages of change model may be viewed as sequential assessments of the balance between resistance and motivation. When difficulty is perceived to exceed the rewards of change, one is unwilling to change; when alternative behaviors are unfamiliar, one is unaware of the possibility of change. Either scenario results in a precontemplative state. With new information or experience, motivation for change may rise as the perceived resistance remains constant. As the gap between the two narrows, one perceives the potential for change, and becomes first contemplative, then preparative. Change is attempted whenever motivation, at least temporarily, exceeds perceived resistance. The behavior change is maintained until or unless resistance overtakes motivation, at which time relapse occurs. More realistic, or at least more practiced, assessments of both resistance and motivation result from unsuccessful attempts at change. These attempts either serve as the necessary preparation for sustainable change, or they lead to frustration.

Virtually all clinical encounters in which behavioral counseling is pertinent may be placed in one of six categories, based on the stages of change. Each scenario indicates the approach to counseling most likely to be of value.

1. The patient is precontemplative, with no prior attempts to change the behavior in question.

Counseling should be directed at raising

motivation. The clinician should attempt to encourage contemplation and preparation for action. Difficulties in achieving and sustaining behavior change should be discussed in anticipation. The focus of counseling is on what the change should be, and why it should occur.

2. The patient is contemplative, or preparative, with no prior attempts to modify the behavior in question.

Generally, in contemplative and preparative stages, motivation and perceived resistance are, or nearly are, balanced. The balance can by tipped by raising motivation slightly, or by addressing any perceived impediments to change and devising strategies to reduce the difficulties involved. The focus of counseling is on both why change should occur, and how change can be achieved.

3. The patient is actively modifying behavior, or

4. The patient is maintaining behavior change.

With sustained effort, motivation tends to wane. Difficulty often rises early, as unanticipated impediments are encountered, and slowly declines, as the new behavioral pattern becomes increasingly familiar. The patient must be encouraged to sustain motivation, and newly encountered difficulties should be discussed to develop tailored strategies. Counseling must be focused on how to maintain changes, in addition to why. As the patient acclimates to the new behavioral pattern, further improvements become possible. More detailed discussion of what additional changes should occur may be indicated.

5. The patient reports a lapse to the prior behavioral pattern.

Lapses occur in any situation where the difficulty involved in sustaining change exceeds motivation. Lapses tend to produce feelings of remorse and to affect self-esteem adversely. Counseling must serve to alleviate remorse, reestablish motivation, and assure the maintenance of an internal locus of control and self-efficacy. Discuss reasons for (re)lapse in the context of the apparent impediments to the particular behavior change. Discuss specific circumstances that lead to (re)lapse, and devise strategies for dealing with such circumstances in the future.

6. The patient is precontemplative, or contemplative, with prior attempts to modify the behavior in question.

Prior, unsuccessful efforts at behavior modification, or relapses following transiently successful efforts, tend to damage self-esteem. Low self-esteem tends to erode perceived self-efficacy and externalize the patient's locus of control. Patients in this group may benefit from counseling directed at raising motivation, but are more in need of counseling directed at raising self-esteem, relieving feelings of failure, and internalizing the locus of control. This can be achieved by explaining the involuntary elements (e.g., environment) influencing behavior and by refuting the concept of personal fault. Patients in this group will be particularly wary of the difficulties involved in changing behavior; counseling efforts should focus on tailored strategies for overcoming specific obstacles. *This stage is probably the most commonly encountered in primary care, and why conventional approaches to counseling are so ineffective.* A preferential focus on motivation in this group is likely to be harmful, exacerbating the patient's perceptions of failure and further eroding self-esteem and self-efficacy.

To apply this model, the discrete components of motivation and difficulty must be identified so that they may be targeted as indicated in counseling efforts. Factors influencing motivation may be summarized in the following relatively short list, although means of enhancing motivation are more subtle and complex (see later).

Factors contributing to motivation for dietary change:

Health beliefs:
  Risks of not changing
  Health benefits of changing
  Body image benefits of change

Social/psychological benefits of change
Social support
Perceived self-efficacy.

Whereas motivation may be inspired by a great many considerations, but is ultimately composed of relatively few, the list of actual or potential barriers to dietary change is virtually endless. Only by working with an individual patient can the salient impediments to dietary modification be identified. There are, however, barriers to dietary change that pertain to the environment, physiology, and pervasive aspects of culture; such barriers, which are apt to be universally relevant, are as follows:

1. Natural preferences for sugar, salt, and fat
2. Natural tendency to "binge" eat
3. Fear of hunger
4. Convenient availability of nonnutritious foods
5. Familiarity of nonnutritious foods
6. Inability to interpret food labels
7. Manipulation by food producers and misleading advertising practices
8. Use of food for purposes other than to satisfy hunger
9. Stress and stress relief
10. Use of food as basis for social gatherings
11. Programmed metabolic efficiency and insulin release
12. Preservation of behaviors learned in childhood
13. Insufficient knowledge to shop for nutritious foods
14. Insufficient knowledge to order nutritious dishes when eating out
15. Insufficient knowledge to prepare nutritious food at home
16. Insufficient knowledge to translate dietary guidelines into eating practices
17. Inconvenience involved in finding, ordering, or preparing nutritious foods
18. Lack of familiarity with dietary guidelines

19. Inappropriate folklore (e.g., hazards of snacking and need to eat breakfast)
20. Unpalatability of unfamiliar, nutritious foods
21. Physiologic adaptation to new foods (e.g., transient gastrointestinal discomfort associated with increased dietary fiber)
22. Genetic heterogeneity (e.g., supertasters)
23. Lack of clearly defined social constraints or societal injunctions specific to diet, such as those imposed on other pleasurable behaviors (e.g., alcohol consumption, sexual activity)
24. Costs, or perceptions regarding costs, of nutritious foods
25. Inconveniences of calorically dilute foods (i.e., need to eat more frequently, greater volume; more frequent bowel movements with higher fiber intake)
26. Sensory-specific satiety and the constant availability of food in both abundance and variety
27. Use of food as a convenient "reward"
28. Modern conveniences and time constraints that limit physical activity
29. Low self-esteem and use of food as punishment
30. Lack of self-efficacy to initiate dietary change due to prior, failed attempts.

Familiarity with a patient's general state of health will permit quick assessment of the potential importance of dietary counseling. When discussion of diet is deemed appropriate in the overall context of care, a brief dietary history should be obtained (see later) to determine how closely the patient's dietary pattern approximates pertinent guidelines. Disparities between the diet described and the diet recommended represent the initial areas of focus for dietary counseling. The patient's experience with the dietary changes of interest then can be quickly assessed to identify the applicable stage from the construct given earlier. On the basis of this classification, a decision can be made to emphasize motivational factors, strategize to overcome impediments to change, or both.

Counseling to Raise Motivation

The traditional role of the physician in promoting lifestyle changes has been to emphasize the hazards of failing to change. Clinicians are certainly well armed to do just this with regard to diet. The evidence linking injudicious dietary patterns to obesity, cardiovascular disease, cancer, metabolic derangements, and premature mortality is overwhelming. Although most of our patients are apt to know that diet is important to health, we are in a position to inform them that it is important to *their* health. The literature consistently indicates that tailored messages, and particularly tailored counseling by a physician, effectively enhance motivation for change (52,53). Consequently, specific reference to a patient's cholesterol, serum glucose, body mass index, or other parameter of individual health risk may serve to enhance motivation. There is evidence that, in general, patients tend to be motivated by personalized risk messages (22). As a result, motivation tends to rise when personal risk is explicit, as in the immediate aftermath of an adverse health event. Such junctures are opportunities for change, frequently referred to in preventive medicine as "teachable moments" (22).

Whereas some patients may be motivated by "bad" news, others respond more favorably to "good" news, i.e., the potential benefits of behavior change (54). Generally, the best results are achieved by providing both, although the relative importance of time spent on each should be assessed jointly with the patient. The advantages of dietary modification include the avoidance of adverse health events, better fitness, better weight control, and possibly longer life. In addition, given the psychological toll and social stigma associated with obesity, dietary change conducive to weight control is apt to confer psychological and even social benefits.

A variety of other considerations pertain to efforts at optimizing patient motivation. Sources of motivation are important, and some are fleeting. For example, motivation for weight loss prior to a special event may be unsustainable after the event; both clinician and patient should plan accordingly. Extrinsic motivation (38), when the patient pursues a behavior to satisfy someone else, tends to be less reliable than intrinsic motivation. Motivation for behavior change predicated on pursuit of a behavioral pattern consistent with health beliefs and personal values tends to be most robust. The clinician's role is to identify and emphasize compatibilities between the patient's priorities and the targeted dietary pattern. At all stages of the process, the patient's autonomy should be cultivated, so that the strategy for raising motivation is as much of the patient's devising as the clinician's (38).

Other aspects of motivation should be addressed based on clinical judgment. In a society where one of two adults is overweight, where obesity is the most common condition seen in primary care, where thinness and fitness are revered, and where the three leading causes of death are all linked to dietary excess, it should come as no surprise that motivation to improve diet is generally substantial. However, many patients lack the requisite knowledge of nutrition and health to relate any particular dietary changes to their personal health goals. When patients are uninformed or misinformed, education, provided by physician or dietitian, is an essential first step in the cultivation of motivation for change. Additional details on motivational interviewing have been published (39,55–57).

When motivation is high, the incremental yield of efforts to further raise motivation is small. In certain patients, such an effort may be harmful, as noted earlier. Therefore, much is to be gained by efforts directed at lowering the difficulty in achieving dietary change. At whatever "level" motivation is maintained, it is more likely to lead to behavior change if the resistance to change can be minimized.

Counseling to Overcome Impediments to Dietary Change

The impediments to dietary change are protean. The single most important element in overcoming such impediments is identifying them. Merely characterizing the following challenges to patients will facilitate a more realistic view of dietary modification, more prudent approaches to dietary health, and greater chances of long-term success.

1. Natural Preferences for Sugar, Salt, and Fat

There are both innate and acquired preferences for certain dietary components that strongly influence preference and behavior. The predilection for sweet, or dietary sugars, is innate in both humans and other mammalian species (see Chapter 36). The preference is enhanced by exposure, apparently even *in utero*. Although preference for dietary fat has not been shown to be innate, it has been shown to be in part involuntary. Activation of endogenous opioid receptors by dietary fat has been demonstrated (58), implicating an addiction-like phenomenon in the struggle to modify diet. The dietary diversity among cultures seems to suggest variability in taste preferences, but modern trends belie that perception. With affluence permitting access to fast food and concentrated dietary fat and sugar, virtually all cultures seem to share these preferences.

Alerting patients to the involuntary component of sugar and fat ingestion is an initial step in confronting the difficulties in modifying such behavior. The virtual ubiquity of these items in the food supply should be discussed. Taste, familiarity, and convenient availability are all powerful determinants of dietary intake (1) and all favor excess consumption of sugar and fat.

Because the ingestion of sugar and fat is pleasurable, and the nature of that pleasure is, at least in part, physiologically akin to addictive drug effects, the concept that pleasure should be constrained is applicable to dietary modification. In attempting to modify diet, most patients feel a sense of sacrifice in foregoing choice foods such as cake or pizza when others are partaking. Two insights should be shared. First, the pleasure derived from such indulgences may not be

worth the cost. Cocaine apparently is highly pleasurable, more so than food, but it is avoided by most people because it is known to be harmful. Similarly, dietary excesses are transiently pleasurable, but they come at a high cost in terms of remorse and, in the long term, are harmful to health. Most people who do not use cocaine feel no sense of sacrifice or self-pity due to this restraint. The avoidance of pleasurable but harmful exposures need not be perceived as sacrifice. The second insight is that the others indulging in what the patient is resisting are themselves subject to the harmful effects and may regret their lack of restraint. A timely reminder that half the adult population in the United States is overweight, 50 million are hypertensive, and 15 million are diabetic may reassure the patient that the need for restraint is not a personal martyrdom.

Although counseling can be effective in reducing the difficulty involved in limiting the intake of sugar and fat, the limitations of this approach should be acknowledged. In a review of methods for modifying sodium intake, Kumanyika (59) concluded that the only true hope was to reduce the salt present in the food supply. The same is almost certainly true of refined sugar and fat in the diet. Natural preferences coupled with ready availability render restraint an extreme challenge. The situation is compounded by deceptive food labeling practices, which have been improved but not abolished by the imposition of Food and Drug Administration regulations over recent years.

In attempting to limit the intake of preferred nutrients, patients should be advised that such changes are most difficult initially and easier with time. The effort involved in scrutinizing food labels, for example, wanes as new foods become familiar. The same is true for food preparation methods. New foods may themselves become preferred once they become familiar. As an example, women in the Women's Health Trial who were assigned to a low-fat diet developed aversions to fatty foods they previously enjoyed (60).

The perception that if food tastes good it

must be harmful, and if it is healthful it must taste bad, is essentially a modern nutritional cliché. The truth in this perception must be disentangled so that patients can make sense of it. There is nothing intrinsically good or bad about taste. Taste is a perception, and as such it is either pleasant or unpleasant. A preference for food that was, in fact, harmful would be incompatible with the survival and success of the species. Our particular food preferences developed exactly because they are healthful and favor survival, or rather were healthful and did favor survival. The dilemma in modern nutrition is that we still prefer the tastes that favored our survival during the prevailing dietary deprivations of our prehistory (61). These foods have only become harmful because we continue to crave them, and now, unlike at any prior time in history, they are readily and constantly available. Foods that taste good are not harmful. Rather, foods that taste good are the foods we tend to eat to the exclusion of others when we can, and suddenly, we can. Although understanding this dynamic does not make dietary modification easy, it may help alleviate the sense of victimization expressed by many patients.

2. Natural Tendency to "Binge" Eat

In addition to naturally prevailing taste preferences, there are natural patterns of dietary behavior. Most relevant of these is the tendency to binge eat or, expressed more moderately, to eat in excess of energy needs. This tendency has implications not only for weight regulation and related chronic disease, but also for the prevalence of eating disorders.

Study of modern-day hunter-gatherers reveals a tendency to binge eat when food is abundantly available (61). This tendency is seen in most carnivorous and omnivorous species for which access to food is intermittent and uncertain. The same tendency is thought to have characterized the dietary patterns of our common ancestry. In an environment where the availability of food is uncertain, two related adaptations are supported. The first is behavioral, namely the tendency to ingest food to the extent possible in anticipation of future shortages, and the second is physiologic, namely the capacity to store excess calories for future use. All available evidence suggests that our ancestors were consistently lean, not as a result of any greater restraint than we now have, but merely due to a very different equilibrium between available and needed calories. Yet even in prehistory, body fat was an essential means of storing energy. Fatty acids stored in the adipose tissue of a lean adult represent sufficient stored energy to last approximately 10 to 60 days. Glycogen, the form in which energy is stored for rapid access without contributing to adiposity, represents an energy supply sufficient for approximately only 10 hours of basal metabolic activity (see Chapters 5 and 10).

As is the case for resisting foods that are enticing, resisting the tendency to overeat is a challenge only partly addressed by recognizing it. Nonetheless, recognizing a problem is a necessary, if not sufficient, step in its resolution. Patients should be encouraged to recognize overeating as a natural tendency rendered maladaptive only by the abundance of the modern food supply. As such, the tendency is not cause for feelings of remorse or self-recrimination. Clearly, however, restraining this tendency is essential to achieve energy balance compatible with optimal health. Strategies for avoiding this tendency include the frequent consumption of nutrient-dense, calorie-dilute snack foods (e.g., fruits, vegetables, dried fruits, whole-grain breads and cereals, nonfat dairy products) to blunt appetite; making decisions about what and how much to eat while away from sources of "tempting" food; avoiding protracted periods without eating; and restricting food choices at home and work to nutritious and appropriate items. Additional strategies for dealing with this impediment are discussed in Chapters 5 and 36.

3. Fear of Hunger

Closely related to the tendency to binge eat, and perhaps of common origin, is a common but often unrecognized fear or anticipation of hunger. Many patients with obesity eat when not hungry. There may be genetic and physiologic factors at work in such situations, including abnormal levels of leptin, enhanced taste perception, or heightened hedonic responses (see Chapters 5 and 36). The tendency to eat despite the absence of hunger is prevalent enough, however, to constitute a cultural phenomenon. Emotional eating is a well-recognized occurrence in both eating disordered and normal populations, and including both lean and overweight (62) (see Chapter 32).

The tendency to eat for reasons other than actual hunger may be an important determinant of energy imbalance. When this tendency is extreme, exploration of the underlying psychological motivators is indicated, and psychotherapy may be required. For the more prevalent, milder tendency to eat in anticipation of hunger, behavioral interventions may prove successful. In particular, establishing a dietary pattern that permits frequent snacking while maintaining appropriate calorie intake may be effective.

4. Convenient Availability of Nonnutritious Foods

The accessibility and convenience of nutrient-dilute, energy-dense foods is a universal experience in the United States. The problem is epitomized in the popularity of the fast-food industry's success. The ultimate solution to this problem is environmental, requiring that healthful food be accessible and convenient enough to compete with the current norm. Such environmental change, advocated in Healthy People 2000 and 2010, is largely driven by market forces and will occur slowly and incompletely, if at all. In the meantime, either directly or indirectly through referrals, health care providers must be prepared to offer counseling that makes the selection of health-promoting foods simple and convenient for dietary modification efforts to succeed.

An important consideration is that people eat meals and snacks, rather than categories of foods. Little is accomplished by advocating increased consumption of fruits and vegetables if that advice is not translated into how to eat out, shop, and/or cook. There is evidence to date that ingredient substitution is among the more successful approaches to modifying nutrient intake, as it allows the basic appearance of the diet to be preserved. This approach only pertains to foods prepared at home, however.

Healthful, calorie-dilute, and nutrient-dense foods are readily available for daytime consumption. Among these are whole-grain breads, fruit, fresh vegetables, dried fruit, whole-grain cereals, and nonfat dairy products. Although such items may not be readily available in restaurants, they are easily prepared at home. One good defense against the convenient availability of poor food choices is to make sure that better food choices are as readily available. Patients should be encouraged to prepare meals and snacks for daytime consumption at home, taking some control over diet away from the environment. Detailed counseling by a dietitian may be helpful to patients uncertain about food choices. Innovative means of enhancing nutrition skills should be developed such as shopping instruction by dieticians in supermarkets. Patients reluctant to prepare food at home should receive advice about choosing restaurant and cafeteria items to promote health. Such advice is available from dietitians, in newsletters, in the media, and on-line. Resources are discussed in Section III. One example of product lines that make healthful food choices relatively easy is Subway's low-fat sandwiches.

5. Familiarity of Nonnutritious Foods

Difficulty in complying with dietary recommendations is driven not only by the familiarity of popular foods, but also by the unfamiliarity of recommended replacements. As noted earlier, one strategy to reduce this difficulty is to encourage preservation of the basic structure and appearance of the diet while changing its nutrient composition. Low-fat, low-salt substitutes can be used in the preparation of baked goods and sauces. Cookbooks and magazines that focus on ingredient substitutions for healthful eating are readily available (see Section III).

Patients should be advised that new foods may be less preferred simply because they are new and, therefore, unfamiliar. An obvious example is skim milk. Individuals accustomed to whole milk find skim milk dilute and unpalatable. This averse reaction fades rapidly, however. Most people find that after 2 weeks of drinking skim milk, its taste and consistency are preferred over whole milk, which suddenly seems too rich. Obviously, there are exceptions, such as patients who cannot adapt their taste preferences to accommodate a recommended food. Such situations call for compromises so that the diet remains pleasurable for the patient, while more closely approximating recommendations. Clearly, in such negotiations, the patient is in charge. Openly acknowledging that the patient's strong preferences will be honored alleviates some of the tension that may otherwise infuse dietary counseling. As the goal of counseling is to improve the overall dietary pattern rather than to introduce or eliminate any particular food, steering discussions around fixed items in the patient's diet is both compatible with clinical goals and conducive to success. Incremental changes in the diet over a protracted period result in gradual acclimation to a new dietary pattern, which, once familiar, becomes as easy to maintain as the diet that it replaced. Patients should be advised that the initial effort in dietary modification is greatest, with the least results to show for it. With time, the effort involved decreases, as the aggregate benefits accrue. A good analogy is mastery of a new language. Learning the rudiments of grammar and an initial vocabulary is labor intensive and tedious, at a time when ability to speak the language is limited. With persistence, fluency is slowly acquired. Once fluent, speaking the language involves little effort, and further advances occur almost naturally. The analogy extends further. For most people, learning a language is a substantial accomplishment, but one that requires considerable effort. The same is true of making meaningful improvements in diet.

6. Inability to Interpret Food Labels

New regulations have resulted in a meaningfully more informative nutrition label on commercial foods than was previously available (63). The utility of the information remains somewhat limited, however. Nutrition labels quantify micronutrient and macronutrient intakes for specified portions, and in reference to a standard diet, but do not help most people improve dietary pattern. In the context of a dietary pattern meeting recommendations, isolated foods high in sugar, salt, or fat need not necessarily be avoided. A diet made up of foods of marginal nutritional value will be poor, no matter how the individual foods contribute to the whole. Few patients keep track of nutrient intake throughout the day or are inclined to approach dinner with not only knife and fork, but also calculator in hand.

To the extent that food label interpretation facilitates healthful food choice, two approaches are recommended. If you have the time, ask the patient to bring in several food labels from foods they eat regularly and assess their ability to interpret the label. If the patient's need for dietary counseling is sufficient to warrant referral, the dietitian will likely include food label interpretation in the counseling and will certainly do so on request.

Once the patient can reliably interpret nutrition labels, the skill should be placed in context. If the diet is made up predominantly of fruits, vegetables, whole grains, fish, lean meats, and nonfat dairy products; and if foods are baked, broiled, grilled, sauteed, and poached but rarely fried, the diet is likely to approximate recommendations. To achieve such a pattern, no calculator is required. The greater the contribution to the diet of processed foods, the greater the need for label interpretation. The best application is in choosing among the many options in a particular food category, where items may differ markedly in fat, sugar, salt, and other nutrient levels. Examples include breakfast cereals, which vary markedly in fat, sugar, salt, fiber, and micronutrient content; soups, which vary markedly in sodium content; and sauces, dips, dressings, and spreads, which vary in fat, trans fat, and sodium content. Patient resources to facilitate product selection are provided in Section III.

7. Manipulation by Food Producers and Misleading Advertising Practices

Health care providers should help patients recognize and resist manipulation by the food industry. The most visible examples of the manipulation are advertisements, which, much like ads for tobacco products, encourage unhealthy practices. Ads, specific for gender, age, or ethnicity, are apt to influence behavior. To date, the manufacturers of nutritious product lines generally lack the resources to compete effectively with more established companies. Although it is unlikely you could find a patient unfamiliar with Frito-Lays chips, few are likely to have heard of Guiltless Gourmet, a producer of only baked snack foods with consistently high nutrition standards (see Section III).

Subtler than advertising practices are the permissible distortions in product labels and the concealed ingredients in many products. Only animal products contain cholesterol, but some vegetable oil bottles are labeled "no cholesterol" as a means of implying the product is health promoting. Product labels on foods containing trans fat from partially hydrogenated oils may declare "contains no tropical oils," implying a health benefit that does not exist (see Chapter 2). The use of terms such as "low-fat," "lite," and "natural" is insufficiently regulated and promotes

products more effectively than understanding.

With regard to composition, few people would suspect that commercial breakfast cereals may contain comparable amounts of salt per serving to potato chips or pretzels. The taste of the salt is concealed by sugar. Only when low-salt cereals are substituted for a period of time does the salt in the popular brand become discernible. In some instances, the addition of concealed ingredients may improve shelf life, but, more importantly, may stimulate greater consumption through the activation of multiple satiety centers (see Chapter 36).

8. Use of Food for Purposes Other than to Satisfy Hunger

Food is consumed to gratify, celebrate, sanctify, pacify, and entertain, as well as nourish. Although eating for reasons other than hunger may be more obvious in some circumstances than others, the practice is nearly universal. In modern society, hunger may be one of the less important determinants of dietary intake. Recognizing the diverse impulses that underlie dietary behavior is essential for both patient and provider in efforts to modify such behavior.

The physician with limited time to devote to dietary counseling may facilitate success by a dietitian if the concept of eating for reasons other than hunger is briefly addressed. Sensitizing patients to this consideration may result in useful insights. The practitioner with time to explore the issue further should ask the patient to compile a food diary indicating not only what and when food was eaten, but also why. This is generally only indicated in patients with either personal or medical indications for calorie restriction, most commonly obesity. When factors other than hunger are identified as consistent antecedents to eating, specific opportunities for behavior modification are generally self-evident. In situations where complex emotional factors underlie dietary patterns, psychotherapy may be indicated.

9. Stress and Stress Relief

Food influences mood. The most dramatic example of this appears to be the tendency for patients with seasonal affective disorder to self-manage with diet (see Chapter 32). Changes in dietary pattern during the menstrual cycle also suggest the use of food to manipulate mood (see Chapter 26). Food often is used in response to psychological stress. This tendency is compounded by the US dietary pattern in which little is eaten during the day, and the large meal is taken in the evening. A typical pattern emerges. Patients working a stressful job go for long periods without eating, or eating little during the day. Food may be avoided during the day in a willful effort to control calorie intake. When such a patient (who may be sounding suspiciously familiar) returns home in the evening, he or she is too hungry to alleviate stress by any means other than eating. Under such circumstances, particularly if the patient prepares the evening meal, food choice is likely to be somewhat compulsive, and portion control is apt to be poor. Dinner is not only the satisfaction of hunger, but also the alleviation of a day's worth of stress and frustration.

Such a pattern, clearly detrimental to dietary health, is perpetuated in part by folklore that seems to be common belief, namely that snacking is bad or harmful. In fact, snacking on appropriate foods may be an ideal way to control appetite and optimize nutrient intake. In particular, a late afternoon snack at work may be the essential prelude to a nutritious and moderate dinner. By snacking in the afternoon, patients are apt to arrive home calmer and less compelled to eat right away. Ideally, after work then becomes a time for physical activity. Physical activity is an effective means of alleviating psychological stress, with a panoply of ancillary health benefits as well. Exercise may actually blunt appetite and tends to encourage more prudent food choices. This scenario clarifies the interconnections among health-promoting behaviors. Exercise prior to dinner may be necessary for dinnertime meals to improve. Snacking in the afternoon may be necessary before a patient will consider exercise before dinner. For dietary counseling to succeed, diet must be addressed in the context of other behaviors and lifestyle considerations. A variety of circumstances, such as small children in the family, may render these recommendations impractical. The general principles still pertain. Working with the patient, an approach to fit some physical activity into the day, and avoid resolving stress primarily with food, generally can be found.

10. Use of Food as Basis for Social Gatherings

One of the more intractable difficulties in modifying diet is the normative pressure exerted by virtually all social gatherings. Throughout history, food has actually been, or at least symbolized, security and comfort (64). In most cultures, food plays a central role in gatherings of social importance. When food is not a significant feature at such events, it is significant by its absence, as in holy days of abstinence and fasting. At almost any time of year there will be events that threaten to disrupt a patient's efforts at dietary modification.

There are two basic approaches to this challenge. The first is to concentrate on establishing a sufficiently healthful dietary pattern so that perturbations due to social gatherings can be tolerated without adverse effect. Obviously, such an approach would require that the social gatherings in question be neither too frequent nor too indulgent. Even in healthy subjects, adverse effects of acute fat ingestion have been demonstrated (40,65) and may be clinically important.

The other approach, important either when the need for dietary modification is great or when social events are frequent, is for the patient to eat before social events and/or set strict limits in advance on food choices and portion sizes. Unlike other potentially harmful substances, diet is not amenable to a "just say no" approach. As difficult as it may be to recover from various addictions, the complexities in establishing a healthful diet are far greater. The same medium that represents a health threat is essential for survival and must be mastered rather than avoided. Simplifying rules are essential to persevere in so complex a struggle.

Such rules should be used, particularly early in efforts to improve diet, to limit temptation and the frequency of lapses. The patient should be reminded that 4 million years of evolutionary pressure are conspiring against adherence to the recommended diet, and frequent challenges to willpower and self-discipline inevitably will end in failure. Rather than permit a "should I or shouldn't I" dilemma to develop at a party or holiday, such choices should be made in advance. If necessary, the patient should formally commit to certain dietary restrictions to someone else who will serve as a social support or at least a goad to conscience. The someone else can be the health care provider, given encounters of sufficient frequency. Such an approach may seem either puerile or pedantic, but it is an effective adjuvant to other behavior modification techniques and important to the success of sustainable dietary change. Once a health-promoting diet becomes an established aspect of lifestyle, such efforts to control occasional indulgences become unnecessary.

11. Programmed Metabolic Efficiency and Insulin Release

As discussed in Chapter 10, the prevalence of type II diabetes and insulin resistance may be ascribed, in whole or in part, to a state of metabolic efficiency (66). Although the theory of metabolic thrift is still a topic of lively debate, the notion that humans have a natural disposition to store excess food energy as body fat is quite clear. Less clear is the temporal sequence in individuals predisposed to insulin resistance (see Chapters 5 and 10). Genetically programmed insulin resistance may contribute to obesity, but the

evidence is at least as good that obesity is the underlying cause of insulin resistance in most cases; certainly, insulin resistance improves with weight loss (see Chapter 10). Thus, dietary counseling to prevent or ameliorate a state of insulin resistance and metabolic efficiency is the same as dietary counseling for weight control.

The single greatest controversy in this context, and one exacerbated by a spate of popular books promoting high-protein or high-fat diets, is whether dietary carbohydrate preferentially promotes weight gain in the context of insulin resistance. In summary, there is no evidence to support this view. Overwhelmingly, the literature on obesity supports the view that energy-dense dietary fat is most strongly associated with body fat. As noted in Chapter 10, the glycemic indexes of various foods are highly variable, unintuitive, and substantively modified by other foods eaten conjointly.

Prudent recommendations for individuals with, or simply concerned about, this impediment to dietary change and weight control include the recommendation that the diet be rich in soluble fiber (67). Good sources include beans and lentils, oats, apples, and citrus fruits. Highly processed carbohydrates should be restricted and not eaten alone (e.g., white bread will raise insulin and glucose levels less if eaten as an accompaniment to whole-grain cereal in the morning, or pasta with beans at dinner; nonetheless, whole-grain bread would be preferable). Physical activity should be routine and consistent. Dietary fat should be restricted as part of an overall effort to control energy intake and prevent/reverse obesity (see Chapter 5). A benefit from substituting monounsaturated fat for refined carbohydrate, provided total calorie intake is not raised in the process, is possible (68). There is accruing evidence to suggest that pharmacotherapy may be of benefit in the prevention of diabetes in cases of overt insulin resistance, although this is not yet standard clinical practice (69–71).

Incremental modifications of diet and lifestyle can facilitate weight control, which in turn can improve insulin sensitivity. With assurances that this impediment to weight control can be overcome, a patient's willingness to engage in dietary modification is apt to increase.

12. Preservation of Behaviors Learned in Childhood

There is strong evidence in both animals and humans that dietary patterns learned in childhood tend to track into adulthood, and that such learning can begin *in utero* or during breast-feeding (see Chapter 25). The composition of breast milk is influenced by the maternal diet and can influence food preferences in childhood. The persistence of early dietary preferences has important implications for counseling.

First, the earlier in life effective nutrition counseling is provided, the better. This is true both because dietary patterns become harder to change with age, and because the sequelae of poor dietary patterns will accrue with time. The difficulty here is that the dietary patterns of children are determined by household patterns and, ultimately, the food selection of adults. Consequently, to promote the dietary health of children requires efforts to promote the dietary health of families. This brings the situation full circle, back to an effort to change the diet of an adult whose preferences were established during their childhood.

Although evidence is lacking and clearly needed in this area, intuition suggests that consistent endorsement of the same basic diet by internists, family practitioners, and pediatricians might help promote optimal nutrition for families. Effective efforts at modifying the dietary patterns of children would show increasing benefit with time, as the children grew up and passed their dietary habits on to their children. When parents with young children are being counseled, they should be reassured that the same basic diet is appropriate for everyone over the age of 2. There is a current trend in the United States to advocate a slow approximation of adult nutritional guidelines between the ages of 2 and 5 (see Chapter 27). Studies in Scandinavia suggest, however, that adult guidelines may be safe even prior to age 2 (see Chapters 6 and 27). Given the low rate of compliance with current dietary guidelines, counseling efforts that encourage households to approximate such guidelines are likely to be beneficial and safe, with little risk of producing extreme responses.

13. Insufficient Knowledge to Shop for Nutritious Foods

14. Insufficient Knowledge to Order Nutritious Dishes when Eating Out

15. Insufficient Knowledge to Prepare Nutritious Food at Home

16. Insufficient Knowledge to Translate Dietary Guidelines into Eating Practices

Most patients have a basic understanding of the fundamentals of a good diet. Some may be confused by the barrage of conflicting information in the news media, but most can distinguish signal from noise. Such knowledge does relatively little to promote national dietary objectives, however (72). There is widespread inability to convert basic dietary recommendations, such as "eat more fruits and vegetables" or "consume no more than 30% of daily calories as fat," into meals. Essentially, the technical skills required to translate dietary recommendations into dietary practices, skills for shopping, ordering out, and cooking, are lacking. Limitations in each of these areas increases the difficulty involved in modifying diet, and together they render dietary change almost impossible.

Research and innovative approaches to redressing these problems on a population basis are needed. Until such innovations occur, technical skills will need to be cultivated through individualized counseling. Such efforts are time consuming and labor intensive, and are best handled by referral to a dietitian. Patients endeavoring to acquire such skills can be aided as well by any of the good cookbooks on the subject, as well as newsletters, magazines, and classes (see Section III). The interventions required to provide cooking, shopping, and restaurant dining skills go well beyond what the clinician can or should address in the office. However, the physician must recognize that offering dietary recommendations without considering the patient's capacity to implement them is apt to be futile. Therefore, sensitivity to this issue on the part of primary care providers, and a willingness to make the needed referrals, can contribute importantly to achieving recommended dietary changes.

17. Inconvenience Involved in Finding, Ordering, or Preparing Nutritious Foods

The common perceptions about nutritious food are that it is difficult to find, inconvenient to prepare, and expensive. All of these views are fallacious. A diet rich in fresh produce and grains is generally less expensive than a diet rich in meat and cheese. Health food stores and health food sections in the major supermarket chains make nutritious products available to almost everyone in the United States. Increasing numbers of fat-, salt-, and/or calorie-reduced products are available to facilitate more healthful shopping and cooking. Often, processed foods touting health advantages are more expensive than generic competitors. Although health food brands tend to be more expensive than the products of larger producers, the price differential is offset if meat makes up a smaller part of the diet.

The principal difficulty in learning to shop, cook, and eat more healthful foods is simply that they are new, and unfamiliar. Preparation time need not increase and could even decrease. Homemade soups and stews can be prepared quickly and allowed to simmer in a pot, with beans instead of meat. A variety of salads can be quickly prepared for summertime dinners. Pasta dishes are less effort to prepare than meat-based meals. Patients must enter into the endeavor, accepting that the steep part of any learning curve is encountered early, and in that phase progress is slow. Mastery of technical skills for nutritious eating can be achieved quickly by a motivated patient. Dietitians can and should be relied on to help impart such skills; written and online resources are available as adjuncts (see Section III).

18. Lack of Familiarity with Dietary Guidelines

Patients for whom knowledge about what to eat is a limiting factor in efforts to modify diet are probably the exception rather than the rule. Such patients will benefit from brief educational efforts in the context of their primary care. Referral to a dietitian is appropriate if substantial nutrition education is indicated. Additional resources for such patients are provided in Section III.

19. Inappropriate Folklore

Certain prevailing assertions about diet and health are misleading and contribute to the difficulty in modifying diet. Most people have heard that health suffers when breakfast is missed. Studies of the adverse health effects of a missed breakfast in the United States were conducted primarily in indigent school children who wanted breakfast but did not get it. Not surprisingly, such children were distracted in school and performed less well than better-fed counterparts. The relevance of these findings to voluntarily missed breakfasts is uncertain (73). There is no evidence that health suffers when one waits to have breakfast until one gets hungry. The first meal of the day, whenever it is, is breakfast. Long periods without eating generally are imprudent, but hunger is an appropriate guide for most people.

Another common adage is that snacking is to be avoided. In fact, what most of us heard in childhood was to avoid snacking so as not to spoil our appetites. Some degree of appetite "spoiling" is desirable for most patients attempting to control calorie intake. Snacks should be nutritious. Portion and calorie control will be poor if snacks are chosen only for pleasure. Few people have the self-discipline to resist chocolate bars if they are hungry and that is what is available. However, by planning ahead, one can be certain to have nutritious snacks available. Eating nutrient-dense foods during the day tends to control appetite, alleviate stress, mitigate psychological factors influencing food intake, make exercise after work more appealing, and possibly confer metabolic benefits such as reduced utilization of insulin (see Chapters 5, 10, and 36).

20. Unpalatability of Unfamiliar, Nutritious Foods

The empirical evidence that the human palate can adapt to a variety of culinary conditions is clear. The variety of cuisines consumed around the globe is testimony to the importance of cultural norms and familiarity in defining dietary preferences. For the same reasons, unfamiliar foods are resisted and often, at first, disliked. Our ancestors apparently struggled with the omnivore's paradox (64), a tendency to be curious about untried food, but an equal tendency to be wary. Such conflicting inclination helped cultivate the necessary dietary diversity, while helping to avoid ingestible toxins.

Provider and patient must recognize that new foods may be unpalatable or relatively so merely because they are new, and that taste perception is likely to change with time. Literature is scant on the time required, but clinical experience suggests that for simple changes, such as whole to skim milk, 1 or 2 weeks generally suffice. More fundamental dietary changes naturally require a longer period of acclimation. Efforts to modify diet must factor in sensory resistance to change. Once overcome, this difficulty becomes an asset. Newly acquired dietary patterns become more satisfying with time as they supplant a previous pattern and become familiar.

21. Physiologic Adaptation to New Foods

Our ancestors are thought to have consumed nearly 100 g per day of dietary fiber, a level few of us could tolerate without unpleasant side effects. Yet, our gastrointestinal tracts certainly are capable of tolerating such a high fiber intake (typical fiber intake among adults in the United States is approximately 10 to 12 g per day, and 30 g per day is recommended). There is clearly physiologic accommodation of a particular dietary pattern, in this instance an alteration in gastrointestinal flora and peristaltic activity in response to differing levels of dietary fiber. If counseling results in a marked increase in dietary fiber, some bloating and discomfort are likely. Clearly this is not a reason to abandon the effort. In such situations, an incremental approach to diet modification spread over weeks to months will permit the necessary physiologic adjustments to occur so that the recommended diet is tolerated without ill effect. Once again, forewarned is forearmed. The patient who suddenly experiences unanticipated abdominal discomfort while attempting to increase cereal, vegetable, and fruit consumption may abandon the effort.

22. Genetic Heterogeneity

There is evidence that dietary preferences may be mediated, at least in part, by sensory and hedonic perceptions mediated by genetic heterogeneity (see Chapter 36). Specifically, variability in the acuity of taste perception has been reported, as have variations in hedonic responses to food of differing composition (see Chapter 36). These traits may facilitate, or more likely impede, efforts at dietary modification. Patients genetically predisposed to derive intense pleasure from fat or sugar in the diet will have particular difficulty modifying their intake of such foods. Assessments of taste perception and/or the activation of the endogenous opioid system by fat or sugar are performed to date only in research settings and are not applied clinically. Whether or not such evaluations will come to guide clinical interventions is unclear. If this difficulty is encountered, there is no evidence base to draw from in designing countermeasures. Reasonable strategies include use of artificial sweeteners to control sugar consumption and use of fat substitutes (see Chapter 38) to modify fat intake. There is an apparent association between obesity and enhanced hedonic responses to food. Therefore, weight management is likely to be an important clinical objective in such patients. Use of pharmacologic agents may be indicated, depending on clinical urgency (see Chapter 5).

23. Lack of Clearly Defined Social Constraints or Societal Injunctions Specific to Diet such as Those Imposed on Other (Pleasurable) Behaviors

The prevalence of obesity in the United States exceeds that in other industrialized countries, although the secular trends are similar. This may be due in part to the deterioration in social constraints on dietary behavior. More and more, food is chosen on the basis of convenience in families where both adults work. Less time for food preparation results in the consumption of more processed and fast food. Frenetic work schedules result in isolated eating, often in an office or car, where social pressures cannot moderate food choice or portion size. Food choices and portions tend to be more moderate in public than in private (72). Patients should be apprised of these threats to self-restraint and encouraged to develop compensatory strategies. Approaches that may be helpful include eating with co-workers during the day, restriction of food choices to those that support nutrition goals, and exertion of control over food choice by preparing food at home to have available during the day. Social support for efforts at improving diet, by both family and friends, can be very important.

Generally, society places boundaries on the pursuit of dangerous pleasures either with legislation or convention. Mind-altering drugs, alcohol, tobacco, recreational vehicles, and sexual activity are all governed to one degree or another by both systems of constraint. Diet, however, is unbound by either system. The probable explanation for this is twofold. First, and simply, diet is essential for life and cannot be avoided. Its governance is too complex to lend itself readily to legislation. Second, and perhaps of greater significance, is the vast human history of dietary deprivation. Most social governance of dietary patterns by convention pertains to food as a scarce commodity. Food is status, as in the "bread" winner, bringing home the "bacon," or making "dough." Health consequences of dietary excess are a modern phenomenon, and one for which we are ill prepared, both individually and collectively.

In counseling patients, the unique position of diet among accessible pleasures should be acknowledged with a specific goal in mind. Although most people accept limits to the pursuit of other pleasures, limits on dietary pleasure-seeking tend to be perceived as self-sacrifice, if not outright martyrdom (discussed earlier). Patients should be advised that widespread public health problems have resulted from the ungoverned pursuit of dietary pleasures, and that applying limits here is no less reasonable than applying them to drug use. Ideally, society will collectively confront dietary excess as a health threat and generate compensatory conventions. Until or unless such changes occur, patients are left to construct such conventions individually. Doing so can effectively overcome this particular difficulty in achieving sustainable dietary change. Failure to do so is a significant threat to sustained change, as the pressure to yield to a sense of sacrifice often is intense.

24. Costs, or Perceptions Regarding Costs, of Nutritious Foods

As noted earlier, the cost associated with nutritious eating need be no higher, and may be lower, than eating a typical American diet. A patient needing extensive help with food selection should be referred to a dietitian.

Resources for choosing foods in accord with recommendations are provided in Section III.

25. Inconveniences of Calorically Dilute Foods

A diet rich in fat and processed carbohydrate is calorie dense. The same diet is naturally low in fiber, minimizing food volume. This caloric density may represent a convenience. Satiety can be achieved with relatively compact meals. Eating may be infrequent and still meet, or more likely exceed, energy needs. An increase in vegetables, fruits, and whole-grain products results in increased fiber intake and increased food volume. In general, a diet meeting recommendations is rather energy dilute. Meeting energy needs with such a diet requires more frequent eating and/or larger meals. Such a diet will naturally tend to increase fecal bulk and, therefore, the frequency of bowel movements. Such an effect is advantageous in terms of health, with a potential reduction in colon cancer risk specifically (74). The inconveniences associated with such changes in diet should be anticipated and accommodated. For example, as discussed earlier, snacking may need to be encouraged to permit satiety when calorically dilute foods are substituted for calorically dense ones. The habit of bringing food from home to work may need to be developed. The inconveniences are relatively minor, but, if encountered without preparation, they may contribute to the aggregate difficulty involved in achieving or sustaining dietary change.

26. Sensory-specific Satiety and the Constant Availability of Food in Both Abundance and Variety

As discussed in Chapter 36, satiety thresholds in the hypothalamus for bitter, salty, sour, and sweet flavors are distinct. Consequently, appetite subsides more readily when food choice is limited and persists when a variety of foods, and flavors, are available. In our society, dietary diversity is available at all times, with diverse flavors contributing to every meal. The activation of multiple satiety centers rather than one is compounded by the addition of largely unperceived flavor enhancers to commercial foods, such as salt in breakfast cereals.

Sensory-specific satiety, the tendency to become satiated with a particular taste but not others, is thought to have conferred a survival advantage in prehistory, when dietary diversity required work and was the key to nutritional adequacy. The trait persists even though, under modern conditions in the United States, it contributes to caloric excess.

Patients should be informed of this tendency, in order to establish pertinent behavioral defenses. For example, snacks should be comprised of one food, or few closely related foods, rather than a greater variety. Meals should be balanced, but should avoid excessive variety. Dessert, when eaten, should be limited to one variety. Commitment in advance to certain protective dietary patterns is essential. Patients should not decide on the spot whether to have one dessert or two, but rather should follow general rules established (by the patient) before "temptation." The rationale here in controlling behavioral responses is similar to the time-honored advice not to shop for food when hungry. Patients should know that an inability to resist dietary temptation is the norm, not the exception. For precisely that reason, the avoidance of such temptation is required.

27. Use of Food as a Convenient "Reward"

As discussed earlier (see also Chapters 32 and 36), food is used as a source of pleasure and gratification. Beyond the physical pleasure associated with food is the psychological role played by food. Tastes and smells evoke memories, foods are associated with occasions, and an abundance of food is strongly linked to a feeling of security and well-being. Parents often use the pleasure of sweets to entice and influence the behavior of children, both dietary behavior (e.g., dessert as a reward for eating other food) or other behavior (e.g., candy as a reward for some accomplishment). Behavioral psychology emphasizes the role of behaviors learned in childhood in subsequent preferences; thus, many of us have learned from early childhood to view the use of food as reward as appropriate.

The use of food for reward tends to contribute to injudicious dietary patterns and excessive intake of total energy. This tendency can be overcome in several ways. To prevent it primarily, clinicians, particularly pediatricians and family practitioners, should discourage the use of nutrient-poor, energy-dense foods as reward or coercion in childhood. The easiest means of achieving this goal is to keep only nutritious foods at hand; even desserts can be relatively low in fat and sugar (see Section III). Nutritious alternatives to most popular snacks are available.

For the adult using food as a reward, two strategies are useful. First is one of harm reduction. To the extent that rewarding foods can be modified to be lower in calories and richer in nutrient value, the less the nutritional harm associated with the reward. Ingredient substitution has been shown to be an effective means of preserving the appealing characteristics of foods and meals, while altering (improving) their nutritional value. The second approach, complementary to the first, is to highlight the "cost" of the reward. The overweight patient who wants to lose weight will to some extent suffer if the use of food for pleasure results in further weight gain. Often, the net discontent exceeds the pleasure; under such conditions, the putative reward has had an effect opposite to that intended. Patients must be guided to see the long view: immediate dietary pleasure may result in net "pain" over the short term, while some degree of immediate restraint may seem like sacrifice at first, but could actually increase net satisfaction. The clinician is well-advised to recognize the powerful role of food in providing gratification and to work with the patient to strategize around this obstacle to the extent required.

28. Time Constraints that Limit Physical Activity

Long-term control of weight without regular physical activity seems virtually unachievable (see Chapter 5). Further, the clustering of health-promoting behaviors suggests that each reinforces the others; physical activity predicts and apparently reinforces good dietary practices. Although dislike of physical activity (or, at least, dislike of anticipated physical activity) may be a common impediment, one of the most widespread excuses for a sedentary lifestyle is lack of time to exercise. Time constraints limiting recreational activity are that much more damaging given an environment in which conveniences increasingly reduce the level of physical activity required in the performance of routine tasks. Drive through restaurants, e-mail, television remote control devices, and computer games are limited examples of influential environmental factors.

There is evidence that clinician counseling is associated with increased physical activity (75). The effect of such counseling is apt to be greater if, in addition to highlighting the benefits of physical activity to health, the clinician takes a realistic view of fitting physical activity into the day. The evidence that, in the aggregate, routine activity is of cardiovascular benefit is now widely accepted. Physical activity counseling should begin with recommended use of the stairs rather than an elevator, parking as far as is reasonable from work or other buildings, and looking for opportunities simply to get up and move during the day.

With regard to actual exercise, the two most available times are before and after work for most adults. There are advantages and disadvantages to each. The morning workout may be facilitated by ease of access to exercise equipment. A home treadmill or Nordic Track, or other such equipment, may be far more practical than membership in a gym one never has time to visit. If the morning workout is kept brief and moderate, it can be energizing rather than draining, and it can help begin the day well. Morning workouts often are precluded when there are young children in the house who wake early. In a two-parent household, some agreement about division of labor may provide time for both parents to get their exercise.

There are particular advantages, and specific impediments, to exercise after work. The principal impediment tends to be hunger. In an effort to control weight, because of an unaccommodating work schedule, or due to the erroneous notion that snacking is invariably bad, many individuals refrain from eating throughout the afternoon and come home from work very hungry. This hunger tends to be compounded by the need to relieve any pent-up frustrations of the day, a need often met with food. However, exercise is an excellent means of alleviating frustration/stress and confers the advantage of burning rather than contributing calories.

For a patient to comply with a recommendation about exercise, other guidance may be required. A late afternoon snack is a good practice that mitigates daytime stress and prevents preoccupying hunger when returning home from work. Physical activity after work then may become feasible, affording additional relief from any residual stress. Dietary behavior following exercise tends to be less compulsive and more moderate, so that a more reasonable dinner is apt to follow. The mere introduction of daytime snacking may facilitate increased physical activity and improved dietary pattern.

Of course, no such simple recommendations can be counted on to work universally. Again, a willingness to work with the individual patient to go beyond what should be done to develop strategies for *how* it can be done is essential for productive counseling.

29. Low Self-esteem and Use of Food as Punishment

30. Lack of Self-efficacy to Initiate Dietary Change due to Prior, Failed Attempt(s)

A common reason for recidivism in efforts to abstain from drugs, alcohol, or tobacco is exposure to the substance in a social context. Obviously, in the case of diet, such exposure is completely unavoidable. Consequently, efforts to modify diet are particularly vulnerable to lapses. A compassionate response on the part of the health care provider is essential.

The evidence of psychological sequelae of dieting efforts is compelling (76). Most patients with reason to modify diet have attempted to do so and failed. In particular, obesity, the most visible evidence of failure to achieve mastery over diet, results in low self-esteem and tends, with time, to erode self-efficacy and externalize the locus of control for behavioral change.

Exacerbating this problem is the tendency for health care practitioners to themselves have an external locus of control for diet, believing they can do little to alter patients' nutrition. Evidence of successful dietary counseling is modest to date, but need not limit future successes. There is nothing to be lost and potentially much to be gained by practitioners acknowledging to patients that dietary change is difficult, but certainly achievable. An important contributor to the limited success of efforts to change diet is likely to be relative inattentiveness to the multiple physiologic, sociologic, anthropologic, and psychological impediments to change outlined here. A patient previously disempowered by failed efforts to improve diet or control weight may be empowered merely by knowing the obstacles faced. A shared recognition of barriers to dietary change between patient and provider(s), and a commitment to design specific, compensatory strategies is empowering to both (all) involved. Failed attempts to modify diet in the past is a weight that should be set down before future attempts ensue. Compassionate and enlightened counseling should permit this weight to be readily laid aside. Without such support, patients, particularly those struggling to control their weight, are apt to use food as punishment for their failed ability to control their diet, a self-perpetuating cycle of failure and despair.

STEPS IN THE DELIVERY OF DIETARY COUNSELING

A systematic approach to diet is an essential first step in effective dietary counseling. The standard outpatient history and physical examination often does not specifically include sections on diet, physical activity, or screening, all of which are fundamental to health promotion and disease prevention. Although putatively components of the social history, diet and physical activity are frequently unaddressed (10). Simply asking a patient to characterize their diet will provide some insights. A patient who does not know what the question means is not likely to be making particular efforts to ensure a prudent diet. Such patients are precontemplative and require motivation to initiate efforts at improving diet. Patients who respond by describing efforts to control fat or sweet intake are in the action stage and are most likely to benefit from "how to" advice.

Ten Steps of Initial Dietary Counseling

The frequency and intensity of dietary counseling in the context of clinical care will vary with the objectives and the patient's disease burden. A healthy patient has little cause to return frequently to the office, and, if they were to do so, insurers would be unlikely to reimburse. Consequently, patients being counseled for health promotion and primary prevention exclusively should receive counseling at the time of the periodic physical examination. Such counseling obviously is less involved, although no less important,

than that given to patients with diet-related pathologies, such as diabetes mellitus or hyperlipidemia, who are returning for regular follow-up.

In either situation, the overriding objective is to modify the patent's diet to promote health and achieve any specific therapeutic goals. The basic steps in achieving that objective are consistently applicable across the spectrum from health promotion to tertiary prevention.

The steps to follow in providing dietary counseling are as follows:

1. Obtain a brief dietary history.
2. Identify any objective indications for dietary change.
3. Obtain, as indicated, a history of prior attempts to modify diet with the rationale and results.
4. Briefly explore the patient's beliefs about dietary change, including their current stage of change, self-efficacy, and locus of control. Specifically address self-esteem in general, and specifically with regard to diet.
5. Discuss the universal difficulty with modifying diet and the shared impediments to dietary change.
6. Explicitly refute individual fault or blame for diet-related medical problems and/or inability to change diet.
7. Emphasize the importance of personal responsibility to sustainable dietary change.
8. Characterize the proper approach to dietary modification and the need to establish lifelong patterns of behavior.
9. Obtain, as indicated, a detailed dietary history, or refer to a nutrition specialist.
10. Deliver tailored advice.

Steps 1 and 2: To modify any patient's diet, the practitioner must know what the current diet is, and whether it warrants changing. Therefore, the first step is to obtain, personally or by referral, an adequate dietary history, and the second step is to identify any objective indications for dietary change. (See "Obtaining a Dietary History" later.) Once a determination has been made that the patient should modify his or her diet, a history of prior attempts to do so is important. The impediments to dietary modification are distinctly different between patients who have not considered issues of nutrition and health and those who have made recurrent attempts to improve diet, often to control weight, resulting in failure or only transient success. The next step is to assess the patient's readiness to change, their understanding and beliefs of the link between diet and health, and the effort they are willing to devote. Patients attempting to control weight, in particular, are apt to suffer from prior failed attempts and low self-esteem.

Steps 3 and 4: The patient for whom dietary change is indicated should be asked about prior attempts to change diet and the outcomes. This should lead to a discussion of the patient's current readiness to accept and act on dietary advice, and his or her sense of self-efficacy with regard to diet. This brief discussion will serve to assign the patient to one of the categories in the pressure system model, indicating whether counseling is likely to benefit most from a focus on motivation or on impediments, as discussed earlier.

Step 5: The next step, especially important for patients discouraged by prior attempts to improve diet, is to describe the pervasiveness of difficulty controlling diet. The prevalence of disease and conditions attributable in whole or in part to dietary excess reveals that struggling with diet is a nearly universal experience in our culture and among our patients. Consequently, a discussion of this struggle almost invariably is the appropriate first element in productive counseling. All of our natural defenses are directed at dietary deficiency: a tendency to binge eat, a preference for fat and sugar, and sensory-specific satiety, to name a few. We have no natural defenses against dietary excess, which is, for the most part, a modern anomaly. Our biologic vulnerabilities are compounded by a manipulative food industry, media hype, lack of opportunity for exercise, and deteriora-

tion of the social constraints on dietary behavior. The result of this constellation of physiologic and sociologic influences is a vulnerability, shared almost universally among populations in developed countries, to overconsume calories with resultant obesity, hypertension, hyperlipidemia, heart disease, and diabetes.

Patients should be informed of the relevance of evolution and natural selection to our dietary tendencies. As discussed in the Chapter 39, much of modern dietary behavior can be explained in an evolutionary context. The human genome has not changed meaningfully in the past 40,000 years; consequently, we remain biologically prehistoric. Our prehistoric environment is responsible for our dietary adaptations, which include a tendency to efficiently store excess energy as body fat. Preferences for dietary sugar and fat are nearly universal and are thought to have conferred a survival advantage during 4 million years of evolutionary history. Foods are preferred based on familiarity, convenient availability, variety, and involuntary aspects of physiology. Both fat and sugar have been shown to activate endogenous opioid receptors. Explaining to patients the obstacles to dietary modification is the first step in overcoming them.

Most patients seeking dietary advice have attempted to modify their diets and failed. This is particularly true of weight control efforts, where the psychological sequelae of recurrent, unsuccessful efforts at dietary mastery have been well described (76). A tendency in American medicine to "blame the victim " (46) has compounded this problem, making patients reluctant to discuss diet with physicians and encumbering them with a sense of inadequacy.

Informing patients of the prevalence of dietary difficulty is essential. Images of perfect bodies on television and in print media cultivate the belief that one's dietary struggles are an anomaly. In fact, some 40% to 60% of the adult population is actively engaged in a weight loss effort during the course of any given year (77), and more than half the adults in the United States are now overweight by National Institutes of Health criteria. By characterizing the prevalence of dietary struggles, both physician and patient readily perceive that such difficulties are not the product of personal failure or lack of will power. Something far more fundamental is at play. Patients with psychological sequelae related to diet are unlikely to succeed in efforts to modify their diets unless such issues are addressed.

Step 6: A population perspective on dietary excess makes it very easy to be a compassionate counselor and help patients renounce the concept of individual failure and fault, which is the next step in effective counseling. There is little to be gained by inferring from the epidemic and endemic state of obesity in the United States that half the adult population suffers from character flaws, such as sloth, gluttony, or lack of will power. These stigmas have been ascribed to obesity, and its victims, by the lay public and health professionals alike. The product has been minimal success in dietary counseling.

Patients would do well to understand the prevailing dietary struggle in which so many are engaged as the product of a toxic nutritional environment. Living in a world of abundant calories, fat, sugar, and salt, creatures that are adapted to crave sugar, salt, and fat and to efficiently store calories fare badly. Our collective nutritional plight is no different from that of polar bears transported to the desert; adapted to store heat where heat is sparse, they would do so no less effectively in an environment where heat abounds.

Step 7: Patients should be guided to discard perceptions of individual blame for dietary difficulties, but not individual responsibility for their resolution; this is the next objective. Although many patients blame themselves for their obesity, when asked, few are willing to blame an individual for his or her diabetes. Yet if the patient with diabetes consistently fails to take prescribed medication or adhere to a recom-

mended diet and winds up repeatedly in the emergency department, most see a breach of responsibility. This paradigm is applicable to all efforts at dietary modification. Patients must be helped to lay aside feelings of personal failure and to embrace responsibility. No effort at dietary modification will succeed if the patient expects the solution to come from without.

Step 8: Most patients with prior attempts at dietary change have made short-term interventions for short-term goals. The "crash diet" as the prelude to a new bathing suit, dress, or suit or to some important occasion is a common experience. Yet this view of weight and diet control is at odds with other chronic conditions. For example, a patient with diabetes may have an elevated blood sugar that falls to normal after a dose of insulin. The diabetes, however, has not been cured despite the normal blood sugar. Similarly, the tendency to store excess calories as body fat, to be hyperlipidemic, hypertensive, or diabetic, does not go away in the aftermath of some transient dietary change. For dietary modification to promote health, it must be permanent, in response to the permanence of the physiology it is intended to accommodate. Clarifying to patients that diet must be approached as an element of lifestyle is the next goal in counseling.

Step 9: Patients for whom nutritional interventions represent a key element in clinical management should provide a detailed dietary history as the basis for individually tailored advice. The acquisition of such a history, and the delivery of such advice, generally are best achieved as a collaborative effort between the primary care provider and a dietitian. Methods for obtaining such a history are described later.

Step 10: The final step in counseling, the delivery of tailored advice, is addressed in Chapters 5–39 and 40.

An unembellished approach to these steps in dietary counseling, with the exception of a detailed history, need not take up more than approximately 10 minutes, even less in uncomplicated patients. Even this modest time commitment may be excessive in the context of a brief, problem-focused encounter, but is an appropriate allocation of time during a longer visit, such as a periodic physical examination. Investing this time in helping patients to understand the broader context of nutritional difficulties is worthwhile whether one will be providing dietary counseling directly and/or referring to a dietitian, or if the patient is to have no further dietary counseling at all.

Obtaining a Dietary History

Obtaining a Preliminary History

Questions about diet and physical activity should be a routine element in the outpatient history and physical examination, and they are often appropriate additions to the inpatient history as well. Obtaining a dietary history is an essential element in assessing chronic disease risk and, therefore, should be included among the screening interventions addressed at the periodic physical examination. The second report of the US Preventive Services Task Force explicitly calls for dietary counseling as a routine aspect of primary care delivery; such counseling presupposes a dietary history. The labor intensiveness of dietary counseling will decline as nutrition is incorporated routinely into the medical interview. Patients with prior experience in recounting their dietary history will do so more fluently and perhaps more accurately; the inclusion of dietary history in the medical record will preclude the need to start from "scratch" with each patient encounter.

A dietary history, as other elements of the history, should begin with open-ended questioning and proceed to more restrictive questions as required. The patient should be asked to describe or characterize his or her overall diet. Generally, patients who respond comfortably to this question are engaged in some effort to control their diet to promote health. Patients not engaged in any particular effort to select a health-promoting diet often

are uncertain how to answer the question. Brief prompting is effective: Do you try to eat a healthy diet; restrict your fat, sugar, or salt intake; eat fruits and vegetables regularly; eat fast food often; eat whatever you feel like without considering health effects? Patients making no effort to choose a healthful diet are best considered to be consuming the "typical American diet," which is a diet deficient in fruits, vegetables, many micronutrients, and fiber, and excessive in total fat, saturated fat, trans fat, salt, refined carbohydrate, simple sugars, and calories. The patient who reports healthful dietary practices only with prompting may be misleading, either intentionally or otherwise. There is evidence that dietary intake often is reported inaccurately (40,78,79).

Time constraints and the goals of dietary counseling will determine the requisite depth, breadth, and accuracy of the dietary history. A minimal history will indicate whether a patient does or does not need encouragement to consider food an important determinant of health outcomes. With only a few questions, the provider can determine whether the patient is engaged in effective efforts to promote health with diet, is attempting to eat a prudent diet but with only partial success, or is not involved in such an effort. The history proceeds based on this determination.

Patients consuming a "typical American" diet and not involved in an effort to improve their nutritional health should be interviewed to determine why. Such patients may feel incapable of improving their diet due to low self-esteem, lack of knowledge, or an external locus of control. Alternatively, such patients may not believe diet represents a potential threat to long-term health, or that dietary modification is an effective means of promoting health. Patients may report being incapacitated by conflicting nutrition reports in the media. The health beliefs of the patient should be elicited to guide counseling. Patients attempting to comply with dietary recommendations but either failing to do so by their own account or based on dietary history (see later) are good candidates for referral to a dietitian. Clinicians should prepare the patient for dietary counseling by specifically endorsing a particular pattern of dietary modification, which should be discussed with the dietitian. Finally, patients apparently succeeding at following a healthful diet should be encouraged to persist. Generally, the effort required to modify and improve one's diet is greatest at the beginning, but wanes with time.

To determine whether a patient engaged in efforts to pursue a healthful diet is or is not succeeding requires a somewhat detailed dietary history. Physicians with insufficient time or interest to obtain such a history themselves may refer to a dietitian at this point. Evidence suggests, however, that the dietitian's efforts will yield greater results if explicitly endorsed by the physician (80). For those who choose to pursue a more detailed history themselves, the recommendations that follow allow for the task to be accomplished efficiently.

Obtaining a Detailed History

Patients reporting efforts to pursue a healthful diet often are inattentive to ingredient labels or food composition; therefore, they are likely to be inaccurate in assessing dietary composition. Such patients are in the action phase of behavior change, and they would benefit from learning how to implement such change (26). In such instances, a detailed history is enlightening for both clinician and patient.

A customary approach to the more detailed history is to ask the patient to describe dietary intake on a typical day. The day prior to the visit is optimal in terms of recall, provided it is representative. Once again, beginning with open-ended questions is preferable. Alternatively, if the dietary history is to be obtained at a follow-up visit, the patient may be asked to compile a 3-day food diary. By referring to such a record, the physician is able to pose detailed questions about the timing, distribution, composition, and size of meals and snacks.

Whether obtained orally or in writing, the food diary serves as a basis for identifying beneficial and detrimental aspects of the patient's dietary behavior and for common misapprehensions. Often, the patient attempting to improve nutrition will achieve greater improvements in the appearance than in the composition of the diet. For example, breakfast is likely to be reported as a bowl of cereal, the common perception being that cereal is "healthy" food, and that a switch from bacon and eggs to cereal inevitably implies better nutrition. The type of cereal should be elicited, however. Cereal can be either low or high in fat, low or high in fiber, low or high in sugar, and low or high in sodium. Many commercial brands contain comparable amounts of salt per serving as potato chips or pretzels, although the salt often is masked by sugar and not readily perceived. Similarly, patients will report the cereal but not the milk. Whole milk is approximately 3.5% fat by weight and provides approximately 50% of its calories from fat, most of which is saturated. In contrast, skim milk is virtually free of fat, and 2% milk contains approximately half the fat of whole milk. A slice of toast or a bagel may be reported; the type of bread and the spread used generally are not. If butter, margarine, or cream cheese is used on bread, the spread may be the dominant source of calories. White bread or plain bagels provide substantially less fiber than do whole-grain counterparts.

Lunch frequently is reported as a sandwich, soup, or salad. Again, more details than are readily offered generally are required to assess the nutritional composition of the meal. For example, a turkey sandwich may be turkey roll (made from processed parts, often including skin, as well as fillers), white bread, mayonnaise, and cheese. In contrast, a turkey sandwich could be sliced turkey breast on whole-grain bread with mustard, lettuce, and tomato. Although perhaps comparable with regard to sodium content, the fat, fiber, calorie, and micronutrient content of the two similarly named sandwiches would differ substantially.

Patients are apt to report eating a salad, but not mention the dressing. With the addition of bleu cheese dressing, a salad can become nutritionally comparable to a cheeseburger. Dinner may be reported as chicken, but the cooking method used may be omitted. Fried chicken with skin is high in both total and saturated fat; baked, broiled, or grilled skinless chicken breast is very low in fat. Throughout the day, snack foods such as chips, nuts, muffins, Danish, or doughnuts are apt to go underreported. Nuts, eaten casually during the day or in the evening, are a dense source of fat and calories, yet are often left out of an initial food diary.

With sufficient prompting, the food diary should serve as the foundation of a detailed dietary history. After reviewing and discussing the food diary or the patient's 24-hour recall for not more than 10 minutes, a reasonably clear picture of the patient's habitual dietary pattern, familiarity with nutrition principles, and understanding of nutrition labels should emerge. Although this information serves as the basis for tailored counseling, merely alerting the patient to misperceptions about his or her customary diet is an important initial counseling effort. For a busy clinician working with a motivated and intelligent patient, much can be achieved merely by asking the patient to compile the diary; there generally are some revelations even for the patient who reviews such a document alone. (See Section III for a dietary intake form for patient use.)

course of clinical care is of universal importance.

Encouraging patients to eat well for the promotion of health and the prevention and/or amelioration of disease should be approached in the context of well-established principles of behavior modification. Some patients will need to be motivated before willing to consider change, others will need help strategizing to maintain change currently under way, and still others will need help overcoming the sequelae of prior failed attempts. This latter group, perhaps predominant, may be harmed by counseling efforts focusing only on motivation. Application of the pressure system model of behavior modification identifies discrete clinical scenarios in which motivational counseling is needed and likely to be productive. Much effort at dietary modification fails due to the diverse and challenging obstacles to a healthy diet in the modern "toxic" nutritional environment. The clinician committed to promoting the nutritional health of patients must commit to devising strategies, tailored to individual patients, over and around such obstacles.

The evidence that dietary counseling in the context of clinical care can change behavior and/or outcomes is limited, but such evidence does exist. The application of methods specifically tailored to the setting of clinical practice should lead to better outcomes than have been described to date. A concerted effort by clinicians to incorporate nonjudgmental dietary guidance into routine clinical care is clearly indicated by the importance, and universal relevance, of diet to health.

SUMMARY

The combination of diet and physical activity pattern together constitute the second leading cause of premature death in the United States (2). Even this dominant role in health may be an underestimate; because everyone eats, the health of every patient seen is influenced, for good, bad, or both, by diet. Therefore, attention to dietary pattern in the

REFERENCES

1. Glanz K, Basil M, Maibach E, et al. Why Americans eat what they do: taste, nutrition, cost, convenience, and weight control concerns as influences on food consumption. *J Am Diet Assoc* 1998;98:1118–1126.
2. McGinnis J, Foege W. Actual causes of death in the United States. *JAMA* 1993;270:2207–2212.
3. US Preventive Services Task Force. *Guide to clinical preventive services,* 2nd ed. Baltimore: Williams & Wilkins, 1996.
4. Davis C. The report to Congress on the appropriate federal role in assuring access by medical students,

residents, and practicing physicians to adequate training in nutrition. *Public Health Rep* 1994; 109:824–826.

5. Bruer R, Schmidt R, Davis H. Nutrition counseling—should physicians guide their patients? *Am J Prev Med* 1994:308–311.

6. Kessler L, Jonas J, Gilham M. The status of nutrition education in ACHA college and university health centers. *J Am Coll Health* 1992;41:31–34.

7. Glanz K. Review of nutritional attitudes and counseling practices of primary care physicians. *Am J Clin Nutr* 1997;65:2016s–2019s.

8. Kushner R. Barriers to providing nutrition counseling by physicians: a survey of primary care practitioners. *Prev Med* 1995;24:546–552.

9. Lazarus K. Nutrition practices of family physicians after education by a physician nutrition specialist. *Am J Clin Nutr* 1997;65:2007s–2009s.

10. Nawaz H, Adams M, Katz D. Weight loss counseling by health care providers. *Am J Public Health* 1999;89:764–767.

11. Brunner E, White I, Thorogood M, et al. Can dietary interventions change diet and cardiovascular risk factors? A meta-analysis of controlled trials. *Am J Public Health* 1997;87:1415–1422.

12. Schectman J, Stoy D, Elinsky E. Association between physician counseling for hypercholesterolemia and patient dietary knowledge. *Am J Prev Med* 1994;10:136–139.

13. Ockene I, Hebert J, Ockene J, et al. Effect of physician-delivered nutrition counseling training and an office-support program on saturated fat intake, weight, and serum lipid measurements in a hyperlipidemic population: Worcester Area Trial for Counseling in Hyperlipidemia (WATCH). *Arch Intern Med* 1999;159:725–731.

14. Kreuter M, Scharff D, Brennan L, et al. Physician recommendations for diet and physical activity: which patients get advised to change? *Prev Med* 1997;26:825–833.

15. Rippe J. The case for medical management of obesity: a call for increased physician involvement. *Obes Res* 1998;6:23s–33s.

16. Calfas K, Long B, Sallis J, et al. A controlled trial of physician counseling to promote the adoption of physical activity. *Prev Med* 1996;25:225–233.

16a. Katz DL. Behavior modification in primary care: the Pressure System Model. *Prev Med* In press.

17. Prochaska J, Crimi P, Papsanski D, et al. Self-change processes, self-efficacy and self-concept in relapse and maintenance of cessation of smoking. *Psychol Rep* 1982;51:989–990.

18. DiClemente C, Prochaska J. Self-change and therapy change of smoking behavior: a comparison of processes of change in cessation and maintenance. *Addict Behav* 1982;7:133–142.

19. Rossi J, Prochaska J, DiClemente C. Processes of change in heavy and light smokers. *J Subst Abuse* 1988;1:1–9.

20. Prochaska J, DiClemente C. Stages of change in the modification of problem behaviors. *Prog Behav Modif* 1992;28:183–218.

21. Abusabha R, Achterberg C. Review of self-efficacy and locus of control for nutrition- and health-related behavior. *J Am Diet Assoc* 1997;97:1122–1132.

22. Jekel J, Elmore J, Katz D. *Epidemiology, biostatistics, and preventive medicine.* Philadelphia: WB Saunders, 1996.

23. Fleury J. The application of motivational theory to cardiovascular risk reduction. *Image J Nurs Sch* 1992;24:229–239.

24. Damrosch S. General strategies for motivating people to change their behavior. *Nurs Clin North Am* 1991;26:833–843.

25. Kelly R, Zyzanski S, Alemagno S. Prediction of motivation and behavior change following health promotion: role of health beliefs, social support, and self-efficacy. *Soc Sci Med* 1991;32:311–320.

26. Mhurchu C, Margetts B, Speller V. Applying the stages-of-change model to dietary change. *Nutr Rev* 1997;55:10–16.

27. Curry S, Kristal A, Bowen D. An application of the stage model of behavior change to dietary fat reduction. *Health Educ Res* 1992;7:319–325.

28. Nigg C, Burbank P, Padula C, et al. Stages of change across ten health risk behaviors for older adults. *Gerontologist* 1999;39:473–482.

29. Velicer W, Hughes S, Fava J, et al. An empirical typology of subjects within stage of change. *Addict Behav* 1995;20:299–320.

30. Prochaska J. Assessing how people change. *Cancer* 1991;67:805–807.

31. Velicer W, Norman G, Fava J, et al. Testing 40 predictions from the transtheoretical model. *Addict Behav* 1999;24:455–469.

32. Ruggiero L, Rossi J, Prochaska J, et al. Smoking and diabetes: readiness for change and provider advice. *Addict Behav* 1999;24:573–578.

33. Strecher V, DeVellis B, Becker M, et al. The role of self-efficacy in achieving health behavior change. *Health Educ Q* 1986;13:73–92.

34. Lynch M, Cicchetti D. An ecological-transactional analysis of children and contexts: the longitudinal interplay among child maltreatment, community violence, and children's symptomatology. *Dev Psychopathol* 1998;10:235–257.

35. Love M, Davoli G, Thurman Q. Normative beliefs of health behavior professionals regarding the psychosocial and environmental factors that influence health behavior change related to smoking cessation, regular exercise, and weight loss. *Am J Health Promot* 1996;10:371–379.

36. AbuSabha R, Achterberg C, Elder J, et al. Theories and intervention approaches to health-behavior change in primary care. *Am J Prev Med* 1999; 17:275–284.

37. Elder J, Ayala G, Harris S. Theories and intervention approaches to health-behavior change in primary care. *Am J Prev Med* 1999;17:275–284.

38. Botelho J, Skinner H. Motivating change in health behavior. Implications for health promotion and disease prevention. *Primary Care* 1995;22:565–589.

39. Miller W. Motivational interviewing: research, practice, and puzzles. *Addict Behav* 1996;21:835–842.

40. Katz DL, Brunner RL, St Jeor ST, et al. Dietary fat consumption in a cohort of American adults, 1985–1991: covariates, secular trends, and compliance with guidelines. *Am J Health Promot* 1998;12:382–390.

41. Kennedy E, Bowman S, Powell R. Dietary-fat in-

take in the US population. *J Am Coll Nutr* 1999;18:207–212.

42. Buttriss J. Food and nutrition: attitudes, beliefs, and knowledge in the United Kingdom. *Am J Clin Nutr* 1997;65:1985s–1995s.

43. Prabhu N, Duffy L, Stapleton F. Content analysis of prime-time television medical news. A pediatric perspective. *Arch Pediatr Adolesc Med* 1996; 150:46–49.

44. Plous S, Chesne R, McDowell AR. Nutrition knowledge and attitudes of cardiac patients. *J Am Diet Assoc* 1995;95:442–446.

45. Wallston B, Wallston K. Locus of control and health: a review of the literature. *Health Educ Monogr* 1978;6:107–117.

46. Lowenberg J. Health promotion and the "ideology of choice." *Public Health Nurs* 1995;12:319–323.

47. Marantz P. Blaming the victim: the negative consequence of preventive medicine. *Am J Public Health* 1990;80:1186–1187.

48. Reiser S. Responsibility for personal health: a historical perspective. *J Med Philos* 1985;10:7–17.

49. Minkler M. Personal responsibility for health? A review of the arguments and the evidence at century's end. *Health Educ Behav* 1999;26.

50. Brownell K. Personal responsibility and control over our bodies: when expectation exceeds reality. *Health Psychol* 1991;10:303–310.

51. Butler C, Rollnick S, Scott N. The practitioner, the patient and resistance to change: recent ideas on compliance. *Can Med Assoc J* 1996;154:1357–1362.

52. Kreuter M, Strecher V. Do tailored behavior change messages enhance the effectiveness of health risk appraisal? Results from a randomized trial. *Health Educ Res* 1996;11:97–105.

53. Brug J, Campbell M, Assema PV. The application and impact of computer-generated personalized nutrition education: a review of the literature. *Patient Educ Counsel* 1999;36:145–156.

54. Rothman A, Salovey P. Shaping perceptions to motivate healthy behavior: the role of message framing. *Psychol Bull* 1997;121:3–19.

55. Berg-Smith S, Stevens V, Brown K, et al. A brief motivational intervention to improve dietary adherence in adolescents. The Dietary Intervention Study in Children (DISC) Research Group. *Health Educ Res* 1999;14:399–410.

56. Smith D, Heckemeyer C, Kratt P, et al. Motivational interviewing to improve adherence to a behavioral weight-control program for older obese women with NIDDM. A pilot study. *Diabetes Care* 1997;20: 52–54.

57. Botelho R, Skinner H, Butler C, et al. The practitioner, the patient and resistance to change: recent ideas on compliance. *Can Med Assoc J* 1996;154: 1357–1362.

58. Drewnowski A. Why do we like fat? *J Am Diet Assoc* 1997;97[Suppl]:s58–s62.

59. Kumanyika S. Behavioral aspects of intervention strategies to reduce dietary sodium. *Hypertension* 1991;17:i90–i95.

60. Kristal A, White E, Shattuck A, et al. Long-term maintenance of a low-fat diet: durability of fat-related dietary habits in the Women's Health Trial. *J Am Diet Assoc* 1992;92:553–559.

61. Eaton S, Konner M. Paleolithic nutrition revisited: a twelve-year retrospective on its nature and implications. *Eur J Clin Nutr* 1997;51:207–216.

62. Somers E. *Food and mood,* 2nd ed. New York: Henry Holt and Company, 1999.

63. Food and Drug Administration. An FDA consumer special report: focus on food labeling. *FDA Consumer* 1993.

64. Tannahill R. *Food in history.* London, England: Penguin Books, 1988.

65. Plotnick GD, Corretti M, Vogel RA. effect of antioxidant vitamins on the transient impairment of endothelium-dependent brachial artery vasoactivity following a single high-fat meal. *JAMA* 1997; 278:1682–1686.

66. Neel J. Diabetes mellitus: A "thrifty" genotype rendered detrimental by "progress"? *Am J Hum Genet* 1962;14:353–362.

67. Mathers J, Daly M. Dietary carbohydrates and insulin sensitivity. *Curr Opin Clin Nutr Metab Care* 1998;1:553–557.

68. Grimm J. Interaction of physical activity and diet: implications for insulin-glucose dynamics. *Public Health Nutr* 1999;2:363–368.

69. Jha R. Thiazolidinediones—the new insulin enhancers. *Clin Exp Hypertens* 1999;21:157–166.

70. Landsberg L. Insulin resistance and hypertension. *Clin Exp Hypertens* 1999;21:885–894.

71. The Diabetes Prevention Program. Design and methods for a clinical trial in the prevention of type 2 diabetes. *Diabetes Care* 1999;22:23–634.

72. Committee on Dietary Guidelines Implementation, Food and Nutrition Board, Institute of Medicine. In: Thomas PR, ed. *Improving America's diet and health: From recommendations to action.* Washington, DC: National Academy Press, 1991.

73. Shaw ME. Adolescent breakfast skipping: an Australian study. *Adolescence* 1998;33:851–861.

74. Bostik R. Diet and nutrition in the etiology and primary prevention of colon cancer. In: Bendich A, Deckelbaum RJ, eds. *Preventive nutrition: The comprehensive guide for health professionals.* Totowa, NJ: Humana Press, 1997.

75. Burton L, Shapiro S, German P. Determinants of physical activity initiation and maintenance among community-dwelling older persons. *Prev Med* 1999;29:422–430.

76. Stunkard A, Sobal J. Psychosocial consequences of obesity. In: Brownell KD, Fairburn CF, eds. *Eating disorders and obesity. A comprehensive handbook.* New York: Guilford Press, 1995, 417–421.

77. Millen B, Quatromoni P, Gagnon D, et al. Dietary patterns of men and women suggest targets for health promotion: the Framingham Nutrition Studies. *Am J Health Promot* 1996;11:42–52.

78. Barr K. To eat, perchance to lie. *New York Times* Aug. 30, 1995.

79. Lichtman S, Pisarska K, Berman E, et al. Discrepancy between self-reported and actual caloric intake and exercise in obese subjects. *N Engl J Med* 1992;327:1893–1898.

80. Hiddink G, Hautvast J, van Woerkum CM, et al. Consumers' expectations about nutrition guidance: the importance of the primary care physicians. *Am J Clin Nutr* 1997;65:1974s–1979s.

BIBLIOGRAPHY

See "Sources for All Chapters."

Thomas B. *Nutrition in primary care.* Oxford, England: Blackwell Science, 1996.

US Preventive Services Task Force. Guide to Clinical Preventive Services, 2nd ed. Alexandria, VA: International Medical Publishing, 1996.

US Department of Agriculture, Agricultural Research Service 1999. USDA Nutrient Database for Standard Reference, release 13. Nutrient Data Laboratory home page, http://www.nal.usda.gov/fnic/foodcomp.

Achterberg C, McDonnel E, Bagny R. How to put the food guide pyramid into practice. *J Am Diet Assoc* 1994;94:1030–1035.

Kritchevsky D. Dietary guidelines—the rationale for intervention. *Cancer* 1993;72:1011–1114.

Department of Agriculture and US Department of Health and Human Services. *Nutrition and your health: dietary guidelines for Americans,* 4th ed. Washington, DC: Department of Agriculture and US Department of Health and Human Services, 1995.

Nutrition Committee, American Heart Association. *Dietary guidelines for healthy American adults. A statement for physicians and health professionals by the Nutrition Committee, American Heart Association. Circulation* 1988;77:721A–724A.

Parcel GS, Edmundson E, Perry CL, et al. Measurement of self-efficacy for diet-related behaviors among elementary school children. *J Sch Health* 1995;65:23–27.

Laforge RG, Greene GW, Prochaska JO. Psychosocial factors influencing low fruit and vegetable consumption. *J Behav Med* 1994;17:361–374.

Rogers PJ. Eating habits and appetite control: a psychobiological perspective. *Proc Nutr Soc* 1999;58:59–67.

Foreyt JP, Poston WS 2nd. The role of the behavioral counselor in obesity treatment. *J Am Diet Assoc* 1998;98[10 Suppl]:s27–s30.

Poston WS 2nd, Foreyt JP. Obesity is an environmental issue. *Atherosclerosis* 1999;146:201–209.

Senekal M, Albertse EC, Momberg DJ, et al. A multidimensional weight-management program for women. *J Am Diet Assoc* 1999;99:1257–1264.

Hark L, Deen D Jr. Taking a nutrition history: a practical approach for family physicians. *Am Fam Physician* 1999;59:1521–1528, 1531–1532.

SECTION III

Tables

TABLE IIIA. *Nutrition formulas of clinical interest*

Biological value of protein
Biological value = Food N − (Fecal N + Urinary N)/(Food N − Fecal N), *where biological value of egg albumin is set at 100 as the reference standard*

Protein chemical score (to measure quality)
Chemical score = (mg of limiting amino acid in 1 gm of test protein/mg of amino acid in 1 gm of reference protein) × 100, *where lysine, sulfur-containing amino acids, or tryptophan are generally the limiting amino acids*

Creatinine height index as a measure of somatic protein status
(Milligram urinary creatinine in 24 hours in the study subject/mg urinary creatinine in 24 hours by normal subject of same height and sex) × 100

Energy units
1 kilocalorie = 4.18 kilojoules

Hamwi equation for ideal body weight
Men: 106 lb/5 ft. + 6 lb/additional inch ± 10%
Women: 100 lb/5 ft. + 5 lb/additional inch ± 10%

Harris-Benedict Equation (energy requirements): [a]
Men: BEE = [66 + (13.7 × W) + (5 × H) − (6.8 × A)] × SF
Women: BEE = [655 + (9.6 × W) + (1.7 × H) − (4.7 × A)] × SF
General: W × 30 kcal/kg/day × SF
W = weight in kg, H = height in cm, A = age in years, SF = stress factor
For weight gain of approximately 1 kg per week, an additional 100 kcal per day should be provided

Representative stress factors:

Alcoholism:	0.9
Burn (>40%):	2.0–2.5
Cancer:	1.10–1.45
Head trauma:	1.35
Long-bone fracture:	1.25–1.30
Mild starvation:	0.85–1.0
Multiple trauma:	1.30–1.55
Peritonitis:	1.05–1.25
Severe infection:	1.30–1.55
Uncomplicated postoperative recovery:	1.00–1.05

Nitrogen balance:
B = I − (U + F + S)
B = balance; I = intake; u = urine; f = feces; s = skin (desquamation)
Alternatively, Nitrogen balance = (Ni/6.25) − Ne + 4
Ni = dietary protein intake in gm/24 hr, Ne = urinary urea nitrogen in gm/24 hr, 4 estimates nonurea nitrogen losses

Percent ideal body weight (BW) = (actual BW/ideal BW) × 100

Percent usual body weight (BW) = (actual BW/usual BW) × 100

Protein requirement in lactation:
Additional protein required = {(750 ml × 0.011 g protein/ml)/0.70 efficiency} × 1.25 variance = 14.7 g/day

Resting energy expenditure by oxymetry:
Metabolic rate (kcal/hr) = 3.9 × VO_2(L/hr) + 1.1 × VCO_2(l/hr), VO_2 = oxygen consumption, VCO_2V = carbon dioxide generation

Units of measure:
1 oz = 28.4 g
1 lb = 454 g
1 kg = 2.2 lb
1 pint (16 oz) = 568 ml
1 liter = 1.76 pints = 0.88 quarts
mg = mmol/atomic weight

[a] See: Frankenfield DC, Muth ER, Rowe WA. The Harris-Benedict studies of human basal metabolism: history and limitations. J Am Diet Assoc. 1998;98:439–445.

TABLE IIIB. *Growth and body weight assessment tables*

TABLE III.B.-1: *Growth chart, 0–36 months, girls*

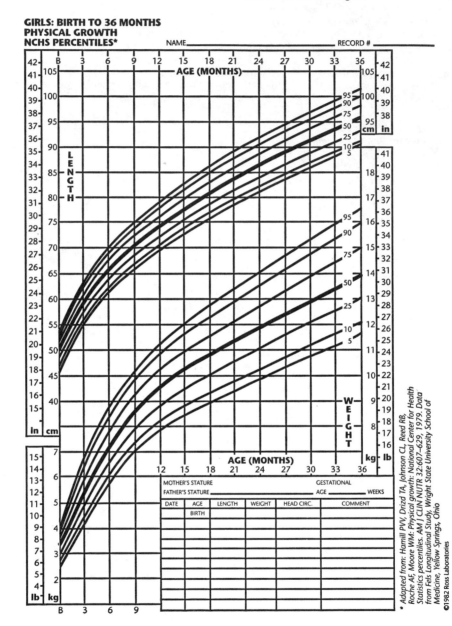

TABLE IIIB.-2: *Growth chart, 0–36 months, boys*

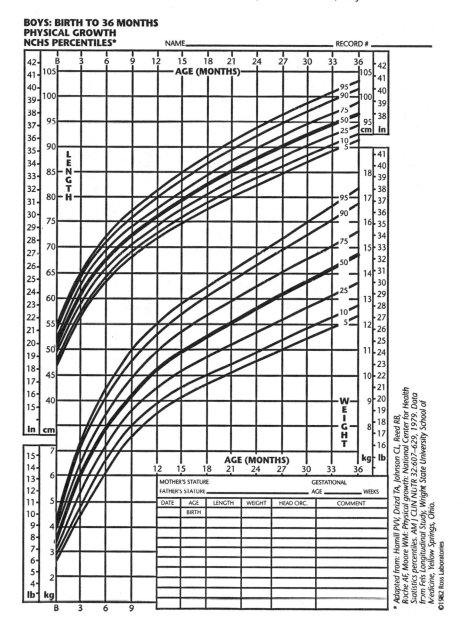

BOYS: BIRTH TO 36 MONTHS
PHYSICAL GROWTH
NCHS PERCENTILES*

TABLE IIIB.-3: *Growth chart, 2–18 years, girls*

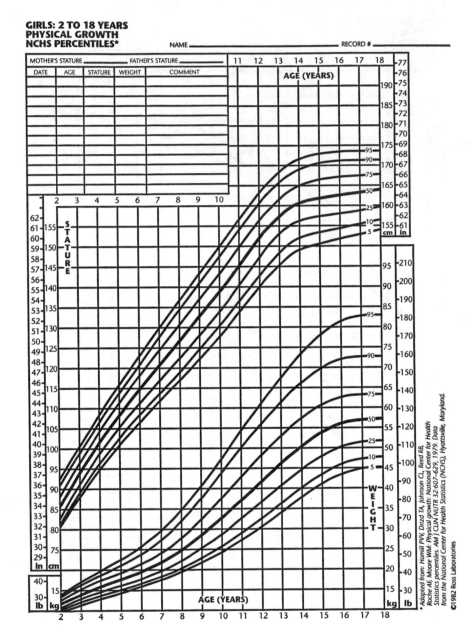

GIRLS: 2 TO 18 YEARS
PHYSICAL GROWTH
NCHS PERCENTILES*

* Adapted from: Hamill PVV, Drizd TA, Johnson CL, Reed RB, Roche AF, Moore WM: Physical growth: National Center for Health Statistics percentiles. AM J CLIN NUTR 32:607–629, 1979. Data from the National Center for Health Statistics (NCHS), Hyattsville, Maryland.

©1982 Ross Laboratories

TABLE IIIB.-4: *Growth chart, 2–18 years, boys*

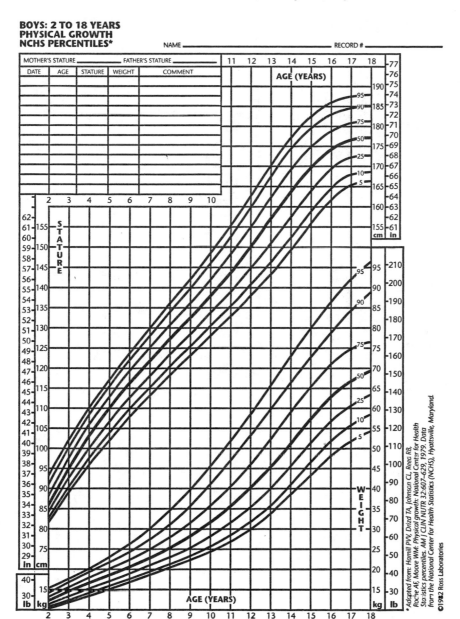

BOYS: 2 TO 18 YEARS
PHYSICAL GROWTH
NCHS PERCENTILES*

*Adapted from: Hamill PVV, Drizd TA, Johnson CL, Reec RB, Roche AF, Moore WM: Physical growth: National Center for Health Statistics percentiles. AM J CLIN NUTR 32:607–629, 1979. Data from the National Center for Health Statistics (NCHS), Hyattsville, Maryland.
©1982 Ross Laboratories

TABLE IIIB.-5: *Body mass index nomogram: adults*

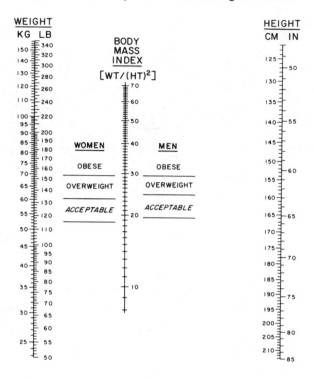

TABLE IIIC. *Dietary intake assessment in the U.S. population*

Dietary intake patterns in the US have been tracked with several surveys of nationally representative samples:

- **National Health and Nutrition Examination Surveys (NHANES)**
  These surveys are conducted by the National Center for Health Statistics of the Centers for Disease Control and Prevention (CDC). Probability samples of the US population are surveyed, using 24-hour recall and food-frequency questionnaire.

NHANES I:	1971–1974	$N = 28,000$
NHANES II:	1976–1980	$N = 25,000$
Hispanic HANES:	1982–1984	$N = 14,000$
NHANES III:	1988–1994	$N = 35,000$

- **Continuing Survey of Food Intakes by Individuals (CFSII)**
  These surveys are conducted by the United States Department of Agriculture (USDA) at 3-year intervals. Probability samples of the US population are surveyed, using one or more 24-hour recall surveys and a 2-day food record.

CFSII:	1985–1986	$N = 9,000$
	1989–1991	$N = 15,000$
	1994–1996	$N = 15,000$

- **Behavioral Risk Factor Surveillance System**
  An annual survey conducted by the CDC of a probability sample of 2000 individuals in each state. Limited information is provided on dietary intake.

For additional information, see Dietary Assessment Resource Manual. The Journal of Nutrition. 1994;124(11s); Kennedy ET, Bowman SA, Powell R. Dietary-fat intake in the US population. J Am Coll Nutr. 1999;18:207–212; Munoz KA, Krebs-Smith SM, Ballard-Barbash R, Cleveland LE. Food intakes of US children and adolescents compared with recommendations. Pediatrics. 1997;100:323–329.

TABLE IIID. *Dietary intake assessment instruments*

Various instruments are available for the assessment of individual dietary intake, each with particular advantages and disadvantages. Standard methods include 24-hour recall; food diaries of varying length, typically from 2 to 7 days; and semi-quantitative food frequency questionnaires. Useful resource materials for identifying or obtaining dietary intake assessment instruments include:

- Dietary Assessment Resource Manual. The Journal of Nutrition. 1994;124(11s)
- United States Department of Agriculture. Center for Nutrition Policy and Promotion. The Healthy Eating Index. USDA Office of Communications. Washington, D.C. 1995
- Olendzki B, Hurley TG, Hebert JR, Ellis S, Merriam PA, Luippold R, et al. Comparing food intake using the Dietary Risk Assessment with multiple 24-hour dietary recalls and the 7-Day Dietary Recall. J Am Diet Assoc. 1999;99:1433–1439

On the following page is a form patients can use for compiling a diet diary. The form is supportive of the counseling goals provided in chapter 41. The patient should be given one copy of the form for each day of intake assessment.

Dietary Intake Form

To the patient: Use the table below to record your dietary intake *during a single day* (indicate the date and day of the week at the top of the table). Make an effort to eat as you usually do, and to record everything in detail. Provide information on what you ate; an estimate of the portion size; when you ate (time); where you ate or the source of the food (e.g., home, car, restaurant, office, vending machine, etc.); and why, whether for hunger, boredom, stress relief, or some other reason. You will be able to review this diary with your doctor, dietitian, or other professional nutrition counselor to identify both what you should change to improve your diet, and how you can implement recommended changes successfully.

Meal/snack	Descriptors	Day of the week:	Date:	Work day? Y/N
Pre-breakfast	What			
	How much			
	When			
	Where			
	Why			
Breakfast	What			
	How much			
	When			
	Where			
	Why			
AM snack(s)	What			
	How much			
	When			
	Where			
	Why			
Lunch	What			
	How much			
	When			
	Where			
	Why			
PM snack(s)	What			
	How much			
	When			
	Where			
	Why			
Dinner	What			
	How much			
	When			
	Where			
	Why			
Evening snack(s)	What			
	How much			
	When			
	Where			
	Why			
Other				

TABLE IIIE. *Nutrient/nutriceutical reference tables: intake range and dietary sources*

The following tables provide detailed information for a representative sample of micronutrients for which there is both current interest in supplementation beyond the traditionally recommended range, and a body of pertinent and controversial research evidence in the literature.

Biotin

BIOLOGICAL FUNCTION(S) IN HUMANS/KEY PROPERTIES: Functions in the transport of carboxyl groups. Essential in carbohydrate and lipid metabolism, and is a cofactor in the metabolic pathways of certain amino acids.

ABSORPTION/SOLUBILITY/STORAGE/PHARMACOKINETICS: Water-soluble. Absorption occurs primarily in the jejunum. Produced by intestinal flora. There is some egestion of biotin in feces; excretion in urine rises with dietary intake. Avidin, a protein found in uncooked egg albumin, binds biotin and prevents absorption.

RATIONALE FOR SUPPLEMENTATION: Advocated to improve insulin sensitivity in diabetes mellitus, to strengthen nails and hair, and for treatment of seborrheic dermatitis.

EVIDENCE IN SUPPORT OF SUPPLEMENTATION BEYOND RDA: Studies of biotin supplementation in humans are limited; animal literature is far more extensive.

Recommended Intake Range (US RDA): Intake in the range of 30–100 μg/day is considered safe and adequate. No formal RDA has been established. An intake of 10 μg/day for formula-fed infants during the first 6 months of life, and 15 μg/day during the second 6 months of life is recommended. Adult levels are recommended for children over the age of 11.

AVERAGE INTAKE, US ADULTS:	28–42 μg/day
ESTIMATED MEAN PALEOLITHIC INTAKE (ADULT)[a]:	Not available
COMMON DOSE RANGE FOR USE AS SUPPLEMENT:	1,000–16,000 μg/day
DO DIETARY PATTERNS MEETING GUIDELINES PERMIT INTAKE IN THE SUPPLEMENT RANGE?:	No
INCLUDED IN TYPICAL MULTI-VITAMIN/MULTI-MINERAL TABLET?:	Yes (dose: 30 μg)

DEFICIENCY
Intake level: Intake threshold for deficiency not established in healthy individuals. Deficiency may be induced after intestinal resection, or with ingestion of large amounts of avidin in raw egg white. Deficiency may be induced by protracted antibiotic use and eradication of normal intestinal flora.
Syndromes: anorexia, nausea, glossitis, dermatitis, depression, alopecia

TOXICITY
Intake level: not established; no toxicity demonstrated at doses up to 10 mg/day
Syndromes: none known

Dietary Sources[b] (Cereal grains contain biotin in amounts ranging from 3–30 μg/100 gm, but with varying bioavailability: most of the biotin in wheat, for example, is bound and not bioavailable. Fruits and meats contain negligible amounts of biotin.):

Food	Serving size (gm)	kcal	Biotin (μg)	Food	Serving size (gm)	kcal	Biotin (μg)
Liver	100	161	100–200	Soy flour	100	436	60–70
Yeast	100	295	100–200	Egg yolk	100	358	16

Effects of Food Preparation and Storage: Not reported to be a generally important determinant of dietary intake levels.

[a] Eaton SB, Eaton SB, III, Konner MJ. Paleolithic nutrition revisited: A twelve-year retrospective on its nature and implications. Eur J Clin Nutr. 1997;51:207–216

[b] The nutrient composition of most foods can be checked by accessing the USDA Nutrient database at: www.nal.usda.gov/fnic/foodcomp/Data/SR 13. Biotin content is not currently provided in USDA reports, and was obtained from the sources cited above.

Sources:
National Research Council. Recommended Dietary Allowances. 10th edition. National Academy Press. Washington, D.C. 1989
Margen S. The Wellness Nutrition Counter. Health Letter Associates. New York, NY. 1997
Murray MT. Encyclopedia of Nutritional Supplements. Prima Publishing. Rocklin, CA. 1996
Shils ME, Olson JA, Shike M (editors). Modern Nutrition in Health and Disease. 8th edition. Lea & Febiger. Philadelphia, PA. 1994
Ziegler EE, Filer LJ, Jr. (editors). Present Knowledge in Nutrition. 7th edition. ILSI Press. Washington, D.C. 1996
Ensminger AH, Ensminger ME, Konlande JE, Robson JRK. The Concise Encyclopedia of Foods and Nutrition. CRC Press, Inc. Boca Raton, FL. 1995
United States Department of Agriculture. USDA Nutrient Database for Standard Reference. Release 11-1. 1997

TABLE IIIE. *Continued (Boron)*

Boron

BIOLOGICAL FUNCTION(S) IN HUMANS/KEY PROPERTIES: Plays a role in the metabolism of calcium, phosphorous, magnesium, steroid hormones, and vitamin D. May play a role in the regulation of cell membrane function. Boron may enhance the effects of estrogen on bone density.

ABSORPTION/SOLUBILITY/STORAGE/PHARMACOKINETICS: Boron in food is rapidly absorbed and excreted predominantly in urine. Boron is distributed throughout the body compartments, but most concentrated in bone, teeth, hair, nails, spleen, and thyroid tissue.

RATIONALE FOR SUPPLEMENTATION: Prevention and treatment of osteoporosis and arthritis. Possibly, prevention of urolithiasis. May lower cardiovascular risks as a result of increasing endogenous estrogen.

EVIDENCE IN SUPPORT OF SUPPLEMENTATION BEYOND RDA: No RDA established. The study of therapeutic effects of supplemental boron is in its infancy. Small human studies, including few randomized, double blind pilot studies, show beneficial effects on bone metabolism and symptoms of osteoarthritis (see chapter 13).

Recommended Intake Range (US RDA): No RDA has been established. A range of 1–10 mg/day is considered safe and adequate daily intake.

AVERAGE INTAKE, US ADULTS:	0.5–3.1 mg/day
ESTIMATED MEAN PALEOLITHIC INTAKE (ADULT)[b]:	Not available
COMMON DOSE RANGE FOR USE AS SUPPLEMENT:	3–9 mg/day
DO DIETARY PATTERNS MEETING GUIDELINES PERMIT INTAKE IN THE SUPPLEMENT RANGE?:	Yes
INCLUDED IN TYPICAL MULTI-VITAMIN/MULTI-MINERAL TABLET?:	Yes (dose: 150 μg)

DEFICIENCY
Intake level: below 0.3 mg/day; possibly, below 1 mg/day
Syndromes: uncertain; may contribute to osteoporosis, and depress both muscle and cognitive function

TOXICITY
Intake level: uncertain; apparently toxic above 500 mg/day
Syndromes: nausea, vomiting, diarrhea, dermatitis, lethargy

Dietary Sources[b]: The boron content of foods is not included in the USDA data base, and is not readily available from other published sources. Noncitrus fruits, leafy green vegetables, nuts, legumes, beer, wine, and cider are abundant in boron. Meat, fish, and dairy products are poor sources.
Effects of Food Preparation and Storage: Not available

---

[a] Eaton SB, Eaton SB, III, Konner MJ. Paleolithic nutrition revisited: A twelve-year retrospective on its nature and implications. Eur J Clin Nutr. 1997;51:207–216
[b] The nutrient composition of most foods can be checked by accessing the USDA Nutrient database at: www.nal.usda.gov/fnic/foodcomp/Data/SR 13.

Sources:
National Research Council. Recommended Dietary Allowances. 10th edition. National Academy Press. Washington, D.C. 1989
Margen S. The Wellness Nutrition Counter. Health Letter Associates. New York, NY, 1997.
Murray MT. Encyclopedia of Nutritional Supplements. Prima Publishing. Rocklin, CA, 1996.
Shils ME, Olson JA, Shike M (editors). Modern Nutrition in Health and Disease. 8th edition. Lea & Febiger. Philadelphia, PA. 1994
Ziegler EE, Filer LJ, Jr. (editors). Present Knowledge in Nutrition. 7th edition. ILSI Press. Washington, D.C. 1996
Ensminger AH, Ensminger ME, Konlande JE, Robson JRK. The Concise Encyclopedia of Foods and Nutrition. CRC Press, Inc. Boca Raton, FL. 1995
United States Department of Agriculture. USDA Nutrient Database for Standard Reference. Release 11-1. 1997

TABLE IIIE. *Continued (Calcium)*

Calcium

BIOLOGICAL FUNCTION(S) IN HUMANS/KEY PROPERTIES: Calcium is the most abundant mineral in the body. It is the principal mineral of bone and teeth. Extraskeletal calcium functions in nerve conduction, muscle contraction, coagulation and hemostasis, and cell membrane permeability.

ABSORPTION/SOLUBILITY/STORAGE/PHARMACOKINETICS: When daily calcium intake is at or near the mean for adults in the US (750 mg), approximately 25–50% is absorbed. Calcium absorption is enhanced when it is ingested with food; gastric acid appears to be a factor. Absorption in the duodenum and proximal jejunum is saturable and vitamin D dependent. Passive, nonsaturable absorption occurs throughout the small bowel, especially in the ileum. Approximately 4% of ingested calcium is absorbed in the large bowel. Calcium in serum is 47.5% ionized and 46% protein-bound; the remainder is stored in various other complexes, both known and as yet unidentified. Ionized calcium is the metabolically active moiety. Serum levels are maintained at or near 10 mg/dl by the actions of parathyroid hormone, calcitonin, and vitamin D. Body stores are 99% skeletal, and 1% exchangeable pool. Calcium regulation is influenced by the actions of glucocorticoids, thyroid hormone, growth hormone, insulin, and estrogen. Renal filtration in the adult is approximately 8.6 gm/day, of which all but 100–200 mg is reabsorbed. Daily fecal losses include 150 mg of calcium in intestinal secretions, as well as unabsorbed dietary calcium; losses therefore vary with intake and approximate 300–600 mg. Small losses in sweat (i.e., 15 mg/day) occur as well. Dietary protein potentiates loss of calcium in urine: for every 50 gm increment in daily protein ingestion, an additional 60 mg of calcium is excreated. Absorption is enhanced by lactose, and blunted by insoluble fiber, phytate, and possibly oxalate.

RATIONALE FOR SUPPLEMENTATION: Women in the US consistently ingest less calcium than the RDA. Intake in males generally approximates recommended levels. Supplementation is particularly advocated for the prevention of osteoporosis in women. Supplemental calcium may lower blood pressure, and may confer some protection against colon cancer. Oyster shell calcium, dolomite calcium, and bone meal calcium supplements should generally be avoided due to the possibility of lead contamination. Preferred supplements include chelated calcium citrate, gluconate, lactate, and fumarate. Calcium carbonate may be slightly less well absorbed, although this appears to be insignificant if ingested with food.

EVIDENCE IN SUPPORT OF SUPPLEMENTATION BEYOND RDA: The literature on both dietary and supplemental calcium is extensive. Evidence is conclusive that supplemental calcium contributes to bone density. Evidence of a modest beneficial effect on blood pressure, particularly systolic blood pressure, as well as on blood pressure in pregnancy, is well substantiated. There is supportive evidence for preventive efficacy against colon cancer. Evidence for other benefits is preliminary.

TABLE IIIE. Continued (*Calcium*)

Recommended Intake Range (US RDA):

	Infancy (0–6 months)	Infancy (6 months–1 yr)	Childhood (age 1–10)	Puberty/adolescence/early adulthood (age 11–24)	Adulthood (age 25–50)	Post-menopause	Senescence	Pregnancy	Lactation
Male	400 mg	600 mg	800 mg	1200 mg	800 mg		800 mg	—	—
Female	400 mg	600 mg	800 mg	1200 mg	800 mg	800 mg	800 mg	1200 mg	1200 mg

Recommended Intake Range (NIH Consensus Statement[a]):

	Infancy (0–6 months)	Infancy (6 months–1 yr)	Childhood (age 1–5)	Childhood (age 6–10)	Puberty/adolescence/early adulthood (age 11–24)	Adulthood (age: 25–65 male 25–50 female)	Post-menopause	Senescence (age > 65)	Pregnancy	Lactation
Male	400 mg	600 mg	800 mg	800–1200 mg	1200–1500 mg	1000 mg	—	1500 mg	—	—
Female	400 mg	600 mg	800 mg	800–1200 mg	1200–1500 mg	1000 mg	On estrogen: 1000 mg; Not on estrogen: 1500 mg	1500 mg	1200–1500 mg	1200–1500 mg

TABLE IIIE. *Continued (Calcium)*

AVERAGE INTAKE, US ADULTS: 750 mg/day
ESTIMATED MEAN PALEOLITHIC INTAKE (ADULT)[b]:   1956 mg/day
COMMON DOSE RANGE FOR USE AS SUPPLEMENT: up to 1200 mg/day
DO DIETARY PATTERNS MEETING GUIDELINES PERMIT INTAKE IN THE SUPPLEMENT RANGE?:   Yes
INCLUDED IN TYPICAL MULTI-VITAMIN/MULTI-MINERAL TABLET?:   Yes (dose: 162 mg)

DEFICIENCY
  Intake level: approximately 550 mg/day
  Syndromes: accelerated osteoporosis

TOXICITY
  Intake level: approximately 2000–2500 mg/day
  Syndromes: constipation; possibly urolithiasis; impaired absorption of iron, zinc, and other micronutrients

Dietary Sources[c]: Abundant in dairy products, tofu, sardines, and leafy green vegetables.

Food	Serving Size	Kilocalories	Calcium (mg)	Food	Serving Size	Kilocalories	Calcium (mg)
Sardines	1 can (370 gm)	659	888	Cheddar cheese	1 slice (1 oz)	114	204
Yogurt, nonfat, plain	1 cup	137	488	Tofu	1/4 block (81 gm)	117	553
Ricotta cheese	1 cup	340	669	Collard greens, boiled	1 cup (190 gm)	49	226
Skim milk	1 cup	86	302	Amaranth	100 gm	374	153
Whole milk	1 cup	150	291	Soybeans	1 cup (172 gm)	298	175
Buttermilk	1 cup	99	285	Almonds	1 oz	167	80
Sesame seeds	1 oz	160	280	Onions	1 medium (110 gm)	42	22
Swiss cheese	1 slice (1 oz)	107	272	Peas, frozen	1/2 cup (72 gm)	30	36
Oatmeal	100 gm	93	98	Figs, dried	1 fig	48	27
Provolone cheese	1 slice (1 oz)	100	214	Celery	1 stalk (40 gm)	6	16

Effects of Food Preparation and Storage: Generally unimportant.

[a] Optimal Calcium Intake. *NIH Consens Statement.* 1994; Jun 6–8; 12(4):1–31.

[b] Eaton SB, Eaton SB, III, Konner MJ. Paleolithic nutrition revisited: A twelve-year retrospective on its nature and implications. Eur J Clin Nutr. 1997;51:207–216

[c] The nutrient composition of most foods can be checked by accessing the USDA Nutrient database at: www.nal.usda.gov/fnic/foodcomp/Data/SR 13. A more extensive list of food sources of calcium is available in: Margen S. The Wellness Nutrition Counter. Health Letter Associates. New York, NY. 1997

Sources:
National Research Council. Recommended Dietary Allowances. 10th edition. National Academy Press. Washington, D.C. 1989
Margen S. The Wellness Nutrition Counter. Health Letter Associates. New York, NY. 1997
Murray MT. Encyclopedia of Nutritional Supplements. Prima Publishing. Rocklin, CA. 1996
Shils ME, Olson JA, Shike M (editors). Modern Nutrition in Health and Disease. 8th edition. Lea & Febiger. Philadelphia, PA. 1994
Ziegler EE, Filer LJ, Jr. (editors). Present Knowledge in Nutrition. 7th edition. ILSI Press. Washington, D.C. 1996
Ensminger AH, Ensminger ME, Konlande JE, Robson JRK. The Concise Encyclopedia of Foods and Nutrition. CRC Press, Inc. Boca Raton, FL. 1995
United States Department of Agriculture. USDA Nutrient Database for Standard Reference. Release 11-1. 1997

Carnitine

BIOLOGICAL FUNCTION(S) IN HUMANS/KEY PROPERTIES: Transports long-chain fatty acids into mitochondria. Carnitine may function in fatty acid synthesis and ketone body metabolism. Carnitine is synthesized in liver and kidney from lysine and methionine; vitamins C, B_6, and niacin are cofactors in carnitine biosynthesis. Carnitine may be an essential nutrient for newborns, who have limited ability to synthesize carnitine. It is present in breast milk at a concentration of 50–100nmol/ml.

ABSORPTION/SOLUBILITY/STORAGE/PHARMACOKINETICS: Water-soluble. Intestinal absorption is both active and passive. Carnitine is rapidly transported into cells, and intracellular stores greatly exceed levels in circulation. Approximately 95% of body stores are in skeletal muscle. Carnitine is filtered in the kidney, and approximately 90% is reabsorbed. With elevated serum levels, reabsorption declines.

RATIONALE FOR SUPPLEMENTATION: Enhancement of exercise tolerance in healthy individuals and performance athletes. Improvement in oxidation metabolism with reduced symptoms in angina and peripheral vascular disease. Improved cardiac function in CHF. Improved cognitive function in Alzheimer's and other forms of senile dementia. Immune enhancement in AIDS.

EVIDENCE IN SUPPORT OF SUPPLEMENTATION BEYOND RDA: An extensive literature on carnitine dates back to the 1970s. Evidence of some benefit in cardiac ischemia, hemodialysis, cardiomyopathy, and dementia is supported by randomized, placebo-controlled trials. Studies have generally been small.

Recommended Intake Range (US RDA): None established. Carnitine is considered a conditionally essential nutrient; dietary deficiency may cause adverse effects under predisposing conditions.

AVERAGE INTAKE, US ADULTS:	100–300 mg/day
ESTIMATED MEAN PALEOLITHIC INTAKE (ADULT)[a]:	Not available; likely higher than current levels due to importance of red meat in the Paleolithic diet.
COMMON DOSE RANGE FOR USE AS SUPPLEMENT:	1500–4000 mg/day in divided doses; available as L-carnitine, L-acetylcarnitine, and L-propionylcarnitine
DO DIETARY PATTERNS MEETING GUIDELINES PERMIT INTAKE IN THE SUPPLEMENT RANGE?:	No
INCLUDED IN TYPICAL MULTI-VITAMIN/MULTI-MINERAL TABLET?:	No

DEFICIENCY

Intake level: No intake level has been specified for healthy adults; deficiency generally results from a genetic defect. Deficiency may occur in newborns, especially premature, on formula not containing carnitine. May be induced by hemodialysis, TPN, or use of valproic acid. Vegetarian diets are likely to be low in carnitine.

Syndromes: Progressive muscle weakness, impaired ketogenesis, and cardiomyopathy.

TOXICITY

Intake level: Not reported. Supplementation with the naturally occurring L stereoisomer is apparently safe; use of the D isomer should be avoided, as it can lead to functional carnitine deficiency.

Syndromes: Not reported. Supplementation with the D isomer may result in deficiency symptoms, particularly muscle pain and reduced exercise tolerance.

TABLE IIIE. *Continued* (*Carnitine*)

Dietary Sources[b]: Red meat, dairy to a lesser extent.

Food	Serving Size (g)	Kilocalories	Carnitine (mg)	Food	Serving Size (g)	Kilocalories	Carnitine (mg)
Beef steak	100	321	95	Chicken breast	100	165	3.9
Ground beef	100	287	94	American cheese	100	375	3.7
Pork	100	226	28	Ice cream	100	216	3.7
Bacon	100	576	23	Whole milk	100	61	3.3
Cod fish	100	105	5.6				

Effects of Food Preparation and Storage: Not reported to be a generally important determinant of dietary intake levels.

[a] Eaton SB, Eaton SB, III, Konner MJ. Paleolithic nutrition revisited: A twelve-year retrospective on its nature and implications. Eur J Clin Nutr. 1997;51:207–216

[b] The carnitine content of foods is not currently included in the USDA Nutrient database. As a gencral rule, carnitine is abundant in meat, and more abundant the redder the meat. Carnitine is present in dairy products; levels in plant foods are negligible. The table is adapted from: Broquist HP. Carnitine. In: Shils ME, Olson JA, Shike M (editors). Modern Nutrition in Health and Disease. 8th edition. Lea & Febiger. Philadelphia, PA. 1994; p. 462. Energy content of foods listed is from the USDA Nutrient database at: www.nal.usda.gov/fnic/foodcomp/Data/SR 13.

Sources:

National Research Council. Recommended Dietary Allowances. 10th edition. National Academy Press. Washington, D.C. 1989

Margen S. The Wellness Nutrition Counter. Health Letter Associates. New York, NY. 1997

Murray MT. Encyclopedia of Nutritional Supplements. Prima Publishing. Rocklin, CA. 1996

Shils ME, Olson JA, Shike M (editors). Modern Nutrition in Health and Disease. 8th edition. Lea & Febiger. Philadelphia, PA. 1994

Ziegler EE, Filer LJ, Jr. (editors). Present Knowledge in Nutrition. 7th edition. ILSI Press. Washington, D.C. 1996

Ensminger AH, Ensminger ME, Konlande JE, Robson JRK. The Concise Encyclopedia of Foods and Nutrition. CRC Press, Inc. Boca Raton, FL. 1995

United States Department of Agriculture. USDA Nutrient Database for Standard Reference. Release 11-1. 1997

TABLE IIIE. *Continued (Carotenoids/Vitamin A)*

Carotenoids/Vitamin A

Biological function(s) in humans/key properties: The essential role of carotenoids in human health as precursors of vitamin A has long been recognized; potential health effects of their antioxidant properties has come under investigation more recently. Vitamin A is essential in cell proliferation and growth, immune function and vision (see Vitamin A). There are more than 500 carotenoids known, of which approximately 50 are known to serve as precursors of retinol, the biologically active form of vitamin A. Of these, all trans β-carotene is the most active. Carotenoids are responsible for the bright pigments in many plants, and are essential to photosynthesis. They apparently act as antioxidants in both plants and animals. Interest in β-carotene is the result of its pro-vitamin A activity; other carotenoids are more powerful antioxidants. The functions of carotenoids other than as antioxidants and vitamin A precursors remain to be elucidated.

Absorption/Solubility/storage/pharmacokinetics: Carotenoids are fat-soluble. Retinol is 70–90% absorbed in the small intestine, while carotenoids are generally 20–50% absorbed. Carotenoid absorption is down-regulated by high intake. Absorption is dependent on the activity of pancreatic enzymes and bile acids, and is enhanced by dietary fat, protein, and vitamin E. Carotenoids are widely distributed in tissues, while β-carotene and ingested retinol are stored in the liver as retinyl esters in subject with adequate vitamin A stores. Inactive metabolites of retinol are 70% egested in stool, 30% excreted in urine. Retinol is slowly released from liver stores to meet metabolic requirements, and circulates in conjunction with a binding protein. Due to hepatic storage capacity, large, intermittent doses of vitamin A or its precursors can prevent deficiency as effectively as consistent dietary intake.

Rationale for Supplementation in RDA range: There is no specific RDA for carotenoids, other than as vitamin A precursors (see vitamin A). Carotenoid intake from dietary sources will be high if the diet is rich in dark green and other brightly colored vegetables and fruits (see dietary sources, below). For individuals with limited intake of vegetables, carotenoid supplementation may be indicated to assure adequate vitamin A status.

Rationale for Megadose Supplementation: The use of carotenoid supplements has been recommended to enhance immune function, to treat photosensitivity, and to prevent both cardiovascular disease and cancer.

Evidence in support of supplementation beyond RDA: Epidemiologic evidence is consistent that high dietary intake and high serum levels of carotenoids are associated with reduced risk of certain cancers[a] and mortality.[b] However, only β-carotene has been studied as a supplement in randomized trials, with consistently negative results. In such trials, β-carotene has been associated with lack of effect on angina or cardiovascular events,[c,d] and either no effect[e] or an adverse effect[c] on cancer incidence. Proponents of carotenoid supplementation argue that antioxidant effects require combination supplements, but evidence of benefit is lacking to data. Preliminary studies of other carotenoids, including lycopene and lutein, are promising.

Recommended Intake Range (US RDA[i]):

	Infancy (age 0–1)	Childhood (age 1–10)	Puberty/ adolescence (age 11–18)	Adulthood (age 19–50)	Post-menopause	Senescence	Pregnancy	Lactation
Male	375 μgRE	400–700 μgRE	1000 μgRE	1000 μgRE	—	1000 μgRE	—	—
Female	375 μgRE	400–700 μgRE	800 μgRE	800 μgRE	800 μgRE	800 μgRE	800 μgRE	1200–1300 μgRE

[i] There is no RDA for carotenoids per se, other than as vitamin A precursors. Recommended intake is therefore expressed as μg of retinol equivalents, or RE. One RE is equal to 1 μg retinol, or 6 μg β-carotene.
[j] Vitamin A supplementation should be avoided during pregnancy; see vitamin A table.

Average Intake, US Adults:	1170–1419 μgRE
Estimated Mean Paleolithic Intake (adult)[h]:	2870 μgRE
Common dose range for use as supplement:	a daily dose of 1000 μgRE for men and 500 μgRE for women; acute doses up to 10,000 μgRE are proposed for use during acute viral illness
Do dietary patterns meeting guidelines permit intake in the supplement range?:	Yes
Included in typical multi-vitamin/multi-mineral tablet?:	Yes (dose: 1000 μgRE)

TABLE IIIE. *Continued (Carotenoids/Vitamin A)*

DEFICIENCY (VITAMIN A)
  Intake level: below 390 μgRE
  Syndromes: xerophthalmia; anorexia; hyperkeratosis; immunosuppression

TOXICITY (CAROTENOIDS)
  Intake level: none for carotenoids; 15,000 μgRE/day vitamin A
  Syndromes: **carotenoids:** none; with extreme doses, reversible skin discoloration may occur
                          vitamin A: hepatotoxicity; bone abnormalities; in pregnancy, birth defects

Dietary Sources[k]:

Food	Serving Size	Kilo-calories	Carotenoid (μg RE)	Food	Serving Size	Kilo-calories	Carotenoid (μg RE)
Apricot, dried	1 cup (130 gm)	309	941	Swiss chard, cooked	1 cup (175 gm)	35	550
Sweet potato, cooked	1 medium (114 gm)	117	2487	Spinach, raw	10 oz (284 gm)	62	1908
Tomato juice	1 cup (243 gm)	41	136	Parsley, raw	1 cup (60 gm)	22	312
Tomato paste	1 can (170 gm)	139	415	Apricots, fresh	1 medium (35 gm)	17	91
Carrots	1 medium (61 gm)	26	1716	Romaine lettuce	1/2 cup (28 gm)	4	73
Kale, raw	1 cup (67 gm)	33.5	596	Broccoli, cooked	1 medium stalk (180 gm)	50	250
Pumpkin, cooked	1 cup (245 gm)	49	265	Cantaloupe	1 medium wedge (69 gm)	24	222
Peppers, yellow	1 large (186 gm)	50	45	Corn, cooked	1 ear (77 gm)	83	17
Peppers, red	1 medium (119 gm)	32	678	Tangerines	1 medium (84 gm)	37	77
Collard greens, cooked	1 cup (190 gm)	49	595	Orange	1 medium (131 gm)	62	28
Saffron	1 tablespoon (2.1 gm)	6.5	1.1	Watermelon	1 wedge (286 gm)	92	106
Paprika	1 tablespoon (6.9 gm)	20	418	Tomato, fresh	1 medium (123 gm)	26	76

Distribution of Carotenoids of Potential Clinical Importance in the Food Supply (leading sources):
  β-carotene: apricots, carrots, sweet potato, collard greens, spinach, kale
  lycopene: tomato juice, tomato paste, guava, watermelon, grapefruit (pink)
  lutein: kale, collard greens, spinach, endive, watercress, swiss chard, romaine lettuce
  α-carotene: pumpkin, carrots, squash, corn, apples, peaches
  β-cryptoxanthin: tangerine, papaya, lemons, oranges, persimmons, corn, green peppers
  zeaxanthin: spinach, paprika, corn

Effects of Food Preparation and Storage: Carotenoids are lipid soluble, and relatively unaffected by food preparation. The bioavailability tends to increase somewhat with cooking. Some carotenoid tends to be lost with freezing.

TABLE IIIE. *Continued (Carotenoids/Vitamin A)*

[a] Zheng W, Sellers T, Doyle TJ, Kushi LH, Potter JD, Folsom AR. Retinol, Antioxidant vitamins, and cancers of the upper digestive tract in a prospective cohort study of postmenopausal women. Am J Epidemiol. 1995;142:955–960

[b] Pandey DK, Shekelle R, Selwyn BJ, Tangney C, Stamler J. Dietary vitamin C and β-carotene and risk of death in middle-aged men. The western electric study. Am J Epidemiol. 1995;142:1269–1278

[c] Rappola JM, Virtamo J, Haukka JK, Heionen OP, Albanes D, Taylor PR, Huttunen JK. Effect of vitamin E and beta carotene on the incidence of angina pectoris. JAMA. 1996;275:693–698

[d] Hennekens CH, Buring JE, Manson JE, Stampfer M, Rosner B, Cook NR, et al. Lack of effect of long-term supplementation with beta carotene on the incidence of malignant neoplasms and cardiovascular disease. N. Engl J Med. 1996;334:1145–1149

[e] Greenberg ER, Baron JA, Tosteson TD, Freeman DH, Beck GJ, Bond JH. A clinical trial of antioxidant vitamins to prevent colorectal adenoma. N Engl J Med. 1994:331:141–147

[f] Alpha-tocopherol, Beta carotene Cancer Prevention Study Group. The effect of vitamin E and beta carotene on the incidence of lung cancer and other cancers in male smokers. N Engl J Med. 1994;330:1029–1035

[g] Omenn GS, Goodman G, Thornquist M, Gizzle J, Rosenstock L, Barnhart S, et al. The β-carotene and retinol efficacy trial (CARET) for chemoprevention of lung cancer in high risk populations: smokers and asbestos-exposed workers. Cancer Research. 1994;54:2038s–2043s

[h] Eaton SB, Eaton SB, III, Konner MJ. Paleolithic nutrition revisited: A twelve-year retrospective on its nature and implications. Eur J Clin Nutr. 1997;51:207–216

[k] The nutrient composition of most foods can be checked by accessing the USDA Nutrient database at: www.nal.usda.gov/fnic/foodcomp/Data/SR13.

Sources:
Ensminger AH, Ensminger ME, Konlande JE, Robson JRK. The Concise Encyclopedia of Foods and Nutrition. CRC Press, Inc. Boca Raton, FL. 1995
Margen S. The Wellness Nutrition Counter. Health Letter Associates. New York, NY. 1997
Murray MT. Encyclopedia of Nutritional Supplements. Prima Publishing. Rocklin, CA. 1996
National Research Council. Recommended Dietary Allowances. 10th edition. National Academy Press. Washington, D.C. 1989
Shils ME, Olson JA, Shike M (editors). Modern Nutrition in Health and Disease. 8th edition. Lea & Febiger. Philadelphia, PA. 1994
United States Department of Agriculture. USDA Nutrient Database for Standard Reference. Release 12. 1998
Ziegler EE, Filer LJ, Jr. (editors). Present Knowledge in Nutrition. 7th edition. ILSI Press. Washington, D.C. 1996

TABLE IIIE. *Continued (Chromium)*

Chromium

BIOLOGICAL FUNCTION(S) IN HUMANS/KEY PROPERTIES: The principal role of chromium is as an insulin cofactor.

ABSORPTION/SOLUBILITY/STORAGE/PHARMACOKINETICS: Chromium absorption is limited, and varies with intake level from a low of 0.5% to a high of 2% of the portion ingested. Chromium accumulates in the lungs with advancing age, while levels in others tissues decline; the significance of this is unclear.

RATIONALE FOR SUPPLEMENTATION IN RDA RANGE: Usual intake in the US is below the recommended intake range of 50–200 μg per day. Chromium deficiency may contribute to insulin resistance.

RATIONALE FOR MEGADOSE SUPPLEMENTATION: Up to 600 μg per day is recommended by some practitioners for treatment of insulin resistance or diabetes, and as an aid in weight loss.

EVIDENCE IN SUPPORT OF SUPPLEMENTATION BEYOND RDA: The literature on chromium supplementation is fairly extensive, but evidence of therapeutic effect in any condition is not more than preliminary. There is evidence of benefit in some groups of diabetics, and in the preferential loss of fat during weight reduction efforts.[a] Arguments against routine supplementation for primary prevention have been raised.[b] Trow and colleagues[c] recently found no evidence of benefit from chromium supplementation in a small group of type II diabetics. Chromium also failed to enhance the beneficial effects of exercise on glucose tolerance in overweight adults.[d] However, corticosteroid-induced DM has been reported to respond to chromium supplementation.[e] High dose supplementation apparently has some potential toxicity[f] although this is generally considerd to be limited. Overall, chromium supplementation is considered promising in diabetes and insulin resistance,[g,h] decidedly less so for weight management.[i] Chromium does not appear to be effective at building muscle mass.[j]

Recommended Intake Range in microns (US RDA): Estimated Safe and Adequate Daily Dietary Intake is provided rather than RDA

	Infancy (age 0–1)	Childhood (age 1–10)	Puberty/ adolescence (age 11–18)	Adulthood (age 19–50)	Post-menopause	Senescence	Pregnancy	Lactation
Male	10–60 μg	20–200 μg	50–200 μg	50–200 μg	—	50–200 μg	—	—
Female	10–60 μg	20–200 μg	50–200 μg	50–200 μg	50–200 μg	50–200 μg	Not available	Not available

AVERAGE INTAKE, US ADULTS: 30–80 μg
ESTIMATED MEAN PALEOLITHIC INTAKE (ADULT)[k]:   not available
COMMON DOSE RANGE FOR USE AS SUPPLEMENT: 50–600 μg
DO DIETARY PATTERNS MEETING GUIDELINES PERMIT INTAKE IN THE SUPPLEMENT RANGE?:   Yes
INCLUDED IN TYPICAL MULTI-VITAMIN/MULTI-MINERAL TABLET?:   Yes (65 μg)

DEFICIENCY
    Intake level: below 50 μg/day
    Syndromes: insulin resistance/glucose intolerance

TOXICITY
    Intake level: uncertain
    Syndromes: none known

Dietary Sources: Chromium is found abundantly in whole grains, brewer's yeast, seafood, potatoes, peanut butter and nuts. Chromium content is not provided in the USDA Nutrient database (www.nal.usda.gov/fnic/foodcomp/Data/SR.13).

Effects of Food Preparation and Storage: Not reported to be a generally important determinant of dietary intake levels.

TABLE IIIE. *Continued (Chromium)*

[a] Preuss HG, Anderson RA. Chromium update: examining recent literature 1997–1998. Curr Opin Clin Nutr Metab Care 1998;1:509–512

[b] Porter DJ, Raymond LW, Anastasio GD. Chromium: friend or foe? Arch Fam Med 1999;8(5):386–390

[c] Trow LG, Lewis J, Greenwood RH, Sampson MJ, Self KA, Crews HM, Fairweather-Tait SJ. Lack of effect of dietary chromium supplementation on glucose tolerance, plasma insulin and lipoprotein levels in patients with type 2 diabetes. Int J Vitam Nutr Res 2000;70:14–18

[d] Joseph LJ, Farrell PA, Davey SL, Evans WJ, Campbell WW. Effect of resistance training with or without chromium picolinate supplementation on glucose metabolism in older men and women. Metabolism 1999;48:546–553

[e] Ravina A, Slezak L, Mirsky N, Bryden NA, Anderson RA. Reversal of corticosteroid-induced diabetes mellitus with supplemental chromium. Diabet Med 1999;16:164–167

[f] Young PC, Turiansky GW, Bonner MW, Benson PM. Acute generalized exanthematous pustulosis induced by chromium picolinate. J Am Acad Dermatol 1999;41(5 Pt 2):820–823

[g] Lukaski HC. Chromium as a supplement. Annu Rev Nutr 1999;19:279–302

[h] Anderson RA. Chromium, glucose intolerance and diabetes. J Am Coll Nutr 1998;17:548–555

[i] Anderson RA. Effects of chromium on body composition and weight loss. Nutr Rev 1998;56:266–270

[j] Clarkson PM, Rawson ES. Nutritional supplements to increase muscle mass. Crit Rev Food Sci Nutr 1999;39:317–328

[k] Eaton SB, Eaton SB, III, Konner MJ. Paleolithic nutrition revisited: A twelve-year retrospective on its nature and implications. *Eur J Clin Nutr.* 1997;51:207–216

Sources:

Ensminger AH, Ensminger ME, Konlande JE, Robson JRK. The Concise Encyclopedia of Foods and Nutrition. CRC Press, Inc. Boca Raton, FL. 1995

Margen S. The Wellness Nutrition Counter. Health Letter Associates. New York, NY. 1997

Murray MT. Encyclopedia of Nutritional Supplements. Prima Publishing. Rocklin, CA. 1996

National Research Council. Recommended Dietary Allowances. 10th edition. National Academy Press. Washington, D.C. 1989

Shils ME, Olson JA, Shike M (editors). Modern Nutrition in Health and Disease. 8th edition. Lea & Febiger. Philadelphia, PA. 1994

United States Department of Agriculture. USDA Nutrient Database for Standard Reference. Release 12. 1998

Ziegler EE, Filer LJ, Jr. (editors). Present Knowledge in Nutrition. 7th edition. ILSI Press. Washington, D.C. 1996

Coenzyme Q₁₀ (Ubiquinone)

BIOLOGICAL FUNCTION(S) IN HUMANS/KEY PROPERTIES: Functions in electron transport and as an antioxidant, quenching free radicals. Involved in the generation of ATP in mitochondria. May contribute to exercise capacity. Can be synthesized endogenously.

SOLUBILITY: lipid

ABSORPTION/STORAGE/PHARMACOKINETICS: uncertain

RATIONALE FOR SUPPLEMENTATION: Generation of ATP in myocardium; antioxidant effects. Recommended for congestive heart failure and coronary disease. May prevent depletion of coenzyme Q10 induced by HMGCoA reductase inhibitors (statins). May be beneficial in a wide range of disease states associated with oxidative injury. Preserves vitamin E levels.

EVIDENCE IN SUPPORT OF SUPPLEMENTATION: Numerous animal and observational studies. There are positive results from double-blind, placebo-controlled studies in humans, in particular for use in congestive heart failure (see chapter 6).

Recommended Intake Range (US RDA): None Established

AVERAGE INTAKE, US ADULTS:	unknown
ESTIMATED MEAN PALEOLITHIC INTAKE (ADULT)[a]:	unknown
COMMON DOSE RANGE FOR USE AS SUPPLEMENT:	50 to 150 mg per day
DO DIETARY PATTERNS MEETING GUIDELINES PERMIT INTAKE IN THE SUPPLEMENT RANGE?:	No
INCLUDED IN TYPICAL MULTI-VITAMIN/MULTI-MINERAL TABLET?:	No

DEFICIENCY
    Intake level: unknown
    Syndromes: unknown

TOXICITY
    Intake level: unknown
    Syndromes: unknown

Dietary Sources: Coenzyme Q₁₀ is known as ubiquinone due to its ubiquitous distribution in nature. While widely distributed in both plant and animal foods, however, dietary sources do not allow for intake in the supplement range. The concentration of ubiquinone in various foods has been studied but not systematically reported. The USDA Nutrient Database does not currently report ubiquinone content.

Effects of Food Preparation and Storage: Not reported to be a generally important determinant of dietary intake levels.

---

[a] Eaton SB, Eaton SB, III, Konner MJ. Paleolithic nutrition revisited: A twelve-year retrospective on its nature and implications. Eur J Clin Nutr. 1997;51:207–216

Sources:
National Research Council. Recommended Dietary Allowances. 10th edition. National Academy Press. Washington, D.C. 1989
Margen S. The Wellness Nutrition Counter. Health Letter Associates. New York, NY. 1997
Murray MT. Encyclopedia of Nutritional Supplements. Prima Publishing. Rocklin, CA. 1996
Shils ME, Olson JA, Shike M (editors). Modern Nutrition in Health and Disease. 8th edition. Lea & Febiger. Philadelphia, PA. 1994
Ziegler EE, Filer LJ, Jr. (editors). Present Knowledge in Nutrition. 7th edition. ILSI Press. Washington, D.C. 1996
Ensminger AH, Ensminger ME, Konlande JE, Robson JRK. The Concise Encyclopedia of Foods and Nutrition. CRC Press, Inc. Boca Raton, FL. 1995
United States Department of Agriculture. USDA Nutrient Database for Standard Reference. Release 11-1. 1997

TABLE IIIE. *Continued (Creatine)*

Creatine

BIOLOGICAL FUNCTION(S) IN HUMANS/KEY PROPERTIES: Creatine is synthesized endogenously from the amino acids glycine and arginine and available methyl groups. Concentrated in skeletal muscle and brain, creatine functions in energy metabolism.

SOLUBILITY: water

ABSORPTION/STORAGE/PHARMACOKINETICS: Largely unknown. Muscle creatine rises with supplementation, apparently to a maximum level of approximately 20% above baseline with supplementation in the range of 3 grams per day.[a] Urinary excretion of creatinine rises with creatine loading.

RATIONALE FOR SUPPLEMENTATION: Enhanced athletic performance. Possibly, improved exercise tolerance.

EVIDENCE IN SUPPORT OF SUPPLEMENTATION: Numerous double-blind, randomized and cross-over studies showing improved work output with creatine supplementation. Most studies have been small and of short duration.[b] Evidence of benefit for sustained activity appears less convincing than evidence for an effect on short-burst activity. The available literature includes both positive and negative studies (see chapter 30).

Recommended Intake Range (US RDA): Unknown

AVERAGE INTAKE, US ADULTS: unknown; daily turnover in an adult male is estimated at 2 gm per day[c]

ESTIMATED MEAN PALEOLITHIC INTAKE (ADULT)[d]: unknown; Paleolithic dietary patterns likely resulted in higher intake than do current patterns

COMMON DOSE RANGE FOR USE AS SUPPLEMENT: approximately 2 gm per day

DO DIETARY PATTERNS MEETING GUIDELINES PERMIT INTAKE IN THE SUPPLEMENT RANGE?: No

INCLUDED IN TYPICAL MULTI-VITAMIN/MULTI-MINERAL TABLET?: No

DEFICIENCY
Intake level: none; creatine can by synthesized endogenously
Syndromes: none known

TOXICITY
Intake level: unknown
Syndromes: unknown

Dietary Sources: Dietary sources of creatine are not systematically reported. Creatine is abundant in red meat and fish.

Effects of Food Preparation and Storage: Not available

[a] Hultman E. Soderlund K, Timmons JA, Cederblad G, Greenhaff PL. Muscle creatine loading in men. J Appl Physiol. 1996;81:232–237

[b] Mujika I, Padilla S. Creatine supplementation as an ergogenic acid for sports performance in highly trained athletes: a critical review. Int J Sports Med 1997 Oct;18:491–496

[c] Balsom PD, Soderlund K, Ekblom B. Creatine in humans with special reference to creatine supplementation. Sports Med. 1994;18:268–280

[d] Eaton SB, Eaton SB, III, Konner MJ. Paleolithic nutrition revisited: A twelve-year retrospective on its nature and implications. Eur J Clin Nutr. 1997;51:207–216

Sources:
National Research Council. Recommended Dietary Allowances. 10th edition. National Academy Press. Washington, D.C. 1989

Margen S. The Wellness Nutrition Counter. Health Letter Associates. New York, NY. 1997

Murray MT. Encyclopedia of Nutritional Supplements. Prima Publishing. Rocklin, CA. 1996

Shils ME, Olson JA, Shike M (editors). Modern Nutrition in Health and Disease. 8th edition. Lea & Febiger. Philadelphia, PA. 1994

Ziegler EE, Filer LJ, Jr. (editors). Present Knowledge in Nutrition. 7th edition. ILSI Press. Washington, D.C. 1996

Ensminger AH, Ensminger ME, Konlande JE, Robson JRK. The Concise Encyclopedia of Foods and Nutrition. CRC Press, Inc. Boca Raton, FL. 1995

United States Department of Agriculture. USDA Nutrient Database for Standard Reference. Release 11–1. 1997

TABLE IIIE. *Continued (Essential Fatty Acids EFA's)*

Essential Fatty Acids (EFA's)

BIOLOGICAL FUNCTION(S) IN HUMANS/KEY PROPERTIES: Essential fatty acids are those polyunsaturated fatty acids required in metabolism that cannot be synthesized endogenously. The two classes of EFA's are n-6 and n-3. Linoleic acid is an essential n-6 fatty acid (C_{18}; i.e., 18 carbons in its chain) that is a precursor to arachidonic acid (C_{20}); when linoleic acid intake is deficient, arachidonic acid becomes an essential nutrient as well. The other EFA is α-linolenic (ALA) acid, a n-3 with 18 carbons. Linolenic acid is a precursor to eicosapentenoic acid (EPA; C_{20}) and docosahexaenoic acid (DHA; C_{22}). However, the efficiency of EPA, and particularly DHA, synthesis from linolenic acid is in question. Animal evidence suggests that supplementation with DHA more effectively raises tissue levels of DHA than does supplementation with ALA.[a,b] EFA's in phospholipids are key structural components of cellular and subcellular membranes. They are metabolic precursors of eicosanoids with a wide range of effects, from inflammatory reactions and immunity to platelet aggregation. DHA is concentrated in the brain and retina.

ABSORPTION/SOLUBILITY/STORAGE/PHARMACOKINETICS: The absorption of ingested fatty acids is highly efficient, ranging from 95% to nearly 100%. Ingested fat releases fatty acids (see chapter 2) that can be utilized immediately as a fuel source, stored as triglyceride in adipose tissue, or used in anabolism. Changes in dietary intake of EFA's is reflected in tissue stores over a period of days to weeks. Animal data suggest that PUFA's, including EFA's, may be preferentially released from adipose tissue in response to catabolic stimuli.[c] Of note, gamma-linolenic acid (GLA) of the ne-6 class bypasses the rate-limiting $\Delta6$ desaturase enzyme, and leads to the generation of metabolic products distinct from other FA's in the n-6 class (see below).

RATIONALE FOR SUPPLEMENTATION IN RDA RANGE: There is no RDA per se for EFA's, and overt deficiency syndromes are exceedingly rare when dietary intake is basically adequate; EFA deficiency is generally associated with abnormal nutriture (e.g., parenteral nutrition, starvation). However, n-6 FA intake in the US is considerably greater than n-3 FA intake, due to the wide distribution of linoleic acid in commonly used vegetable oils. Approximately 7% of the energy in a typical diet in the US is derived from linoleic acid. In contrast, the distribution of linolenic acid is narrow, and intake levels are low. A predominance of n-6 over n-3 fatty acids in the diet fosters preferential synthesis of the products of n-6 FA metabolism, as EFA's of both classes utilize the same enzyme systems. With the exception of γ-linolenic acid (GLA), the products of n-6 FA metabolism tend to be pro-inflammatory leukotrienes and prostaglandins that promote platelet aggregation, while the products of n-3 fatty acid metabolism generally have opposite effects. Thus, an imbalance in EFA intake in favor of the n-6 class may contribute to inflammation and a pro-thrombotic tendency. Gamma-linolenic acid (GLA), although of the n-6 class, uniquely bypasses the rate-limiting enzyme ($\Delta6$ desaturase) in EFA metabolism, and as a result preferentially leads to the synthesis of prostaglandins in the 1 series, which have antiinflammatory and antiplatelet effects, as well as the suppression of pro-inflammatory cytokine synthesis.[d,e,f,g] GLA is found in evening primrose oil, borage seed oil, and black currant seed oil.

RATIONALE FOR MEGADOSE SUPPLEMENTATION: Unlike most nutrients with nutriceutical applications, fatty acids are ingested at a macro level, contributing appreciably to energy intake. Therefore, there is no rationale per se for 'megadosing' of any fatty acid, and such a practice would carry with it the risk of excess energy intake and weight gain. The underlying rationale for supplementation of either n-3 FA's or GLA is to reduce the synthesis of inflammatory cytokines and platelet-stimulating prostaglandins, and preferentially support the synthesis of anti-inflammatory cytokines, by shifting the distribution of FA's in the diet.

EVIDENCE IN SUPPORT OF SUPPLEMENTATION BEYOND RDA: There is not RDA for EFA's. There is suggestive evidence for the therapeutic use of supplemental EFA's in a wide range of inflammatory conditions, and convincing evidence in the aggregate for shifting the distribution of EFA's from the now prevailing pattern in the US to a more balanced distribution of n-3's and n-6's to promote health. The typical diet in the US provides n-6 to n-3 FA's in a ratio of at least 11:1, with roughly 7% of calories derived from EFA's. An intake ratio of n-6 to n-3 of between 4:1 and 1:1 is thought to be preferable and health-promoting, although conclusive evidence is not available. There is no clear evidence that total EFA intake should be increased, although a shift in fat calories from saturated and trans fatty acids to MUFA and PUFA is strongly supported by both epidemiologic and intervention studies (see chapters 6, 10 and 12). Total PUFA intake in the range of 10–15% of calories is consistent with evidence for diet and general health promotion (see chapter 39). Relatively greater intake of n-3 fatty acids is supported by studies of cognitive development and visual acuity in infants (see chapters 25 and 27); by studies of chronic inflammatory conditions (see chapters 15, 18, and 22); by studies of cardiovascular disease (see chapter 6); and to a lesser extent, by the cancer prevention literature (see chapter 12). A recent (2000) supplement of the *American Journal of Clinical Nutrition* provides reviews of evidence for EFA supplementation and various health outcomes. Convincing evidence is available of benefit from n-3 FA supplementation at a daily dose of 3 g of EPA and DHA in combination in rheumatoid arthritis.[h] A similar benefit has been suggested in inflammatory bowel disease, but the evidence is less consistent, and therefore must be considered preliminary.[i] Supplementation of the maternal diet with DHA during pregnancy has theoretical support, and is unlikely to be harmful, but is as yet not supported by conclusive outcome studies.[j,k] Evidence of benefit of DHA in infant nutrition is convincing with regard to visual acuity,[l] and suggestive in the area of cognitive development.[m] In the aggregate, evidence of cardiovascular benefit from fish oil supplementation is convincing[n] (see chapter 6). The immunologic effects of n-3 FA's are convincingly favorable in inflammatory states, but may be disadvantageous in relatively immuno-compromised individuals; concurrent vitamin E supplementation may prevent attendant immunosuppression.[o] A potential beneficial role in inflammatory diseases of the lung (e.g., asthma, bronchitis) has been suggested[p] (see chapter 14). There is some evidence that n-6 FA's may act as promoters in carcinogenesis, while n-3 FA's have the opposite effect. Therapeutic applications of GLA are supported by diverse sources of evidence as well. A recent (2000) study demonstrated an accelerated clinical response in patients with endocrine receptor-positive breast cancer treated with GLA (2.8 g/day) in addition to tamoxifen, as compared to tamoxifen alone.[q] Inhibition of atherogenesis with GLA has been demonstrated in vitro, and in animal studies.[r] A therapeutic role for GLA in atopic eczema is convincingly supported by available evidence.[s] A benefit of GLA in rheumatologic conditions[t] and diabetic neuropathy[u] is suggested.

Recommended Intake Range (US RDA): There is no RDA for EFA's. The Food and Nutrition Board of the Institute of Medicine (IOM) at the National Academy of Sciences has a standing committee evaluating guidelines for macronutrient intake; recommendations, including dietary reference intakes for EFA's, are projected for September, 2001. Updated guidelines can be accessed from the IOM website: http://www4.nationalacademies.org/iom/iomhome.nsf.

The best available data to date suggest that an intake of PUFA in the range of 10–15% of calories is optimal, with total fat representing approximately 25% of calories. EFA should comprise approximately 10% of total calorie intake, with n-6 to n-3 in a ratio of between 4:1 and 1:1. In a 2000 kcal/day diet, this pattern would call for the ingestion of 22 g of EFA per day, with at least 5–6 g of n-3 and the remainder n-6. The optimal distribution of ALA to EPA and DHA in the diet is uncertain, but a mixture of these may be advantageous. To achieve this, total fat intake generally requires restriction, with particular attention to restriction of saturated and trans (commercially hydrogenated) fat; and consistent intake of fish, oils rich in n-3 FA, or use of a supplement is required.

TABLE IIIE. *Continued (Essential Fatty Acids)*

AVERAGE INTAKE, US ADULTS: Total EFA: approximately 7–10% of calories; n-6 to n-3 ratio: between 11 : 1 and 20 : 1

ESTIMATED MEAN PALEOLITHIC INTAKE (ADULT)[av]:   Total EFA: approximately 7–10% of calories; n-6 to n-3 ratio: between 4 : 1 and 1 : 1

Paleolithic intake of n-3 FA's is thought to have been considerably greater than that in most industrialized countries in part because the meat of wild ungulates is low in total fat (roughly 10% of calories) relative to domestic cattle (roughly 45% of calories), yet proportionately rich in n-3 fatty acids. Thus, the paleolithic diet is thought to have provided n-3 FA's from sources other than marine animals.

COMMON DOSE RANGE FOR USE AS SUPPLEMENT: Fish oil: 3–20 g/day (generally a combination of EPA and DHA)
ALA: approximately 10 g/day
GLA: approximately 1.5–3g/day

DO DIETARY PATTERNS MEETING GUIDELINES PERMIT INTAKE IN THE SUPPLEMENT RANGE?: Generally no; possibly, if intake of certain fish (e.g., salmon, mackerel) is unusually high. Of note, the n-3 FA content of fish is derived from the algae and phytoplankton the fish ingest. Fish raised commercially tend to have a much reduced n-3 FA content in their diet, and therefore a much lower n-3 content in their flesh (much like what has occurred with the domestication of cattle). While the efficiency of conversion of ALA to EPA and especially DHA is questionable, dietary supplementation with ALA appears to provide most of the health benefit of directly ingesting the longer chain n-3's. Given the potential importance of EFA's in health promotion, a general recommendation for dietary supplementation with ALA is reasonable. The recommended dose of approximately 10 g/day can be obtained by using *1–2 tablespoons of flaxseed (flax) oil daily.* Flaxseed oil (e.g., Barlean's brand) is available in health food stores. It can be used on salads and in cold dishes, but is not suitable for cooking. Vitamin E requirements rise with intake of PUFA's, and therefore vitamin E supplementation in conjunction with regular EFA ingestion is not unreasonable (see Vitamin E). With the addition of flaxseed oil to the diet, other sources of fat (particularly saturated and/or trans fat) should generally be restricted to avoid increasing total fat intake.

INCLUDED IN TYPICAL MULTI-VITAMIN/MULTI-MINERAL TABLET?:   No

DEFICIENCY
   Intake level: EFA's < 1% of calories
   Syndromes: dry skin; hair loss; immunosuppression

TOXICITY
   Intake level: variable; dependent in part on the ratio of n-6 to n-3
   Syndromes: pro-oxidant effects; cancer promotion; bleeding diathesis/platelet dysfunction

Dietary Sources[b]:

α-linolenic acid (ALA) Dietary Sources[w]:

Food	Serving Size	Energy (kcal)	ALA (g)
Canola oil	1 tbsp (14 g)	124	1.3
Flax (flaxseed) oil	1 tbsp (11 g)	110	6.2
Kale	1 cup (130 g)	36	0.1
Soy bean oil	1 tbsp (13.6 g)	120	0.9
Spinach	1 cup (180 g)	41	0.2

TABLE IIIE. *Continued* (*Essential Fatty Acids*)

Docosahexenoic acid (DHA) Dietary Sources:[w]

Food	Serving Size	Energy (kcal)	DHA (g)
Mackerel (Atlantic)	1 fillet (88 g)	231	0.6
Oysters (cooked)	6 medium (42 g)	57	0.2
Salmon (Atlantic)	1/2 fillet (154 g)	280	2.2
Sardines (canned in oil)	1 can (92 g)	191	0.5
Scallops (raw)	3 oz (85 g)	313	0.09

Eicosapentenoic acid (EPA) Dietary Sources:[w]

Food	Serving Size	Energy (kcal)	EPA (g)
Mackerel (Atlantic)	1 fillet (88 g)	231	0.4
Oysters (cooked)	6 medium (42 g)	57	0.2
Salmon (Atlantic)	1/2 fillet (154 g)	280	0.6
Sardines (canned in oil)	1 can (92 g)	191	0.4
Scallops (raw)	3 oz (85 g)	75	0.08

δ-linolenic acid (GLA) (Medicinal Oils)

Food	Dose	Energy (kcal)	GLA (g)
Black currant seed oil	1 tbsp (13.6 g)	120	2.3
Borage seed oil	1 tbsp (13.6 g)	102	3.0
Evening primrose oil	1 tbsp (13.6 g)	120	1.2

Linoleic acid Dietary Sources:[w]

Food	Serving Size	Energy (kcal)	Linoleic Acid (g)
Corn Oil	1 tbsp (13.6 g)	120	7.9
Flax (flaxseed) oil	1 tbsp (11 g)	110	1.8
Safflower oil	1 tbsp (13.6 g)	120	2.0
Sunflower Oil	1 tbsp (13.6 g)	120	8.9

For more information see: Goodman J. The Omega solution. Prima Publishing. Rocklin, Ca. In press.
Effects of Food Preparation and Storage: Expeller-pressing is the preferred extraction method for oil. Hydrogenation enhances the commerical properties of PUFA's at the expense of their health effects; "partial hydrogenation" produces trans stereoisomers. PUFA's are susceptible to degradation when exposed to light and/or heat; opaque, plastic packaging is preferred. Oils rich in n-3 FA's are particularly heat intolerant, and generally cannot be used for cooking.

TABLE IIIE. *Continued (Essential Fatty Acids)*

---

[a] Abedin L, Lien EL, Vingrys AJ, Sinclair AJ. The effects of dietary alpha-linolenic acid compared with docosahexaenoic acid on brain, retina, liver, and heart in the guinea pig. Lipids 1999;34:475-82

[b] Su HM, Bernardo L, Mirmiran M, Ma XH, Corso TN, Nathanielsz PW, Brenna JT. Bioequivalence of dietary alpha-linolenic and docosahexaenoic acids as sources of docosahexaenoate accretion in brain and associated organs of neonatal baboons. Pediatr Res 1999;45:87-93

[c] Conner WE, Lin DS, Colvis C. Differential mobilization of fatty acids from adipose tissue. J Lipid Res 1996;37:290-8

[d] Dirks J, van Aswegen CH, du Plessis DJ. Cytokine levels affected by gamma-linolenic acid. Prostaglandins Leukot Essent Fatty Acids 1998;59:273-7

[e] Villalobos MA, De La Cruz JP, Martin-Romero M, Carmona JA, Smith-Agreda JM, Sanchez de la Cuesta F. Effect of dietary supplementation with evening primrose oil on vascular thrombogenesis in hyperlipemic rabbits. Thromb Haemost 1998;80:696-701

[f] Wu D, Meydani M, Leka LS, Nightingale Z, Handelman GJ, Blumberg JB, Meydani SN. Effect of dietary supplementation with black currant seed oil on the immune response of healthy elderly subjects. Am J Clin Nutr 1999;70:536-43

[g] Fan YY, Chapkin RS. Importance of dietary gamma-linolenic acid in human health and nutrition. J Nutr 1998;128:1411-4

[h] Kremer JM. n-3 fatty acid supplements in rheumatoid arthritis. Am J Clin Nutr 2000;71(1 Suppl):349S-51S

[i] Belluzzi A, Boschi S, Brignola C, Munarini A, Cariani G, Miglio F. Polyunsaturated fatty acids and inflammatory bowel disease. Am J Clin Nutr 2000;71(1 Suppl):339S-42S

[j] Al MD, van Houwelingen AC, Hornstra G. Long-chain polyunsaturated fatty acids, pregnancy, and pregnancy outcome. Am J Clin Nutr 2000;71(1 Suppl):285S-91S

[k] Makrides M, Gibson RA. Long-chain polyunsaturated fatty acid requirements during pregnancy and lactation. Am J Clin Nutr 2000;71(1 Suppl):307S-11S

[l] Neuringer M. Infant vision and retinal function in studies of dietary long-chain polyunsaturated fatty acids: methods, results, and implications. Am J Clin Nutr 2000;71(1 Suppl):256S-67S

[m] Morley R. Nutrition and cognitive development. Nutrition 1998;14:752-4; Innis SM. Essential fatty acids in infant nutrition: lessons and limitations from animal studies in relation to studies on infant fatty acid requirements. Am J Clin Nutr 2000;71(1 Suppl):238S-44S

[n] Nestel PJ. Fish oil and cardiovascular disease: lipids and arterial function. Am J Clin Nutr 2000;71 (1 Suppl):228S-31S

[o] Wu D, Meydani SN. n-3 polyunsaturated fatty acids and immune function. Proc Nutr Soc 1998;57:503-9

[p] Schwartz J. Role of polyunsaturated fatty acids in lung disease. Am J Clin Nutr 2000;71(1 Suppl):393S-6S

[q] Kenny FS, Pinder SE, Ellis IO, Gee JM, Nicholson RI, Bryce RP, Robertson JF. Gamma linolenic acid with tamoxifen as primary therapy in breast cancer. Int J Cancer 2000;85:643-648

[r] Fan YY, Ramos KS, Chapkin RS. Modulation of atherogenesis by dietary gamma-linolenic acid. Adv Exp Med Biol 1999;469:485-91

[s] Horrobin DF. Essential fatty acid metabolism and its modification in atopic eczema. Am J Clin Nutr 2000;71 (1 Suppl):367S-72S

[t] Belch JJ, Hill A. Evening primrose oil and borage oil in rheumatologic conditions. Am J Clin Nutr 2000;71 (1 Suppl):352S-6S

[u] Vinik AI. Diabetic neuropathy: pathogenesis and therapy. Am J Med 1999;107:17S-26S

[v] Eaton SB, Eaton SB, III, Konner MJ. Paleolithic nutrition revisited: A twelve-year retrospective on its nature and implications. Eur J Clin Nutr. 1997;51:207-216.

[w] The nutrient composition of most foods can be checked by accessing the USDA Nutrient database at: www.nal.usda.gov/fnic/foodcomp/Data/SR 13.

Sources:
Ensminger AH, Ensminger ME, Konlande JE, Robson JRK. The Concise Encyclopedia of Foods and Nutrition. CRC Press, Inc. Boca Raton, FL. 1995

Margen S. The Wellness Nutrition Counter. Health Letter Associates. New York, NY. 1997

Murray MT. Encyclopedia of Nutritional Supplements. Prima Publishing. Rocklin, CA. 1996

National Research Council. Recommended Dietary Allowances. 10th edition. National Academy Press. Washington, D.C. 1989

Shils ME, Olson JA, Shike M (editors). Modern Nutrition in Health and Disease. 8th edition. Lea & Febiger. Philadelphia, PA. 1994

United States Department of Agriculture. USDA Nutrient Database for Standard Reference. Release 12.1998

Ziegler EE, Filer LJ, Jr. (editors). Present Knowledge in Nutrition. 7th edition. ILSI Press. Washington, D.C. 1996

Sardesai VM. Introduction to Clinical Nutrition. Marcel Dekker, Inc. New York. 1998

TABLE IIIE. *Continued (Fiber)*

Fiber

BIOLOGICAL FUNCTION(S) IN HUMANS/KEY PROPERTIES: Fiber is by definition indigestible plant material, generally categorized along with carbohydrate. Soluble fiber dissolves in water. Dissolution of soluble fiber in the gastrointestinal tract causes delayed absorption of glucose and fatty acids, blunting postprandial rises. Soluble fiber has lipid-lowering properties, and attenuates postprandial insulin release. Soluble fibers of relative importance include guar gum, psyllium, pectin, and β-glucan. Insoluble fibers, such as lignins, celluloses, and hemicelluloses, reduce GI transit time and increase fecal bulk. Both categories of fiber may increase the satiating capacity of food.

ABSORPTION/SOLUBILITY/STORAGE/PHARMACOKINETICS: By definition, fiber is not digested, and therefore neither absorbed nor stored.

RATIONALE FOR SUPPLEMENTATION IN RDA RANGE: There is no RDA for dietary fiber, although current dietary guidelines call for an intake of approximately 30 gm/day. A specific guideline for soluble fiber is elusive; based on the guideline for total fiber, a daily intake of 10–15 gm is advisable.

RATIONALE FOR MEGADOSE SUPPLEMENTATION: Intake of soluble fiber at levels above the prevailing average in the US is associated with reductions in lipid and insulin levels. Intake of insoluble fiber at levels above the prevailing average in the US is generally associated with reduced risk of diverticular disease and colon cancer. However, gastrointestinal intolerance tends to be dose limiting so that "mega-dosing" of fiber is not practical.

EVIDENCE IN SUPPORT OF SUPPLEMENTATION BEYOND RDA: Soluble fiber supplementation is effective in lowering serum lipids even when the diet is already fat-restricted.[a] Soluble fiber also can improve glycemic control in diabetes.[b] Increased intake of insoluble fiber is effective in the management of constipation, and relatively high intake of insoluble fiber is associated with reduced risk of diseases of the large bowel, from diverticulosis to cancer (see chapters 12 and 22).

Recommended Intake Range (US RDA): There is no RDA for either total or soluble fiber. An intake of 20–30 g/day of total fiber is recommended for adults.

AVERAGE INTAKE, US ADULTS:	12 g/day total fiber
ESTIMATED MEAN PALEOLITHIC INTAKE (ADULT)[c]:	104 g/day total fiber
COMMON DOSE RANGE FOR USE AS SUPPLEMENT:	3–15 g/day soluble fiber
DO DIETARY PATTERNS MEETING GUIDELINES PERMIT INTAKE IN THE SUPPLEMENT RANGE?:	Yes
INCLUDED IN TYPICAL MULTI-VITAMIN/MULTI-MINERAL TABLET?:	No

DEFICIENCY
  Intake level: Variable
  Syndromes: Constipation

TOXICITY
  Intake level: Variable
  Syndromes: Gastrointestinal intolerance; micronutrient malabsorption

Dietary Sources[d]: Insoluble fiber is abundant in whole grains, especially wheat; soluble fiber is abundant in fruits, oats, lentils, and beans.

Food [e]	Serving Size	Energy (kcal)	Fiber (g)	Food [f]	Serving Size	Energy (kcal)	Fiber (g)
Wheat bran (raw)	1 cup (58 g)	125	25	Oat bran (raw)	1 cup (94 g)	231	14.5
Bulgur wheat	1 cup (182 g)	151	8.2	Raspberries	1 cup (123 g)	60	8.4
Barley, pearled	1 cup (157 g)	193	6	Lentils	1 cup (198 g)	230	15.6
Bread, whole wheat	1 slice (28 g)	69	2	Chick peas	1 cup (164 g)	269	12.5
Brown rice	1 cup (195 g)	218	3.5	Apples	1 medium (138 g)	81	3.7
Pasta	1 cup (140 g)	197	2.4	Carrots	1 medium (61 g)	26	1.8

Effects of Food Preparation and Storage: Health effects of fiber are generally unaffected by food preparation and storage under normal conditions.

TABLE IIIE. *Continued* (*Fiber*)

[a] Jenkins DJ, Kendall CW, Vidgen E, Mehling CC, Parker T, Seyler H, et al. The effect on serum lipids and oxidized low-density lipoprotein of supplementing self-selected low-fat diets with soluble fiber, soy, and vegetable protein foods. Metabolism. 2000;49:67–72

[b] Wursch P, Pi-Sunyer FX. The role of viscous soluble fiber in the metabolic control of diabetes. A review with special emphasis on cereals rich in beta-glucan. Diabetes Care. 1997;20:1774–1780

[c] Eaton SB, Eaton SB, III, Konner MJ. Paleolithic nutrition revisited: A twelve-year retrospective on its nature and implications. Eur J Clin Nutr. 1997;51:207–216

[d] The nutrient composition of most foods can be checked by accessing the USDA Nutrient database at: www.nal.usda.gov/fnic/foodcomp/Data/SR 13.

[e] Good sources of insoluble fiber. Values for all grains are reported for cooked portions unless otherwise stated.

[f] Good sources of soluble fiber.

Sources:

Ensminger AH, Ensminger ME, Konlande JE, Robson JRK. The Concise Encyclopedia of Foods and Nutrition. CRC Press, Inc. Boca Raton, FL. 1995

Margen S. The Wellness Nutrition Counter. Health Letter Associates. New York, NY. 1997

Murray MT. Encyclopedia of Nutritional Supplements. Prima Publishing. Rocklin, CA. 1996

National Research Council. Recommended Dietary Allowances. 10th edition. National Academy Press. Washington, D.C. 1989

Shils ME, Olson JA, Shike M (editors). Modern Nutrition in Health and Disease. 8th edition. Lea & Febiger. Philadelphia, PA. 1994

United States Department of Agriculture. USDA Nutrient Database for Standard Reference. Release 12. 1998

Ziegler EE, Filer LJ, Jr. (editors). Present Knowledge in Nutrition. 7th edition. ILSI Press. Washington, D.C. 1996

TABLE IIIE. *Continued (Flavonoids)*

Flavonoids

BIOLOGICAL FUNCTION(S) IN HUMANS/KEY PROPERTIES: Flavonoids are brightly colored phenolic compounds in plants. While the class contains over 4000 known compounds, interest to date has focused on proanthocyanidins (procyanidolic oligomers; PCO), quercetin, a group of bioflavonoids in citrus (hydroxyethylrutosides; HER), and polyphenolic compounds in tea. Some proprietary products, such as pycnogenol, are patented combinations of purified bioflavonoids. Flavonoids are not known as essential nutrients in humans, however their deficiency may contribute to the manifestations of scurvy; some consider them 'semi-essential'. Flavonoids play an important role as antioxidants. They chelate divalent cations, and by doing so may preserve levels of ascorbate (vitamin C). An effect on capillary permeability under experimental conditions may be direct, or may be mediated via ascorbate.

ABSORPTION/SOLUBILITY/STORAGE/PHARMACOKINETICS: Flavonoids are water soluble; their metabolism is similar to that of ascorbate. They are in general efficiently absorbed in the upper small bowel; however, absorption may vary between food sources and supplements. Excretion is in the urine, and storage is limited. The typical American diet provides between 0.15 and 1 g of mixed flavonoids daily.

RATIONALE FOR SUPPLEMENTATION IN RDA RANGE: None; there is no RDA for flavonoids.

RATIONALE FOR MEGADOSE SUPPLEMENTATION: Supplements of various flavonoids in varying doses are used by natruopathic practitioners for health promotion and for the treatment of venous insufficiency and inflammatory conditions. PCO is advocated for its antioxidant effects at a dose of approximately 50 mg/day, and for therapy of venous insufficiency or retinopathy at a dose of up to 300 mg/day. A dose of 100 mg quercetin daily is advocated for chronic inflammatory conditions such as asthma, rheumatoid arthritis, or atopy. HER is recommended at a dose in the range of 1 g/day for conditions of venous insufficiency. Up to 400 mg/day of green tea polyphenols is recommended for cancer prevention.

EVIDENCE IN SUPPORT OF SUPPLEMENTATION BEYOND RDA: The protean health benefits of a diet rich in fruits and vegetables are established conclusively; flavonoids may contribute to these benefits, but whether that is so, and if so to what extent, is uncertain. Most of the evidence in support of flavonoid supplementation remains preliminary, derived from animal and in vitro studies.[a] The role of flavonoids in green tea in cancer prevention is supported by animal and cell culture studies, but only observational data based on tea consumption patterns in humans.[b] However, evidence of benefit with flavonoid supplementation in venous insufficiency is convincing, if not definitive.[c]

Recommended Intake Range (US RDA): There is no RDA for flavonoids, nor is there an obvious source for a generalizable recommendation for an intake range for all adults. On the basis of various lines of evidence from diverse sources, an argument could be made that total flavonoid intake in the range of 1–2 g/1000 kcal would likely offer health benefits without any appreciable risk relative to the typical American intake of <500 mg/100 kcal.

TABLE IIIE. *Continued (Flavonoids)*

AVERAGE INTAKE, US ADULTS:	<1g/day
ESTIMATED MEAN PALEOLITHIC INTAKE (ADULT)[d]:	uncertain; likely in the range of 3–6/day
COMMON DOSE RANGE FOR USE AS SUPPLEMENT:	varies with particular com pound; from 50 mg to 1 g
DO DIETARY PATTERNS MEETING GUIDELINES PERMIT INTAKE IN THE SUPPLEMENT RANGE?:	Yes
INCLUDED IN TYPICAL MULTI-VITAMIN/MULTI-MINERAL TABLET?:	No

DEFICIENCY
Intake level: none known with certainty
Syndromes: vascular permeability

TOXICITY
Intake level: none known with certainty
Syndromes: pro-oxidant effects

Flavonoids Dietary Sources[e]:   The flavonoid content of specific foods is not readily available.[f] Flavonoids are concentrated in the brightly colored outer layers, skin, or peel of many fruits and vegetables. Concentrated sources include citrus fruits; berries; grapes; peaches; tomatoes; red cabbage; onion; peppers; beans; sage; green tea; and red wine.

Effects of Food Preparation and Storage: Flavonoids are relatively heat-resistant. Food processing is not thought to substantially alter flavonoid content or activity.

---

[a] Croft KD. The chemistry and biological effects of flavonoids and phenolic acids. Ann N Y Acad Sci 1998;854:435-42

[b] Yang CS. Tea and health. Nutrition 1999;15:946-9; Bushman JL. Green tea and cancer in humans: A review of the literature. Nutr Cancer 1998;31(3):151-9.

[c] Struckmann JR. Clinical efficacy of micronized purified flavonoid fraction: an overview. J Vasc Res 1999;36 Suppl 1:37-41.

[d] Eaton SB, Eaton SB, III, Konner MJ. Paleolithic nutrition revisited: A twelve-year retrospective on its nature and implications. Eur J Clin Nutr. 1997;51:207-216

[e] The nutrient composition of most foods can be checked by accessing the USDA Nutrient database at: www.nal.usda.gov/fnic/foodcomp/Data/SR 13. As of 3/2000, flavonoid content is not reported.

[f] Kuhnau J. The flavonoids: A class of semi-essential food components. World Review of Nutrition and Diet. 1976;24:117-191).

Sources:
Ensminger AH, Ensminger ME, Konlande JE, Robson JRK. The Concise Encyclopedia of Foods and Nutrition. CRC Press, Inc. Boca Raton, FL. 1995
Margen S. The Wellness Nutrition Counter. Health Letter Associates. New York, NY. 1997
Murray MT. Encyclopedia of Nutritional Supplements. Prima Publishing. Rocklin, CA. 1996
National Research Council. Recommended Dietary Allowances. 10th edition. National Academy Press. Washington, D.C. 1989
Shils ME, Olson JA, Shike M (editors). Modern Nutrition in Health and Disease. 8th edition. Lea & Febiger. Philadelphia, PA. 1994
United States Department of Agriculture. USDA Nutrient Database for Standard Reference. Release 12. 1998
Ziegler EE, Filer LJ, Jr. (editors). Present Knowledge in Nutrition. 7th edition. ILSI Press. Washington, D.C. 1996

TABLE IIIE. *Continued (Folate)*

Folate

Biological function(s) in humans/key properties: Folate, also referred to as folic acid or folacin, is apart of the B vitamin complex, and functions in the transfer of single carbon fragments. Folate is an essential cofactor in amino acid and nucleic acid synthesis, and is thus fundamental to all cell replication.

Absorption/Solubility/storage/pharmacokinetics: Folate is water soluble, and absorbed efficiently with saturation kinetics in the jejunum. Approximately 5-10 mg is stored in the average adult, half of which is in the liver. Excretion is in both urine and bile.

Rationale for Supplementation in RDA range: The usual intake of folate in the US is thought to be approximatley 280–300 μg per day in men, and less in women. While these levels exceed the 1989 RDA (200 μg per day for men and 180 μg per day for women), there is now widespread consensus that folate intake should be at least 400 μg per day to prevent neural tube defects in infants (see chapters 25 and 27) and vascular injury due to elevated homocysteine levels in older adults (see chapter 6). The dietary reference intake for folate is due to be published in 2000.[a] While compliance with guidelines for fruit and vegetable intake could lead to the recommended level of folate in the diet, there is evidence that between 80% and 90% of adults in the US consume less than the recommended level of folate. Nominal folate deficiency is considered the most common nutritional deficiency in the US. Thus, routine supplementation is indicated. This has been addressed through fortification of the food supply (grain products). However, fortification is expected to add 100 to 200 μg of folate to the daily diet of the average woman in the US. Further, absorption of folate in supplement form is more complete than of that in food. Therefore, routine use of a multivitamin formula (containing, on average, 400 μg folate) by at least women of child-bearing age and older adults is appropriate.

Rationale for Megadose Supplementation: Generally, none. A very limited literature suggests that folate in the range of 10 mg per day (25 times the current recommended intake level) may be beneficial in cervical dysplasia, and that a dose of 15 mg per day may be beneficial in depression. In neither case is the literature adequate to support routine clinical application.

Evidence in support of supplementation beyond RDA: The evidence that intake of at least 400 μg of folate per day around the time of conception can reduce the risk of neural tube defects is conclusive, and is the basis for fortification of the US food supply. Prenatal vitamins typically contain 1000 μg of folate. Evidence that folate intake can influence the risk of cardiovascular disease via effects on serum homocysteine (see chapter 6) is also strong[b,c] although not considered conclusive.[d] Beneficial effects of folate supplementation on vascular reactivity (endothelial function) have been demonstrated.[e]

Recommended Intake Range (US RDA): *N.B.* The 1989 RDA for folate should be considered outdated; the updated recommendation is therefore provided as well.

	Infancy (age 0–1)	Childhood (age 1–10)	Puberty/ adolescence (age 11–18)	Adulthood (age 19–50)	Post-menopause	Senescence	Pregnancy	Lactation
Male	25–35 μg	50–100 μg	150–200 μg update: 150–400 μg	200 μg update: 400 μg	—	200 μg update: 400 μg	—	—
Female	25–35 μg	50–100 μg	150–180 μg update: 150–400 μg	180 μg update: 400 μg	180 μg update: 400 μg	180 μg update: 400 μg	400 μg	260–280 μg update: 400 μg

TABLE IIIE. *Continued (Folate)*

AVERAGE INTAKE, US ADULTS:	150-300 µg/day before grain fortification; estimated 250-400 µg/day at present
ESTIMATED MEAN PALEOLITHIC INTAKE (ADULT)[f]:	360 µg/day
COMMON DOSE RANGE FOR USE AS SUPPLEMENT:	400-1000 µg/day
DO DIETARY PATTERNS MEETING GUIDELINES PERMIT INTAKE IN THE SUPPLEMENT RANGE?:	Yes
INCLUDED IN TYPICAL MULTI-VITAMIN/MULTI-MINERAL TABLET?:	Yes (dose: 400 µg; prenatal vitamin dose: 1000 µg)

DEFICIENCY
Intake level: 100 µg per day to prevent overt deficiency; 400 µg per day to prevent nominal deficiency
Syndromes: megaloblastic anemia; neural tube defects; hyperhomocysteinemia

TOXICITY
Intake level: intake at the RDA can mask B12 deficiency; doses in excess of 10 mg/day (25 times DRI) may be toxic
Syndromes: neurologic sequelae of B12 deficiency; seizures in susceptibles with mega-dosing

Folate Dietary Sources[g:] Green vegetables, beans, legumes and whole grains; to a lesser extent, fruit and fruit juice.

Food	Serving Size	Energy (kcal)	Folate (µg)	Food	Serving Size	Energy (kcal)	Folate (µg)
Lentils	1 cup (198 g)	230	358	Orange juice	1 cup (248 g)	112	75
Kidney beans	1 cup (177 g)	225	229	Radishes	1 medium (4.5 g)	0.9	1.2
Asparagus	4 spears (60 g)	14	88	Peas	1 cup (160 g)	134	101
Avocado	1 whole (201 g)	324	124	White beans	1 cup (179 g)	249	144
Wheat germ	1 cup (115 g)	414	323	Wild rice	1 cup (164 g)	166	43
Pinto beans	1 cup (171 g)	234	294	Banana	1 medium (118 g)	109	23
Chickpeas	1 cup (164 g)	269	282	Endive	1 head (513 g)	87	728
Lima beans	1 cup (188 g)	216	156	Broccoli	1 medium stalk (180 g)	50	90
Spinach	1 cup (180 g)	41	262	Brussel sprouts	1/2 cup (78 g)	30	47
Oatmeal	100 g	93	76	Lettuce (butterhead)	1 head (163 g)	21	119

Effects of Food Preparation and Storage: Not reported to be a generally important determinant of dietary intake levels.

[a] Dietary Reference Intakes for Thiamin, Riboflavin, Niacin, Standing Committee on the Scientific Evaluation of Dietary Reference Intakes, Institute of Medicine. Vitamin B6, Folate, Vitamin B12, Pantothenic Acid, Biotin, and Choline. National Academy Press. Projected publication: 2000.; see: http://books.nap.edu/catalog/6015.html

[b] Christensen B, Landaas S, Stensvold I, et al. Whole blood folate, homocysteine in serum, and risk of first acute myocardial infarction. Atherosclerosis 1999;147:317-26.

[c] Bunout D, Garrido A, Suazo M, et al. Effects of supplementation with folic acid and antioxidant vitamins on homocysteine levels and LDL oxidation in coronary patients. Nutrition 2000;16:107-10.

[d] Eikelboom JW, Lonn E, Genest J Jr, et al. Homocyst(e)ine and cardiovascular disease: a critical review of the epidemiologic evidence. Ann Intern Med 1999;131:363-75.

[e] Woo KS, Chook P, Lolin YI, et al. Folic acid improves arterial endothelial function in adults with hyperhomocystinemia. J Am Coll Cardiol 1999;34:2002-6.

[f] Eaton SB, Eaton SB, III, Konner MJ. Paleolithic nutrition revisited: A twelve-year retrospective on its nature and implications. Eur J Clin Nutr. 1997;51:207–216

[g] The nutrient composition of most foods can be checked by accessing the USDA Nutrient database at: www.nal.usda.gov/fnic/foodcomp/Data/SR 13.

Sources:

Ensminger AH, Ensminger ME, Konlande JE, Robson JRK. The Concise Encyclopedia of Foods and Nutrition. CRC Press, Inc. Boca Raton, FL. 1995

Margen S. The Wellness Nutrition Counter. Health Letter Associates. New York, NY. 1997

Murray MT. Encyclopedia of Nutritional Supplements. Prima Publishing. Rocklin, CA. 1996

National Research Council. Recommended Dietary Allowances. 10th edition. National Academy Press. Washington, D.C. 1989

Shils ME, Olson JA, Shike M (editors). Modern Nutrition in Health and Disease. 8th edition. Lea & Febiger. Philadelphia, PA. 1994

United States Department of Agriculture. USDA Nutrient Database for Standard Reference. Release 12. 1998

Ziegler EE, Filer LJ, Jr. (editors). Present Knowledge in Nutrition. 7th edition. ILSI Press. Washington, D.C. 1996

TABLE IIIE. *Continued* (*Lycopene*)

Lycopene

BIOLOGICAL FUNCTION(S) IN HUMANS/KEY PROPERTIES: Lycopene is a non-provitamin A carotenoid with 11 carbons arranged linearly in conjugated double bonds, and no ionone ring. Antioxidant capacity of carotenoids is related to the number of conjugated double bonds; thus, the antioxidant capacity of lycopene is the greatest of known carotenoids, and exceeds that of β-carotene by a factor of 2. Lycopene is thought to serve as a potent quencher of oxygen free radicals within cells and on the inner surfaces of cell membranes; other functions in human physiology remain to be elucidated. Lycopene is not known to be an essential nutrient.

ABSORPTION/SOLUBILITY/STORAGE/PHARMACOKINETICS: In general, carotenoids are protein bound and lipid soluble. Heating foods can cause dissociation of such complexes, and enhance carotenoid bioavailability. Carotenoids in general, and lycopene in particular, are more efficiently absorbed when ingested with a lipid source, such as oil. Nonabsorbable lipids, such as olestra, are likely to decrease absorption. Lycopene is hydrophobic, and transported predominantly near the core of lipoprotein particles, in particular LDL; levels are lower in small, dense than in normal LDL particles. Serum concentrations vary over a wide range, from 50 to 900 nM/L. Serum lycopene changes gradually in response to varied intake, with a plasma depletion half-life of between 12 and 33 days; levels in chylomicrons are a better marker of short-term change. Lycopene is prominently stored in the adrenal glands, testes, liver, and prostate. Storage in adipose tissue varies with as yet undetermined factors.

RATIONALE FOR SUPPLEMENTATION IN RDA RANGE: No RDA has been established for lycopene.

RATIONALE FOR MEGADOSE SUPPLEMENTATION: None known. Studies of supplements have not been reported to date. Supplements are available in the form of "tomato extract with lycopene" but have not been studied in comparison to natural sources. The rationale for increasing lycopene intake is enhanced antioxidant activity, and possible protection against gastrointestinal and prostate cancers. Protection against myocardial infarction has also been suggested.[a]

EVIDENCE IN SUPPORT OF SUPPLEMENTATION BEYOND RDA: None; not pertinent.

Recommended Intake Range (US RDA): None

AVERAGE INTAKE, US ADULTS:	3–4 mg/day
ESTIMATED MEAN PALEOLITHIC INTAKE (ADULT)[b]:	Not known. Paleolithic intake may have been low, given that tomatoes are the predominant source of lycopene, and tomatoes entered the human diet only recently; the tomato plant was originally discovered as a weed in fields of maize and beans in Central America.[c]
COMMON DOSE RANGE FOR USE AS SUPPLEMENT:	Internet sites advertise supplements providing between 5 and 10 mg lycopene.
DO DIETARY PATTERNS MEETING GUIDELINES PERMIT INTAKE IN THE SUPPLEMENT RANGE?:	Yes, provided tomato and tomato-product intake is high.
INCLUDED IN TYPICAL MULTI-VITAMIN/MULTI-MINERAL TABLET?:	No

DEFICIENCY
  Intake level: None known
  Syndromes: None known

TOXICITY
  Intake level: None known
  Syndromes: None known

TABLE IIIE. *Continued (Lycopene)*

Lycopene Dietary Sources[b]:

Food	Serving Size	Energy (kcal)	Lycopene μg	Food	Serving Size	Energy (kcal)	Lycopene μg
Tomatoes, raw	100 gm	21	2937	Apricot, dried	100 gm	238	864
Tomatoes, fresh, cooked	100 gm	27	3703	Grapefruit, pink	100 gm	30	3362
Tomato sauce, canned	100 gm	30	6205	Guava	100 gm	51	5400
Tomato paste, canned	100 gm	82	6500	Watermelon	100 gm	32	4100
Tomato juice, canned	100 gm	17	8580	Papaya	100 gm	39	2000– 5300
Tomato catsup	100 gm	104	9900	Rosehip, puree, canned	100 gm	—	780

Effects of Food Preparation and Storage: Heating foods, particularly in the presence of oil, enhances the absorption and bioavailability of lycopene. Freezing preserves lycopene content.

[a] Kohlmeier L, Kark JD, Gomez-Garcia E, et al. Lycopene and Myocardial Infarction Risk in the EURAMIC Study. Am J Epidemiol. 1997;146:618–626

[b] Eaton SB, Eaton SB, III, Konner MJ. Paleolithic nutrition revisited: A twelve-year retrospective on its nature and implications. Eur J Clin Nutr. 1997;51:207–216

[c] Tannahill R. Food in History. Three Rivers Press. New York. 1988

[d] Lycopene content is derived from: Gerster H. The Potential role of Lycopene for Human Health. J Am College Nutr. 1997;16:109–126. The nutrient composition of most foods can be checked by accessing the USDA Nutrient database at: www.nal.usda.gov/fnic/foodcomp/Data/SR 13. At present, the lycopene content of foods is not reported in the Nutrient database.

Sources:
Clinton SK. Lycopene: chemistry, Biology, and Implications for Human Health and Disease. Nutr Rev. 1998;56:35–51

Ensminger AH, Ensminger ME, Konlande JE, Robson JRK. The Concise Encyclopedia of Foods and Nutrition. CRC Press, Inc. Boca Raton, FL. 1995

Gerster H. The Potential role of Lycopene for Human Health. J Am College Nutr. 1997;16:109–126

Margen S. The Wellness Nutrition Counter. Health Letter Associates. New York, NY. 1997

Murray MT. Encyclopedia of Nutritional Supplements. Prima Publishing. Rocklin, CA. 1996

National Research Council. Recommended Dietary Allowances. 10th edition. National Academy Press. Washington, D.C. 1989

Shils ME, Olson JA, Shike M (editors). Modern Nutrition in Health and Disease. 8th edition. Lea & Febiger. Philadelphia, PA. 1994

Stahl W, Sies H. Lycopene: a biologically Important Carotenoid for Humans? Archives of Biochemistry and Biophysics. 1996;336:1–9

United States Department of Agriculture. USDA Nutrient Database for Standard Reference. Release 12. 1998

Ziegler EE, Filer LJ, Jr. (editors). Present Knowledge in Nutrition. 7th edition. ILSI Press. Washington, D.C. 1996

TABLE IIIE. *Continued (Magnesium)*

Magnesium

BIOLOGICAL FUNCTION(S) IN HUMANS/KEY PROPERTIES: Magnesium is known to function in over 300 enzyme systems in the human body, impacting virtually all aspects of metabolism.

ABSORPTION/SOLUBILITY/STORAGE/PHARMACOKINETICS: Roughly 33% of ingested magnesium is absorbed in the upper small bowel. Poorly understood homeostatic mechanisms generally maintain a plasma Mg concentration of between 1.4 and 2.4 mg/dl (0.65-1.0 mM/L). Excretion is in the urine; when serum Mg begins to fall, the kidney compensates by reabsorbing most filtered Mg. Approximately 20-28 g of Mg is stored in the body of an adult, with slightly more than half (60%) in the skeleton and slightly less than half in muscles and soft tissue; 1% of body stores is distributed in extracellular fluid. Thiazide diuretics and alcohol increase urinary losses.

RATIONALE FOR SUPPLEMENTATION IN RDA RANGE: The RDA for magnesium is 420 mg/day for adult men and 320 mg/day for adult women. Average intake in the US is estimated to be below this level. Therefore, the risk of nominal magnesium deficiency exists with typical American dietary patterns. Supplementation is a reasonable means of precluding such deficiency.

RATIONALE FOR MEGADOSE SUPPLEMENTATION: Doses up to approximately twice the RDA are advocated for the treatment of myocardial ischemia; cardiac dysrhythmia; congestive heart failure; hypertension; claudication; osteoporosis; fibromyalgia; osteoporosis; and premenstrual syndrome. Supplementation during pregnancy has been advocated to reduce the risk of preeclampsia.

EVIDENCE IN SUPPORT OF SUPPLEMENTATION BEYOND RDA: Evidence supporting intake of Mg at approximately the RDA is considerable, and in the aggregate represents the rationale for the particular recommendations made. To the extent that supplementation is required to achieve the RDA, supplementation is therefore of likely benefit. Evidence of benefit from supplementation beyond the RDA is generally suggestive at best. Magnesium depletion may accompany diuretic use in CHF, and there is some evidence of acute[a] and sustained[b] suppression of ventricular dysrhythmias in such patients. There is inconsistent evidence of increased bone density with magnesium supplementation.[c,d] Magnesium has generally not been found effective in the treatment of hypertension (see chapter 7) or the prevention of preeclampsia.[e] Magnesium deficiency is associated with insulin resistance; whether magnesium supplementation is of benefit in insulin resistance not associated with deficiency is uncertain.

Recommended Intake Range (US RDA[f]):

	Infancy (age 0–1)	Childhood (age 1–10)	Puberty/ adolescence (age 11–18)	Adulthood (age 19–50)	Post- menopause	Senescence	Pregnancy	Lactation
Male	40–60 mg	80–200 mg	240–410 mg	400–420 mg	—	420 mg	—	—
Female	400–60 mg	80–200 mg	240–360 mg	310–320 mg	320 mg	320 mg	350–400 mg	310–360 mg

TABLE IIIE. *Continued* (*Magnesium*)

AVERAGE INTAKE, US ADULTS: 250-350 mg/day

ESTIMATED MEAN PALEOLITHIC INTAKE (ADULT)[f]: Not available; given the distribution of Mg in the food supply, paleolithic intake would have been considerably greater than current intake, as is true for potassium (see chapters 7 and 39)

COMMON DOSE RANGE FOR USE AS SUPPLEMENT: 100-1000 mg/day

DO DIETARY PATTERNS MEETING GUIDELINES PERMIT INTAKE IN THE SUPPLEMENT RANGE?: Yes

INCLUDED IN TYPICAL MULTI-VITAMIN/MULTI-MINERAL TABLET?: Yes (dose: 100 mg)

DEFICIENCY
Intake level: variable; deficiency is often due to malabsorption, alcoholism, or use of diuretics
Syndromes: weakness, muscle tremors, cardiac dysrhythmia, mental status changes

TOXICITY
Intake level: variable, depending on renal function; toxicity of oral Mg is limited
Syndromes: nausea, vomiting, hypotension; if extreme, respiratory depression and asystole

Magnesium Dietary Sources[g]: Magnesium is abundant in leafy green vegetables, grains, legumes, certain fish, nuts, seeds, and chocolate.

Food	Serving Size	Energy (kcal)	Magnesium (mg)	Food	Serving Size	Energy (kcal)	Magnesium (mg)
Sunflower seeds	1 oz (28 g)	175	37	Soybeans	1 cup (172 g)	298	148
Wild rice	1 cup (164 g)	166	52	White beans	1 cup (179 g)	249	113
Wheat germ	1 cup (115 g)	414	275	Peaches	1 medium (98 g)	42	7
Halibut	1/2 fillet (159 g)	223	170	Bulgur	1 cup (182 g)	151	58
Avocado	1 medium (201 g)	324	78	Navy beans	1 cup (182 g)	258	107
Mackerel	1 fillet (88 g)	231	85	Oatmeal	100 g	93	35
Almonds	1 oz (28 g)	169	81	Lettuce (butterhead)	1 head (163 g)	21	21
Chocolate (semi-sweet)	1 oz (28 g)	136	33	Banana	1 medium (118 g)	109	34
Spinach	1 cup (180 g)	41	157	Buckwheat	1 cup (168 g)	155	86
Cashews	1 oz (28 g)	163	74	Swiss chard	1 cup (175 g)	35	150

Effects of Food Preparation and Storage: Not reported to be a generally important determinant of dietary intake levels.

[a] Ceremuzynski L, Gebalska J, Wolk R, et al. Hypomagnesemia in heart failure with ventricular arrhythmias. Beneficial effects of magnesium supplementation. J Intern Med 2000;247:78-86.

[b] Bashir Y, Sneddon JF, Staunton HA, et al. Effects of long-term oral magnesium chloride replacement in congestive heart failure secondary to coronary artery disease. Am J Cardiol 1993;72:1156-62.

[c] Martini LA. Magnesium supplementation and bone turnover. Nutr Rev 1999;57:227-9;

[d] Doyle L, Flynn A, Cashman K. The effect of magnesium supplementation on biochemical markers of bone metabolism or blood pressure in healthy young adult females. Eur J Clin Nutr 1999;53:255-61.

[e] Mattar F, Sibai BM. Prevention of preeclampsia. Semin Perinatol 1999;23:58-64.

[f] Eaton SB, Eaton SB, III, Konner MJ. Paleolithic nutrition revisited: A twelve-year retrospective on its nature and implications. Eur J Clin Nutr. 1997;51:207–216.

TABLE IIIE. *Continued (Magnesium)*

---

g The nutrient composition of most foods can be checked by accessing the USDA Nutrient database at: www.nal.usda.gov/fnic/foodcomp/Data/SR 13.

Sources:

Ensminger AH, Ensminger ME, Konlande JE, Robson JRK. The Concise Encyclopedia of Foods and Nutrition. CRC Press, Inc. Boca Raton, FL. 1995

Margen S. The Wellness Nutrition Counter. Health Letter Associates. New York, NY. 1997

Murray MT. Encyclopedia of Nutritional Supplements. Prima Publishing. Rocklin, CA. 1996

National Research Council. Recommended Dietary Allowances. 10th edition. National Academy Press. Washington, D.C. 1989

Shils ME, Olson JA, Shike M (editors). Modern Nutrition in Health and Disease. 8th edition. Lea & Febiger. Philadelphia, PA. 1994

United States Department of Agriculture. USDA Nutrient Database for Standard Reference. Release 12. 1998

Ziegler EE, Filer LJ, Jr. (editors). Present Knowledge in Nutrition. 7th edition. ILSI Press. Washington, D.C. 1996

TABLE IIIE. *Continued* (*Phosphorous*)

Phosphorous

BIOLOGICAL FUNCTION(S) IN HUMANS/KEY PROPERTIES: Phosphorous is an essential dietary mineral. Most (85%) of the 800–850gm stored in the body of an adult is incorporated in the hydroxyapatite matrix of bone in a ratio of 1:2 with calcium. Phosphorous is essential to the hardening of both bone and tooth mineral. Phosphorous participates in the regulation of blood pH. It is present as a component of lipid particles (phospholipids), and in the molecular structure of carbohydrates nad proteins. Phosphorous is a key component of many chemical messengers, including cyclic-AMP (adenosine monophosphate), cyclic GMP (guanine monophosphate), and 2,3-diphosphoglyecerate. Renal calcitrol production is in part mediated by serum phosphate levels. Phosphorous also plays a role in the transport of many nutrients into cells, and is required for the synthesis of DNA and RNA. Phosphate bonds in adenosine triphosphate (ATP) are the principal source of energy for metabolism.

ABSORPTION/SOLUBILITY/STORAGE/PHARMACOKINETICS: Phosphorous absorption takes place in the small intestine by a mechanism independent of calcium and vitmain D; by a mechanism dependent on both calcium and vitamin D; and by a mechanism dependent on vitamin D, but independent of calcium. Nearly 90% of phosphorous in human milk is absorbed by infants. Adults absorb more than 50% of ingested phosphorous, with absorption rising as habitual intake falls. The skeleton is the principal storage depot for phosphorous. Virtually all phosphorous lost from the body is excreted in the urine.

RATIONALE FOR SUPPLEMENTATION IN RDA RANGE: Phosphorous deficiency does not normally occur, but can be seen with extensive use of phosphate binding antacids (i.e., aluminum based) by adults, or in premature infants. In infants, phosphorous deficiency leads to hypophosphatemic rickets, while in adults it induces bone loss, weakness, and malaise.

RATIONALE FOR MEGADOSE SUPPLEMENTATION: There appears to be no rationale for megadosing of phosphorous.

EVIDENCE IN SUPPORT OF SUPPLEMENTATION BEYOND RDA: None

TABLE IIIE. *Continued (Phosphorous)*

Recommended Intake Range in May (US RDA):

	Infancy (age 0–0.5)	Infancy (age 0.5–1)	Childhood (age 1–10)	Puberty/ adolescence/ (age 11–18)	Adulthood (age 19–50)	Post-menopause	Senescence	Pregnancy	Lactation
Male	300 mg	500 mg	800 mg	1200 mg	800 mg	—	800 mg	—	—
Female	300 mg	500 mg	800 mg	1200 mg	800 mg	800 mg	800 mg	1200 mg	1200 mg

TABLE IIIE. *Continued* (*Phosphorous*)

AVERAGE INTAKE, US ADULTS: Approximately 1500 mg per day for adult men, 1000 mg per day for women.

ESTIMATED MEAN PALEOLITHIC INTAKE (ADULT)[a]: Not available.

COMMON DOSE RANGE FOR USE AS SUPPLEMENT: NA

DO DIETARY PATTERNS MEETING GUIDELINES PERMIT INTAKE IN THE SUPPLEMENT RANGE?: Not routinely used as a supplement; Yes.

INCLUDED IN TYPICAL MULTI-VITAMIN/MULTI-MINERAL TABLET?: Yes (approximately 48 mg; 5% of RDA)

DEFICIENCY
Intake level: Uncertain; a 1:1 ratio with ingested calcium is the recommended minimum.
Syndromes: Hypophosphatemic rickets in neonates; osteopenia and malaise in adults. Acute hypophosphatmia can cause myopathy, cardiomyopathyy and rhabdomyolysis. When the product of calcium ion and phosphate ion (the double product) is less than 0.7 mmol/L, there is likely to be a bone mineralization defect.

TOXICITY
Intake level: More than twice the intake level of calcium.
Syndromes: High intake of phosphorous does not appear to be toxic when calcium and vitamin D intake are adequate. When either calcium or vitamin D intake are marginal, high phosphorous intake may induce hypocalcemia. Neither this, nor the hyperparathyroidism induced in laboratory animals, are clinical entities that ordinarily occur. Acute hyperphosphatemia can cause hyocalcemic tetany. When the calcium phosphate ion double product is greater than 2.2 mmol/L, soft tissue calcification is likely.

Phosphorous Dietary Sources[b]:

Food	Serving Size	Energy (kcal)	Phosphorous (mg)
Wheat germ	1 cup (113 g)	432	1295
Sunflower seeds	1 cup (134 g)	829	1552
Sardines	1 can (92 g)	191	451
Wild rice	1 cup (164 g)	166	134
Pumpkin seeds	1 cup (64 g)	285	59
Salmon	1/2 fillet (154 g)	280	394
Tuna, canned	1 can (165 g)	191	269
Flounder/sole	1 fillet (127 g)	149	367
Skim milk	1 cup (245 g)	85	247
Yogurt, non-fat	1 cup (245 g)	137	383

Effects of Food Preparation and Storage: Phosphorous is relatively unaffected by food processing.

TABLE IIIE. *Continued (Phosphorous)*

[a] Eaton SB, Eaton SB, III, Konner MJ. Paleolithic nutrition revisited: A twelve-year retrospective on its nature and implications. Eur J Clin Nutr. 1997;51:207–216

[b] The nutrient composition of most foods can be checked by accessing the USDA Nutrient database at: www.nal.usda.gov/fnic/foodcomp/Data/SR 13.

Sources:

Ensminger AH, Ensminger ME, Konlande JE, Robson JRK. The Concise Encyclopedia of Foods and Nutrition. CRC Press, Inc. Boca Raton, FL. 1995

Margen S. The Wellness Nutrition Counter. Health Letter Associates. New York, NY. 1997

Murray MT. Encyclopedia of Nutritional Supplements. Prima Publishing. Rocklin, CA. 1996

National Research Council. Recommended Dietary Allowances. 10th edition. National Academy Press. Washington, D.C. 1989

Shils ME, Olson JA, Shike M (editors). Modern Nutrition in Health and Disease. 8th edition. Lea & Febiger. Philadelphia, PA. 1994

Standing Committee on the Scientific Evaluation of Dietary Reference Intakes, Food and Nutrition Board, Institute of Medicine. Dietary Reference Intakes for Calcium, Phosphorous, Magnesium, Vitamin D, and Fluoride. National Academy Press. Washington, D.C. 1997

United States Department of Agriculture. USDA Nutrient Database for Standard Reference. Release 12. 1998

Ziegler EE, Filer LJ, Jr. (editors). Present Knowledge in Nutrition. 7th edition. ILSI Press. Washington, D.C. 1996

TABLE IIIE. *Continued (Selenium)*

Selenium

BIOLOGICAL FUNCTION(S) IN HUMANS/KEY PROPERTIES: Selenium is a mineral that functions as a component of glutathione peroxidase, an essential antioxidant system. It is involved in the metabolism of vitamin E, and in thyroid function.

ABSORPTION/SOLUBILITY/STORAGE/PHARMACOKINETICS: Selenium is generally well absorbed in the small bowel, and is transported in circulation bound to protein. The mineral is concentrated in liver and kidney, and to a lesser extent myocardium. Excretion is primarily in the urine, secondarily in stool. An adult of average size stores approximately 15 mg of selenium.

RATIONALE FOR SUPPLEMENTATION IN RDA RANGE: Selenium is supplemented in the RDA range to assure its function as an antioxidant. However, the typical diet in the US provides well in excess of the RDA for selenium. Supplementation is indicated to prevent deficiency syndromes in parts of the world where the soil is selenium deficient. Selenium deficiency has been most extensively evaluated in rural areas of China with selenium-poor soil, and little access to outside food sources. Under such conditions, selenium supplementation in the range of the RDA is indicated to prevent overt deficiency, manifested as Keshan disease, a cardiomyopathy[a,b] and Kashin-Beck Syndrome, a form of arthritis,[c] as well as to reduce cancer risk.[d,e]

RATIONALE FOR MEGADOSE SUPPLEMENTATION: Selenium supplementation is advocated for putative benefits in cancer prevention, cardiovascular disease prevention (especially the prevention of events in those with established CAD), immune enhancement, rheumatoid arthritis, cataract prevention, and the prevention of sudden infant death syndrome (SIDS). However, the evidence for most of these effects is either limited to conditions of selenium deficiency, or is highly speculative. As selenium toxicity is well established at a dose 1 mg (1000 μg) per day, there is no rationale for "mega" dosing.

Evidence in support of supplementation beyond RDA: None.

Recommended Intake Range (US RDA):

	Infancy (age 0–1)	Childhood (age 1–10)	Puberty/ adolescence (age 11–18)	Adulthood (age 19–50)	Post-menopause	Senescence	Pregnancy	Lactation
Male	10–15 μg	20–30 μg	40–50 μg	70 μg	—	70 μg	—	—
Female	10–15 μg	20–30 μg	45–50 μg	55 μg	55 μg	55 μg	65 μg	75 μg

TABLE IIIE. *Continued (Selenium)*

AVERAGE INTAKE, US ADULTS:	approximately 100 μg/day
ESTIMATED MEAN PALEOLITHIC INTAKE (ADULT)[f]:	Not available
COMMON DOSE RANGE FOR USE AS SUPPLEMENT:	50–200 μg/day
DO DIETARY PATTERNS MEETING GUIDELINES PERMIT INTAKE IN THE SUPPLEMENT RANGE?:	Yes
INCLUDED IN TYPICAL MULTI-VITAMIN/MULTI-MINERAL TABLET?:	Yes (dose: 20 μg)
DEFICIENCY	
Intake level:	<10–20 μg/day
Syndromes:	cardiomyopathy (Keshan disease); arthritis (Kashin–Beck Syndrome); immunosuppression; increased susceptibility to cancer
TOXICITY	
Intake level:	>1000 μg/day
Syndromes:	nausea and vomiting; neuropathy; alopecia

Selenium Dietary Sources[g]: Organ meats, fish, and shellfish are generally selenium-rich. The selenium content of grains varies with the soil content.

Food	Serving Size	Energy (kcal)	Selenium (μg)	Food	Serving Size	Energy (kcal)	Selenium (μg)
Tuna	1 can (165 g)	191	133	Yogurt (nonfat)	1 cup (245 g)	137	9
Oysters	6 medium (42 g)	58	30	Skim milk	1 cup (245 g)	86	5
Flounder (or Sole)	1 fillet (127 g)	149	74	Peanut butter	2 tbsp (32 g)	190	2.4
Wheat germ	1 cup (115 g)	414	91	Pecans	1 oz (28 g)	196	2
Turkey	1/2 breast (306 g)	413	98	White bread	1 slice (27 g)	79	8.4
Chicken	1/2 breast (86 g)	142	24	Egg	1 large	101	14
Farina	1 cup (233 g)	116	21	Almonds	1 oz (28 g)	169	2.2
Shrimp	4 large (22 g)	22	9	Walnuts	1 oz (28 g)	185	1.3
Mushrooms	1/2 cup (78 g)	21	9	Mozzarella (part skim)	1 slice (28 g)	79	4.6
Barley	1 cup (157 g)	193	14	Swiss cheese	1 slice (28 g)	107	3.6

Effects of Food Preparation and Storage: Not known to be a significant factor.

[a] Neve J. Selenium as a risk factor for cardiovascular diseases. J Cardiovasc Risk 1996;3:42-7.

[b] Hensrud DD, Heimburger DC, Chen J, et al. Antioxidant status, erythrocyte fatty acids, and mortality from cardiovascular disease and Keshan disease in China. Eur J Clin Nutr 1994;48:455-64.

[c] Moreno-Reyes R, Suetens C, Mathieu F, et al. Kashin-Beck osteoarthropathy in rural Tibet in relation to selenium and iodine status. N Engl J Med 1998;339:1112-20.

[d] Blot WJ, Li JY, Taylor PR, et al. The Linxian trials: mortality rates by vitamin-mineral intervention group. Am J Clin Nutr 1995;62(6 Suppl):1424s-1426s.

[e] Taylor PR, Li B, Dawsey SM, et al. Prevention of esophageal cancer: the nutrition intervention trials in Linxian, China. Linxian Nutrition Intervention Trials Study Group. Cancer Res 1994;54(7 Suppl):2029s-2031s.

[f] Eaton SB, Eaton SB, III, Konner MJ. Paleolithic nutrition revisited: a twelve-year retrospective on its nature and implications. Eur J Clin Nutr. 1997;51:207–216.

[g] The nutrient composition of most foods can be checked by accessing the USDA Nutrient database at: www.nal.usda.gov/fnic/foodcomp/Data/SR 13.

Sources:

Ensminger AH, Ensminger ME, Konlande JE, Robson JRK. The Concise Encyclopedia of Foods and Nutrition. CRC Press, Inc. Boca Raton, FL. 1995

Margen S. The Wellness Nutrition Counter. Health Letter Associates. New York, NY. 1997

Murray MT. Encyclopedia of Nutritional Supplements. Prima Publishing. Rocklin, CA. 1996

National Research Council. Recommended Dietary Allowances. 10th edition. National Academy Press. Washington, D.C. 1989

Shils ME, Olson JA, Shike M (editors). Modern Nutrition in Health and Disease. 8th edition. Lea & Febiger. Philadelphia, PA. 1994

United States Department of Agriculture. USDA Nutrient Database for Standard Reference. Release 12. 1998

Ziegler EE, Filer LJ, Jr. (editors). Present Knowledge in Nutrition. 7th edition. ILSI Press. Washington, D.C. 1996

TABLE IIIE. *Continued (Vitamin B$_6$)*

Vitamin B$_6$

BIOLOGICAL FUNCTION(S) IN HUMANS/KEY PROPERTIES: The several forms of Vitamin B$_6$, pyridoxine, pyridoxal, and pyridoxamine function in a variety of metabolic pathways, especially transamination, decarboxylation, and racemization of amino acids. B$_6$ is vital to protein metabolism, the manufacture of neurotransmitter production, gluconeogenesis, and glycogenolysis. B$_6$ requirements vary directly with protein intake.

ABSORPTION/SOLUBILITY/STORAGE/PHARMACOKINETICS: Water-soluble. Intestinal absorption is nonsaturable. Storage occurs primarily in plasma in a complex with albumin, and in erythrocytes.

RATIONALE FOR SUPPLEMENTATION IN RDA RANGE: Intake below the RDA is apparently widespread, especially among the elderly and both pregnant and lactating women. Low B$_6$ intake is associated with elevated plasma homocysteine, a risk factor for cardiovascular disease.

RATIONALE FOR MEGADOSE SUPPLEMENTATION: Claims have been made for therapeutic roles in asthma, immunodepression, carpal tunnel syndrome, pregnancy-induced nausea, and pre-menstrual syndrome, among other conditions.

EVIDENCE IN SUPPORT OF SUPPLEMENTATION BEYOND RDA: There is consensus that supplementation to meet the RDA is appropriate among groups at risk of deficiency. In addition, low levels are widespread among smokers, women taking oral contraceptives, and during pregnancy and lactation; supplementation is recommended for these groups. Supplementation in the form of a multivitamin tablet generally provides up to 150% of the RDA for adults. The use of megadose supplements for certain conditions is supported by randomized trials[a,b], but these are mostly small, and there is lack of consensus. Doses of up to 250 mg per day are considered safe.

TABLE IIIE. *Continued (Vitamin B₆)*

Recommended Intake Range (US RDA):

	Infancy (age 0–1)	Childhood (age 1–10)	Puberty/ adolescence (age 11–18)	Adulthood (age 19–50)	Post-menopause	Senescence	Pregnancy	Lactation
Male	0.3–0.6 mg	1.0–1.4 mg	1.7–2.0 mg	2.0 mg	—	2.0 mg	—	—
Female	0.3–0.6 mg	1.0–1.4 mg	1.4–1.5 mg	1.6 mg	1.6 mg	1.6 mg	2.2 mg	2.1 mg

TABLE IIIE. *Continued* (*Vitamin B₆*)

AVERAGE INTAKE, US ADULTS:	1.16–1.87 mg
ESTIMATED MEAN PALEOLITHIC INTAKE (ADULT)[c]:	unknown
COMMON DOSE RANGE FOR USE AS SUPPLEMENT:	50–100 mg per day
DO DIETARY PATTERNS MEETING GUIDELINES PERMIT INTAKE IN THE SUPPLEMENT RANGE?:	No
INCLUDED IN TYPICAL MULTI-VITAMIN/MULTI-MINERAL TABLET?:	Yes (dose: 2.0 mg)

DEFICIENCY
Intake level: below 0.016 mg B_6 per gram dietary protein
Syndromes: dermatitis, anemia, seizures

TOXICITY
Intake level: above 250 mg per day for extended periods (months)
Syndromes: ataxia, myalgia, peripheral neuropathy, irritability

Vitamin B₆ Dietary Sources[b]:

Food	Serving Size	Kilocalories	Vitamin B₆ (mg)	Food	Serving Size	Kilocalories	Vitamin B₆ (mg)
Tuna, yellowfin, cooked	3 oz	118	0.88	Carrot juice	1 cup	94	0.51
Avocado, Florida	one	340	0.85	Snapper	3 oz	109	0.39
Potato, with skin	one	115	0.36	Beef, sirloin	3 oz	211	0.36
Banana	One (medium)	92	0.68	Sweet potato	One (medium); 114 gm	117	0.28
Salmon	3 oz	155	0.80	Halibut	3 oz	119	0.34
Chicken	1/2 breast 86 gm)	142	0.52	Swordfish	3 oz	132	0.32
Chickpeas	1 cup	269	0.23	Tuna, canned	3 oz	109	0.18
Turkey	117 gm	184	0.63	Peppers (green)	One (medium)	32	0.30
Prune juice	1 cup	182	0.56	Lentils	1 cup	230	0.35
Sunflower seeds	1 oz	175	0.23	Walnuts	1 oz	182	0.16

Effects of Food Preparation and Storage: Freezing and processing of meats, grains, fruits, and vegetables can result in losses of up to 70% of native B_6.

---

[a] Vutyavanich T, Wongra-ngan S, Ruangsri R. Pyridoxine for nausea and vomiting of pregnancy: A randomized, double-blind, placebo-controlled trial. Am J Obstet Gynecol. 1995;173:881–884
[b] The nutrient composition of most foods can be checked by accessing the USDA Nutrient database at: www.nal.usda.gov/fnic/foodcomp/Data/SR 13. A more extensive list of food sources of vitamin C is available in: Margen S. The Wellness Nutrition Counter. Health Letter Associates. New York, NY. 1997
[c] Eaton SB, Eaton SB, III, Konner MJ. Paleolithic nutrition revisited: A twelve-year retrospective on its nature and implications. Eur J Clin Nutr. 1997;51:207–216

Sources:
Ensminger AH, Ensminger ME, Konlande JE, Robson JRK. The Concise Encyclopedia of Foods and Nutrition. CRC Press, Inc. Boca Raton, FL. 1995
Margen S. The Wellness Nutrition Counter. Health Letter Associates. New York, NY. 1997
Murray MT. Encyclopedia of Nutritional Supplements. Prima Publishing. Rocklin, CA. 1996
National Research Council. Recommended Dietary Allowances. 10th edition. National Academy Press. Washington, D.C. 1989
Shils ME, Olson JA, Shike M (editors). Modern Nutrition in Health and Disease. 8th edition. Lea & Febiger. Philadelphia, PA. 1994
United States Department of Agriculture. USDA Nutrient Database for Standard Reference. Release 12. 1998
Ziegler EE, Filer LJ, Jr. (editors). Present Knowledge in Nutrition. 7th edition. ILSI Press. Washington, D.C. 1996

TABLE IIIE. *Continued (Vitamin C)*

Vitamin C (Ascorbic Acid)

BIOLOGICAL FUNCTION(S) IN HUMANS/KEY PROPERTIES: An essential co-factor for 8 known enzymes; functions as an electron donor. Facilitates hydroxylation reactions. Vital for a range of metabolic pathways. Cannot be synthesized by humans.

ABSORPTION/SOLUBILITY/STORAGE/PHARMACOKINETICS: Water-soluble. Absorbed via sodium-dependent transport mechanism in small intestine. Body stores are largely intracellular, and saturate in adults at a level of approximately 3 grams. Steady state levels rise minimally with intakes exceeding 200 mg/day, and are maximized at an intake level of 500 mg/day.[a]

RATIONALE FOR SUPPLEMENTATION: Vitamin C is a potent water-soluble antioxidant. Megadosing is touted to prevent cancers, heart disease, respiratory infections, and a wide range of other health problems. Doses up to 10 gram per day have been advocated to the public.

EVIDENCE IN SUPPORT OF SUPPLEMENTATION BEYOND RDA: Available evidence derives predominantly from observational studies, and is based primarily on vitamin C in whole foods rather than supplement form. No evidence from randomized trials is available to date to support dosing in excess of 200 mg per day.

TABLE IIIE. *Continued* (*Vitamin C*)

Recommended Intake Range (US RDA):

	Infancy (age 0–1)	Childhood (age 1–10)	Puberty/ adolescence (age 11–18)	Adulthood (age 19–50)	Post-menopause	Senescence	Pregnancy	Lactation
Male	30–35 mg	40–45 mg	50–60 mg	60 mg	—	60 mg	—	—
Female	30–35 mg	40–45 mg	50–60 mg	60 mg	60 mg	60 mg	70 mg	90–95 mg

TABLE IIIE. *Continued* (*Vitamin C*)

AVERAGE INTAKE, US ADULTS:	84–109 mg
ESTIMATED MEAN PALEOLITHIC INTAKE (ADULT)[b]:	604 mg
COMMON DOSE RANGE FOR USE AS SUPPLEMENT:	500 mg to several grams
DO DIETARY PATTERNS MEETING GUIDELINES PERMIT INTAKE IN THE SUPPLEMENT RANGE?:	Yes
INCLUDED IN TYPICAL MULTI-VITAMIN/MULTI-MINERAL TABLET?:	Yes (dose: 60 mg)

DEFICIENCY
Intake level: below 10 mg per day in adults
Syndromes: scurvy

TOXICITY
Intake level: above 1000 mg per day in adults
Syndromes: diarrhea (uncommon); pro-oxidant effects

Vitamin C (Ascorbic Acid) Dietary Sources[c]:

Food	Serving Size	Kilocalories	Vitamin C (mg)	Food	Serving Size	Kilocalories	Vitamin C (mg)
Acerola (West Indian cherry)	1 cup (98 gm)	31	1644	Cantaloupe	1 cup (156 gm)	55	66
Sweet red peppers, raw	1 cup (149 gm)	40	283	Red cabbage, raw	1 cup (70 gm)	19	40
Sweet green peppers, raw	1 cup (149 gm)	40	133	Peas, boiled	1/2 cup (80 gm)	34	38
Orange juice, fresh	1 cup (248 gm)	112	124	Tomatoes, raw	One (123 gm)	26	23
Orange juice, frozen concentrate	1 cup (248 gm)	112	97	Raspberries	1 cup (123 gm)	60	31
Grapefruit juice	1 cup (247 gm)	96	94	Sweet potato, baked	One (114 gm)	117	28
Strawberries	1 cup (152 gm)	46	86	Potato with skin, baked	One (202 gm)	220	26
Broccoli	1 cup (88 gm)	25	82	Salsa	1/2 cup (130 gm)	29	26
Oranges, navel	One (140 gm)	64	80	Avocado, Florida	One (304 gm)	340	24
Kiwi	One (76 gm)	46	75	Onions, raw	1 cup (160 gm)	32	19

Effects of Food Preparation and Storage: Not reported to be a generally important determinant of dietary intake levels.

TABLE IIIE. *Continued (Vitamin C)*

[a] Blanchard J, Tozer TN, Rowland M. Pharmacokinetic perspectives on megadoses of ascorbic acid. Am J Clin Nutr 1997;66:1165–1171

[b] Eaton SB, Eaton SB, III, Konner MJ. Paleolithic nutrition revisited: A twelve-year retrospective on its nature and implications. Eur J Clin Nutr. 1997:51:207–216

[c] The nutrient composition of most foods can be checked by accessing the USDA Nutrient database at: www.nal.usda.gov/fnic/foodcomp/Data/SR 13. A more extensive list of food sources of vitamin C is available in: Margen S. The Wellness Nutrition Counter. Health Letter Associates. New York, NY. 1997.

Sources:

National Research Council. Recommended Dietary Allowances. 10th edition. National Academy Press. Washington, D.C. 1989

Margen S. The Wellness Nutrition Counter. Health Letter Associates. New York, NY. 1997

Murray MT. Encyclopedia of Nutritional Supplements. Prima Publishing. Rocklin, CA. 1996

Shils ME, Olson JA, Shike M (editors). Modern Nutrition in Health and Disease. 8th edition. Lea & Febiger. Philadelphia, PA. 1994

Ziegler EE, Filer LJ, Jr. (editors). Present Knowledge in Nutrition. 7th edition. ILSI Press. Washington, D.C. 1996

Ensminger AH, Ensminger ME, Konlande JE, Robson JRK. The Concise Encyclopedia of Foods and Nutrition. CRC Press, Inc. Boca Raton, FL. 1995

United States Department of Agriculture. USDA Nutrient Database for Standard Reference. Release 11-1. 1997

TABLE IIIE. *Continued (Vitamin E)*

Vitamin E (alpha tocopherol)

BIOLOGICAL FUNCTION(S) IN HUMANS/KEY PROPERTIES: Vitamin E refers to a group of compounds, collectively known as tocopherols and tocotrienols. The most abundant and biologically active is α-tocopherol. Vitamin E functions as a lipid antioxidant, protecting and preserving the integrity of cellular and subcellular membranes.

ABSORPTION/SOLUBILITY/STORAGE/PHARMACOKINETICS: Absorption of vitamin E is relatively inefficient, ranging from 20% to 80% of that amount ingested. Vitamin E is lipid soluble, and transported along with lipoprotein particles. It is stored preferentially in liver and organs with high lipid content, such as the adrenals.

RATIONALE FOR SUPPLEMENTATION IN RDA RANGE: Prevailing, average intake levels in the US are in close approximation to the RDA, and therefore many individuals, particularly those with low intake of polyunsaturated fat, may have intake below the recommended level. Vitamin E is included in multivitamin tablets at a dose of approximately 30 IU (approximately 20 mg α-TE).[a]

RATIONALE FOR MEGADOSE SUPPLEMENTATION: The antioxidant effects of vitamin E are thought to be of benefit in the prevention of a variety of chronic diseases, including cardiovascular disease and cancer. Antioxidants are thought to have an anti-aging effect as well. Increasingly, evidence suggests that antioxidant benefit is greatest when lipid-soluble (such as vitamin E) and water-soluble (such as vitamin C) antioxidants are combined.

EVIDENCE IN SUPPORT OF SUPPLEMENTATION BEYOND RDA: The evidence for benefit of high-dose (up to 800 IU per day) supplementation of vitamin E is strongest for cardiovascular disease prevention. However, the evidence remains equivocal to date, with negative evidence from the most definitive studies. Data from the Cambridge Heart Antioxidant Study surggest a benefit of supplemental vitamin E in the prevention of second MI, although evidence of a mortality benefit was not found.[b] Beneficial effects of acute vitamin E supplementation on endothelial function have been reported. However, in the GISSI-Prevenzione trial, patients with recent MI (n = 11,324) randomly assigned to vitamin E supplementation (300 mg) did not do better than those assigned to placebo with regard to MI or death.[c] Similarly, the HOPE trial demonstrated no significant benefit of vitamin E supplementation (400 IU) with regard to both MI and death in high-risk coronary patients.[d]

TABLE IIIE. *Continued (Vitamin E)*

Recommended Intake Range (US RDA):

	Infancy (age 0–1)	Childhood (age 1–10)	Puberty/ adolescence (age 11–18)	Adulthood (age 19–50)	Post-menopause	Senescence	Pregnancy	Lactation
Male	3–4 mg α-TE	6–7 mg α-TE	10 mg α-TE	10 mg α-TE	—	10 mg α-TE	—	—
Female	3–4 mg α-TE	6–7 mg α-TE	8 mg α-TE	8 mg α-TE	8 mg α-TE	8 mg α-TE	10 mg α-TE	11–12 mg α-TE

TABLE IIIE. *Continued* (*Vitamin E*)

AVERAGE INTAKE, US ADULTS:	7–11 mg α-TE
ESTIMATED MEAN PALEOLITHIC INTAKE (ADULT)[e]:	33 mg α-TE
COMMON DOSE RANGE FOR USE AS SUPPLEMENT:	200–800 IU (133–533 mg α-TE)
DO DIETARY PATTERNS MEETING GUIDELINES PERMIT INTAKE IN THE SUPPLEMENT RANGE?:	No
INCLUDED IN TYPICAL MULTI-VITAMIN/MULTI-MINERAL TABLET?:	Yes

DEFICIENCY
  Intake level: Intake below RDA and/or fat malabsorption for years
  Syndromes: Neurologic dysfunction/neuropathy

Toxicity
  Intake level: Uncertain; in excess of 1200 IU/day
  Syndromes: diarrhea, headache, coagulopathy

Vitamin E Dietary Sources[b]:

Food	Serving Size	Energy (kcal)	Vitamin E (mg α-TE)	Food	Serving Size	Energy (kcal)	Vitamin E (mg α-TE)
Wheat germ oil	1 tablespoon (13.6 g)	120	26	Canola oil	1 tablespoon (14 g)	124	3
Sardines	1 can (92 g)	191	0.3	Corn oil	1 talespoon (13.6 g)	120	3
Almonds	1 oz (28 g)	169	7.5	Avocado	1 medium (201 g)	324	2.7
Peanut butter	2 tablespoons (32 g)	190	3.2	Flounder	1 fillet (127 g)	149	2.4
Blueberries	1 cup (145 g)	81	1.4	Swiss Chard (boiled)	1 cup (175 g)	35	3.3
Tuna	1 can (165 g)	191	0.9	Broccoli	1 spear (31 g)	9	0.5
Tomato puree	1 cup (250 g)	100	6.3	Nectarines	1 medium (136 g)	67	1.2

Effects of Food Preparation and Storage: Vitamin E will be lost if fat or oil is removed during cooking or preparation.

TABLE IIIE.   *Continued (Vitamin E)*

[a] Vitamin E is commonly measured in both mg α-TE (mg alpha tocopherol equivalents) and international units. One α-TE is approximately equal to 1.5 IU.

[b] Stephens NG, Parsons A, Schofield PM, Kelly F, Cheeseman K, Mitchinson MJ, Brown MJ. Randomized controlled trial of vitamin E in patients with coronary disease: Cambridge Heart Antioxidant Study (CHAOS). Lancet. 1996;347;781–786.

[c] GISSI-Prevenzione Investigators. Dietary supplementation with n-3 polyunsaturated fatty acids and vitamin E after myocardial infarction: results of the GISSI-Prevenzione trial. Lancet. 1999;354;447–455

[d] The Heart Outcomes Prevention Evaluation Study Investigators. Vitamin E supplementation and cardiovascular events in high-risk patients. N Engl J Med. 2000:342:154–160.

[e] Eaton SB, Eaton SB, III, Konner MJ. Paleolithic nutrition revisited: A twelve-year retrospective on its nature and implications. Eur J Clin Nutr. 1997;51:207–216

[f] The nutrient composition of most foods can be checked by accessing the USDA Nutrient database at: www.nal.usda.gov/fnic/foodcomp/Data/SR13.

Sources:

Ensminger AH, Ensminger ME, Konlande JE, Robson JRK. The Concise Encyclopedia of Foods and Nutrition. CRC Press, Inc. Boca Raton, FL. 1995

Margen S. The Wellness Nutrition Counter. Health Letter Associates. New York, NY. 1997

Murray MT. Encyclopedia of Nutritional Supplements. Prima Publishing. Rocklin, CA. 1996

National Research Council. Recommended Dietary Allowances. 10th edition. National Academy Press. Washington, D.C. 1989

Shils ME, Olson JA, Shike M (editors). Modern Nutrition in Health and Disease. 8th edition. Lea & Febiger. Philadelphia, PA. 1994

United States Department of Agriculture. USDA Nutrient Database for Standard Reference. Release 12. 1998

Ziegler EE, Filer LJ, Jr. (editors). Present Knowledge in Nutrition. 7th edition. ILSI Press. Washington, D.C. 1996

TABLE IIIE. *Continued (Zinc)*

Zinc

BIOLOGICAL FUNCTION(S) IN HUMANS/KEY PROPERTIES: Zinc functions in nearly 100 enzyme systems with prominent roles in CO_2 transport and digestion. Zinc also influences DNA and RNA synthesis, immune function, collagen synthesis, olfaction, and taste. Recent interest in zinc has focused on its role in immune function. Zinc lozenges and sprays have been studied for the treatment of upper respiratory infection, and zinc has been found to confer some benefit in lower respiratory infections.[a,b] Evidence of benefit is inconsistent, however, and refuted by the results of some trials.[c,d]

ABSORPTION/SOLUBILITY/STORAGE/PHARMACOKINETICS: The efficiency of zinc absorption varies inversely with body stores. The absorption of zinc is impeded by fiber phytates, and influenced by the stores and dietary intake of other minerals. Zinc is stored in bone and muscle, but these stores do not readily exchange with the circulation, and therefore cannot compensate rapidly for dietary deficiency.

RATIONALE FOR SUPPLEMENTATION IN RDA RANGE: The typical American diet provides approximately 5 mg of zinc per 1000 kcal. An intake of 15 mg per day is recommended for men, 12 mg per day for women. Older adults in particular are unlikely to take in sufficient calories to meet the RDA for zinc without supplementation.

RATIONALE FOR MEGADOSE SUPPLEMENTATION: Supplementation in the range of 15 to 60 mg per day is advocated to enhance immune function; improve pregnancy outcomes; improve male sexual function and fertility; and to provide a therapeutic effect in rheumatoid arthritis, acne, Alzheimer's dementia, and macular degeneration. Zinc supplementation may be beneficial in Wilson's disease, a state of copper overload, because zinc interferes with copper absorption.

EVIDENCE IN SUPPORT OF SUPPLEMENTATION BEYOND RDA: Targeted dosing of zinc to the upper airway has shown benefit in some studies of viral infections, but not in others.[d] Evidence of other benefits of zinc supplementation is largely anecdotal, or derived from small and unreplicated studies. Overall, the evidence available to date would support supplementation in adults at a level of approximately 15 mg/day (provided in multivitamin/mineral preparations), but generally fails to support supplementation at higher doses other than under particular and carefully monitored circumstances.

TABLE IIIE. *Continued (Zinc)*

Recommended Intake Range (US RDA):

	Infancy (age 0–1)	Childhood (age 1–10)	Puberty/ adolescence (age 11–18)	Adulthood (age 19–50)	Post-menopause	Senescence	Pregnancy	Lactation
Male	5 mg	10 mg	15 mg	15 mg	—	15 mg	—	—
Female	5 mg	10 mg	12 mg	12 mg	12 mg	12 mg	15 mg	16–19 mg

TABLE IIIE. Continued (Zinc)

AVERAGE INTAKE, US ADULTS:	7–15 mg/day
ESTIMATED MEAN PALEOLITHIC INTAKE (ADULT)[e]:	43 mg/day
COMMON DOSE RANGE FOR USE AS SUPPLEMENT:	15–60 mg/day
DO DIETARY PATTERNS MEETING GUIDELINES PERMIT INTAKE IN THE SUPPLEMENT RANGE?:	Yes
INCLUDED IN TYPICAL MULTI-VITAMIN/MULTI-MINERAL TABLET?:	Yes

DEFICIENCY
Intake level: Below RDA
Syndromes: impaired taste and smell; impaired immune function

TOXICITY
Intake level: >20 mg/day
Syndromes: impaired copper status; at higher intake levels, reduced HDL and impaired hematopoiesis

Zinc Dietary Sources[f]: Zinc is found abundantly in shellfish, red meat, legumes and nuts.

Food	Serving Size	Energy (kcal)	Zinc	Food	Serving Size	Energy (kcal)	Zinc
Oysters	6 medium (42 g)	58	76	White beans	1 cup (179 g)	249	2.5
King crab	1 leg (134 g)	130	10.2	Almonds	1 oz (28.3 g)	169	1
Wheat germ	1 cup (115 g)	414	14	Avocado	1 medium (201 g)	324	0.8
Sardines	1 can (92 g)	191	1.2	Barley, pearled	1 cup (157 g)	193	1.3
Lamb	3 oz (85 g)	219	3.7	Chick peas	1 cup (164 g)	269	2.5
Turkey breast	1/2 breast (306 g)	413	5.3	Lentils	1 cup (198 g)	230	2.5
Cashews	1 oz (28.3 g)	163	1.6	Chicken breast	1/2 breast (86 g)	142	0.9
Swordfish	1 piece (106 g)	164	1.6	Oat bran	1 cup (219 g)	88	1.2
Tofu	1/2 cup (126 g)	97	1.3	Oatmeal	100 g	93	0.8

Effects of Food Preparation and Storage: Not reported to be a generally important determinant of dietary intake levels.

[a] Sazawal S, Black RE, Jalla S, Mazumdar S, Sinha A, Bhan MK. Zinc supplementation reduces the incidence of acute lower respiratory infections in infants and preschool children: a double-blind, controlled trial. Pediatrics 1998;102(1 Pt 1):1–5.

[b] Marshall S. Zinc gluconate and the common cold. Review of randomized controlled trials. Can Fam Physician 1998;44:1037–42.

[c] Macknin ML, Piedmonte M, Calendine C, Janosky J, Wald E. Zinc gluconate lozenges for treating the common cold in children: a randomized controlled trial. JAMA 1998;279:1962–7.

[d] Macknin ML. Zinc lozenges for the common cold. Cleve Clin J Med 1999;66:27–32.

[e] Eaton SB, Eaton SB, III, Konner MJ. Paleolithic nutrition revisited: A twelve-year retrospective on its nature and implications. Eur J Clin Nutr. 1997;51:207–216

[f] The nutrient composition of most foods can be checked by accessing the USDA Nutrient database at: www.nal.usda.gov/fnic/foodcomp/Data/SR 13.

Sources:
Ensminger AH, Ensminger ME, Konlande JE, Robson JRK. The Concise Encyclopedia of Foods and Nutrition. CRC Press, Inc. Boca Raton, FL. 1995
Margen S. The Wellness Nutrition Counter. Health Letter Associates. New York, NY. 1997
Murray MT. Encyclopedia of Nutritional Supplements. Prima Publishing. Rocklin, CA. 1996
National Research Council. Recommended Dietary Allowances. 10th edition. National Academy Press. Washington, D.C. 1989
Shils ME, Olson JA, Shike M (editors). Modern Nutrition in Health and Disease. 8th edition. Lea & Febiger. Philadelphia, PA. 1994
United States Department of Agriculture. USDA Nutrient Database for Standard Reference. Release 12. 1998
Ziegler EE, Filer LJ, Jr. (editors). Present Knowledge in Nutrition. 7th edition. ILSI Press. Washington, D.C. 1996

TABLE IIIF. *Nutrient composition of foods*

On-line:
The nutritional composition of virtually any food can be detailed using the USDA Nutrient Database for Standard Reference (as of 2/00, Release 13): *http://www.nal.usda.gov/fnic/cgi-bin/nut search.pl.* At this address, simply enter the name of the food of interest. A list of food choices within the pertinent category will be displayed. Once a specific food is chosen, portion size options are displayed. Once the portion is selected, a table of nutrient composition is displayed.

In print:
Margen S. The Wellness Nutrition Counter. Health Letter Associates. New York, NY. 1997
• *Produced by the University of California at Berkeley, this text provides detailed nutritional information for over 6,000 foods.*

Morrill JS, Bakun S, Murphy SP. Are You Eating Right?: Analyze Your Diet Using the Nutrient Content of More Than 5,000 Foods. 4th edition. Orange Grove Publishers. Menlo Park, CA. 1997
• *A user-friendly guide to the nutrient composition of over 5000 foods. Nutrient content is displayed in measures comparable to those appearing on food labels.*

TABLE IIIG. *Diet–drug interactions*

Examples:

Alcohol

Alcohol increases the potential hepatotoxicity of many drugs, acetaminophen being a noteworthy example (Sinclair J, Jeffery E, Wrighton S, Kostrubsky V, Szakacs J, Wood S, Sinclair P. Alcohol-mediated increases in acetaminophen hepatotoxicity: role of CYP2E and CYP3A. Biochem Pharmacol 1998;55:1557–1565).

Folate

Phenytoin depletes folate, and folate facilitates the maintenance of steady-state phenytoin levels. Folate (400 μg per day) should be supplemented when phenytoin is prescribed (Lewis DP, Van Dyke DC, Willhite LA, Stumbo PJ, Berg MJ. Phenytoin-folic acid interaction. Ann Pharmacother. 1995;29:726–735).

Grapefruit Juice

Grapefruit juice inhibits the cytochrome P450 enzyme CYP3A4, thereby potentially affecting the levels of the many drugs metabolized in the P450 system (Dresser GK, Spence JD, Bailey DG. Pharmacokinetic-pharmacodynamic consequences and clinical relevance of cytochrome P450 3A4 inhibition. Clin Pharmacokinet. 2000;38:41–57).

Vitamin K

Warfarin (coumadin) is opposed by dietary vitamin K. Dark green vegetables are rich sources of vitamin K, but distribution in the food supply is wide. If anticoagulation is difficult, a dietary assessment is indicated (Booth SL, Centurelli MA. Vitamin K: a practical guide to the dietary management of patients on coumadin. Nutr Rev. 1999;57(9 pt 1):288–296).

Reference Materials:

On-line:

http://vm.cfsan.fda.gov/~lrd/advice.html
   This site, maintained by Food and Drug Administration Center for Food Safety and Applied Nutrition, includes a selection on diet/drug interactions listed by category of illness for which the medication would be taken.

In print:

Books:

Holt GA (Editor). Food and Drug Interactions: A Guide for Consumers. Bonus Books. Chicago, IL. 1998
Lininger SW (ed), Austin S, Gaby AR, Brown DJ, Batz F. The A-Z Guide to Drug-Herb and Vitamin Interactions. Prima Publishing. Rocklin, CA. 1999

Other:

Jefferson JW. Drug and diet interactions: avoiding therapeutic paralysis. J Clin Psychiatr. 1998;59 suppl 16:31–39
• *Review article of drug/diet interactions in psychiatry, particularly the treatment of depression.*

Thomas JA. Drug-nutrient interactions. Nutr Rev. 1995;53:271–282
William L, Holl DP Jr., Davis JA, Lowenthal DT. The influence of food on the absorption and metabolism of drugs: an update. Eur J Drug Metab Pharmacokinet. 1996;21:201–211
Barrett B, Kiefer D, Rabago D. Assessing the risks and benefits of herbal medicine: an overview of scientific evidence. Altern Ther Health Med. 1999;5:40–49
Cupp MJ. Herbal Remedies: adverse effects and drug interactions. Am Fam Physician. 1999;59:1239–1245
Yamreudeewong W, Henann NE, Fazio A, Lower DL, Cassidy TG. Drug-food interactions in clinical practice. J Fam Pract. 1995;40:376–384
Singh BN. Effects of food on clinical pharmacokinetics. Clin Pharmacokinet. 1999;37:213–255

TABLE IIIH. *Nutrient remedies for common conditions: patient resources*

On-line resources:
http://www.Drkoop.com/wellness/nutrition/condition/
  Condition-specific nutrition information is accessible from the Dr. Koop website.

Print Resources:
Lininger SW (editor), Austin S, Lininger S, Wright JW, Brown D, Gaby A. The Natural Pharmacy: From the Top
  Experts in the Field, Your Essential Guide to Vitamins, Herbs, Minerals and Homeopathic Remedies. Prima
  Publishing. Rocklin, CA. 1998
Craig SY, Haigh J, Harrar S (editors). The Complete Book of Alternative Nutrition. Rodale Press, Inc. Emmaus,
  PA. 1997
Murray MT. Encyclopedia of Nutritional Supplements. Prima Publishing. Rocklin, CA. 1996
Tyler VE & The Editors Of Prevention Health Books. The Doctors Book of Herbal Home Remedies: Cure Yourself
  With Nature's Most Powerful Healing Agents: Advice from 200 Experts for More Than 150 Conditions. Rodale
  Press. 2000

TABLE IIII. *Print and web-based resource materials for professionals*

PRINT RESOURCE MATERIALS:

Books:
See "Sources for All Chapters."

Newsletters:
Nutrition and the MD. University of California, San Diego. Lippincott, Williams & Wilkins. Hagerstown, MD.
Phone: (410) 528-8572
e-mail: *adyson@lww.com*
website: *www.lww.com*
Highlights of recent, clinically-relevant advances in nutrition.

Nutrition Research Newsletter. John Wiley & Sons, Inc.
Phone: (201) 568-4744
Website: *www.wiley.com/technical insights*
Essentially, a nutrition "journal watch."

Other:
Foreyt JP, Poston WS 2nd. The role of the behavioral counselor in obesity treatment. J Am Diet Assoc. 1998;98(10 suppl):s27–s30.

WEB-BASED RESOURCE MATERIALS:

www.healthfinder.gov
A site of use to both professional and lay users, *healthfinder* is maintained by the U.S. Department of Health and Human Services and serves as a directory to credible sources of health information on the web. A search engine allows for easy identification of nutrition sites of interest.

www.navigators.tufts.edu
Maintained by the Tufts University School of Nutrition Policy and Science, this site serves as a directory to other nutrition sites for both professional and lay users.

www.nal.usda.gov/fnic/foodcomp/index.html
This site provides access to the USDA Nutrient Data Laboratory. The nutrient composition of virtually any food can be found in the database. To determine the nutrient composition of a food, click on "Search the Database," then type in the name of the food.

http://www.aoa.dhhs.gov/factsheets/enp.html
The Administration on Aging maintains this website detailing the Elderly Nutrition Program, an assistance program for older adults. The information is of use in efforts to provide nutrition to older patients with limited ability to maintain a balanced diet.

http://www.fns.usda.gov/cnd/Contacts/StateDirectory.htm
The USDA maintains this site indexing food assistance program offices for children by state.

http://www.cdc.gov/nchs/nhanes.htm
This site is maintained by the National Center for Health Statistics at the Centers for Disease Control and Prevention, and provides access the dietary intake data from the National Health and Nutrition Examination Surveys.

http://www.eatright.org/find.html
This site is maintained by the American Dietetic Association and provides information about the services of dietitians, as well as a search engine to find a local dietitian listed with the Association.

http://vm.cfsan.fda.gov/~dms/aems.html
This site, maintained by the U. S. Food and Drug Administration Center for Food Safety and Applied Nutrition, Office of Special Nutritionals, provides updated information on the reporting of adverse health events associated with use of nutritional products.

http://www.niddk.nih.gov/health/nutrit/nutrit.htm
Updated information on diet and obesity, maintained by the National Institute of Diabetes, Digestive and Kidney Disease (NIDDK) at the NIH.

http://www.ars.usda.gov/dgac/
Updated dietary guidelines, maintained by the USDA.

http://www.nhlbi.nih.gov/health/prof/heart/index.htm
This site, maintained by the National Heart, Lung, and Blood Institute at the NIH provides the professional links to information on the management of cardiovascular risk factors, including hypertension, obesity, and hyperlipidemia.

TABLE IIIJ. *Print and web-based resource materials for patients*

PRINT RESOURCE MATERIALS

Newsletters/Magazines/Articles

Eating Well. The Smart Magazine of Food & Health. Hachette Filipacchi Magazines. Charlotte, VT. {Subscriptions: (303) 604–1464; *hachette@neodata.com*}
A magazine about both food and health, with excellent recipes.

Kostas G. Low-fat and delicious: Can we break the taste barrier? J Am Diet Assoc. 1997;97(suppl):s88–s92
A discussion of methods for translating nutrition guidelines into actual cooking and eating; appropriate reading for patients as well as providers.

Nutrition Action Health Letter. Center for Science in the Public Interest. 1875 Conn Ave., N. W./Suite 300, Washington, D.C. 20009
Fax: (202) 265-4954
e-mail: *circ@cspinet.org*
Consumer advocacy; inside information on commercial food and nutrition practices with implications for consumer health.

Tufts University. Health and Nutrition Letter. 10 High Street, Suite 706, Boston, MA 02110 Phone: (800) 274-7581
e-mail: *healthletter@tufts.edu*
website: *www.healthletter.tufs.edu*
Sound nutrition advice for the lay person from a leading school of nutrition.

University of California, Berkeley Wellness Letter. PO Box 420148, Palm Coast, Florida 32142 Phone: (904) 445-6414
Excellent and credible advice on health promotion, including nutrition, fitness, and lifestyle.

Cookbooks

(Books listed below are considered particularly helpful, but are a representative sample only; books to guide nutritious cooking are available by virtually every category of cuisine and health condition. The patient with a specific interest not addressed below should be referred to an actual or on-line bookstore.)

Food Intolerance/Allergy

Hagman B. The Gluten-Free Gourmet Cooks Fast and Healthy: Wheat-Free With Less Fuss and Fat. Henry Holt. 1997

Pannell M (ed). Allergy Free Cookbook (Healthy Eating). Lorenz Books. New York. 1999

Diet and Health

American Heart Association. American Heart Association Low-Fat, Low Cholesterol Cookbook: Heart-Healthy, Easy-To-Make Recipes That Taste Great. Times Books. New York. 1998
Castelli WP, Griffin GC. Good Fat, Bad Fat: How to Lower Your Cholesterol and Reduce the Odds of a Heart Attack. Fisher Books. Tuscon, AZ. 1997
D'Agostino J. Convertible Cooking for a Healthy Heart. Healthy Heart. Easton, PA. 1991
Editors of the Wellness Cooking School, University of California at Berkeley. The Wellness Lowfat Cookbook. Rebus, Inc. New York, NY. 1993
Editors of the Wellness Cooking School, University of California at Berkeley. The Simply Healthy Lowfat Cookbook. Rebus, Inc. New York, NY. 1995
Lund JM, Alpert B. Cooking Healthy With the Kids in Mind: A Healthy Exchanges Cookbook. Putnam Publishing Group. 1998
Lund JM. The Diabetic's Healthy Exchanges Cookbook (Healthy Exchanges Cookbooks). Perigee. New York. 1996
Melina V, Forest J, Picarski R. Cooking Vegetarian: Healthy, Delicious, and Easy Vegetarian Cuisine. John Wiley & Sons. 1998
Nigro N, Nigro S. Companion Guide to Healthy Cooking: A practical Introduction to Natural Ingredients. Featherstone Inc. Charlottesville, VA. 1996
Nixon DW, Zanca JA, DeVita VT. The Cancer Recovery Eating Plan: The Right Foods to Help Fuel Your Recovery. Times Books. New York. 1996
Pensiero L, Olivieria S, Osborne M. The Strang Cookbook for Cancer Prevention. Dutton. New York, NY. 1998
Ponichtera BJ. Quick & Healthy Recipes and Ideas: For People Who Say They Don't Have Time to Cook Healthy Meals Scaledown. The Dalles, OR. 1991
Ponichtera BJ. Quick & Healthy Volume II: More Help for People Who Say They Don't Have Time to Cook Healthy Meals. Scaledown. The Dalles, OR. 1995
Rosso J. Great Good Food. Crown/Turtle Bay Books. New York, NY. 1993

TABLE IIIJ. *Continued*

Starke RD, Winston M (eds). American Heart Association Low-Salt Cookbook: A Complete Guide to Reducing Sodium and Fat in the Diet. Times Books. New York. 1990

Wood R. The New Whole Foods Encyclopedia: A Comprehensive Resource for Healthy Eating. Penguin Books. New York. 1999

Other Books of Interest

Alleman GP. Save your child from the fat epidemic. Prima Publishing. Rocklin, CA. 1999

Craig SY, Haigh J, Harrar S (editors). The Complete Book of Alternative Nutrition Rodale Press, Inc. Emmaus, PA. 1997

Dietz WH, Stern L. (eds). American Academy of Pediatrics Guide to Your Child's Nutrition. Villard Books (Random House, Inc.) New York, NY. 1999

Margen S. The Wellness Nutrition Counter. Health Letter Associates. New York, NY. 1997

Margen S (editor) and the Editors of the University of California at Berkeley Wellness Letter. The Wellness Encyclopedia of Food and Nutrition. Rebus. New York, NY. 1992

Murray MT. Encyclopedia of Nutritional Supplements. Prima Publishing. Rocklin, CA. 1996

Rinzler CA. The New Complete Book of Food. A Nutritional, Medical, and Culinary Guide. Facts on File, Inc. New York, NY. 1999

Rothfield GS, LeVert S. Natural Medicine for Heart Disease. Rodale Press, Inc. 1996

Somer E. Food & Mood. 2nd edition. Henry Holt & Company. New York, NY. 1999

Tamborlane WV (ed). The Yale Guide to Children's Nutrition. Yale University Press. New Haven, CT. 1997

Werbach M. Healing with Food. HarperPerennial. New York, NY. 1993

WEB-BASED RESOURCE MATERIALS:

www.healthfinder.gov
A site of use to both professional and lay users, *healthfinder* is maintained by the U.S. Department of Health and Human Services and serves as a directory to credible sources of health information on the web. A search engine allows for easy identification of nutrition sites of interest.

http://www.nal.usda.gov:8001/py/pmap.htm
http://www.nalusda.gov/fnic/Fpyr/pyramid.gif
These sites allow access to images of the USDA Food Guide Pyramid.

http://www.navigator.tufts.edu/
Maintained by the Tufts University School of Nutrition Policy and Science, this site serves as a directory to other nutrition sites for both professional and lay users.

www.nal.usda.gov/fnic/foodcomp/index.html
This site provides access to the USDA Nutrient Data Laboratory. The nutrient composition of virtually any food can be found in the database. To determine the nutrient composition of a food, click on "Search the Database," then type in the name of the food.

http://www.deliciousdecisions.org/
This site, maintained by the American Heart Association, provides a wealth of information about heart-healthy eating and cooking, including detailed recipes.

http://www.noah.cuny.edu/wellness/nutrition/nutrition.html
The New York Online Access to Health (NOAH) web site provides health information in both English and Spanish. The nutrition index is extensive, and very user friendly.

http://www.ama-assn.org/insight/gen_hlth/nutrinfo/nutrinfo./htm
The *Personal Nutritionist* Website maintained by the American Medical Association allows for individual dietary assessment on-line, as well as on-line calculation of BMI from height and weight.

http://vm.cfsan.fda.gov/~dms/wh-nutr.html
Essays on topics in nutrition and health by the U. S. Food and Drug Administration's Center for Food Safety and Applied Nutrition.

http://www.aoa.gov/aoa/webres/wellness.htm
Maintained by the Administration on Aging, this site provides advice on diet and physical activity for health promotion that is tailored to older adults.

http://ificinfo.health.org/infosn.htm
This site, maintained by the International Food Information Council, provides consumer-oriented information on food safety.

http://vm.cfsan.fda.gov/label.html
This site, maintained by U. S. Food and Drug Administration Center for Food Safety and Applied Nutrition, provides detailed information on the interpretation of food labels, including their use for specific health goals.

TABLE IIIJ. *Continued*

---

http://www.eatright.org/find.html
This site is maintained by the American Dietetic Association and provides information about the services of dietitians, as well as a search engine to find a local dietitian listed with the Association.

http://www.kidshealth.org/parent/nutrition_fit/
A private foundation, the Nemours Center for Children's Health Media, maintains this website that offers detailed information on nutrition for the newborn. The site is listed on the *healthfinder* website. Information on diet and nutrition for older children, through adolescence, is easily accessible from this site.

http://www.niddk.nih.gov/health/nutrition.htm
This site is maintained by the National Center for Diabetes, Digestive and Kidney Diseases (NIDDK) at the National Institutes of Health, and provides extensive references on cooking and nutrition in the management of diabetes.

http://www.mayohealth.org/mayo/recipe/htm/maintoc.htm
This site provides a "virtual cookbook" maintained by the Mayo Foundation for Medical Education and Research of the Mayo Clinic. Patients can select from a variety of recipes, and see the nutritional composition for "standard" and "modified" recipes side by side.

http://www.niddk.nih.gov/health/nutrit/pubs/quitsmok/index.htm
This site, maintained by the National Center for Diabetes, Digestive and Kidney Diseases (NIDDK) at the National Institutes of Health provides information to patients on how to avoid weight gain during smoking cessation.

http://cancernet.nci.nih.gov/peb/eating/hints/index.html
This site is maintained by the National Cancer Institute at the NIH and provides detailed information on diet tailored for patients with cancer.

http://vm.cfsan.fda.gov/~lrd/advice.html
This site, maintained by the Food and Drug Administration Center for Food Safety and Applied Nutrition, provides the consumer information on safe food handling and preparation.

http://www.tops.org/
This is the home page for *Take Off Pounds Sensibly,* an international club providing information and support for sensible weight loss.

http://www.nhlbi.nih.gov/health/public/heart/obesity/lose_wt/wtl&lawbar;prog.htm
This site, maintained by the National Heart, Lung, and Blood Institute at the NIH, provides guidance in choosing a safe and reasonable weight loss program.

http://www.niddk.nih.gov/health/nutrit/pubs/choose.htm
This site, maintained by the National Institute of Diabetes, Digestive and Kidney Diseases at the NIH, provides guidance in choosing a safe and reasonable weight loss program.

Index